W9-AHA-138

Chicago Public Library

Form 178 rev. 11-00

# WORLD *of* COMPUTER SCIENCE

# WORLD *of* COMPUTER SCIENCE

Brigham Narins, *Editor*

## Volume 2

### M-Z

**General Index**

**GALE GROUP**

**THOMSON LEARNING**

Detroit • New York • San Diego • San Francisco
Boston • New Haven, Conn. • Waterville, Maine
London • Munich

# GALE GROUP STAFF

Brigham Narins, *Editor*

Maria Franklin, *Permissions Manager*
Margaret A. Chamberlain, *Permissions Specialist*
Shalice Shah-Caldwell, *Permissions Associate*

Mary Beth Trimper, *Manager, Composition and Electronic Prepress*
Evi Seoud, *Assistant Manager, Composition and Electronic Prepress*
Dorothy Maki, *Manufacturing Manager*
Rhonda Williams, *Buyer*

Michelle DiMercurio, *Senior Art Director*
Michael Logusz, *Graphic Artist*

Barbara J. Yarrow, *Manager, Imaging and Multimedia Content*
Robyn Young, *Project Manager, Imaging and Multimedia Content*
Dean Dauphinais, *Senior Editor, Imaging and Multimedia Content*
Kelly A. Quin, *Editor, Imaging and Multimedia Content*
Leitha Etheridge-Sims, Mary K. Grimes, Dave Oblender, *Image Catalogers*
Pam A. Reed, *Imaging Coordinator*
Randy Bassett, *Imaging Supervisor*
Robert Duncan, *Senior Imaging Specialist*
Dan Newell, *Imaging Specialist*
Luke Rademacher, *Imaging Specialist*
Christine O'Bryan, *Graphic Specialist*
Indexing provided by Linda Kenny Sloan of Information Universe
Illustrations created by Electronic Illustrators Group, Morgan Hill, California

ISBN: 0-7876-4960-0 (set)
ISBN: 0-7876-5066-8 (Volume 1)
ISBN: 0-7876-5067-6 (Volume 2)

Printed in the United States of America
10 9 8 7 6 5 4 3 2 1

I(T)P™

Library of Congress Control Number: 2001096880

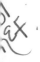

# Contents

# INTRODUCTION

Welcome to the *World of Computer Science*. We hope you will find this collection interesting and useful. The nearly 800 individual entries in this volume provide an up-to-date overview of computer science and its related disciplines. The entries explain in concise, detailed, and jargon-free language some of the most important topics, principles, and recent discoveries in the computer and information sciences. Biographies of the people who made those discoveries and shaped our understanding of the field are also included.

From Ada, B-tree, and C to X-Windows, Y2k bug, and Zone punch, this book covers a broad spectrum of the most significant concepts, historical events, programming languages, devices, software, and people in computational history. *World of Computer Science* has been designed and written with the student and non-expert in mind. In so doing, we have compiled a vast array of entries that will be useful to students who need accessible and concise information for school-related work, as well as to others who want reliable and informative introductions to the numerous aspects of the world of computer science.

In this increasingly wired and virtual world, it has become necessary for all citizens to have a practical, theoretical, and historical understanding of computers and the major issues regarding information and communication technology—how computers work; who invented them, and why; and the issues and problems that arise from their rapid growth and the diffusion of high technologies into the lives of individuals. We hope that the essays and articles contained in this book will help you understand some of these important issues and how they affect you and the world in which you live.

## How to Use the Book

This first edition of *World of Computer Science* has been designed with ready reference in mind.

- **Entries are arranged alphabetically**, rather than by chronology or scientific field.
- **Boldfaced terms** direct reader to related entries.
- **Cross-references** at the end of entries alert the reader to related entries that may not have been specifically mentioned in the body of the text.
- A **Sources Consulted** section lists many worthwhile print and electronic materials encountered in the compilation of this volume. It is there for the inspired reader who wants more information on the people and concepts covered in this work.
- The **Historical Chronology** includes over 500 important events in the history of computer science and related fields spanning the period from around 1500 B.C. through 2001.
- A **comprehensive general index** guides the reader to all topics and persons mentioned in the book. Boldface page references refer the reader to the term's full entry.

## Advisory Board

In compiling this edition, we have been fortunate in being able to call upon the following people—our panel of advisors—who contributed to the accuracy of the information in this premier edition of *World of Computer Science,* and to them we would like to express sincere appreciation:

**Robert E. Beck**
*Professor, Computing Sciences*
Villanova University Villanova, Pennsylvania

**William I. Grosky**
*Professor of Computer and Information Science*
University of Michigan-Dearborn

**Ian Parberry**
*Professor, Department of Computer Sciences*
University of North Texas

**Edmond Schonberg**

*Professor, Department of Computer Science*

Courant Institute of Mathematical Sciences

New York University

The editor would like to thank the advisors for all of their good work reviewing and compiling the entry list and for their patience and good will answering my many questions. Thanks are also due to all the writers who contributed their expertise to this book: William Arthur Atkins, Aner Ben-Artzi, Ramola D., Mike DeAndrea, John Forrest Engle, Kim Masters Evans, Paula Ford-Martin, Surya Ganguli, Larry Clifford Gilman, Mark Godfrey, Brian Hoyle, Denise Hurd, Donn Le Vie Jr., Adrienne Wilmoth Lerner, Brenda Wilmoth Lerner, K. Lee Lerner, Lee Wilmoth Lerner, W. Eric Martin, Cara Mia Massey, Debbie Merz, Elisabeth Morlino, Otto Östergård, Ian Parbury, Antonio Parmigganni, Jonathan Parry-McCulloch, Shrisha Rao, Kimno Rathikainen, Gordon Rutter, Elja Sosialon-Soinnen, Lisa Tallman, Christina Tolliver, David Tulloch, Susan Thorpe-Vargas, Jarhi Verijalainen, Patrick Worden, and Christopher Wyckoff.

Larry Clifford Gilman deserves another nod for his excellent writing, his invaluable reviewing and copyediting of some troublesome material, and for his consistent good humor in the face my many e-mail messages. And Bill Atkins and Shrisha Rao deserve additional recognition for writing so much and so well.

Finally, special thanks go to K. Lee Lerner and Brenda Wilmoth Lerner who provided great help, advice, reassurance, hard work, and talent when it was needed most; some day, godfather—and I hope that day does come—I'll do you a service in return.

[Note: Portions of the entries "Chomsky, Noam" and "Chomsky and computer science" originally appeared as "Noam Chomsky," by Sandra L. Haarsager, in *Dictionary of Literary Biography, Volume 246: Twentieth-Century American Cultural Theorists.* A Bruccoli Clark Layman Book. Edited by Paul Hansom. The Gale Group, 2001. pp. 50-63.]

# ACKNOWLEDGMENTS

Abacus, indicating upper and lower deck with beads on rods, enclosed within a frame, illustration created by Electronic Illustrators Group. Gale Group.—Allen, Paul., Dallas, Texas, photograph. AP/Wide World Photos. Reproduced by permission.—An Wang, photograph. Corbis. Reproduced by permission.—Atanasoff, John, photograph. AP/Wide World Photos. Reproduced by permission.

Babbage, Charles, engraving. The Library of Congress.—Babbage's "difference engine," photograph. The Granger Collection, New York. Reproduced by permission.—Bardeen, John, photograph. AP/Wide World Photos. Reproduced by permission.—Berners-Lee, Tim, photograph. AP/Wide World Photos. Reproduced by permission.—Binary arithmetic equations, illustrations created by Electronic Illustrators Group. Gale Group.—Boole, George, illustration. The Library of Congress.

Brattain, Walter Houser, photograph. The Library of Congress.—Bush, Vannevar, photograph. The Library of Congress.—Chomsky, Noam, photograph. © Donna Coveney. Reproduced by permission of South End Press.—Computer chip on display, photograph. AP/Wide World Photos. Reproduced by permission.—Cray, Seymour, photograph. AP/Wide World Photos. Reproduced by permission.—Dot operator equation, illustration created by Electronic Illustrators Group. Gale Group.

Eckert, J. Presper and John W. Mauchly, photograph. AP/Wide World Photos. Reproduced by permission.—Eckert, J. Presper, photograph. AP/Wide World Photos. Reproduced by permission.

Emeagwali, Philip, photograph. Reproduced by permission.—ENIAC (first electronic calculator, six people working it), photograph. Corbis. Reproduced by permission.—Gates, Bill, photograph by David A. Cantor. AP/Wide World Photos. Reproduced by permission.—Hannibal (Attila II) MIT Artificial Intelligence Lab, photograph by Bruce Frisch/ S.S. Photo Researchers, Inc. Reproduced by permission.—Hollerith, Herman, photograph. The Library of Congress.—Hopper, Grace Murray, photograph. UPI/Corbis. Reproduced

by permission.—Jacquard, Joseph Marie, photograph. Archive Photos. Reproduced by permission.—Jobs, Steven, photograph. Archive Photos/Reuters/Sell. Reproduced by permission.—Joy, Bill, photograph. AP/Wide World Photos. Reproduced by permission.—Karp, Richard, photograph © 1996 Mary Levin/University of Washington. Reproduced by permission of Richard Karp.—Kemeny, John G., photograph. The Library of Congress

Kurtz, Thomas E., photograph. Reproduced by permission.—La Pascaline, calculating machine designed by Blaise Pascal in 1642, illustration. The Library of Congress.—Lanier, Jaron, photograph © 1990 Peter Menzel. Reproduced by permission.—Leibniz, Gottfried Wilhelm von, photograph. The Library of Congress.—Light micrograph of a silicon wafer microchip, photograph by Astrid & Hanns-Frieder Michler. Photo Researchers, Inc. Reproduced by permission.—Mark I, designed by Howard Aiken in 1943, photograph. The Library of Congress.—McCarthy, John, photograph. The Library of Congress.—Micro wires, silicon chip, photograph by Andrew Syred. The National Audubon Society Collection/ Photo Researchers, Inc. Reproduced by permission.—Minsky, Marvin, photograph. AP/Wide World Photos. Reproduced by permission.—Mitnick, Kevin, photograph. Reuters/The News and Observer-Jim/Archive Photos. Reproduced by permission.—Napier, John, illustration. The Library of Congress.—Napier's Bones, a multiplying machine built by Samuel Morland in 1672, illustration. The Library of Congress.—Napier's rods, illustration created by Electronic Illustrators Group. Gale Group.—Neumann, Dr. John Von, photograph by United Press Photo. UPI/Corbis. Reproduced by permission.—Noyce, Robert, photograph. AP/Wide World Photos. Reproduced by permission.—Pascal, Blaise, painting. The Library of Congress.—Rifkin, Stanley Mark, photograph. UPI/Corbis. Reproduced by permission.—Schockely, Dr. William, photograph. AP/Wide World Photos. Reproduced by permission.—Shockley, William, photograph. The Library of Congress.

Simon, Herbert Alexander, photograph. AP/Wide World Photos. Reproduced by permission.—Slide rule illustrations, created by Electronic Illustrators Group on behalf of the Gale Group.—Stallman, Richard, photograph. Free Software Foundation. Reproduced by permission.—Torvalds, Linus, photograph by Paul Sakuma. AP/Wide World Photos. Reproduced by permission.—Torvalds, Linus, photograph. © Reuters Newmedia Inc./Corbis. Reproduced by permission.—Turing, Alan, photograph. Photo Researchers, Inc. Reproduced by permission.—Two men working a UNIVAC computer, photograph. Corbis. Reproduced by permission.—Watson, Thomas John, Sr., photograph. The Library of Congress.—Wiener, Norbert, photograph. UPI/Corbis. Reproduced by permission.—Wozniak, Steve, photograph. AP/Wide World Photos. Reproduced by permission.

# M

## M-ary tree

An m-ary **tree** is a **data structure** employed to improve external **sorting** in which for every **node** in the tree there are no more than m child nodes. Binary trees are a specific implementation of an m-ary tree where there are m = 2 child nodes for every node on the tree. This type of **data** tree is particularly important when in certain computing scenarios sorting must be done with the majority of the data remaining on auxiliary storage devices. An external sorting strategy, called the Hillsort, in combination with the m-ary tree architecture allowed the development of the Ternary Hillsort. This combinational sorting method is superior in its performance over the pure external sorting and the pure ternary tree since it executes faster and the parent-child and sibling relationships are easily calculated.

A tree is a type of organizational structuring of classes of elements, **databases**, or directory files that has a type of generalization or hierarchical architecture. This type of structure looks like a tree with its different branches and nodes. Also there is a unique path between any pair of nodes on the tree. The top of the file structure is called the root node and each entry on a different branch is called a **child node** of the **parent**. An m-ary tree is a particular type of tree where there are no more than m child nodes for every node in the tree. When m = 2 the tree is called a binary tree. This means that for each node on the tree that there are exactly two links to two other trees or subtrees where the two subtrees are often referred to as the left and right subtrees. This particular type of m-ary tree is the most commonly used type of tree data structure. If there are exactly m or zero child nodes for each node in the tree then the tree is called a full binary tree.

There is a simple formula for counting the number of nodes of an m-ary tree. If an m-ary tree has depth n and m > 1 then the number of nodes is given by:

$$\sum_{k=0}^{0} m^k = (m^{n+1} - 1)/(m-1).$$

## Machine architecture

The term architecture refers to a **design**. In the case of computers, architecture can be thought of as the architecture of the machine, as well as the architecture of the machine's ability to link to other computers or **peripherals**.

The functional machine may have what is termed an **open architecture**, where the knowledge of the design of **hardware** and software is sufficiently public to permit the easy installation of devices and programs from many vendors. In contrast, a computer with a closed architecture has a proprietary design, and can accommodate only select connections, often from the same vendor.

Machine architecture can refer to hardware or software, or to a combination of hardware and software. Furthermore, machine architecture can consider different levels of detail. The architecture of a system always defines that system's broad outlines, and may also define precise mechanisms operating within the system.

The central part of machine architecture is the **central processing unit**, or **CPU**. The CPU controls the functioning of a computer. In turn, central to the **operation** of the CPU is the ability to store information in **memory**. Basically, there are two kinds of memory, **Read-Only Memory** (RAM), and the **hard drive**. The rule for hard drives is simple—the bigger the better. The bigger the storage capacity of the hard drive, the more information a computer is capable of storing. Now, the average computer is approaching a hard drive size of one gigabyte. A gigabyte is one billion bytes of information. In an office analogy, RAM would be a worker's desktop and the hard drive would be a file cabinet in which all the company information was housed. As the desktop is used to handle portions of the total information, so RAM allows the computer to **access** and work with bits of the total stored information. Being able to deal with a portion of the total information is more efficient. But, conversely, insufficient RAM means that task requiring large portions of information can only be done in a series of small operations, which slows the task. Thus, an efficient machine architecture has suitable RAM available to permit large-scale tasks to be performed.

A vital part of machine architecture is the ability to convey information to portable **data storage** systems. Floppy disks, CD-ROMs, and tape drives are three examples of portable **data** storage systems. Other types of storage systems, with much greater data storage capacity, are on the horizon. **Holographic storage** is an example.

Another vital component of machine architecture is the ability of a computer to remotely communicate with other computers and devices. In the past, such communication was achieved through the use of the portable data storage systems. A floppy disk would be physically removed from the **disk drive** of one computer, installed in the disk drive of another computer, and the desired information retrieved from the disk, for example. Now, the **Internet** and hard wiring of computers together in networks has made the direct communication between machines possible. Two hardware components that are essential for this electronic communication to occur are a **modem** and an ethernet card. A modem is the intermediary that translates digitizes electronic information, and visa versa, enabling information to be transmitted over telephone lines and then converted into a form that is understandable to a computer. Whereas a modem tells a computer how to talk to another computer over a phone line, an ethernet card tells a computer how to act like a computer on a network.

For information to be useful to a user, it must be presented in a form that is recognizable. For many functions, a visual presentation of the information is required. Thus, a monitor—a display screen where text or **graphics** can be displayed—is a key architectural component. Increasingly, audio and video (moving images) are being used to convey information. Speakers and digital cameras are thus becoming more popular hardware components.

Yet another vital aspect of machine architecture is a means to convey information "on paper". A keyboard provides a user with the means of expressing information in a textual manner that can subsequently be printed. There is a wide range of printers, both in terms of price and print quality.

The hardware components are an important part of machine architecture, as is thee ability to control the operation of these components, both in isolation and in a coordinated fashion. Various software programs are responsible for these functions. As well, various **programming** languages allow data or graphical images on a screen to be connected together, facilitating analysis of data or the efficient operation of a program.

*See also* Computer architecture; Data storage; DOS; Open architecture; Software architecture

# MACHINE CODE

Machine **code** is the sequence of binary-coded machine instructions specifically written to be used within **machine language**. *Machine language* is the low-level **programming** language that is directly read and interpreted by a computer's

**central processing unit** (**CPU**) in order for it to perform its functions. The *instructions* within machine code are binary strings that may be either all the same size (e.g., one 32-bit word) or of different sizes (where the size of the instruction is determined from the first word or **byte**). For instance, when a CPU is set-up to use 32-bit words, it realizes that it only needs to scan that particular sequence of bits in order to perform all of its instructions.

Many of the computer programs "coded" by mathematical programmers from the mid-1940s to the late-1950s were written in the binary (base 2) numbering system—while some were written in octal (base 8) or hexadecimal (base 16)—using low-level machine languages. Programs in machine code were not usually very large, only consisting of hundreds or thousands of separate instructions that were very simple in structure when compared to modern high-level programs. These machine codes were written specifically for a particular machine, until the first high-level programming language **FORTRAN** (**Formula Translator**) became available in 1958.

A program in machine code normally consists of sequences of binary digits, or bits, which are represented by 1s and 0s that make up the machine instructions. These bits, the smallest piece of information used by the CPU, form the basic instructions that direct the **operation** of a computer. When computer programs were written in machine code, it was difficult for programmers to read and follow the language because the instructions appeared as sequences of bits (i.e., zeros and ones). Because of this, errors were very difficult to detect within the numerous rows and columns of zeros and ones. Today errors are much easier to detect with the use of alphanumeric words for **commands** within high-level code. In addition, writing programs in machine code consumed much time and effort because computer programmers had to organize each specific **bit** in an instruction; and with thousands or millions of lines of code, those tasks became quite daunting.

Execution of machine code may be permanently hard-wired into the CPU (as in personal computers) or the execution may be controlled by microcode. A microcode is a technique for implementing the **instruction set** of a **microprocessor** as a sequence of instructions ("microinstructions"), each of which typically consists of a large number of bit fields and the address of the next microinstruction to execute. (The collection of all possible instructions for a particular computer is known as its "instruction set".) The fundamental execution cycle of machine code consists of (1) grabbing the next instruction from main **memory**, (2) decoding it (determining the operation that it specifies and the location of any independent variables), (3) executing it by opening various gates (electronic switches that allow **data** to flow from main memory into a CPU memory **register**), and (4) enabling functional units (subsystems within the CPU that perform certain distinct functions). The specific set of instructions that constitutes a machine code depends on the make and model of the microprocessor (the computer's CPU) inside a particular computer. For instance, the machine code for the Motorola 68000 microprocessor differs from that used in the **Intel** Pentium® microprocessor.

These days almost all computer programmers use assembly (intermediate) languages or high-level languages when programming for computers (instead of machine language). An **assembly language** contains a one-to-one correspondence with the resulting machine code instructions, but the instructions and variables possess familiar names instead of being just numbers. Like assembly languages, all high-level languages must first be translated into machine code before a computer can run them. To accomplish this, programmers use various types of utility programs (such as compilers, assemblers, linkers, and debuggers) that help them translate **high-level language** into machine code. The computer code used to write a program is called source code before being translated into machine code, which is called object code. Thus, machine code is the ultimate result of the compilation of assembly language or any high-level language.

*See also* Bit; Central processing unit (CPU); High-level language; Intermediate languages; Machine language; Object-oriented programming

# MACHINE LANGUAGE

Machine language is the **programming** language the computer understands; its native tongue. Machine language instructions are written with binary numbers, 0 and 1. The 0 and 1 represent electrical off and on states. All other programming languages must be compiled or translated into binary **code** to be recognized and used by the **central processing unit** (**CPU**). Machine language, therefore, is the lowest level computer language, executable without prior software translation.

Machine language instructions correspond to the **instruction set** of a particular **hardware** architecture and are machine dependent. Different computers use different machine languages, but every machine language includes instructions for basic operations such as addition and subtraction. The instructions are patterns of 0s and 1s in lengths of 16, 24, 32, or 64 bits (*binary digits*). Each instruction has two parts: an **operator** and an operand. The operator is the first few bits of the instruction. It specifies the **operation** to be performed, such as movement of **data** between **memory**, the storage address, and the CPU. The remaining bits constitute the operand. The operand is usually an address, or location, of the data to be operated on. Each address is 8-bits long and referred to as a word.

Each machine language instruction is very simple and by itself accomplishes very little. However, the cpu has the ability to execute millions of instructions per second.

## Binary

Computers use electrical impulses to represent numbers. Electrical impulses can exist in two states: off and on. This makes binary the ideal system for computers. Binary is a base-two number system—it has two digits, 0 and 1, representing the states off and on or true and false. Groups of binary digits represent instructions. Each instruction is a pattern or series of 0s and 1s with a precise meaning. For example, the binary digits 1000 could represent the instruction ADD.

Binary instructions accomplish simple tasks, such as adding and moving data. Although ideal for computers, binary numbers are difficult for programmers to understand. To ease translation, binary-coded decimals (**BCD**) are used.

## Binary-coded Decimal

A binary-coded decimal is a system for encoding decimal numbers in binary form. Decimal is the base-ten number system, digits 0 through 9, that we are accustomed to using. There are two reasons why BCD is used. First, BCD avoids the rounding and conversion errors that occur with the use of binary numbers. Second, BCD allows for larger numbers to be used. In binary, the highest number that can be represented by the 8-bit words computers use is 256. Using BCD, decimal numbers larger than 256 can be used. In BCD each decimal digit is coded separately as a four-digit binary number. For example, the decimal number 5,270 is represented by the binary code for 5, 2, 7, 0, which translates into 0101 0010 0111 0000.

The following is a list of the numbers 0 through 9 in binary and decimal:

```
0000 = 0
0001 = 1
0010 = 2
0011 = 3
0100 = 4
0101 = 5
0110 = 6
0111 = 7
1000 = 8
1001 = 9
```

## Why Higher-Level Languages?

Though machine language is the most efficient programming language in terms of execution, it has various drawbacks. Programming in machine language is tedious and error-prone. The use of numeric codes to represent instructions is difficult and makes programming a complex, arduous task. This complexity results in programs that are difficult to read and even more difficult to debug.

In addition to being tedious, machine language requires the programmer to keep track of where individual bits of data are stored in the computer's memory. Inserting new instructions or changing the address of one **bit** of data affects the **correctness** of the program and the subsequent memory addresses used in the rest of the program. Machine language programs are very long since each instruction only accomplishes a small task. For example, to multiple two numbers could require more than 10 instructions in machine language. These drawbacks make programming in machine language slow and far from cost effective. To combat these and other difficulties, other languages were developed. Higher-level programming languages allow the programmer to concentrate more fully on the problem, not how the computer software and hardware interact to solve the problem. These programs are designed for ease and reliability, while machine language is designed for efficient execution.

With the advent of higher-level languages most programmers have very little use for machine language to write programs. However, programmers still need to understand machine language. For programmers responsible for maintaining machine language code and creating assemblers, knowledge of machine language is essential. Additionally, there are still tasks best accomplished using machine language.

*See also* BCD; Binary number system; Programming languages, types

# MACRO

A macro is a name or **identifier** that represents a (usually larger) combination of other names, identifiers, or symbols. Typically these represented identifiers will be a list of **commands** or program **code**. Macros have two similar but subtly different interpretations, and which one is used depends chiefly on the program interpreting it.

The simplest kind of macro is what might be called a "substitution macro." This type of macro is found in **programming** languages like **C** and **C++**, which support a "pre-processor" stage immediately before the **compiler** proper takes over to turn the computer program into a form the computer can understand. In these languages a macro is defined like this:

```
#define MY_MACRO printf("this is my macro!");
```

This line tells the pre-processor to replace every occurrence of the text "MY_MACRO" it finds in the code with the **expression** printf("this is my macro!"). This means that if the macro is used like this

```
if(printing == TRUE) {
MY_MACRO
}
```

the compiler will see the code

```
if(printing == TRUE) {
printf("this is my macro!");
}
```

after the pre-processor has finished. It is also possible to create macros that behave like functions. The macro

```
#define MY_MACRO(a) printf("this is my %s!," a)
```

when invoked like this

```
if(printing == TRUE) {
MY_MACRO("macro")
}
```

will generate the code

```
if(printing == TRUE) {
printf("this is my macro %s!," "macro");
}
```

The C and C++ pre-processor is a complex and powerful utility, and it has many more features than are discussed above. Nevertheless, using macros is generally frowned upon and used as a last resort by programmers; for not only do

macros make **debugging** code harder (it is hard to tell what is going on without constantly referring back to the macro definition), but macros that take parameters are not type-checked by the compiler even though their substituted code is. A result of this is that messages reporting errors on the line of code containing the macro use the name of the *function* the macro calls rather than the name of the macro. This can be very confusing.

The second type of macro is a "function macro." This type is more like a sequence of commands (which can be run by using a single name or keystroke) than a simple fragment of text to be substituted. In many ways they are akin to simple programs themselves, and, indeed, so-called "macros" in some complex software have developed into full-blown programming languages (for example Microsoft's "VBA" or "Visual Basic for Applications").

Today, any self-respecting word processor or spreadsheet will have a macro facility in it. Suppose, for example, that a writer is using a word processor and wants to indent every other line by eight spaces. In a word-processor that supports macros it would be possible to tell it to carry out the following commands and to run them by pressing a unique combination of keys or by typing a single command:

1. move the cursor to start of the first line
2. move the cursor down by two lines
3. insert eight spaces
4. repeat from step 2

Most word processors will allow the user to write these actions like a programmer, or even record them by doing the actions while in a special mode.

Macros can also be used to insert words and phrases that are used often, like names and addresses or salutations for letters. In this case the behavior of the macro (replacing a section of text with something else) behaves very much like the C and C++ macros do.

# MAGNETIC-CORE MEMORY

Magnetic-core **memory** (often called simply "core memory") is a class of computer memory devices, which consists of a series of small doughnut-shaped masses of hard ferromagnetic material strung on a wire matrix that can be magnetized in either of two directions. Such computer memory is associated with the **central processing unit** (**CPU**) where **data** is stored for periods of time ranging from a small fraction of a second to days, weeks or even longer before being retrieved for further processing. Magnetic-core memory refers to physical main memory that is internal to the computer. Today, however, other types of main memory devices have replaced magnetic-core memory.

The word main is used to distinguish main memory from external (secondary) mass storage devices such as disk drives. Another term for main memory is **random access memory** (RAM). Before magnetic-core memory, main memory consisted of vacuum tubes. For example, the **ENIAC**, the world's first general purpose, electronic, digital computer, used vacuum tubes in the 1940s for main memory. The **EDVAC**, **EDSAC**, and other historically important computers (all of which came after ENIAC) used so-called mercury delay lines for main storage. Magnetic-core memory came into use within computers in the early to mid-1950s. Today main memory consists of integrated circuits, each of which contains thousands of **semiconductor** devices. Where each vacuum tube or magnetic core represented one **bit** and the total memory of most computers were measured in thousands of bytes (or kilobytes, KB), each semiconductor device now represents millions of bytes (or megabytes, MB) and the total memory of many computers is measured in billions of bytes (or gigabytes, GB).

American electrical engineer Jay Wright Forrester (1918–) invented and patented the Multicoordinate Digital Information Storage Device in the late 1940s (using the basic concept of core memory patented by **An Wang** of Harvard University along with independent work performed by John Presper Eckert on the ENIAC project) while working on Project Whirlwind, a strategic defense computer developed at the Massachusetts Institute of Technology. This technology later became magnetic-core memory; a precursor to RAM that became the standard in central information storage for digital computers. **International Business Machines (IBM)** Corporation commercially developed magnetic core memory in the early 1950s. At that time, magnetic core memory consisted of tiny rings of magnetic material interspersed into a mesh of thin wires. When a computer sent a current through a pair of wires that were perpendicular to one another, the ring at their intersection became magnetized either clockwise or counterclockwise depending on the direction of the current; one orientation of magnetization represented a 0, while the opposite magnetization represented a 1. Computer manufacturers first used core memory in production computers in the 1950s, at about the same time that they began to replace vacuum tubes with transistors. Magnetic core memory was used through most of the 1960s and into the 1970s.

*See also* Bit; Byte; Disk drive; EDSAC (Electronic Delay Storage Automatic Calculator); EDVAC (Electronic Discrete Variable Automatic Computer); ENIAC (Electronic Numerical Integrator and Computer); Random-access memory (RAM)

# MAINFRAME

In the broadest sense, any large computer—large in the sense of computing capacity, that is, not in physical size—can be classified as a "mainframe" computer. Other classes of computer include **supercomputers**, minicomputers, and personal computers. Although there is no precise formula for what differentiates a mainframe computer from other types, there are some basic guidelines. Generally speaking, in a multi-user environment a mainframe computer is capable of supporting more users than a minicomputer. Like the typical mainframe computer, a supercomputer is a large and powerful device but, unlike the more general-purpose mainframe, usually serves a few users or only one, and is usually dedicated to solving complex computational problems (such as those found in

advanced engineering or scientific applications), rather than to general-purpose use.

The term "mainframe computer" had its genesis in the early days of the commercial computer industry. The major components of the electronic computers produced in the 1950s and early 1960s were mounted on racks or *frames*. In order to keep the lengths of cables interconnecting a computer's components to a minimum (thereby maximize processing speed), a computer's **central processing unit** (**CPU**) and main **memory** were most often housed together in a single frame, which came to become called the computer's *main frame*. Other frames of the computer housed peripheral devices, such as the secondary memory.

The first commercial electronic computers were physically huge machines that used vacuum tubes to perform their computations. By the late 1950s, mainframe computers appeared with transistors completely replacing vacuum tubes. Although transistors used considerably less space and power than vacuum tubes, the first all-transistor computers remained large mainframe machines. The advent of the **integrated circuit** in the 1970s meant that computers could be greatly reduced in size while still possessing adequate processing power for many tasks.

Mainframe computers have often been applied to multiuser and **multitasking** environments. In a multi-user environment, the mainframe computer can allocate computational resources to multiple users, conversing with each user through a different input/output **terminal**. Multitasking is a feature provided by a computer's operating system which allows multiple tasks to be performed concurrently.

Unlike personal computers, a mainframe is managed and maintained by professional programmers and system operators. Early mainframe computers were often used in a batch-processing mode with "jobs" being submitted by users using "dumb" terminals (i.e., machines with no built-in logic circuits, capable only of exchanging information with the mainframe computer). The mainframe computer executed the jobs submitted to it and returned the results to the appropriate terminal. As computer technology evolved, mainframe computers became an integral part of distributed processing systems. In such systems many smaller computers, such as minicomputers, are linked together in a system controlled by a host computer, often a mainframe computer.

Since the early 1980s personal computers have become increasingly powerful. Today, these smaller computers are able to perform many tasks once associated with mainframes. For example, personal computers are capable of performing sophisticated **graphics** and video-rendering tasks that at one time were solely the domain of mainframe computers or even supercomputers. Moreover, for the cost of a single mainframe an organization can purchase many smaller computers. Software costs, too, are usually higher for mainframes than for personal computers. This is because commercial software packages and tools have been extensively developed for personal computers, whereas the system and application software for mainframe computers is often custom-written. Because of these and other factors, it seemed a foregone conclusion to many industry analyts of the early 1990s that mainframes would soon be completely replaced by smaller, more versatile computers.

However, mainframe systems continue to be utilized for a variety of reasons. In government, military, and corporate environments, mainframe computers are often seen as having several advantages. First, a single mainframe computer may require less maintenance than a network of smaller computers. Another beneficial aspect of mainframes is security and system control. Because mainframe processing and memory storage are centralized, mainframes are often seen as providing a more secure environment than, say, a collection of workstations, each with its own memory and **microprocessor**. **Access** to the mainframe can be monitored more effectively than access to a multitude of distributed computers. Finally, organizations are sometimes reluctant to forego their tried-and-true mainframe systems for a new approach (such as multiple workstations) that may have unforeseen impacts on operations.

Mainframe computer systems have been enhanced with new capabilities. **Internet** software tools, for instance, add new capabilities. Additionally, over the past decade the new disciplines of data warehousing and data mining have provided another useful role well for the mainframe. A **data** warehouse is a collection of historic data; oftentimes corporations or government agencies archive huge amounts of data for later analysis, or even just on the off chance that it might come in handy some day. To handle such huge data bases requires correspondingly muscular computers. **Data mining** (sometimes called "knowledge discovery") is a data-processing function designed to uncover new and useful information from collections of data such as those stored in data warehouses.

*See also* Data mining; Integrated circuit; Multitasking; Personal computer; Supercomputers

# MASK

A mask is a pattern of bits used as a filter to selectively accept or reject bits in a set of **data**. (A bit is the smallest piece of information used by modern electronic computers and consists uniquely of the binary digits 0 and 1.) For example, when defining the field of a database, a mask is assigned to indicate what type of **value** the field should contain (such as only alphabetic characters). Values that do not conform to the mask requirements cannot be entered into the database.

The binary image of a mask, commonly called a *bit mask*, is used to selectively reject or accept certain corresponding bits in a data value when the mask is used in an **expression** with a logical **operator**. When a mask is used in this way, the areas with **bit** values of "1" are accepted while the areas with bit values of "0" are rejected (or "masked") in the calculations. A logical (or Boolean) operator (such as AND, OR, XOR, and NOT) is used to match a mask of 0s and 1s with a **string** of data bits (a data value). When a "1" bit occurs in the mask, the bit in the data value remains the same, but when a "0" bit occurs in the mask, the bit in the data value is switched from 1 to 0 (while a 0 remains a 0). For example, the mask 00111111, when used with the AND operator, removes (or

"masks off") the two uppermost bits (those on the far left) in a data value (such as 11010101) but does not affect the rest of the value. Thus, in the expression "11010101 AND 00111111" the mask (00111111) takes off the "11" from the uppermost (left side) of the data value (11010101), resulting in the value 00010101.

**Hardware** interrupts are often enabled and disabled with software that contains masking, with each **interrupt** assigned a bit position in a mask **register** (a set of bits used to store data). A hardware interrupt is a signal that tells a computer program that an event has occurred. When a program receives an interrupt signal, it takes a specified **action** (either to accept or reject the signal). Interrupt signals can cause a program to suspend itself temporarily to service the interrupt. Various interrupt signals exist, such as individual keystrokes that generate an interrupt signal, and interrupts that are generated by devices (such as printers). A maskable interrupt is any hardware interrupt that can be temporarily disabled (masked) during periods when a program needs almost the entire capacity of the **microprocessor**.

*See also* Bit; Boolean algebra; Logical operations

# MAUCHLY, JOHN WILLIAM (1907-1980)
*American computer engineer*

John William Mauchly, a physicist and computer engineer, is widely credited with co-inventing two of the most important early computers. With J. Presper Eckert, Mauchly invented the first general-purpose digital electronic computer, the **Electronic Numerical Integrator and Computer** (**ENIAC**). Also with Eckert, Mauchly developed the first commercial digital electronic computer, the **Universal Automatic Computer** (**UNIVAC**). Their work together effectively began the commercial computer revolution in America and throughout the world.

Mauchly was born on August 30, 1907, in Cincinnati, Ohio, to Sebastian J. Mauchly and Rachel Scheidemantel Mauchly. His father was an electrical engineer who, in 1915, moved the family east to accept a position as head of the Section of Terrestrial Electricity and Magnetism at the Carnegie Institute in Washington, D.C. Mauchly attended the Johns Hopkins University from 1925 to 1927, when he was admitted to the graduate school there without an undergraduate degree. He received a Ph.D. in physics from Johns Hopkins in 1932. He spent another year there as a research assistant, and then in 1933 he was appointed head of the physics department at Ursinus College, near Philadelphia.

Mauchly had a strong early interest in meteorology, but he found studying the weather to be particularly difficult because it took so much time to coordinate all the **data**. Computations could only be done by hand or with the primitive calculating machines then available. Interested in using statistics to prove the effect of sun flares on the weather, he began trying to develop a better machine for calculating. During the late 1930s, Mauchly began to experiment with vacuum tubes in place of the slower gears and wheels used in mechanical computing devices.

Mauchly did not publish anything on his experiments until December of 1940, when he gave a paper to the American Association for the Advancement of Science on using computing machines to solve meteorology problems. After presenting his paper, he was approached by **John Atanasoff**, a professor at Iowa State University, who told him he was building an electronic computer. In June of 1941, Mauchly went to Iowa State to see Atanasoff's computer—a visit which was later used against his patent claim that he and Eckert had invented the first computer. Atanasoff said later that Mauchly had been fascinated by it; Mauchly said that seeing the computer had been of little **value**. It had run slowly and had only done simple arithmetic functions.

When the United States entered World War II, Mauchly agreed to study electrical engineering at the Moore School of Engineering at the University of Pennsylvania in order to further the war effort. It was there he met Eckert and they began their famous collaboration. The Moore School had already developed one of the most advanced electro-mechanical computational devices in the world, the differential analyzer. At the beginning of the war, the United States Army had awarded the school a contract to compute the tables of trajectories for artillery shells. Both Mauchly and Eckert became deeply involved in this project.

Mauchly and Eckert were both fascinated with the idea of using vacuum tubes to create an electronic digital computer. They used vacuum tubes, photoelectric cells, and other devices to make the existing mechanical computer at the Moore School work ten times faster. In August of 1942, Mauchly wrote a five-page memo to an administrator at the school, John Grist Brainerd. The memo, "The Use of High-Speed Vacuum Tube Devices for Calculating," outlined how vacuum tubes could be used to add, subtract, multiply, and divide much more rapidly than mechanical calculators. Brainerd, Herman H. Goldstine, and Oswald Veblen saw the potential for an electronic computer, and in April of 1943 the Moore School got permission from the army to go ahead with what is now called the ENIAC.

Eckert and Mauchly designed and built the ENIAC with a team of fifty other people at the Moore School, overcoming a number of technical and logistical obstacles. Unfortunately for the war effort, the ENIAC did not run its first full-scale test until December of 1945, several months after World War II had ended. After the war, ENIAC was used to solve trajectory problems and compute ballistics tables at the army's Aberdeen Proving Ground. Later, it performed calculations for the development of the hydrogen bomb.

Mauchly and Eckert applied for a patent on the ENIAC in 1947. By then, they had resigned from the Moore Engineering School and had begun their own corporation, the Eckert and Mauchly Computer Corporation. They assigned their patent to their corporation, where they developed the first commercial computer, the UNIVAC. Eckert took care of the engineering functions, and Mauchly ran the business. Neither Mauchly nor Eckert, however, was a good businessman. Mauchly was very easy going and jovial, but he was also

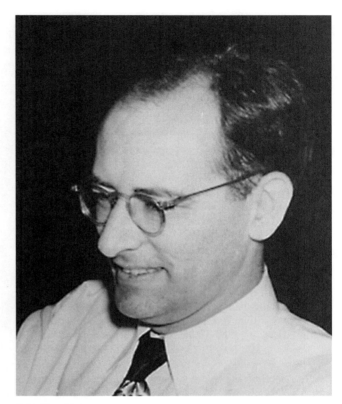

**John Mauchly**

unconventional. When he and Eckert visited **IBM** and its famous president, **Thomas Watson**, Sr., Mauchly flopped down on the couch and put his feet up on the coffee table. Eckert and Mauchly eventually ran into financial troubles, and in 1950 they sold their company along with their computer patents to Remington Rand. Sperry Rand later bought out Remington. Mauchly worked for Remington and Sperry until 1959, when he left to form his own consulting corporation, Mauchly Associates. In 1968, he founded a second computer consulting corporation, which he called Dynatrend.

In February 1964, after seventeen years, the ENIAC patent was finally issued to one of Sperry Rand's subsidiaries, Illinois Scientific Developments. The patent, however, was very broad and vaguely written. When Sperry Rand sued the Honeywell Corporation in 1967 for infringing the ENIAC patent, Honeywell countersued. Honeywell claimed, among other things, that the patent was a fraud and that Eckert and Mauchly did not invent the first general-purpose digital electronic computer. Honeywell's suit claimed that Atanasoff was the real inventor. There was a lengthy trial, and each side presented thousands of pages of documents to support its arguments. In October, 1973, Judge Earl Larson of Minneapolis issued his judgment, which made Honeywell the winner. Judge Larson's decision to invalidate the patent was based primarily on the facts that the patent on the ENIAC was filed after the computer had been in use for over a year and that information about the ENIAC had already been published, making the technology "prior art" and thus unpatentable.

In his decision, the judge also held that Atanasoff was the real inventor of the electronic digital computer. This last reason especially bothered Mauchly. Atanasoff had never considered himself the originator of the electronic digital computer until an IBM lawyer mentioned the idea to him in 1954. Atanasoff never even built a working electronic computer; he attempted a prototype but he could not get all the parts to work together before he abandoned it. His computer was also highly specialized and could only compute linear equations, whereas the ENIAC could add, subtract, multiply, divide, extract square roots, compare quantities, and perform other functions. Many people who have studied the case believe that Mauchly and Eckert were wronged by Judge Larson's decision. Mauchly himself believed he had been wronged, and the patent decision left him bitter. Even though he won many awards for his accomplishments, including the Howard N. Potts Medal in 1949, the John Scott Award in 1961, and the Harry Goode Award in 1966, Mauchly never ceased to feel he had been denied full credit for his role in the development of the computer.

Mauchly had married Mary Augusta Walzl in 1930. They had two sons. But in September of 1946, while they were swimming in the Atlantic, his wife was swept out to sea and drowned. On February 7, 1948, Mauchly married Kathleen R. McNulty, who had been one of the programmers on the ENIAC. He had five more children with her, four daughters and a son. Mauchly suffered all his life from a hereditary genetic disease called hemorrhagic telangiectasia, which caused bloody noses and internal bleeding, among other symptoms. In his later life he had to carry around oxygen to breathe properly. He died on January 8, 1980, of complications from an infection.

# McCarthy, John (1927-   )

*American computer scientist*

John McCarthy coined the term **artificial intelligence** (AI) and is recognized as the father of AI research. He founded two of the most important AI laboratories in the world and wrote the primary computer **programming** language for AI research, **List Processing** Language (**LISP**). While his quest for an intelligent machine has yet to be fulfilled, his work in computers has produced a number of other important advances, including interactive time-sharing, computer semantics, and one of the first proposals to link home computers to a public network.

The oldest of two brothers, McCarthy was born in Boston, Massachusetts, on September 4, 1927. His father, John Patrick McCarthy, was an Irish immigrant and working-class militant. His mother, Ida Glatt, was a Jewish Lithuanian active in the suffrage movement. Both were members of the Communist party in the 1930s, so McCarthy is what is known among political activists as a "red diaper" baby. John Patrick McCarthy worked as a carpenter, a fisherman, a union organizer, and also as an inventor. He held two patents, one for a ship caulking machine and the other for a hydraulic orange juice squeezer. Young John McCarthy and his brother Patrick

were raised to think politically and logically, and although McCarthy eventually decided that Marxism was hardly scientific, he never renounced science, logic, or politics.

McCarthy was a bookish lad whose health problems eventually spurred his family's move to Los Angeles. He attended public school and skipped three grades before entering the California Institute of Technology (Cal Tech) in 1944 with plans to become a mathematician. After several interruptions, including a stint as an army clerk, he graduated in 1948. From Cal Tech, McCarthy went to Princeton University, where he earned his doctorate in mathematics and took his first academic job as an instructor in mathematics in 1951. Two years later he became an acting assistant professor of mathematics at Stanford University before moving to Dartmouth College in 1955. While at Dartmouth in the summer of 1956, he was the principle organizer of the first conference on modeling intelligence in computers and coined the term artificial intelligence for the conference proposal. McCarthy was working on a chess-playing computer program at the time. In order to limit the moves the computer had to consider, McCarthy invented a search strategy and mathematical **method** that is now called the alpha-beta heuristic, which allowed the computer to eliminate any moves that permit the computer's opponent to quickly gain an advantage.

In 1958 McCarthy moved to the Massachusetts Institute of Technology (MIT), where he became an associate professor and founded the first AI laboratory. It was here that McCarthy constructed the computer programming language called List Processing Language, or LISP, which is still the most common computer language used in AI research. He also began work on the idea of giving a computer "common sense"—a difficult problem that became the focus of many AI researchers in the late 1980s—and developed the first means of interactive time-sharing on computers which allows hundreds, or even thousands, of people, to use one large computer at the same time. During his tenure at MIT, McCarthy married for the first time and had the first of his two daughters, Susan Joanne. In 1962 he moved his family to Stanford to take up a professorship in computer science and start a second AI laboratory. He has two other children, Sarah Kathleen and Timothy Talcott.

While at Stanford McCarthy continued to contribute to AI research in a number of ways, from mentoring many of the best young scientists in the field, to clarifying the different roles played by mathematical logic and common sense (called nonmonotonic reasoning by McCarthy) in AI. But his greatest contribution has been in the area of artificial languages, especially semantics. Philip J. Hilts, in his book *Scientific Temperaments,* quotes one mathematician on LISP: "The new expansion of man's view of the nature of mathematical objects, made possible by LISP, is exciting. There appears to be no limit to the diversity of problems to which LISP will be applied. It seems to be a truly general language, with commensurate computing power." In addition, McCarthy has speculated on machines that could make copies of themselves (automata) as well as artificial intelligence smarter than its creator.

McCarthy's adventurous impulses have not been confined to academic speculations. He has been a rock climber, a pilot, and he has even made a dozen parachute jumps. After

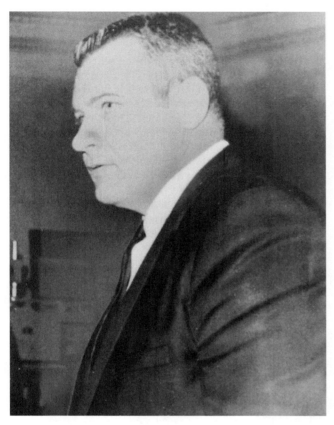

**John McCarthy**

McCarthy's first marriage ended in divorce in the 1960s, he married Vera Watson, a computer programmer and a world-class mountain climber. She was the first woman to solo the 22,800-foot Aconcagua peak in the Andes, and for a number of years she and McCarthy climbed lesser peaks together. Tragically, Watson died while a member of the women's expedition attempting to scale Annapurna peak in the Himalayas.

Politics have always been important to McCarthy, as they were to his parents. While he has called himself a reactionary because of his rejection of Marxism, in many ways his views defy simple categories. In the 1960s he was involved in many political campaigns and projects, such as the Free University in Palo Alto, California, but he eventually became disillusioned by the methods of some of the leftist groups with which he worked. Still, he felt that his own work on computer technology could benefit democracy by allowing people easy access to information. The danger of authoritarian control over computer technology led him to propose an extension of the Bill of Rights to cover electronic **data** and communications, an idea that became part of the national debate on computer networks in the 1990s. Specifically, McCarthy called for limiting control of public data files and allowing each person the right to read, correct, and limit access to his or her own files.

In 1971 McCarthy won the prestigious Alan Mathison Turing Award from the Association for Computing Machinery, of which he is a member. In addition, he is a former president of the American Association for Artificial Intelligence. He also received the Kyoto Prize in 1988 and the National Medal of Science in 1990. In 1987 he assumed the Charles M. Pigott chair of the Stanford University School of Engineering and became a professor in Stanford's Computer Science Department and director of the Stanford Artificial Intelligence Laboratory.

McCarthy has argued that making artificially intelligent robots that are more intelligent than human beings is quite possible, since (according to McCarthy) intelligence is made up of logic and common sense that can be mathematically represented. Despite his optimism in the goal of constructing intelligent machines, McCarthy has been one of the most rigorous critics of AI research. In a survey conducted in the 1970s and reprinted in his collection of essays, *Formalizing Common Sense,* McCarthy concluded that "artificial intelligence research has so far been only moderately successful; its rate of solid progress is perhaps greater than most social sciences and less than many physical sciences. This is perhaps to be expected, considering the difficulty of the problem."

## MECHANICAL COMPUTATION

Mechanical computation refers to the use of moving parts in a machine to perform mathematical operations upon numbers. The vast majority of modern computers perform their computations electronically, by manipulating the movement of electrons, and not through the movement of the parts of a machine. An example of the difference between the mechanical versus the electronic representation and manipulation of numbers is that of timekeeping devices. At one time, watches used springs, cogs, gears, etc. to "compute" and track time. Today, mechanical watches have largely been replaced by electronic versions in which no moving parts are used.

One of the first devices used for mechanical computations was the **abacus**. Abacuses, which are still used in some parts of the world today, usually consist of a rectangular frame enclosing rods on which balls or beads are moved. A person moves the beads to perform arithmetic calculations. Versions of the abacus have been around since at least 3,000 B.C. The Renaissance brought about revolutionary advances in science and technology, including the creation of new computing devices. In 1617 Scotsman **John Napier** (1550–1617) showed how logarithms could simplify the operations of multiplication and division, as well as aid in calculating square roots and powers. Napier developed a calculating tool utilizing logarithms that consisted of numbered rods. Called **Napier's rods**, the device would eventually be transformed into the modern logarithmic-scale **slide rule**, which was an essential calculating device used by engineers and scientists until the 1970s.

In 1623 German mathematician and clergyman Wilhelm Schickard (1592–1635) developed a "computing clock" to perform the four basic arithmetic operations (addition, subtraction, multiplication and division). Schickard's **calculator** incorporated aspects of Napier's rods, but added wheels and gears. Unfortunately, Schickard's computing clock was destroyed in a fire, and Schickard died shortly thereafter. After Schickard, **Blaise Pascal** (1623–1662) and Gottfried Wilhelm von Leibniz (1646–1716), developed their own hand-operated calculating machines. In 1642, at the age of eighteen, **Pascal** devised a "numerical wheel calculator." Pascal's calculator (called the Pascaline) was contained in a small rectangular box and featured eight movable dials for entering numbers up to eight digits long. The **Pascaline** added decimal numbers (i.e., numbers expressed with the digits 0 through 9). The Pascaline could not perform subtraction, multiplication or division. About thirty years after Pascal's invention, Leibniz created a calculating machine based upon the Pascaline that he called the Stepped Reckoner (also called Leibniz's wheel). Like the Pascaline, Leibniz's calculator employed a system of dials and gears; a hand crank powered the device. Leibniz incorporated a "stepped-drum gear" (hence the name "stepped reckoner") that allowed his calculator to perform not only addition (like the Pascaline), but multiplication as well. Mechanical problems plagued Leibniz's calculator, thereby limiting its usefulness.

An important distinction in computing is highlighted by the devices discussed above: they may be analog or digital. A digital process or machine proceeds in discrete steps, as in the case of the abacus. Computations with the abacus entail moving singular objects (beads or balls) from one location to another. By contrast, an analog process or machine involves a continuous movement or "flow"; in the case of the slide rule, components slide past one another in a continuous movement, not in the discrete "jumps" of a digital process. Although numbers (which by definition are discrete entities) are inscribed on a slide rule, the **operator** must "estimate" the computational results from the juxtaposition of the slide rule's parts.

In spite of the calculating machines introduced in the seventeenth and eighteenth centuries, it was only in the nineteenth century that sophisticated computational machines were widely used. The **Arithmometer**, invented in 1818 by Frenchman Charles Xavier Thomas (1785–1870), is generally considered the first calculating machine to be commercially mass-produced. The Arithmometer could add, subtract, multiply and divide numbers up to 30 decimal digits. Users "dialed" numbers onto a set of wheels and then used a hand crank to perform the calculations. By 1830 some fifteen hundred Arithmometers had been sold.

One of the most influential and famous inventors of computational machines was Englishman **Charles Babbage** (1792–1871). Around the time that the Arithmometer was being introduced, Babbage began a project (with British government funds) to build a "difference engine." Babbage's **difference engine** was designed to determine the values of algebraic expressions called "polynomials." The difference engine was to compute those values using a system of gears, shafts, etc., to be driven by a steam engine. Babbage never completed more than small portions of the difference engine; however, he moved on to a more ambitious calculating device, called the "Analytical engine" that possessed many features of modern computers. **Programming** and **data** was to be supplied by punch cards. Conditional branching (i.e., "if-then" statements) was to be supported. There was a "store" that held data

for processing, which today would be called the computer's primary **memory**. An addition was to be done in 3 seconds and a multiplication or division in two to four minutes. Unfortunately, the British government cancelled funding for both Babbage machines, and they were never completed (however, in the mid-1800s a Swedish father-son team did complete and sell at least two difference machines based on Babbage's plans).

Other important developments in computing at the end of the nineteenth century include the American Dorr E. Felt (1862–1930), who in 1885 built the "Comptometer," which was the first calculator wherein numbers were entered by pressing keys as opposed to using dials or similar methods. In 1889 Felt invented the first desk calculator with a built-in **printer**. Another important American inventor was **Herman Hollerith** (1860–1929), who developed a punch card machine for tabulating the 1890 United States census figures.

The apex of gear-driven computers may have been the analog "integraph" of **Vannevar Bush** (1890–1974), completed in 1930. The integraph was a large, mechanical computer that employed gears, chains, shafts, etc. that solved solutions through "integration." To "reprogram" the machine meant that it had to be physically dismantled and the gears, shafts, etc. reoriented to solve a new problem. The integraph worked successfully for many years in solving equations with engineering and scientific applications.

The 1930s witnessed the displacement of the purely mechanical computing device by "electromechanical" and "electronic" computers. *Electromechanical computers* (sometimes called *relay computers*) can be thought of as a **transition** between the earlier mechanical computers and modern electronic computers. Electronic computers perform their calculations through the movement of electrons instead of moving parts, and so are not classified as mechanical computers. Like electronic computers, electromechanical computers performed computations through the control of electrons (or current flow), but that control depended on the movement of parts (i.e., relays) that were opened and closed. Examples of electromechanical computers were the series of **Bell Laboratories relay computers**. First operational in 1939, Bell relay computers were used throughout the 1940s and into the 1950s, when they gave way to the modern electronic computer. The first electronic computers created in the 1940s used vacuum tubes; by the mid-1950s the vacuum tubes were being replaced by transistors.

*See also* Abacus; Analog vs. digital computing; Analytic engine; Arithmometer; Bell Laboratories relay computers; Felt's comptometer; History of computer science; Leibniz's mechanical multiplier; Napier's rods; Pascaline

# MEMBER FUNCTION

A member **function** is a component of objects. Objects are miniature programs, which consist of both **code** and **data** (data members). The code is comprised of a series of member functions. It is these functions that are called on by a user, also described as sending the **object** a **message**, in order to use the object. For example, calling an object's Draw function can also be described as sending the object the Draw message. Calling a member function invokes the function on the object.

A member function allows some of an object's behavior or contents to be retrieved. Thus, it forms one of the underpinnings of the **programming** of object-oriented languages such as C++.

Member functions can be classified according to their purpose. Examples of some types of member functions in C++ are "getters", "setters", "command methods", and "factory methods." Also, classification based on the properties of member functions is possible. Examples of these include "primitive or composed method", "hook or **template** method", "class or instance method", or a "convenience method."

*See also* C++; Object-oriented programming

# MEMORY

Memory is basically any form of electronic storage. For example, a light switch has memory, as it is able to memorize position 0 and 1 in order to turn a light on and off. Practically, memory is most often used to designate fast and temporary forms of storage. This is electronic memory. Other forms of memory are magnetic core memories and optical memories (such as **CD-ROM**).

There are two main categories of memory, volatile and nonvolatile. Volatile memory loses the **data** when the system is turned off. Most types of RAM are volatile. In contrast, nonvolatile memory does not lose its data when the system or the device is turned off. **ROM** is a familiar example of nonvolatile memory.

The electronic memory systems designed for temporary storage of data are vital to a computer's efficient performance. A **central processing unit** operates much more swiftly by using data kept in memory than if the **CPU** had to acquire every piece of information from the **hard drive**. A computer disk is also a memory system, being capable of information storage.

There is an array of solid-state electronic memory **hardware** available in a computer. The following is a brief summary.

- Flip-flop—the basic memory cell, capable of either a 0 or 1 state. It is used as a basic building block in circuits.

- Register—a small set of flip flops arranged in parallel, used in complex chips.

- SRAM (Static Random Access Memory)—an array of flip flops, often used in cache applications.

- DRAM (Dynamic Random Access Memory)—an array of storage cells, used for main computing data storage.

- ROM (Read Only Memory)—an array of wired cells, which are set up by the manufacturer. There are still other types of ROM available, but these are relevant to users with specialized needs, or for whom extremely fast computational speeds are necessary

The CPU in a computer is constantly using memory during **operation**. As an illustration, the following occur sequentially when a computer is turned on and used. First, data is loaded from **read-only memory** (ROM) and a power-on self test (POST) is done to ensure that all major components are working. A memory controller checks for errors in memory chips. Next, the basic input/output system (**BIOS**) is loaded from ROM, to provide information about certain computer functions. The operating system (OS) is loaded from the hard drive into the system's **random access memory** (RAM). As long as the computer is on, information critical for its operation is maintained in RAM, to provide the CPU with immediate access to the information. When an application is opened, it is loaded into RAM, either all at once, or the information needed to commence operation is loaded followed by the remaining information as needed. As files are opened, they too are loaded into RAM. Finally, when the file is closed, the information is written to the specified storage device and then deleted from RAM.

RAM is central to a computer's function. Each time something is loaded or opened, it is placed into RAM. RAM is a storage area, which the CPU can use to obtain data. The CPU requests the data it needs from RAM, processes it and writes new data back to RAM. This cycle occurs continuously, millions of times each second, during operation of the computer.

In addition to the memory associated with the CPU and RAM, a computer also has so-called caches of memory, **virtual memory**, and memory associated with **disk storage**. This plethora of memory allows for the management of memory, and helps make high-speed computing possible. Modern CPUs running at speeds such as 1 gigahertz are massive consumers of data—billions of bytes per second. If the data flow is not fast enough, the CPU literally stops and waits for data to arrive. The amount of memory necessary to keep up with a 1 gigahertz CPU was often prohibitively expensive. Computer engineers solved this problem by "tiering" memory—using expensive memory in small quantities and then backing it up with larger quantities of less expensive memory.

Hard disk memory is the least expensive form of memory. While inexpensive, hard disk memory operates slowly. It can take up to a second to read a megabyte of information off of a hard disk. The next level of hierarchy is RAM. Data can be transmitted to the CPU faster by means of hardware called a **bus**. This hardware alone is not sufficient to keep up with the demands of the CPU. For that, caches are required.

Caches make data used most often by the CPU instantly available. This is achieved by building a small amount of memory, primary, or level 1 cache, right into the CPU. Level 1 cache is small, normally between 2K and 64K. The secondary or level 2 cache, ranging in size from 256K to 2MB, typically resides on a memory card near the CPU. Some higher performance computers have the level 2 cache built directly onto the CPU board. The caches service the CPU almost 95 percent of the time.

*See also* Allocation and deallocation of memory; Magnetic core memory; Physical and virtual memory; Protonic memory; Separation of memory; Solid-state memory storage technology; Ultrasonic memory

# MENU BAR

A menu bar is a horizontal menu, or a list of the task options, which usually appears at the top of a window in a graphical user environment. This type of menu can also be called a moving bar menu, as the various options are highlighted as the mouse-directed bar or box is moved from one option to another. The bar is designed such that the clicking of the **mouse** on a selected option triggers the appearance of a popup or pull-down menu (which can also be called a cascading menu), which lists further sub-options. Highlighting a desired option using the mouse and clicking the relevant mouse key or pad will trigger the functioning of the option.

The menu bar contrasts with the so-called command-driven system, in which the command must be explicitly entered, rather than chosen from a list of possible **commands**. A menu-driven system, and the menu bar in particular, is intended to be simpler and easier to learn than a command-driven system. However, a command-driven system retains greater flexibility in terms of interaction with programs.

*See also* Graphical user interface (GUI); Windows

# MESSAGE

Messages are usually text based displays designed to update the computer user on system status or to issue warnings regarding specific operations.

Messages that contain numerical **data** usually have the numerical data converted to **string** format prior to display. Most messages are programmed responses to certain default conditions or sets of **programming** flags. Other messages provide standard warnings against the **deletion** of files or the opening of insecure documents. **Internet** messages often update the user on the status of a page search (e.g., "Page not found messages") or warn against the sending of information over an insecure link.

Although often similar in appearance, messages differ from dialog boxes in that messages do not require a user response. Modified message formats may ask the user to acknowledge the message by pressing a prompt key before the message is removed from the screen and operations or programs proceed.

Programming or software objects also communicate via messages, and these messages become a vital part of program **operation**. Because of this, programming objects do not need to be in the same program, process or physical machine—as long as there is an establishable communication link between the objects. A program may set a certain number of flags (indirect message) or send a direct message to a **subroutine** to execute a certain portion of a program. The sending **object** is, in a

programming sense, sending a message to the second object so that the second object performs a specific operation.

Although messages may have multiple components or parameters, almost all messages contain at least three vital components. First, the message must contain the address of the object to which it is directed. Second, the message must contain sufficient information to direct the receiving object what to do when the message is received. Finally, the message must contain any information required to perform the desired operation(s).

*See also* Computer-Assisted Instruction (CAI); Control structure; Default condition; Hash table; Input and output; Protocols; String

# MESSAGE-PASSING

One of the most basic paradigms in distributed computing is that of **message** passing. For computing nodes in a distributed system to be able to communicate effectively and share their work and information, it is necessary for them to either be able to write to and read from some common area of **memory**, or else for nodes to be able to send messages to one another. A distributed system that uses the first method is said to be following the shared-memory model, while one that uses the second is said to be using message-passing. The shared memory model is used in **parallel processing** with a small number of processors, while the message-passing model is used in larger systems with many processors.

In a message-passing system, nodes or processors communicate by sending messages over links or communication channels which provide bidirectional connectivity between pairs of nodes. The pattern of connections provided by the channels defines the topology (geometric structure) of the distributed system. The topology of such a system is usually represented by an undirected graph in which each computing node is represented by a **node**, and an edge is present between two nodes if and only if there is a communication link between the computing nodes that they represent. The collection of communication links is also often called a network.

In order to use message-passing effectively on real systems, it is necessary to have well-defined and meaningful **algorithms**. An algorithm usable on a message-passing system with a certain topology specifies the behavior of each node on the system. The processor at that node is able to perform local computation as well as send and receive messages from its immediate neighbors in the network. Nodes that are not immediate neighbors must rely on the **action** of intermediate nodes acting as relays, to convey messages to one another.

A message-passing system is said to be asynchronous if there is no fixed upper bound on how long it might take for a message to be delivered. Another measure thought to denote asynchronicity is the lack of bounds on the speeds of individual computing nodes in the network. A common example of an asynchronous system is the Internet, where **e-mail** and other messages can sometimes take days to arrive (though at other times they arrive within minutes of being sent). The computing power of individual nodes on the **Internet** may also vary widely, and there is no universal performance or speed guarantee that could be made. In most smaller practical message-passing systems (such as Intranets) there is some kind of upper bound on message delays and processor speeds, but these upper bounds can be quite large, may be subject to change arbitrarily with **hardware** and software upgrades, maintenance and outages, and may be reached rarely. Therefore, it is often desirable to avoid making references to information about such bounds, even if they exist, in designing message-passing algorithms. Those who **design** and work with asynchronous systems, which are the most common kinds of message passing systems there are, prefer to design and implement algorithms that are largely, if not totally, free of any particular timing information.

The other kind of message-passing system, although rarely seen in larger contexts, is the synchronous system. In this case the processors at all the nodes must execute in lockstep, and the execution is partitioned into "rounds." In each round, nodes may send messages to other nodes, all messages sent are delivered, and the processor at each node performs local computations based on the information it has, including any messages it has just received. This model is extremely convenient when it comes to designing algorithms, as in this case there is little scope for uncertainty. However, it is very difficult to implement this model in practice, which is why it remains largely confined to the realm of theory.

One measure of the complexity of a message-passing algorithm is its message-complexity—which is defined as the maximum number of messages sent, over all the possible reasonable executions of the algorithm. This definition of message complexity is valid in asynchronous as well as synchronous systems. In the specific case of synchronous systems, another measure of complexity applies—the time complexity. This is simply the number of rounds it takes the algorithm, under any possible reasonable execution, to terminate. Measuring the time delay in an asynchronous system is much more difficult—in this case, we may make a convenient assumption that the message delay in every instance is one, and simply count the delay in any execution of the algorithm. The time complexity thus measured is then reasonable to the extent that the assumption about the message delays is accurate. In the literature, such systems which offer partial guarantees about message delays and are thus not truly asynchronous, are called partially synchronous systems.

In a true asynchronous message-passing system, determining which event happened when tends to become a tricky matter also. Work by Lamport in the 1970s has shown that there cannot be a global sense of time in such a system, and that a "logical clock" which may be able to order the relative (though not absolute) times of two events, is the best that can be achieved. Likewise, a famous 1985 paper by Lynch (writing with co-authors) has shown that in a true asynchronous system, it is not possible to achieve **consensus** if even one single processor is faulty.

*See also* Consensus; Distributed Systems; Graphs; Internet; Parallel Processing

# METALANGUAGE

If a native English speaker who knows no other language has to take an introductory class to learn French, the instructor will of course have to begin the discussion in English. The French language will be introduced to the native speaker of English, through the medium of his own. This is a real-world approximation of the concept of metalanguage—applicable in linguistics, philosophy, computer science, and formal logic, to name but a few fields. In the situation given, English is the metalanguage, and French is the **object** language. The metalanguage is one which is used to describe and discuss the properties of the object language. Another common example of a metalanguage would be an English grammar, which is used to describe and analyze the correctness of spoken and written English.

The prefix meta- (of Greek origin) is often added to words to give them similar special meanings. Similar to the above, for instance, one can speak of a metatheory that is used to describe a theory; or a metacommunication that is a communication about a communication; or a metasyntax, or metadata—reasoned about similarly. The meaning of the prefix meta- as applied here comes from analytic philosophy—in literature it is used to denote opposition or error, as in metachronism, the error of incorrect temporal ordering (such as placing a person in history before the time of his or her parents). The renowned mathematician David Hilbert (1862-1943) was the first to use the prefix meta- in metalanguage, metatheory, and now metasystem. He even introduced the term metamathematics to denote a mathematical theory of mathematical proof.

An elementary example of a formal metalanguage is the algebraic notation that we all learn in high school. Algebra may be thought of as a metatheory with respect to the theory of arithmetic, and its formal language of **expression** is a metalanguage with respect to the language of arithmetic. For instance, using basic arithmetic one can do the most elementary calculations such as finding the sum of two and two, but using algebra, it is possible to take one step up, such as to discover that there are an infinite number of primes (a result traditionally attributed to the Greek mathematician Euclid).

However, high school algebra is not the highest up one can get. Modern algebra is for the most part a metatheory for high school algebra, and one can go even higher (as do some research mathematicians). Thus, at the most basic level, there is the simple language of numbers that a child is first introduced to; then there is the language of arithmetic, which manipulates those numbers and expresses results about them, and is thus a metalanguage for the language of numbers. High school algebra is in turn a metalanguage for the language of arithmetic, and modern algebra is a metalanguage for high school algebra. Each of these languages has a distinct role and power—it would take an infinite number of arithmetical statements and derivations to make up a single proof from high school algebra.

Thus, it is important to understand that a meta- object is different in a formal sense from the object(s) it describes, and is immensely more powerful in its expression. In the real world this might not be intuitively obvious, since one can learn French in English or English in French, so that either could be the metalanguage for the other, but in formal systems, it is erroneous to consider the metalanguage and the object language as equivalent. A well-known piece of mathematics called Russell's paradox, named after its discoverer Bertrand Russell (1872-1970), illustrates this for metasets. A metaset cannot be the same as a set, because if it were, then the metaset that consists of all sets that do not contain themselves, must both contain itself and not contain itself, simultaneously.

In contemporary logic research, a metalanguage is used to express proofs about the statements of the object language. The metalanguage may be rigorously defined, but is more often a mixture of human language and some mathematical notation. There are also other specifically defined metalanguages that are used to describe or reason about formal languages. For instance, **XML** (**Extensible Markup Language**) is the key to creating markups that can be used by any number of applications such as web browsing and others. XML is a metalanguage: it defines and describes the language, much like a grammar (with terms such as subject, verb and object) describes the English language. This metalanguage is an offshoot of GML (Generalized Markup Language) and its standardized descendant, **SGML**, which was invented in the 1960s and let users—particularly large government agencies, including the IRS and Department of Defense—define their own markups.

Because it's a metalanguage, XML is not meant to replace **HTML**. HTML, which is a specific implementation of SGML, focuses on the presentation, rather than the description, of **data**. Unlike XML, HTML cannot be used to define other languages. Rather, XML enables users to define their own languages, with tags that have specific meaning within the context of their documents.

*See also* Computer science and mathematics; HTML; SGML; XML

# METCALFE, ROBERT M. (1946-    )
## *American computer scientist and writer*

Robert Metcalfe is best known for his development of Ethernet and **LAN** technology as well as for founding the 3Com company.

Robert Metcalfe was born in Brooklyn, New York, in 1946, although he grew up on Long Island. By the age of 10 he knew he wanted to attend the Massachusetts Institute of Technology (MIT) to study electrical engineering. He achieved this aim and graduated from MIT with a bachelor's degree in electrical engineering and business management in 1969. Metcalfe then moved to Harvard University where he received a master's degree in applied mathematics. He remained at Harvard, initially failing his Ph.D. in computer science in 1972. Metcalfe's thesis was on **packet switching** in ARPANet (Advanced Research Projects Agency Network). In 1972 Metcalfe wrote a booklet detailing a range of uses for ARPANet and a brief outline of how it worked. He then gave a demonstration of ARPANet using packet switching to a

number of officials from AT&T. The system crashed, confirming to the AT&T officials their belief that circuit switching was still the way of the future. In 1972 Metcalfe took a position at Xerox Palo Alto Research Center (**Xerox PARC**) as a network expert. (He was advised that he could finish his doctoral studies at a later date.) At Xerox two problems were given to Metcalfe. First, Xerox had just invented the laser **printer** but they wanted to make a single printer accessible to all computers at the site. Second, Xerox had two large computers connected to ARPANet, but they wanted all of their computers to have **access**. The same solution was the answer to both problems—a system that could connect all of the computers within the complex, which would allow access to the larger computers, and hence ARPANet, and also to the laser printer. The solution was a local area network, or LAN, system. All of the local computers were connected together, which in turn were connected to the two larger computers, which were connected to ARPANet. This system allowed everyone access to ARPANet with only two connections. Metcalfe developed this system with the assistance of David R. Boggs and they called it Ethernet. One of the innovations of this system was that the information was sent in small packets with two-way communication between the computers. This meant a computer knew when another one was able to accept material, reducing the chance of collisions; when they did occur, only a small packet of information had to be resent, rather than a whole document. This system of limiting the number of collisions by assessing the level of traffic became the thrust of Metcalfe's new Ph.D. thesis and he was awarded his doctorate in 1973. In 1975 Metcalfe was made a consulting associate professor of electronic engineering at Stanford University, a position he kept along with his other duties until 1983 when he relinquished it. In 1976 Metcalfe and Boggs published *Ethernet: Distributed Packet Switching for Local Computer Networks*, which defined many of the operational parameters of Ethernet and LAN. This allowed the system to be readily adopted by any who wanted it.

In 1976 Metcalfe moved within Xerox to start work in the Xerox Systems Development Division. While in this position he was responsible for the development of the Xerox Star Workstation; this was the first **personal computer** to include a **mouse**, WYSIWYG ("What You See Is What You Get") **word processing**, and the Ethernet, along with software to allow text and **graphics** in the same document. In 1979 Metcalfe left Xerox to found his own company, the 3Com Corporation (the 3 "Com"s stand for Computers, Communication, and Compatibility). The aim of 3Com was to get Ethernet accepted as an industry standard in LAN. This aim was unsuccessful but it has become the most widely used LAN, with the system being adopted by such companies as **Intel**, Xerox, and **Digital Equipment Corporation**. In 1990 Metcalfe retired from 3Com and became a visiting fellow at Wolfson College, Cambridge University, England. After one year Metcalfe returned to the United States where he took to journalism, writing for a number of technology and computer magazines. In 1993 Metcalfe became the vice president of the International **Data** Group.

The same packet communication work that led to Ethernet also made a major contribution to the **TCP/IP** protocol, of which Metcalfe was a co-creator. In 1993 Metcalfe was credited with formulating Metcalfe's law (first published in *Forbes* magazine) which states that "The **value** of a network increases with the square of the number of people connected to it."

Robert Metcalfe has developed a number of innovations that have made the **Internet** of today possible. For these he has been granted a number of awards including the Institute of Electrical and Electronics Engineers Medal of Honor, the Alexander Graham Bell Award, and the Association of Computer Machinery (ACM) Grace Murray Hopper Award. Metcalfe now divides his time between writing, organizing conferences, and his vice president position at the International Data Group. Robert Metcalfe also endowed the Robert Metcalfe Professorship in Writing at MIT in 1986.

*See also* ARPANet; Ethernet; Internet; LAN; Packet switching; TCP/IP protocol; Xerox PARC

# METHOD

A method is fundamentally a **function**, a self-contained block of **code** that performs some **action** and returns a **value**. It is identical in all respects to a normal function except that a method always belongs to an **object** or **class**. **C++** supports conventional functions and methods, but in **Java** every function is a method.

Methods can be declared with the visibility modifiers "private," "protected," or "public," and these determine what methods other program entities can invoke on the object. The behavior of an object is fully defined by all the methods it supports; but the interface to an object is defined only by the public methods it supports because this will determine how the object appears to other program entities.

When a method on an object is invoked it is often described as "sending a **message** to the object." This can be confusing terminology to programmers new to **object-oriented programming**, but its use is prevalent in the discipline. Methods in languages that support function **overloading** and **overriding** can of course be overloaded and overridden, thus also supporting **polymorphism**.

Methods can in Java and C++ be declared as "static," which means they are characteristic of the class rather than of instances or objects of the class. The chief difference is that a **static** method can be invoked even if no objects of the type exist in the program, whereas a non-static method must always be invoked on an object. As an example, consider a payroll system that has an Employee class. Each object of this type will uniquely identify an employee, but it may also be desirable to keep track of how many employees there are on the payroll. This can be done using a static method:

```
#include <string.h>
#include <iostream.h>
class Employee {
public:
Employee(const char* name) : _name(strdup(name)) {
_employeeCount++;}
static int getEmployeeCount() { return
employeeCount; };
const char* getName() const { return _name; }
private:
static int _employeeCount;
char* _name;
};
int Employee::_employeeCount = 0; // have to initial-
ize static member variables
int main() {
count << "employee: << "no one") << ," #" <<
Employee::getEmployeeCount();
Employee fred("Fred");
count << "employee: << fred.getName() << ," #"
<< Employee::getEmployeeCount();
Employee bill("Bill");
count << "employee: << bill.getName() << ," #"
<< Employee::getEmployeeCount();
return 0;
}
```

This code when compiled and run will give the following printout:

    employee: no one, #0

    employee: Fred, #1

    employee: Bill, #2

This is because the name of each Employee is unique to each object, but the number, _employeeCount, belongs to the class as whole. It is entirely legal to **call** Employee::getEmployeeCount() even before any Employee objects have been created.

While the term "method" has a specific meaning in object-oriented **programming**, its use does somewhat depend on which language is being discussed. In Java and Smalltalk methods are almost always called methods, but in C++ the most commonly used term is "member function." The two terms have identical meanings.

# MICROPROCESSOR

At the core of every computer is a microprocessor, a device that has been called the greatest invention of the century. The dictionary defines the microprocessor as "a **semiconductor central processing unit** usually contained on a single **integrated circuit** chip." More important than what a microprocessor is, is what a microprocessor can do.

The microprocessor is also known as a central processing unit, or **CPU**. The CPU actually runs the programs in a device, be it a computer, personal digital assistant (PDA), or cell phone; but the CPU depends on instructions from other microcomponents to tell it what to do. These instructions usually come from a software program that is stored in **memory**.

The CPU directs computer operations by sending control signals, memory addresses, and **data** from one area of the

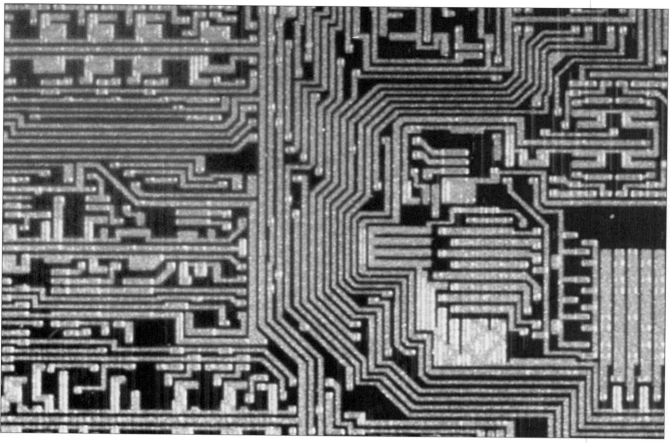

**Microchip**

computer to another by using interconnected pathways called a *bus*. At locations along the **bus** are **input and output** ports that other components, such as memory and support chips, or co-processors, are attached. Data traveling to and from the CPU to other parts of the computer passes through these input/output (I/O) ports.

The manufacture of microprocessors begins with creation of a nearly pure (99.999999 percent pure) silicon nugget that serves as a nucleus for the growth of a cylinder of silicon called an ingot. The silicon ingot is grown in such a way that electricity flows through it in a predictable way. The ingot is cut into 8-inch or 12-inch diameter wafers, where each wafer is polished to a mirror-like finish and coated with an insulating material in preparation for building microprocessors.

Each 8-inch silicon wafer can yield hundreds of individual microprocessors. Many manufacturers, such as **Intel**, are retooling their microprocessor labs for 12-inch wafers. The microprocessor yield is much higher on a 12-inch wafer, meaning there is less scrap, or unused area of the wafer. Such a retooling effort is very expensive, costing hundreds of millions or even billions of dollars.

The millions of tiny transistors on these microprocessors are created using layers of conductive and insulating materials through a photolithography process that uses light and light-

sensitive materials to yield layers of etched and printed lines of insulating and conducting material. Current technology is fast approaching line widths of 0.13 microns; one micron is one-millionth of a meter, or about 1/300th the thickness of a human hair. The vertical thickness of layers is measured in angstroms, where one angstrom is the average width of an atom. Some layers today measure just a few angstroms thick.

Once the individual microprocessors have been cut from the wafer, they undergo a wafer sort to separate the functioning microprocessors from those that are defective. The next major step is to package the microprocessor in way that allows it work in a PC or other device. Microprocessor packaging protects the microprocessor from moisture, scratches, and contamination, and provides the electrical contacts so the microprocessor can communicate with other components of the device. An automated wire-bonding process establishes electrical connections between the microprocessor and the package pins that connect the chip to the computer or other device.

Microprocessor packaging can come in several configurations in plastic and ceramic. "Plastic quad flat packaging," also known as PQFP, is a type of packaging used with many types of microprocessors, is soldered directly to a PC or device printed circuit board (direct solder is also known as "surface mount technology"). "Ceramic pin grid array" (PGA) technology is better suited to higher speed microprocessors because of ceramic's excellent thermal and electrical properties. This packaging technology is very expensive as it uses gold pins to enhance the electrical connections between the microprocessor and the PC or other device. The pins plug into a printed circuit board-mounted socket, making it easy to upgrade to faster microprocessors within the same family.

Gordon Moore, one of the founders of Intel, discovered that every new process technology doubles the number of available transistors for a given wafer size (Moore's Law). Today, 0.13 micron process technology is available, and microprocessors can reach speeds of 2 gigahertz (GHz). Microprocessor process technology of the future must be able to find a way to overcome the limitations submicroscopic wires impose on electron speed, clock frequencies, heat dissipation, and power consumption. Experiments have been carried out with surface-emitting microlasers, which can transfer encoded data at the speed of light. Such technology is not only ultrafast and energy efficient, it consumes far less power than silicon-based chips. Some experts predict that the next microprocessor process technology will be a revolution, and require a leap in physics, perhaps to **nanotechnology** and molecular computing. Should that occur, then perhaps Moore's Law will have to be restated.

# MICROSOFT

Microsoft is a United States–based company that develops and sells a wide variety of software products and services for business and personal computing. Microsoft is the world's largest supplier of operating systems (OSs) and other software for IBM-compatible personal computers. The Microsoft **Windows** OS is the most widely used OS in the world. Microsoft operates subsidiary and sales offices in more than 50 countries and employs nearly 44,000 people worldwide, but performs nearly all of its research and development at its corporate headquarters in Redmond, Washington.

Microsoft's best-known products include Microsoft Disk Operating System (MS-DOS), Microsoft Windows, and Windows NT. Its popular programs Word (a word processor), Excel (a spreadsheet), PowerPoint (for business presentations), and Access (for **databases**) are sold individually and also bundled together as Microsoft Office (a suite of integrated office software). The company also makes such software programs as BackOffice (an integrated set of server products), Microsoft **Internet** Explorer (a web **browser**), **LAN** Manager (an OS/2-based network operating system), SQL Server (a relational-database management system), ODBC (Open **Data** Base Connectivity, providing access to databases), and MS Mail (the Windows **e-mail** program). Among its other products are **programming** languages, reference **applications** (e.g., Encarta Encyclopedia), games, financial software, input devices (e.g., keyboards and mice), and computer-related books. Microsoft operates the Microsoft Network (MSN), an Internet web site featuring news, information, finance, travel, and entertainment. Microsoft and television network NBC together operate MSNBC, an around-the-clock news, talk, and information cable-television channel and Internet web site.

In 1975, the magazine *Popular Electronics* reported the advent of the **Altair** 8800, the first **personal computer**. This prompted **Bill Gates** and **Paul Allen** (high school friends interested in programming the **DEC** PDP-10 computer) to adapt **BASIC** (a popular **mainframe** programming language) for use with the Altair. The two young men licensed the software to Altair's manufacturer, Micro Instrumentation and Telemetry Systems. Gates and Allen soon formed a company they called "Micro-soft" (for MICROcomputer SOFTware) on April 4, 1975, in Albuquerque, New Mexico, to develop versions of BASIC for other computer companies. They later renamed the company Microsoft. In 1977 Microsoft sold its second programming language, Microsoft **FORTRAN**, and later released new versions of BASIC for the Intel-8080 and Intel-8086 microprocessors.

The company moved to Bellevue, Washington, in January 1979, a Seattle suburb that was Gates's and Allen's home town. In 1980 **International Business Machines Corporation (IBM)** asked Microsoft to write the OS for its first personal computer, the IBM PC. Having no suitable operating system ready to hand, Microsoft purchased QDOS (Quick and Dirty Operating System) from Seattle programmer Tim Paterson and renamed it MS-DOS (Microsoft Disk Operating System). In August 1981 the IBM PC, running the operating system MS-DOS, was introduced to the commercial market. As part of the IBM contract, Microsoft was allowed to license the OS to other companies. Microsoft was incorporated on June 25, 1981. By 1984 Microsoft had licensed MS-DOS 1.0 to 200 PC manufacturers. By the early 1990s Microsoft had sold more than 100 million copies of all versions of MS-DOS, and in the process had squeezed out most of its competition.

During this time, Microsoft began to develop business PC applications. In 1983 it released the word-processing program Word. In 1984 Microsoft was one of the few established software companies to develop applications for **Apple** Computers' Macintosh computer. Microsoft's early support for the Macintosh resulted in tremendous success for its Macintosh application software, including Word, Excel, and Works (an integrated software suite).

In 1985 Microsoft released Windows, an operating system that extended the features of MS-DOS and introduced a **graphical user interface (GUI)** modeled on the Macintosh GUI, which improved the PC's user-friendliness. In 1986 Microsoft moved to its current headquarters in Redmond, Washington and became a publicly owned company. Windows 2.0, released in 1987, improved performance and appearance. In 1990 Microsoft introduced its most complex version to that date, Windows 3.0, which swiftly went through versions Windows 3.1 and 3.11. These OSs usually came preinstalled on new PCs and quickly became the world's most used operating systems. By 1993 Windows 3.0 and later versions were selling at a rate of one million copies per month, with nearly 90% of the world's PCs running on a Microsoft OS.

In 1991 Microsoft and IBM ended their partnership; IBM pursued the OS/2 operating system while Microsoft chose to stick with Windows. In 1993 Apple lost a copyright-infringement lawsuit against Microsoft that claimed Windows was an illegal copy of Macintosh's GUI. Apple had granted a license to Microsoft in 1985 to use Apple's windows-and-icons motifs in the development of Windows 1.0, as Microsoft had threatened to cease development of software for the Macintosh unless the license was granted. Apple sued Microsoft for breaching the term of the license when Microsoft 2.0 was released in 1987, but finally lost its case in 1993. Microsoft thus retained its exclusive rights to Windows.

In 1993 Microsoft released Windows NT, an OS that effectively networked PCs within business environments. In August 1995, the company released Windows 95, which for the first time fully integrated MS-DOS with Windows. It featured a simplified interface, **multitasking**, and graphical improvements that nearly matched the elegance of Apple's Macintosh OS. About 7 million copies of Windows 95 were sold worldwide within seven weeks of its release. During this period Microsoft also became the leader in productivity software (i.e., word-processing and **spreadsheet programs**).

In 1996 Microsoft introduced Windows CE, an OS for handheld PCs. The next year Microsoft bought the company WebTV Networks, a manufacturer of low-cost devices that connected televisions to the Internet. Soon afterwards Microsoft invested in cable-television **operator** Comcast Corporation in order to expand into the high-speed Internet. In June 1998, Microsoft released Windows 98, which featured integrated Internet capabilities. By first giving away its Internet Explorer web browser, and then packaging it into Windows 98, Microsoft managed to make IE the most popular access Internet browser. In February 2000, the company released Windows 2000, the latest version of the Windows NT operating system.

As Microsoft's influence grew in the market for PC operating systems, Microsoft was criticized for monopolistic business practices. These claims have been investigated several times by the United States Justice Department. These investigations have resulted in numerous rulings that have been contested by Microsoft over the years, with some settled and others still open as of this writing.

*See also* Apple; Windows

# MINSKY, MARVIN (1927-  )

*American computer scientist*

Marvin Lee Minsky is an educator and computer scholar at Massachusetts Institute of Technology and a pioneer in the field of **artificial intelligence**. Since the early 1950s, he has attempted to define and explain the thinking process and **design** a machine that can duplicate it. His 1987 book, *The Society of Mind,* put forward a detailed and mechanistic theory of how the mind works, and how it might be artificially duplicated. For his original and outstanding achievements in science and technology, Minsky was awarded the Japan Prize in 1990. Marvin Lee Minsky was born in New York City on August 9, 1927, to Dr. Henry Minsky and Fannie Reiser. His father was an eye surgeon and an artist. His mother was active

in the Zionist movement. For the most part, Minsky attended private schools during his childhood, where his intelligence and later his interest in electronics and chemistry were nurtured. He learned early that he was most comfortable in the intellectually stimulating world of academia. This perception was enhanced in 1945, when, following his high school graduation, he enlisted in the United States Navy. He took his basic training at the Great Lakes Naval Training Center north of Chicago, with about one hundred and twenty other recruits. He later told Jeremy Bernstein, an interviewer for the *New Yorker,* that "they provided my first, and essentially my last, contact with nonacademic people."

Minsky enrolled at Harvard University in 1946, majoring in physics, but his eclectic interests kept him attending classes in a wide variety of subjects, including genetics, mathematics, and the nature of intelligence. He associated briefly with the researchers in the psychology department, but questioned the prevailing theories of what happens deep inside the mind. He confided to Bernstein in a *New Yorker* interview that he found B. F. Skinner's theories unacceptable "because they were an attempt to fit curves to behavior without any internal ideas." Skinner had enjoyed considerable success in conditioning animal behavior using these hypotheses, but Minsky felt there must be a better explanation. Minsky switched his major to mathematics in his senior year, and graduated in 1950.

From Harvard, Minsky moved to Princeton to begin his doctoral studies. In the same environment in which mathematician **Alan Turing** had constructed the first electrical multiplier just prior to World War II, Minsky applied his budding theories of mentation to the construction of a learning machine which he called the Snarc, whose purpose was to learn how to traverse a maze using forty "agent" components and a system to reward success. However, Minsky's accomplishments with the Snarc were limited; although he felt himself on the right track with the "reward" principle, it was not versatile enough for Minsky's purposes.

Minsky began to explore how a machine might use **memory** to use past experience. This thought is elaborated on in his doctoral dissertation, in which he tries to show ways that a learning machine can predict the results of its behavior, based on its knowledge of past actions. There was some question at the time whether this line of inquiry properly belonged in a program that was ostensibly about mathematics. This is a recurring problem for Minsky, whose interests typically draw from so many disciplines that it becomes difficult to determine exactly what to label them. After receiving his Ph.D., Minsky accepted a three-year junior fellowship at Harvard, where, as he later said, he had no obligations except to pursue his theories about intelligence.

In 1958 Minsky joined the staff at the Massachusetts Institute of Technology's Lincoln Laboratory. He became an assistant professor of mathematics, and, in 1959, he and a colleague, John Mc Carthy, founded the MIT Artificial Intelligence Project. This project eventually became the Artificial Intelligence Laboratory, of which Minsky was the director from 1964 until 1973. In 1974, he was promoted to Donner professor of science in the department of electrical engineering and computer science. In 1989, he moved to

MIT's media laboratory, where he became Toshiba Professor of Media Arts and Sciences.

Minsky has made it his life's work to finalize an overall theory of how minds work. He has disturbed, and perhaps alienated, many of his co-researchers by insisting that what we think of as "consciousness" or "self-awareness" is actually a myth—a convenient fallacy which allows us to function as a society. According to Minsky's theory (which he has outlined in *The Society of Mind* as well as in numerous articles in popular magazines), there is no difference between humans and machines, because, he believes, humans are machines whose brains are made up of many semi-autonomous but unintelligent "agents," but who mistakenly consider themselves intelligent individuals. According to Eugene F. Mallove in a *Tech Talk* article, "it is Minsky's view that hundreds of specialized 'computers' make up the human brain—or any other large brain for that matter. Many of these are at work cooperatively and unconsciously." Some have expressed concern that Minsky's mechanistic view of how minds work flies in the face of much established knowledge in the fields of biology and psychology, and contradicts what we seem to perceive about ourselves. But Minsky dismisses such objections, maintaining that most research on how the mind works has been crippled by researchers who simply ask the wrong questions.

Although Minsky still holds a professorship at the Artificial Intelligence Laboratory, most of the recent activity there has gone in directions that do not fully support his theories. For the past few years, Minsky has devoted himself to private research, fleshing out his Society of Mind theory. His professional writings are not prolific, but he writes often in such publications as *Omni* and *Discover,* and has co-authored a science fiction novel (not surprisingly based on his theory) with Harry Harrison titled *The Turing Option.* Artificial intelligence itself is a field in stasis; no major steps toward developing—or even defining—a truly intelligent machine have been made in decades. Minsky believes this could change if more researchers would pay attention to his theory. Whether or not that turns out to be true, it is very likely that when the field of artificial intelligence does move forward, Minsky will be somewhere nearby, giving it a push.

Minsky married Gloria Rudisch, a doctor, in 1953. The couple has three children: Margaret, Henry, and Juliana. Minsky has won many honors for his pioneering work: the Donner professorship, the Turing award in 1970, and the prestigious Japan award in 1990.

# MITNICK, KEVIN D. (1965-    )

*American computer programmer and hacker*

Kevin D. Mitnick made a name for himself by **hacking** his way into telephone networks and vandalizing corporate, government, and university computers. For a while, according to assistant United States attorney Kent Walker, "He was arguably the most wanted computer hacker in the world."

Kevin D. Mitnick was born in 1965 and grew up in the San Fernando Valley near Los Angeles, California. After his

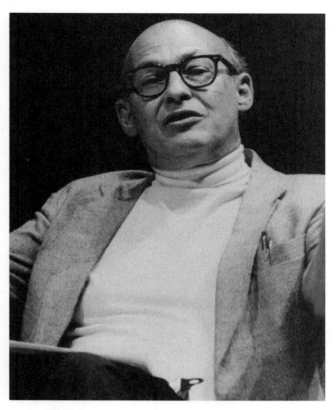

**Marvin Minsky**

parents divorced when he was three years old, he lived with his mother, who worked long hours as a waitress at a delicatessen. As a youth he had few friends. He rarely saw his father and grew up lonely and isolated.

While in his teens, Mitnick got into phone "phreaking," using electronic techniques to gain illegal **access** to telephone services. He became friends with other phone phreaks and often hung out with a group that met at a pizza parlor in Los Angeles to plot ways to break into local computer and communications systems. Together with other phone phreak friends—such as a young woman who called herself Susan Thunder and a young man who went by the name of Roscoe—he searched the dumpsters behind phone company offices for manuals that would provide vital information about company computers.

Mitnick first got into trouble with the law during his teens. As a student at Monroe High School in North Hills, California, he broke into the computer system of the Los Angeles Unified School District. He could have changed students' grades, but he did not. He also reportedly hacked his way into the military's North American Air Defense Command computers in Colorado just for fun. When Mitnick, just seventeen years old, was caught stealing valuable technical manuals from the Pacific Bell Telephone Company, a judge sentenced him to probation (a trial period to test his good behavior). In spite of his brush with the law, Mitnick returned to hacking.

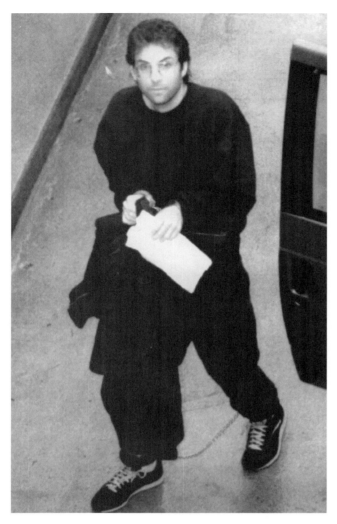

**Kevin D. Mitnick**

After he was caught breaking into computers at a local university, he was sentenced to six months in jail.

When Mitnick was twenty-three, he met Bonnie Vitello, who worked for the phone company. A short while later, Mitnick and Vitello were married. Mitnick's computer hacking created a strain on the relationship, and the couple eventually divorced.

Mitnick attracted the attention of security experts in December 1988, when he was charged with breaking into MCI telephone computers and stealing long-distance codes. By secretly reading the electronic mail of security officials at MCI and **Digital Equipment Corporation**, Mitnick discovered how the companies' computers and phone equipment were protected against hackers. In July 1989, he was convicted and sentenced to one year in federal prison at Lompoc, California—followed by a period at a rehabilitation center. One of Mitnick's defense attorneys had managed to convince the judge that his client was "addicted" to computers—and that, like an alcoholic, he was not able to control his behavior.

Following his release from federal prison, Mitnick was sent to Beit T'Shuvah, a residential program designed to help addicts overcome their addictions. (The program's name is Hebrew for "house of repentance.") There he followed a 12-step program modeled after Alcoholics Anonymous. He spent six months at the rehabilitation center—during which time he was forbidden to use a computer or a **modem**.

Mitnick was released early from Beit T'Shuvah, in the spring 1990. One of the conditions of his parole specified that he was forbidden to use computers until he could demonstrate that he was able to control his behavior. Mitnick returned to Los Angeles in early 1992, following the death of his half brother. He was employed for a while with his father, Alan, who was a general contractor. When that did not work out, he took a job with a private investigation agency called Tel Tec Investigations.

In September 1992, federal officials, armed with a search warrant, raided Mitnick's apartment. Mitnick, who was suspected of breaking into a Pacific Bell computer, was nowhere to be found. But coded disks and documents provided proof of his activities. In November, a federal judge issued a warrant for the hacker's arrest. Mitnick had violated the conditions of his parole. Aware that the heat was on, Mitnick went into hiding.

For more than two years, Mitnick managed to elude federal officials. But on Christmas Day 1994, he committed a fatal mistake. Mitnick broke into the home computer of Tsutomu Shimomura, a computational physicist who worked as a computer security expert at the Supercomputer Center in San Diego. Using a modem, Mitnick "spoofed" his way into Shimomura's networked **databases**. "Spoofing" involves fooling a computer into thinking that it is communicating with a friendly computer. Mitnick took over a computer that was "friendly" to the computer he wanted to enter. Once inside the target computer, he stole hundreds of documents and software programs that contained sensitive information about computer security. The attack lasted from 2:00 P.M. on Christmas Day until 6:00 P.M. the following evening.

Shimomura was on his way to Lake Tahoe, California, for a ski vacation, when he was informed that someone had broken into his databases. He returned home and immediately set out to discover the identity of the intruder. On December 27, he received a mocking **message** on his office voice mail. A man's computer-altered voice said: "My technique is the best. Damn you. I know send-mail technique. Don't you know who I am? Me and my friends, we'll kill you." Next, another voice said, "Hey, boss, my kung fu is really good." Before the end of the month, Shimomura had received another message: "Your technique will be defeated," the voice said. "Your technique is no good."

After Shimomura made the voice messages available on the **Internet** (in computer audio files), he received yet another message. This time, the computer-altered voice said, "Ah Tsutomu, my learned disciple. I see that you put my voice on the Net. I'm very disappointed my son." The messages provided little information about the intruder's identity. But they indicated that he viewed the situation as a game of wits.

For most of the following month, no new clues appeared. On January 27, 1995, Bruce Koball, a computer programmer, received notice from an online service called WELL. The notice informed him that his account was taking up too much disk space: Koball's account suddenly claimed hundreds of millions of bytes of storage space. But Koball had not been using his account. When he looked at the files in his account, he found Shimomura's name. The next day, when he read a newspaper story about the theft of files from a computer expert named Shimomura, he realized what had happened. The computer thief had stashed Shimomura's files in his account. And that was not all. The WELL account included secret codes for various companies, **password** files, and more than twenty-one thousand credit card numbers.

Shimomura and a few other computer experts formed a surveillance team at the WELL headquarters in Sausalito, California, in order to track the hacker's online movements. Using sophisticated programs, they were able to monitor every keystroke the intruder made. By February 8, the team had determined that their subject was gaining access to WELL through Netcom, another Internet provider. The team of cyber sleuths moved to Netcom's headquarters in San Jose, California. There, they monitored the intruder's modem calls. Using Shimomura's complicated security programs, they unraveled the tangled computer connections that allowed the hacker to connect to the Internet without being identified.

But the intruder's identity was slowly coming to light. Mitnick was already a well-known hacker—whose habits and interests were familiar to computer security experts such as Shimomura. Like Mitnick, the intruder was a night owl who often remained online into the early morning. What's more, the information stashed in the WELL accounts included software that controls the operations of cellular phones made by various manufacturers—exactly the sort of information that interested Mitnick.

Working with government investigators, Shimomura's team compared telephone company records with records of the intruder's activity on the Internet. Soon, they determined that the hacker was using a telephone switching office in Raleigh, North Carolina, to reroute phone calls—making it difficult to trace calls from his cellular phone modem. On Sunday, February 12, Shimomura flew to Raleigh, where he met a Sprint cellular technician. The pair drove through the streets of suburban Raleigh with hightech scanning and homing equipment designed to locate the origin of the cellular modem activity. By early Monday morning, Shimomura and the technician concluded that the calls originated from an apartment complex near the Raleigh airport.

Earlier that month, a man who identified himself as Glenn Thomas Case had rented a one-bedroom apartment at the Players Club complex. When federal agents knocked on the door of apartment 202 at 2:00 A.M. on February 15, they found Kevin Mitnick. Although it took him five minutes to open the door to his apartment, Mitnick surrendered without a struggle. As he waited to be charged in a North Carolina jail, he was allowed a few phone calls—to his attorney, his mother, and his grandmother. All of his calls were monitored. Charged

with computer fraud and illegal use of telephone-access devices, Mitnick faced up to thirty-five years in prison.

## MIXED-MODE OPERATION

Mixed-mode **operation** is a term that refers to a **programming** feature known as the domain controller. The function of the domain controller is to provide directory-like and administrative functions, such as **password** administration, to the operating environment. Additionally, in mixed-mode operation, the domain controller is able to run two operating systems in the same domain. Features from the operating systems are enabled or disabled so as to make the two operating systems compatible and, as much as possible, invisible to the user.

Mixed-mode operation allows files that were created and stored in one operating system to be read and manipulated in a normal fashion in the other operating system. In essence, the systems become transparent.

The ability to operate in mixed-mode is a ubiquitous feature of operating systems. For example, mixed-mode enables controller servers running on **Microsoft Windows** NT 4.0 and servers responsible for **message** functions running on Windows 2000 to communicate seamlessly with one another. As another example, the mixed-mode manager in the Macintosh operating system is designed to both permit the running of two operating systems and to hide, as much as possible, these dual operating environments from the user.

*See also* Operating systems, types

## ML

ML, or Meta-Language, is a family of **programming** languages that are functional in nature. **Functional programming** is a programming style that is based on the evaluation of expressions rather than execution of **commands**. Functional programming is concerned with what needs to be done instead of how it is to be accomplished.

### History

ML was first designed and implemented in the 1970s at the University of Edinburgh's Laboratory for Foundations of Computer Science. As the ML developed further in the 1980s, a common dialect and a base set of features was standardized. In 1990 the Standard ML (SML) was released. In 1997 the standard was revised as SML'97. SML is the most common implementation of ML.

In addition to SML, the ML family of languages includes Standard ML of New Jersey (SML/NJ), Extended ML (EML), Moscow ML, CAML, and others. ML is portable, and it has been implemented on a variety of platforms, including PCs, workstations, mainframes, and **supercomputers**. Most ML implementations provide an interactive system for writing programs, compiling and linking programs, and executing the programs. Some implementations also provide extensive libraries as well as sophisticated development tools.

### The SML Implementation

SML was developed by the research community and is most widely used in academic settings. It is particularly useful in metaprogramming, or writing programs that manipulate other programs. In this context SML is used in compilers and interpreters. SML imposes strict semantics, hierarchical structure, and a modular manner of programming. These help enforce **abstraction** of reusable components.

In a pure functional language, all computation is done via functions. Programmers declare functions and references to values. **Function** calls are nested inside each other to build up complex expressions. SML encourages functional programming where appropriate, but it allows imperative programming if necessary. Because it does not meet all the requirements of a pure functional language, SML is considered an extended functional language.

Some of the defining characteristics of SML include the use of type inference, type checking, **polymorphism**, and **pattern matching**. Type inference means that many **variable** types do not have to be specified programmatically; instead SML can interpret basic types and also offers a mechanism for a programmer to extend variable types as needed. ML uses the context of an **expression** to determine the types of the operands. Using this mechanism it can infer the types of the arguments and the type of the return result. The basic SML types include integer, real, **string**, character, and Boolean.

SML also does type checking, meaning that the type is verified before an expression is evaluated. A type **constructor** mismatch error occurs when operators are paired with arguments of the incorrect type. The benefits of type checking include reduced **debugging**, as mistakes can be caught earlier in the development process, and faster execution.

SML supports polymorphism of **data** types and functions. A declaration of data type list could be used to represent lists of strings, integers, or characters. Similarly, a declaration of function order_list could be used to order lists of strings, integers, or characters. Polymorphism supports reuse since the same data type or function can be extended for multiple uses.

Pattern matching simplifies the definition of functions in SML. Pattern matching allows functions to be defined in a case format, which uses a format of clauses to indicate possible structures. When evaluating the expression, each clause is tried in the order of presentation. The first successful match is taken if more than one matches.

Additional features of SML include an error and **exception handling** mechanism and a portable standard basis **library** that defines a rich collection of common types and routines. This library contains functions for data manipulation, string handling, and interfacing with the operating system.

SML can be used interactively from the command line or in a program that has been written and saved to a file. When SML commands are entered, the interpreter knows to begin evaluating the expressions when it sees a semicolon. The interpreter returns the **value** of the result.

### Other Implementations of ML

There are two other implementations of ML that are similar to SML. Moscow ML is a lightweight implementation of SML, meaning that it contains some of the features of SML but is less complex. EML is an extension of SML; it has most of the characteristics of SML plus some additional features. In practice both Moscow ML and EML programs look very similar to SML programs.

*See also* Programming languages, types

# MODEM

The word modem is an acronym for modulator-demodulator. Its name describes its function. A modem is a device or program that enables computers to send **data** over telephone lines. Computer data is digital, capable of distinguishing between zero and one. The opposite of digital is analog—the infinite smooth gradation between numbers. A modem converts the data supplied by a computer in digital form to a modulated analog waveform that is able to travel over telephone lines. A modem can also work in reverse—accepting an incoming modulated analog wave and converting it to digital form, which can then be passed on to a computer. A modem is thus the communication bridge between computers.

Modems can be located inside a computer, or can be an external attachment. An internal, or onboard, modem is a type of printed circuit board called an expansion card. An external modem is a piece of **hardware**, which is connected to the computer via an RS-232 **port**. These ports are virtually standard, so almost all personal computers can accommodate an external modem. An external modem also requires an operating interface between itself and the computer. This interface, called RS-232, is also standard.

Different models of modems operate at different speeds, with respect to the speeds at which information can be transmitted and received. At slow rates, modems are measured in baud rates. A baud is the number of signaling elements occurring each second, and is named after J.M.E. Baudot, the inventor of the Baudot telegraph **code**. At higher speeds, modems are measured in terms of bits per second (bps). The fastest modems can run at about 56,000 bps. Higher transmission speeds are possible for modems that are capable of compressing the data. Higher transmission speeds decrease the time that a phone line is occupied and makes transmission of large blocks of data realistic in terms of time. The selection of a modem should be made in recognition of its intended usage. For example, if data is being sent to a 56,000 bps modem by a modem operating at 2,400 bps, then the slower rate is the determiner of the transmission speed. Also, a modem capable of **data compression** must be connected to a modem capable of decompressing the data for that feature to work.

The 56,000 bps modems operate differently from other, slower modems. **Internet** Service Providers provide digital connections to the telephone company. Because the modem itself is digital, the digital-to-analog-to-digital conversion can be eliminated at the provider's site. The result is the ability to download data into a **personal computer** at a faster speed—the Integrated Services Digital Network. Similar technology is being increasingly utilized to provide people with high-speed Internet **access** via cable modems. Here, the modem is connected to the television cable. Finally, simultaneous phone service and Internet access, called Digital Subscriber Line, can enable data transmission speeds of up to 1.5 Mbps.

Modern modems can have other ancillary features, in addition to data compression. Voice/data enables a modem to function as either a telephone or as a modem. Auto answer enables a modem to accept transmissions automatically, in the absence of an **operator**. Some modems have flash **memory** instead of **ROM**. This enables updates to be accomplished easily, in some cases by simply inserting a new memory card in the modem. Finally, modems can also send and receive fax transmissions.

*See also* Analog versus digital computing; Baudot code; Dataflow

# MODULA

Modula is a Pascal-based **programming** language. Unlike **Pascal**, which was designed primarily as a teaching language, Modula was designed to be used for designing and running production systems. Modula can be considered a superset of the Pascal programming language.

Modula retained the strongest features of Pascal while adding a module system and **hardware** device interfaces. Modules allow a programmer to encapsulate subprograms and **data**. Interfaces to hardware devices are accomplished through low-level programming constructs within Modula.

Modula-1 was developed in the late 1970s by Dr. **Niklaus Wirth**, the inventor of Pascal. Modula-2, the most common implementation of the Modula language, was introduced in the early 1980s. Modula-2 was used as the system language for the Lilith workstation.

Modula-3 is an object-oriented derivative of Modula-2. It adds support for generics, objects, and garbage collection to the Modula-2 implementation. With Wirth's blessing, Modula-3 was developed by a team at the Digital Systems Research Center and the Olivetti Research Center. Rather than extending Modula-2, the team designed and developed Modula-3 from the ground up, keeping the basic concepts of Modula-2. Modula-3 was published in 1988.

*See also* Encapsulation; Object-oriented programming; Pascal

# MODULARITY

The only reason large, complex artifacts such as automobiles, aircraft, houses, and ships can be constructed by people who individually can only do so much, is that there is a meaningful way to split large tasks into small ones. The large, extremely complex task that is often even impossible for a single person to comprehend fully, can be divided into small parts that can be completed by a single person or by a small group of people, and there is a well-defined procedure by which all those small parts can then be put together to produce the final, large artifact.

Although the notion of splitting a large task into smaller parts is certainly as old as recorded history—if not more so—the scientific analysis of the notion and its application to computer science are recent. The name given to the concept is "modularity," and any **design** of a large, complex artifact along these lines is called "modular design." The fragments of the large task or structure that are involved are called "modules."

Because the word "modularity" is used in different senses by neural scientists, linguists, biologists, and others, perhaps it is accurate to specify the meaning of the word as used in computer science and related disciplines like information technology, as "compositional modularity." The longer phrase is sometimes used in the literature of computing sciences and **programming**, just for this reason. However, programmers and other computing professionals often prefer the shorter phrase even with its lack of clarity, and thus "modularity" is a jargon word that means the same thing—many computer scientists and programmers are even unaware that there is any other meaning to the word.

Modular design has certain simple but important objectives and principles. First of all, a module should be an entity that has a clearly defined objective, taking a single input and delivering a single output. Such clarity is essential for reasoning how modules fit together to form the total artifact or system. Another important principle of modular design is encapsulation—the module should not be liable to outside interference in any form other than through its legitimate input. A closely related concept is information hiding—the module should conceal the details of its inner workings from outside users, and should be capable of being reasoned about just in terms of its input-output relationship. It may not be obvious why information hiding is essential in a good module, but lots of empirical and anecdotal evidence exists to show that it is—having to worry about the details of the workings of a module do not allow users to use it very well.

Modularity facilitates extensive reuse and systematic upgrades of software. In a non-modular system, the interactions between different parts of the system are not clearly defined, and it is often uncertain what the effects of changing one part will be on other parts of the total system. Using modularity enables each module to be upgraded, maintained, repaired, installed, or removed separately; replacements can be made of specific modules with the confidence that as long as the specification of the module with respect to its input-output relationship is maintained as required by the overall system design, the rest of the system will continue to function.

Modular design also facilitates nesting and hierarchical composition of systems. This means that a complete system at a certain level can itself be thought of as a module for a larger meta-system, and so on. At each level of description and reasoning, we have modules that join together to form a system, which itself may be a module in a larger system. The behavior of modules is specified at the appropriate level. Any problems that occur can then be dealt with by a suitable analysis at the appropriate level of description. Whenever a module is found to be faulty, it can then be treated as a system, and its components (themselves modules at the lower level of description) can be analyzed, and so on. This approach allows for the exact source of any faults or bugs to be found in the shortest possible time, and hence is of great use.

While modular designs of software can, in principle, be implemented in any programming language, such implementation is much easier if the programming language used offers tools that allow for the easy achievement of modular goals. These include permitting the encapsulation of **code** and **data** structures. The mechanisms that are important for this are: the procedure (or function) having locally scoped variables and **argument** list (useful in encapsulating code); a user-defined datatype (useful in encapsulating data); and dynamic memory allocation, which allows subroutines and subprograms to access memory without having to go to the calling programs each time. The features listed here are supported in modern programming languages such as **Java** and **C++**, but not in older or less refined languages like Fortran and **COBOL**.

*See also* Object-oriented programming; Program design; Structured programming

## MOLECULAR SWITCHES

Molecular switches are a part of the discipline of nanotechnology—making operational machines of atomic dimensions. Specifically, a molecular switch is composed of atoms of material that function as a switch, or a **logic gate**. A logic gate is a necessary computing component, used to represent ones and zeros, the binary language of digital computing. Molecular switches would permit an atomic form of random **access** memory—a key computer **operation** that allows users to store and manipulate information.

To date, molecular switches remain more a possibility than a reality, although several research groups have manufactured atomic sized complexes that are capable of conducting electricity. In 1999, researchers from Rice University in Houston, Texas used chemical methods to manufacture a molecular switch that cold be turned on and off in a reversible manner. The chemical switch is some one million times smaller than the current silicon switches, creating the potential for further miniaturization of computers. Another research team from the Center for Nanoscale Science at the University of Liverpool, United Kingdom, has been able to control the current flowing through another type of molecular switch constructed of a gold particle six millionths of a meter in diameter linked to wires made of organic molecules strung together. By applying voltage, the electrical current flowing through the wires to the gold particle can be turned on and off. Others have been able to demonstrate electrical conductance through tubes of carbon that are smaller than a filament of DNA. Finally, a research team from UCLA has constructed two interlocked rings of a molecule called a catenane. Electrically-induced rearrangement of the rings in a reversible manner allows electron flow

The promise of such molecular switches depends on the ability to organize the tiny structures into functional devices, and then to marry these devices to electrical contacts so those machines of atomic dimensions can be built. Not only would the machines be appreciably smaller than anything possible at present, but such molecular computers would be far more powerful than those available now using silicon-based logic gates.

*See also* Architecture (hardware); Binary number system; Nanotechnology; Random access memory (RAM)

## MOOS AND MUDS

MOOs and MUDs were developed by aficionados of **computer games** in order to make the games more interactive. The first such environments, developed by Stephen White, were called Multiple User Dragons, or MUDs. Later, these environments were enhanced and renamed. The most widely used of the second generation MUDs are the Multiple User Dragons, **Object** Oriented, or MOO.

MOOs and MUDs allow users to communicate with each other by writing messages. They are similar to a chat room. However, the other inhabitants of the programmed environment may not be human. They may, for example, be robots designed by the programmer of the particular MOO or MUD, that will interact with the user and other inhabitants of the room in programmed ways. In Dungeons and Dragons, for example, the MUD was a text-based description of an alternate reality where those who had logged on to the game met creatures who were, in fact, other players that were also participating in the game.

MOOs and MUDs are no longer restricted to computer games. Their utility as on-line interactive chat room-like environments has been developed for a wide range of academic and social uses. For example, on-line classes and conferences are held in MOO seminar rooms. MUDs are now also known as 3-D worlds and chat worlds, reflective of their importance as non-gaming electronic meeting places.

*See also* Computer games

## MOSAIC

Mosaic was the first readily available and widely distributed program to provide a multimedia, **graphical user interface (GUI) browser** to the **World Wide Web** (WWW or Web). A GUI Web browser is graphics-based software that easily allows users to view **HTML** (HyperText Markup Language) documents and **access** files and software associated to those documents within the Web through images such as icons, dialog boxes, and menus. (Mosaic is often used as the generic term for any graphical browser.) During the early 1990s the National Center for Supercomputing and Applications (NCSA) within the University of Illinois at Champaign-Urbana developed Mosaic. Mosaic, whose copyrighted name is NCSA Mosaic, helped to ignite the enormous interest in the

Web during its first decade of existence. Mosaic is usually considered to be the software that introduced the World Wide Web (and the **Internet**) to a worldwide audience.

British physicist and computer scientist **Timothy Berners-Lee** developed the Web in the early 1980s, and introduced it to the scientific world in 1989; it quickly became popular at universities and research centers around the world. Realizing the possibilities of the Internet now that it contained the widely popular Web, **Marc Andreessen, Eric Bina**, and other members of the NCSA team researched the emerging Internet technologies, and eventually designed and programmed Mosaic to be used in association with different operating systems. An **operating system**, such as **Microsoft Windows**, is software that controls the various operating aspects of computer **hardware** resources such as main **memory**, central processing times, disk space, and peripheral devices.

During the first part of the 1990s Mosaic was released in several versions that allowed the Macintosh, Windows, and **UNIX** operating systems to be accessible to Mosaic. Thus, Mosaic became the first Web browser that could be used on computers running the three popular operating systems. Because of this common interface, the development of Mosaic helped to initiate the popularity of the Web. Throughout its lifetime Mosaic has been distributed as freeware (copyrighted software given away for free by the owner). In 1994 NCSA licensed the commercial development of an enhanced version of Mosaic to a company called Spyglass, headquartered in Naperville, Illinois. Then in 1997 NCSA announced that it was ceasing development of the Mosaic browser. Today, versions of Mosaic are available both as freeware and for sale. The source-code to Mosaic has been licensed by several companies, and there are several other web browsers as good or better than Mosaic, such as Netscape Navigator and Microsoft Explorer. Generally, Mosaic is distinguished from other early Web browsers by its ease of use and its addition of graphical images to Web documents.

*See also* Browser; Graphical user interface (GUI); HTML (HyperText Markup Language); Hypertext; Internet; World Wide Web (WWW)

# MOTHERBOARD

A motherboard is the physical arrangement, typically used in smaller computers such as personal computers (PCs), that links together the basic circuitry and components of the computer. It consists of a main printed circuit board containing the primary electronic components of a computer system, such as the (1) **microprocessor**, (2) main **memory**, (3) **random access memory** (RAM), (4) basic input/output system (**BIOS**) that contains the basic set of instructions required to control the computer when it is first turned on, (5) expansion boards and slots, (6) integrated circuitry controls for such things as the **mouse**, keyboard, and monitor, (7) mass storage interfaces for such things as the hard disk, floppy disk, and **CD-ROM** drives, (8) **bus** controllers and connectors, and (9) other electronic components that give additional functions to the computer. The motherboard, sometimes called the system board, is critical to the **operation** of the computer because it provides its main computing capability and controls all built-in and add-on **peripherals**. Because the motherboard contains the most essential components of the computer, it is sometimes said to be the "heart" of the computer system.

On the typical motherboard, the electrical circuitry (called the "traces") is imprinted (or affixed) to the surface of a sturdy, flat surface and is usually manufactured in a single step. A commonly used motherboard **design** in personal computers is the AT, based on the **International Business Machines** (**IBM**) Corporation's IBM AT motherboard. The ATX is a more recent motherboard specification that improves on the AT design. The AT, ATX, LPX, and NLX are frequently used motherboards. The most important component of the motherboard is the microprocessor. Within PCs the microprocessor is called the **central processing unit** (**CPU**). The microprocessor is sometimes not permanently attached to the motherboard but, rather, plugged into a socket so it can be easily removed and upgraded. However, to add additional features, the motherboard may need to be entirely replaced with another, more advanced motherboard.

Motherboards also contain other important microprocessor components, such as different types of memory microprocessors (i.e., RAM and cache memory) and logic microprocessors (that control many parts of the computer's function). Together, all of these microprocessors (or "chips") that reside on the motherboard are known as the motherboard's chipset.

Sometimes peripherals may not be directly attached (i.e., soldered) onto the motherboard. If not attached, they are considered "independent" controllers that are plugged into an expansion slot on the motherboard. Such daughterboards (i.e., expansion and input/output boards) are attached through the bus connector. For instance, expansion boards are inserted into expansion slots on the motherboard in order to increase the capability of the computer. Expansion slots on motherboards, standard with essentially all PCs, can offer better communications with other computers, faster speeds, and enhanced audio/video capabilities. Expansion slots are manufactured in either half or full size, and can normally transfer 8 or 16 bits (one **bit** is the smallest units of information that a computer can process) at a time, respectively.

The pathways that carry **data** on the motherboard are called buses. The amount of data that can be transmitted at one time between a device, such as a scanner or monitor, and the microprocessor affects the speed at which programs run. For this reason, bus architecture has been enhanced to increase data **throughput**. To work properly, expansion boards must conform to certain bus standards, such as integrated drive electronics (IDE), Extended Industry Standard Architecture (EISA), or small computer system interface (SCSI).

*See also* BIOS (Basic Input/Output system); Bus; Central processing unit (CPU); Microprocessor; Random-access memory (RAM)

# MOUSE

A *mouse* is a small pointing device that a user manipulates in order to input information into a computer. By moving a mouse over a surface such as a mouse pad, a user controls an on-screen pointer in order to select, move, and activate various items. The mouse's actions are electronically registered by software called a "mouse driver" and passed on to any active application that is designed to receive such input.

Computer scientist Douglas Engelbart invented the first mouse in 1963 while at the Stanford Research Institute. In 1970 he received a patent on his invention. Engelbart described his patent as an "X-Y position indicator for a display system," and nicknamed it a "mouse" because its connecting cable suggested a mouse's tail. Xerox Corporation brought the mouse to the commercial market, but it first became a widely used computer tool when **Apple** Computer made it a standard part of their Macintosh **personal computer**.

The basic characteristics of a mouse are: (1) a flat-bottomed metal or plastic housing that is gripped by one hand and moved about on some flat surface; (2) a rubber or plastic-coated ball set into the housing's underside; (4) a detection device to keep track of the ball's motions; (4) one or more buttons on the housing's upper surface; and (5) a cable (or wireless transmitter) that conveys information from the mouse to the computer.

The conventional mouse has one or two buttons. On a two-button mouse, the left-hand button is the primary button because it is used most frequently, and is operated with the index finger to select and activate objects represented on a screen. For example, a user may "click" once to send a "select" indication that a particular **object** has been chosen for further **action**. The next click, or two clicks in quick succession (often called a "double click"), causes a particular action to be performed on the selected object. These signals allow a user to call up menus, select items, open files, modify selections, copy or delete text and **graphics**, choose **commands**, and activate programs or bring different **applications** to the foreground. The right-hand button has different functions depending on operating systems and graphical user interfaces. For example, the right-hand button may allow the user to click on a Web page image to see a popup menu that allows a choice of actions such as saving an image to disk.

The five most common actions performed with the mouse are (1) pointing, that is, placing a pointer over an on-screen item; (2) clicking; (3) double-clickng; and (5) dragging, that is, holding down the button while moving the mouse in order to shift text, move an **icon**, resize a window, or make some other spatial change on the screen.

The conventional roller-ball mouse possesses a rubber or plastic-coated ball sticking out from the housing's underside and rolling on a flat surface. The ball's motions are communicated to a pair of spring-loaded rollers inside the mouse. The rollers divide the ball's movement into separate vertical and horizontal components which interior sensors measure and electronically transfer to the computer through the connecting cable.

The mouse's **design** continues to evolve, with new ways to point or position a cursor on a display being developed. An optical mouse uses a pair of light-emitting diodes (LEDs), optical sensors, and digital signal processing to detect the mouse's motion by sensing changes in reflected light, instead of the motions of a ball. The two LEDs are of different colors, and the special (light sensing) mouse pad contains a grid of lines in the same colors, one color for vertical lines and another for horizontal lines. Light detectors paired with the LEDs sense when a colored light passes over a line of the same color, indicating the direction of movement. Another type of mouse is a cordless mouse that uses a radio signal to transmit information to the computer. An optomechanical mouse translates motion into directional signals through a combination of optical and mechanical means. The optical portion includes pairs of LEDs and matching sensors, while the mechanical portion consists of rotating wheels with cutout slits. When the mouse is moved, the wheels turn and the light from the LEDs either passes through the slits and strikes a light sensor or is blocked by the solid portions of the wheels. Because the sensors are slightly out of phase with one another, the direction of movement may be determined by which sensor is the first to regain light contact. An optomechanical mouse eliminates the need for many of the wear-related repairs and maintenance necessary with purely mechanical mice, which inevitably draw dirt up into their mechanism, and does not require the special operating surfaces associated with optical mice.

# MULTIMEDIA AND HYPERMEDIA

Information interchange between humans and computers has long been restricted to the media of typescript and displayed text. Some graphic elements have been introduced over the years though they are quite rudimentary in comparison with the standards for free exchange among mature humans. Even with the addition of **graphics**, the fact remains that much information that is transmitted from a computer to a human uses only one human perceptive sense, that of vision. The other four senses (olfaction, audition, gustation, and taction) are not fully utilized. This creates an imbalance between online media of information, and real-life media of information.

A relatively new concept called multimedia addresses this difficulty. Although there is no precise definition for multimedia, it is generally agreed that the term applies to any situation where one has a computer presentation of information using two or more human senses. Most commonly, the senses of vision and audition are applied, but in special circumstances, others might be as well. In a looser sense, sometimes the term multimedia is applied even when text and moving graphics are both present but sound is not. In the sense described, multimedia is certainly an everyday experience since even television can qualify as conveying information through two human senses. To avoid such trivial cases, 'multimedia' is generally restricted to those cases where there is a certain interactivity rather than a fixed presentation. This is sometimes clarified by the use of the compound phrase, 'interactive multimedia,' where a user has some ability to choose a path through the presentation offered.

The success of the **World Wide Web** is at least in part due to the fact that it allows for interactive multimedia. Websites can be viewed as attempting to convey a multimedia presentation of their contents. In addition to the usual text and graphics, websites also offer animation, sounds, and videos. The Web's enhanced text feature called **hypertext** gives the user the option of customizing her online experience, much more so than a **static** presentation of the same content. Therefore, and also because the Web is now—and is likely to stay—the default technology for widespread online communication, the marriage of multimedia with the Web has resulted in hypermedia. In a certain sense, hypermedia is to multimedia what hypertext is to regular text. By allowing the user to customize her path through the Web, using the same principle as hypertext, but on graphics and moving pictures (i.e., by allowing the user to click on different parts of a graphic to access different information), a rich experience is created.

Multimedia is big business—more billions of dollars are spent each year on development of multimedia **applications**, than are spent on research to fight diseases like cancer. Multimedia applications are often user applications where simple text output will not do, and fierce competition with industry rivals and increased expectation from users demands that a rich multimedia experience be created. It is possible to argue that just about any application can be considered a candidate in this sense, but some are more established as multimedia targets than others. The best-known multimedia application in the civilian world is video games, where increasingly lifelike graphics, sounds, and the like are the norm. Another civilian application that has attracted much attention in recent years is computer based education (CBE), sometimes also called computer based training (CBT).

Multimedia applications are used by the military—and to a far lesser extent by others—for training and **simulation** purposes. A virtual environment (formerly called "virtual reality") is a special case of a multimedia application which is "immersive," i.e., where the user is meant to become engrossed in the multimedia presentation to such an extent that it dominates her consciousness; she has no significant interaction with and awareness of the real world, for the duration of the presentation. Such applications are used by the military for safe simulation of combat action—soldiers can be trained in maneuvers, and can learn the cost of certain mistakes without actually having to pay for them. Similarly, certain experiments in the behavioral sciences, such as studies in teenage driving habits, or on the influence of distractions on driving performance, and the like, can be safely investigated.

Until recent times, computer **hardware** used on PCs and other generic equipment did not include items necessary for multimedia presentations, but such items—sound cards, speakers, **CD-ROM** drives, et cetera—are standard these days. The processor chips used in computers formerly were also largely unequal to the task of producing high-quality multimedia presentations, because tasks like rendering moving graphics in real time are highly computation-intensive. With the growth in

processor speeds and performance in recent years, however, this is not a problem any longer. In fact, leading chip manufacturers like **Intel** often encourage research and development in multimedia applications, because they know that the widespread use of such applications will create an increasing demand for their fast, high-priced chips. It is in a chip manufacturer's interest, for instance, for a user to create a multimedia communication with moving pictures and sound to send a greeting or to make another communication, even when a simple two-line text **message** would have achieved the same purpose but with considerable economy of computational resources.

*See also* Computer architecture; CPU; HTML; Human-computer interaction; Virtual reality; World Wide Web

# MULTIPLE INHERITANCE

**Inheritance** is a feature of some but not all object-oriented computer **programming** languages. Inheritance describes the situation when a programmer creates a new **class** and bases it on an old one. The new class is said to be a "derived class" or "subclass" of the old one, which is often termed the "base class" or the "superclass."

In languages that support inheritance, the **derived class** is said to be a "kind of" the **base class** in an "is a" relationship. And by being a "kind of" the base class, the derived class includes all the **data**, methods, and characteristics of its base class; the programmer's job is then to refine the behavior of the base class to make it more like the thing it represents.

For example, if a Mastiff class is derived from a Dog class, then a Mastiff is a "kind of" Dog, in a clear "is a" relationship. The basic Dog class will have four legs, probably a tail, and will know how to bark, eat, and do all the typically doggy things we expect of Man's best friend. The derived Mastiff class will "inherit" the generic doggy behavior and then extend it into behavior typical of the Mastiff: slow, friendly, big, slobbering, lazy, loyal, and extremely protective of its family. A different kind of dog, like a Yorkshire Terrier, for example, would extend the common doggy behavior in different ways and be more like the irascible yappy creature that the Yorkie is. Different languages have different **syntax** for expressing inheritance, but the principle is the same.

Inheritance in **C++** is expressed like this:

```
class Dog {
public:
virtual int getAge() const { return _age; }
virtual void bark() const { }; // does nothing
private:
int _age;
};
class Mastiff : public Dog {
virtual void bark() const { }; // woofs
};
class Yorkie : public Dog {
```

```
virtual void bark() const { }; // yaps
};
```

And in **Java**, like this:

```
class Dog {
public:
int getAge() const { return _age; }
void bark() const { }; // does nothing
private:
int _age;
};
class Mastiff extends Dog {
void bark() const { }; // woofs
};
class Yorkie extends Dog {
void bark() const { }; // yaps
};
```

The C++ programming also supports "multiple inheritance." Multiple inheritance is a form of inheritance where the derived class has more than one class as its base class. As an example, a breeder might cross a Mastiff with a Yorkshire terrier to produce a Morkie. The **class declaration** might look like this:

```
class Morkie : public Mastiff, public Yorkie {
}
```

But this can lead to ambiguities when objects of the class are actually used. For example, assume that the Dog class has a bark() **method** that the programmer has overridden in both subclasses so the Mastiff "Woofs" and the Yorkie "Yaps." If the programmer writes **code** like this:

```
Morkie* pooch = new Morkie();
pooch→bark();
```

The **compiler** will not know which version of bark() to use, the Mastiff one or the Yorkie one. Does the Morkie woof or yap? If the programmer knows ahead of time, he can explicitly **call** the Mastiff's woof like this:

```
pooch→Mastiff::bark();
```

or the Yorkie yap like this:

```
pooch→Yorkie::bark();
```

If the Morkie has a bark all of its own, a "yoof" or a "wap," perhaps, the programmer would override the bark() method in the Morkie class so the ambiguity would never arise.

Another potential problem arises in this case because both Mastiff and Yorkie derive from the same base class. This means that hidden from the programmer the compiler creates both a Mastiff and a Yorkie when it creates a Morkie; and this in turn means that it creates two Dog objects. The problem this causes occurs when the programmer uses a **function** that refers to a **data member** in the Dog **object**, the Dog's getAge() function, perhaps. Which base object should the compiler use?

To resolve this, the programmer would have to override the getAge() method in the Morkie class explicitly to use one or other of the base objects' methods. Either of the below would be acceptable:

```
class Morkie : public Mastiff, public Yorkie {
```

```
int getAge() const { return Mastiff::getAge();}
}
class Morkie : public Mastiff, public Yorkie {
int getAge() const { return Yorkie::getAge();}
}
```

It is possible to remove this problem entirely by using what is called "virtual inheritance," which makes Dog a "virtual base class" of both Mastiff and Yorkie. The **declarations** might look like this:

```
class Mastiff : virtual public Dog {
virtual void bark() const { }; // woofs
};
class Yorkie : virtual public Dog {
virtual void bark() const { }; // yaps
};
```

Usually, a class's **constructor** will initialize its own variables and its base classes, but with virtual inheritance only the last derived class in the chain (the most derived class) initializes virtually inherited objects. Thus, Dog is initialized not by Mastiff or Yorkie, but only by Morkie. Morkie no longer has explicitly to call getAge() and it is free to inherit it immediately from Dog.

While multiple inheritance offers a number of advantages over single inheritance it does pose some potential hazards. Not only that, but a lot of compilers do not support it properly, it plays havoc with some debuggers, and, most important, it is possible to do most everything that can be done with multiple inheritance without it.

Java does not support multiple inheritance, largely because of the concerns above. However, multiple inheritance does offer some real advantages in certain circumstances. What Java supports instead is the concept of "interfaces." An interface definition is basically a list of functions, and when it is applied to a class declaration it is essentially saying "this class will implement this method." Indeed, the compiler enforces this very strictly and will report an error if it finds a method missing in a class that has been promised by an interface. A class in Java can extend only one class, but it can implement an unlimited number of interfaces.

Thus it is possible with careful thought to abstract functionality into interfaces that classes can then implement to get multiple-inheritance-like effects. For example, if "fish" and "supermodel" are two interfaces that contain the functions swim() and lookGorgeous(), respectively, then it would be possible to do this:

```
class Mermaid extends MythicalBeast
implements fish, supermodel {
void swim();
void lookGorgeous();
}
```

and so declare a Mermaid class that could both swim and look gorgeous, all without using multiple inheritance and thus avoiding the problems it can pose.

# MULTITASKING

Multitasking is a technique of most of today's operating systems in which a computer's **microprocessor** is able to safely and efficiently run several independent tasks (such as the **operation** of many application programs) at the same time without any noticeable delays to the user. As an example, a computer user is able to open a Web **browser** in order to "surf" the **Internet**, while also opening and using a **word processing** program. The first multitasking operating systems were designed in the early 1960s. Multitasking is referred to by several other names, including "multiprocessing," "multiprogramming," "concurrency," and "process scheduling."

The number of programs that can be effectively multitasked depends on such things as the type of multitasking performed, the speed of the **central processing unit** (**CPU**), and the amount of available main **memory**. Multitasking is accomplished because the computer's CPU is able to switch from one task to another so quickly that is appears to the user that all programs are operating at the same time. Programs can be run in parallel within the computer because of the differences between input/output (I/O) and processing speed. That is, while one program is waiting for input, instructions in another program can be executed. During the milliseconds that one program waits for **data** to be read from a disk, millions of instructions in another program can be executed. The ability to perform multitasking does not mean, however, that an unlimited number of tasks can be indefinitely switched back and forth. Each task consumes a certain amount of system storage and other resources, and as more tasks are started, the operating system slows down or begins to run out of shared storage.

Multitasking can be either classified as cooperative or preemptive. In cooperative multitasking the operating system allows the currently running task to voluntarily give up control to another task. One or more secondary tasks are then given processing time during idle times of the primary task; that is, if the currently running (primary) task allows such processing transfer. The **Apple** Macintosh operating system uses cooperative multitasking as its primary mode of multitasking. In *preemptive* multitasking (generally considered more common than cooperative) the operating system periodically determines which task receives priority. It is sometimes called "time-slice" multitasking because one task is only allowed to run for a fixed period known as a "time-slice" so that one program is prevented from monopolizing the system over other programs. The **Microsoft Windows** and **UNIX** operating systems use preemptive multitasking.

*See also* Input and output; Memory; Microprocessor; Operating systems, types; Time slice

# MULTITHREADED OPERATION

The traditional operating system perspective of a process is as one entity that pursues a single activity. However, in the context of **distributed systems**, and also in the context of uniprocessor systems that required **concurrency**, this traditional view was found, starting in the early 1980s, to be obsolete and inadequate. The traditional model of a process thus had to be enhanced so that it could be associated with multiple activities in the computer system taking place at once.

Nowadays, therefore, a process is considered to be an environment of execution, together with one or more threads—a **thread** being an **abstraction** for a "thread of execution" of a certain activity within the operating system. The execution environment is a collection of local resources managed by the operating system kernel, to which the threads have **access**. An execution environment has to consist of:

- an address space;
- thread management resources—semaphores or other primitives for synchronization and communication;
- other resources, including higher-level ones such as files.

Threads can be created and destroyed at run-time, as necessary. The purpose of having more than one thread is to make possible a high level of concurrency between operations—thus causing processing to take place simultaneously with input and output—and also to allow the use of more than one processor at the same instant. Having multiple threads can reduce bottlenecks in servers—for instance, one thread in the server process can process a new request while another thread waits for an I/O device to let the old one complete.

The structure of the execution environment provides the threads with protection from other threads belonging to other processes; any sharing of resources has to be conducted in an orderly way. Lacking this protection, it would come to pass that threads would continually invade each other's domains, causing all manner of disarray.

We may summarize the advantages of multiple threads—as against multiple processes—as follows:

- Creating a new thread with the same execution environment is easier than creating a new process with a new execution environment.
- Switching to a new thread within the same process is easier, as it does not usually involve context-switching by the CPU.
- Threads, for the reason of their belonging to the same execution environment, are able to share **data** and resources more easily than are processes.

As older, traditional operating systems and models allow only one thread per process, it is not uncommon to find authors who speak of "multi-threaded process" or "multi-threaded operation" for clarity or emphasis. A somewhat unsavory analogy for threads and execution environments was proposed in a posting to the comp.os.mach newsgroup by Chris Lloyd. According to this, an execution environment may be thought of as a jar with a tight lid, containing air and some food. Initially, there is one fly—a thread—inside it. This fly can produce other flies, and can also kill them off, and the same applies to the progeny. Any fly can use any resource (food or air) in the jar. Flies may work in cooperation for orderly exploitation of resources, or else they may act in an unstructured fashion and produce unpredictable results, including possible harm to themselves and their environment. Flies may communicate with other flies in their own jar, but no outside fly may enter it, nor may one within it leave. In this model, the traditional operating system analogy of a process would be a jar with a single sterile fly in it.

Multithreaded **operation** has certain distinct benefits in a client-server system. A server may function using a pool of more than one thread, each of which dequeues a request from the server's request **queue** and processes it. Under this arrangement it is possible for a thread to function while another is blocked for input or output. This allows the server to continue handling service requests without having to make all requests wait while one is blocked waiting. Similarly, a client process may also create multiple threads; for example, when a complex web page with several images, as well as text and possibly other data, is downloaded, the client **browser** program uses several threads, one each to download a significant **object** making up the page. In this way, the user can view some quick content such as text, while larger material like images are being downloaded slowly.

There are several possible architectures that are in common use for multiple-threaded operation. The architecture that has just been described above is called the worker pool architecture, for example, where a pool of worker threads successively dequeues and handles incoming requests. However, in case there are priorities among the requests (which is possible in corporate networks, for instance), a simple worker pool approach is considered insufficient. This situation can be handled using multiple queues of varying priorities, and by creating a protocol where entries from higher-priority queues are handled first, but doing this is cumbersome. Another architecture, called the thread-per-request architecture, is able to handle this situation much better. In this architecture, a central supervisor thread creates a new thread for each request received, and the new thread terminates after its request is serviced. In this system, the handling of priorities is left to the supervisor rather than to contending worker threads. Similar to this architecture, there are other ones called thread-per-connection and thread-per-object (the last for object-based models and systems).

*See also* Client-server system; Operating system (theory); Parallel processing; Semaphores

# MULTIWAY SELECTION

Multiway selection is a term that is relevant to **programming** in computer science. Languages such as C++ employ multiway selection. Specifically, multiway selection is a style of **code** writing that allows the testing of a **variable** against a list of possible values. The different values will affect the variable in different ways. Thus, multiway selection allows a programmer to assess the influence of values on the desirable or undesirable function of a variable, and to program in various options for a given variable.

Multiway selection operates by the use of what is termed the switch statement. A switch statement is what per-

mits many possibilities to be presented, along with the criteria for their selection.

The following is an example of multiway selection:

```
switch (lottery win) {
case (10): <tab>cout << "Get 5 more lottery tickets"<< endl;
break;
case (25): <tab>cout << "Get expensive meal in a restaurant" << endl;
break;
case (100): <tab>cout <&lr; "Weekend at local Bed and Breakfast" << endl;
break;
case (1000): <tab>cout << "Cruise around the world" << endl;
break;
case (10000): <tab>cout << "Stop writing and retire" << endl;
break;
default: <tab>cout << "Put winnings in the bank." << endl;
} // end of switch
```

As illustrated above, a multiway selection invokes a default **action** as well as a number of actions that are dependent on the changeable nature of the variable (in this case the size of the lottery winning). In a real case, the computer would look at the **value** of the **data** point and then jump to appropriate case in the switch statement. After executing the 'cout' statement a 'break' statement would be encountered. The computer would then jump to the end of the switch statement. If the data point does not match any of the listed cases, the default clause would be invoked, if present. A **default condition** is not mandatory. But it is often useful.

The multiway selection builds more flexibility into a program. This is particularly important when the variable is inherently complex in its behavior. Invoking a single option for a variable that is capable of multiple behaviors would be inappropriate.

*See also* Programming

# MUTATOR

A mutator is a **function** or **method** that changes the state of the **object** it belongs to; this is in contrast to an "accessor," which only "reads" the state of the object it belongs to.

In object-oriented programs, the program's **data** typically comprises "objects" that represent things or concepts in the real world. Objects not only have data, sometimes called "state" or "identity"; but they also have behavior, or things that they can do, either on their own data or data given to them by other objects. An object that represents an egg-timer might contain data about how long to boil an egg, and it might have a function to ring a bell once the egg has been boiling for long enough.

When a function that is associated with an object actually changes some of the data in the object, the function is referred to as a "mutator function" because it quite literally "mutates" the object into a different state.

As an example, consider a simple **C++** eggTimer class:

```
class eggTimer {
public:
eggTimer() : _hasBeenSet(false), _timeVal(0) { } // constructor
void setTimer(int t) { _timeVal = t;} // mutator
int getTimer() const { _hasBeenSet = true; return _timeVal;} // accessor
private:
int _timeVal;
mutable bool _hasBeenSet; // can be changed in a const function
};
```

In the above **code**, the function setTimer() is a mutator function because it changes the data in the eggTimer object by setting its _timeVal member to a given **value**. But the setTimer() function is an accessor function because it does not change anything about the object.

To make the **compiler** enforce this, getTimer() has been declared as "const," which means that if a programmer mistakenly did something in writing the function that did change the object, the compiler would detect this and issue an error.

The interesting thing to note is that even though getTimer() has been declared "const," the member **variable** _hasBeenSet is being changed. This is allowed because _hasBeenSet has been declared as "mutable," which tells the compiler that it is allowed to change the value of _hasBeenSet in a "const" function.

# MUTUAL EXCLUSION

There are certain situations where processes can be competing for a shared resource in a system, where it is important for only one process to be allowed to **access** the resource. This is also called the critical section problem, and it is important in the context of operating systems and distributed computing. One easy example of the need for mutual exclusion is in an office or school environment with multiple computers hooked up to a shared **printer**. Print jobs must be scheduled so that when a certain print job is under execution, all others have to wait. It would be grossly unacceptable for pages from different jobs to be mixed up in printing, or for lines from different jobs to be mixed up on the same page. Multiprocessor cache-coherence **protocols** are another good example where mutual exclusion is needed—a cache cannot be read at the same time as it is being updated, as that might result in invalid or stale values being read. Thus, mutual exclusion between a process that wishes to write to a cache, and any other process that wishes to read, is required.

The implementation of mutual exclusion also has to address other concerns—chiefly, the concern that there be no **deadlock** or starvation. A deadlock would involve two or more processes waiting forever to access the critical section, such as by having only one lock each while two locks by one process are required to access the shared resource. Starvation would occur if a certain process was never allowed to use the resource while others were. This would be unfair to that process, but would seemingly preserve the basic condition of mutual exclusion.

Thus, if we consider that desirable qualities in a system's behavior or functioning can be divided along the lines suggested by Lamport into safety and liveness properties, then the basic condition of mutual exclusion is a safety property—that no two processes may simultaneously access the resource is a specification that something bad must not be allowed to happen. That all processes who wish to access the shared resource succeed eventually is a liveness property, as it is saying that something good will eventually happen. Another issue is fairness—the order in which the processes are allowed to use the shared resource. Ideally, processes should be granted access to the resource in the same order as their requests for it. However, in the absence of a global real-time clock (lacking in asynchronous **distributed systems**) there is no way to accurately determine the global ordering of all request events. A useful approximation for the **fairness** condition is that of determining the order based on Lamport's "happens-before" relation, i.e., to fix the events on a logical time-scale that may or may not correspond to the ordering in real time.

Many practical solutions to the distributed mutual exclusion problem rely on the use of a central server or coordinator that receives requests for access to the shared resource, and grants such access to one process at a time. This server can be a special processor specifically tasked for such application, or it may be one of the processors on the system running a special process to serve this purpose. Any process that wishes to use the resource sends a request to the coordinator, which sends that process an acknowledgement when the resource is available for its use. Upon finishing with the resource, the process then sends a release **message** to the server, which is then able to allocate it to another requesting process.

Although the central server solution is simple and intuitive, it is not necessarily usable in practice—having a single server to process requests creates a single point of failure for the whole system; should the server fail, no process can access the shared resource. Such a single server also can cause communication bottlenecks in the system, or itself may get bogged down if required to handle a large numbers of requests. For these reasons, such a solution is not always practical. De-centralized **algorithms** that achieve mutual exclusion without need for a server are thus often preferred.

The first such published algorithm is by Lamport. It assumes that channels for delivering messages are FIFO (first-in, first-out). Each process in the system maintains its own private request-queue Q. The algorithm is described by the following rules:

- To request access to the shared resource, each process sends a timestamped request message to every other process, and logs it in Q behind the previous entry.

- When a process receives a request from another process, it logs it in Q behind the previous entry. If it is not already accessing the shared resource, it sends a timestamped acknowledgement to the requesting process; else, it defers such acknowledgement until it finishes using the shared resource.

- A process accesses the resource when its own entry in Q is ahead of all others, and when it has received acknowledgements from every other process in response to its current request.

- After a process is done accessing the resource, it deletes its entry from Q, and sends a timestamped release message to all other processes.

- When a process receives a release message, it deletes the corresponding entry from Q.

It is an interesting exercise to try to understand Lamport's algorithm for mutual exclusion, and it is not hard to convince oneself that it satisfies all three conditions: safety, liveness, and fairness. An improvement over Lamport's algorithm was given by Ricart and Agrawala, with another improvement subsequently being made by Maekawa. Although the earlier algorithms had all assumed the existence of a completely connected network (since every processor should be able to send messages to every other), subsequent work has relaxed this unrealistic restriction, and much work has also been done on reducing the message complexity (the number of messages that are required to be passed).

***See also*** Concurrent programming; Deadlock; Dining philosophers; Distributed computing; Fairness

# N

## NANOTECHNOLOGY

Nanotechnology refers to the construction and use of atomic machines—functioning consortia of atoms that are less than about 1,000 nanometers in size. A nanometer is one billionth of a meter. The technology is relevant to computer science as it could potentially be used to construct molecular computers, which could be smaller than the size of a bacterial cell and capable of performance exceeding technology currently in use.

Molecular machines are in the early developmental stages. Several reports have described the physical rearrangement of atoms into a desired configuration, such as the use of a scanning tunneling microscope by International Business Machine researcher John Foster to push xenon atoms around to spell "IBM." Other reports have described the atomic assembly of crude interlocking gears. And, in 1999, a molecular electronic research team successfully constructed a "molecular wire" circuit based on a polyphenylene polymer and a functional molecular switch.

In the future, it may be possible to use atomic assemblers—robotic arms analogous in function to a construction crane—to position atoms. This is called positional assembly. There is precedent for molecular positional assembly. Ribosomes, which position and link together amino acids in a specified sequence to form a specific protein, are biological assemblers. Atomic assemblers would be capable of assembling atoms into three-dimensional configurations and attaching the atoms together by a variety of chemical means. Assemblers would theoretically also be capable of constructing copies of themselves, or replication. Self-replication at the atomic scale was first studied by John von Neuman in the 1940's.

The construction of molecular computers hinges on the refinement of techniques of molecular electronics, in which chemistry is used to assemble circuit components, such as the building of the polyphenylene circuit. Molecular electronics began with the realization that molecules comprised of long chains of atoms could conduct electricity. Individual electrons hop from one molecule to the next in the chain. This movement differs from conventional current, which results from the bulk movement of electrons through the material of the wire. To harness the molecular current, it is necessary to have controllable "gates."

Several gating designs exist. One feasible **design** for a molecular computer is based on sliding rods that act to block or unblock one another's sliding action as they interact at certain sites, or locks. The controlled interaction of the locks would allow information—electrical or otherwise—to pass from rod to rod. It has been calculated that the number of locks necessary to build a simple 4-bit or 8-bit general-purpose computer would occupy only a few nanometers of space. Another design is to attach a molecular "side chain" to a molecular wire. The molecule could both accept and donate electrons. Control of these processes would allow for the controlled movement of electrons through the molecular gate. A functional molecular gating device has been constructed at Bell Labs.

The next goal is to find a chemical means to construct what is called a three-terminal **transistor**. These would enable electricity to flow in a web-like pattern, rather than in a straight line. In turn, complex logic devices could then be made. Current research is exploring the use of chemical processes to construct the transistors, rather than the use of atomic assemblers.

A drawback to nanotechnology is the problem of random defects. While molecular structures self-assemble very accurately, compared with human-directed assembly processes, perfection is impossible, and defects in assembly will occur in a random way. For a molecular wire, which requires molecular **precision**, such imperfections are lethal to the function of the wire. The question of how molecular defects will be handled is an important design constraint. The focus is to find circuit architectures that will be able to function with fidelity even with defects present. Perhaps circuit design will incorporate the presence of a certain number of defects. Or, analogous with biological systems, perhaps parallel redundant molecular wires could be used. Also, molecular computers may be designed to operate similarly to the human brain, where networks of neurons permit information flow, even with abnormally functioning neurons.

Shrinking computers to atomic size would allow computerized control of processes inside many currently inaccessible niches, such as the human body. Medical treatment could potentially be revolutionized. If chemical reactions can be harnessed to create the logical electrical pathways needed for computer operations, then molecular computers could become a reality.

*See also* Molecular switches; von Neuman architecture

# NAPIER, JOHN (1550-1617)
## *Scottish mathematician*

John Napier is best remembered as the inventor of the first system of logarithms. A logarithm is the power to which a number, called the base, must be raised to produce a given number. Napier's work with logarithms was described in two Latin treatises, *Mirifici logarithmorum canonis descriptio* (1614; "A Description of the Wonderful Canon of Logarithms") and *Mirifici logarithmorum canonis constructio* (1619; "The Construction of the Wonderful Canon of Logarithms"). This work was immediately recognized by other mathematicians as a great advance. Three hundred years later, in an essay marking the publication anniversary of the *Descriptio*, P. Hume Brown wrote that Napier's most notable achievement "has given him a high and permanent position in the history of European culture."

Napier, the eighth laird of Merchiston, was born in 1550 at Merchiston Castle near Edinburgh, Scotland. He came from a line of influential noblemen and statesmen. His father, Sir Archibald Napier, was a prominent public figure who was allied with the Protestant cause. Among other roles, Sir Archibald served for more than 30 years as Master of the Mint. Sir Archibald's first wife and Napier's mother, Janet Bothwell, was the daughter of an Edinburgh burgess.

Napier entered the University of St. Andrews at age 13, which was typical of wellborn boys of the time. However, he was a dropout, staying at the university for only a short while. It is likely that Napier then traveled to the European continent to continue his studies, although little is known of this period. By 1571, however, he had returned to Scotland and was living at Gartnes, where he built a castle. In 1572 Napier married Elizabeth Stirling. The couple had two children, Archibald and Joanne, before Elizabeth's death in 1579. Napier later married Agnes Chisholm, with whom he had ten children. These included a son named Robert, who eventually served as his father's literary executor. The family stayed in Gartnes until 1608, when Napier inherited Merchiston Castle upon Sir Archibald's death.

Napier lived an active life as a Scottish landowner. He was an amateur scientist who never held a professional post. Nevertheless, his varied accomplishments earned him the nick-

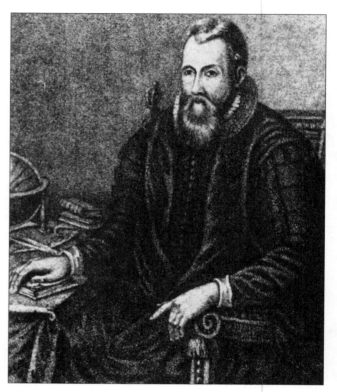

**John Napier**

name of "Marvelous Merchiston." He experimented with fertilizers to improve his land, and he invented a hydraulic screw and revolving axle that could be used to remove water from flooded coal pits. Not surprisingly, Napier was also intrigued by the religious and political controversies of his day. A staunch Protestant, he published *A Plaine Discovery of the Whole Revelation of St. John* in 1593. This book, a virulent attack on Catholicism that concluded the Pope was the Antichrist, was read widely and translated into several languages.

Napier's preoccupation with defending his faith and country prompted him to **design** various weapons. These included burning mirrors for setting enemy ships on fire, an underwater craft, and a tank–like vehicle. He invested much time and money in these projects, even building prototypes in some cases. In one instance, Napier was said to have built and tested an experimental rapid–fire gun that he claimed would have killed 30,000 Turks without the loss of a single Christian.

Astronomywas another of Napier's passions, and it was this pursuit that led to his greatest discovery. Napier's astronomy research required him to do a number of tedious calculations involving trigonometric functions. Over the course of more than two decades, he gradually developed and refined new ideas for speeding such calculations through the use of logarithms. The *Descriptio*briefly explained his invention and presented the first logarithmic tables. The *Constructio*, published after his death, described how the tables had been computed.

The *Descriptio* attracted the attention of English mathematician Henry Briggs, who traveled to Edinburgh to discuss the new tables. Napier and Briggs worked on such improvements as using the base 10. The result was Briggs's development of a standard form of logarithmic table that remained in common use until the advent of calculators and computers. Thanks to his efforts, logarithms were quickly adopted by mathematicians throughout Europe.

Napier made other advances in spherical trigonometry. The so–called "Napier's analogies" were formulas for solving spherical triangles. "Napier's rules of circular parts" were ingenious rules for stating the interrelationships of the parts of a right spherical triangle. In addition, Napier pioneered the use of the decimal point to separate the whole number part of a number from its fractional part. As one of the first to use decimal fractions, he helped to popularize them.

Napier's contributions to mathematics did not end there, however. His concern with simplifying calculations led him to invent mechanical aids for doing arithmetic, described in *Rabdologia* (1617). Among these aids were rods with numbers marked off on them, often known as "Napier's bones" because they were usually made of bone or ivory. Using the rods, multiplicationbecame a process of reading the appropriate figures and making minor adjustments. In addition, Napier invented other types of rods for extracting square roots and cube roots.

It is not clear when Napier first began to dabble in mathematics. However, some early writings, dealing mainly with arithmetic and algebra, seem to date from the period just after his first marriage. These writings were collected and transcribed after Napier's death by his son Robert. They were first published in 1839 by descendant Mark Napier under the title *De arte logistica*, revealing the keenness of Napier's mathematical ruminations. Among other subjects, it appears that he investigated imaginary roots of equations.

During his lifetime, Napier was reputed to be not only a mathematician, but a magician as well. It was rumored that he possessed supernatural powers, and that he owned a black rooster as a spiritual familiar. Given his wide–ranging interests, Napier was almost never idle. A combination of overwork and gout finally led to his death at Merchiston on April 4, 1617. His burial place is uncertain, but it is probably at the old church of St. Cuthbert's parish in Edinburgh.

In 1914, the 300th anniversary of the publication of the *Descriptio* was commemorated by the Royal Society of Edinburgh. In his inaugural address, Lord Moulton lauded Napier as one who "stands prominent among that small band of thinkers who by their discoveries have substantially increased the powers of the human mind as a practical agent." In 1964 Napier University, named for the mathematician, was founded in Edinburgh. Among its campuses is one at Merchiston, which houses courses in science, technology, and design.

## NAPIER'S RODS

*Napier's rods* (or *bones*) were a set of graduated rods used as a mechanical aids to calculation beginning in the early seven-

teenth century. Scottish mathematician **John Napier** (1550–1617) invented the rods named after him in order to speed up arithmetic calculations. Napier published his *Rabdologia* in 1617, in which he discussed various methods for abbreviating calculations. One method of multiplication and division (and of determining squares roots and powers) that Napier described in his *Rabdologia* was the ingenious system of numbered rods eventually called Napier's rods or bones (see figure). It was a major improvement on the ancient system of counters then in use, and today Napier's rods are considered the forerunner of the **slide rule**.

Multiplication can be reduced to simple addition with Napier's rods by using an "index" rod (i.e., a rod with "index" written across the top or sometimes, as shown in the figure, with no number at the top) and other rods with specific numbers appearing at the top of each. The index rod is laid to the left of specifically numbered rods for multiplication. For example, to multiply 6 by 7, first locate the index rod (the left-most rod in Figure 1), and also the rod marked "7" at the top. Next, look right from "6" across the index rod, and then down from the 7 rod until the two meet. The result appears on the 7 rod: 42.

Multiplication of a number (i.e., 6) by larger numbers (i.e., 467) can also be quickly calculated. As shown in Figure 1, place the 4, 6, and 7 rods in sequence next to each other, and place the index rod to the right of all three. The row on the "index" rod that contains numeral "6" gives the result of 6 × 467 when the products with the units 7 rod (6 × 7 = 42), the tens 6 rod (6 × 60 = 360), and the hundreds 4 rod (6 × 700 = 2,400) are added together: 42 + 360 + 2,400 = 2,802. Multiplying even larger numbers is accomplished by inserting the necessary rods for thousands, ten thousands, hundred thousands, and so forth.

*See also* Slide rule

# NETWORK APPLICATIONS

Network **applications** may be defined as software applications used in networks that require or substantially benefit from the presence of networked computers. Networks essentially are created in order to connect users and facilitate the performance of tasks. Networks therefore exist for applications. Without applications software, users can do little on a network. Network application software allows users to tap the power of networks in increasingly creative ways.

Networked applications came into being with the advent of the client-server model in the 1980s and 1990s, when LANS (Local-Area Networks) and WANs (Wide-Area Networks) proliferated, and corporations increasingly began to rely on centralized computer programs for all business functions. This meant that robust data-handling applications were placed on central network servers, rather than on desktop workstations. Networked users then used thin-client interfaces at their desktops to connect with network applications and perform business tasks such as accounting, querying for **data**, data analysis, and reporting. This model was found to be cost- and resource-effective. Soon, cost and infrastructure efficiencies dictated the use of sophisticated back-end network applications for all corporate needs including networked **e-mail**, scheduling, **data storage**, and data back-ups. This reliance increased as the use of networks expanded and the **Internet** gained visibility and significance. Locally **networked computing** began to make the switch to Internet computing, with users now relying for applications on large central servers accessible over the Internet. Currently the drive toward hosted applications has led Internet service providers and web site hosting servers to offer bundled services that include messaging, web e-mail and instant messaging, scheduling, content management, directory services, newsgroups, listservs, **authentication**, and other services as part of the Internet access and application package.

**Telnet**, Email, MajorDomo, and FTP are examples of early network applications that have continued to maintain their significance; and other complex and newer applications continue to crowd the market. Telnet is a **UNIX** program using **TCP/IP** (Transmission Control Protocol/Internet Protocol) that allows computers to connect remotely to other hosts or from a client to a server on the network as if connected directly. The most common usage of Telnet today is to allow users to log into remote computers on which they have an account and perform various functions such as editing and processing of email. Email or electronic mail programs such as **Microsoft** Outlook, Netscape Mail, Eudora, or Lotus Notes allow users to send electronic text, image, or multimedia messages to single or group computer-users on a local network or over the Internet. MajorDomo is a list server management program that allows users to automatically set up and manage e-mail discussion lists called listservs.

FTP or File Transfer Protocol is a TCP/IP program that allows users on computers to connect to remote servers or hosts and download or upload files, explore and organize directories, and manage files on the remote **host system** from a distance. Interestingly FTP was the standard means for transfer of files on the Internet before the advent of the **HyperText Transfer Protocol** (**HTTP**) and the **World Wide Web**. Although many FTP functions have been taken over by HTTP, FTP is still used extensively for file transfer on the Internet, especially by webmasters making updates to Web sites.

Currently network applications can be classified into three kinds— network-ignorant, network-aware, and network-intrinsic. Network applications can also include programs written for network administration and management such as NetWare's SYSCON, as well as **printer** and disk management utilities. Increasingly utilities are included in network operating systems.

Network-ignorant applications are essentially stand-alone applications that can be hosted on a single file server and be made available to all users on a network. Users can run the application on their desktops and make changes on files available through the application. However, there is no **concurrency** control, which means that if more than one user works on the same file over the network, changes made will always override the existing copy of the file, and will not discretely reflect the input of all users. Also, if two users try to use the application simultaneously, data can be lost or corrupted.

Network-aware applications are very similar to network-ignorant applications in that they too offer single copy hosting on a server, and access by multiple users over a network. However, the difference is concurrency control. Network-aware applications such as Paradox offer the advantages of record- or file-locking, which locks down a **record** or file in use by any user on a network, thus preventing overwrites by other users. The specific database record or word-processing file in use is locked down for every other user and becomes available only when the first user relinquishes control by closing the record or file. These programs have been created or modified expressly to allow usage by multiple concurrent users. Database applications, word-processing programs, communications software, and electronic mail are all network-aware applications. Most client-server applications today are network-aware applications. Their primary **value** lies in using the network to extend the abilities of a PC and to share network resources.

However, network-aware applications do not fully harness the power of networks since they use the network only as a peripheral sharing device. Although the file server hosts the program and data, it does not do any processing. All processing is done by individual users' computers, including all concurrency control. This is being replaced today by network-intrinsic applications, which share or distribute processing power among network computers, and is also known as distributed computing. Application programs of this kind have multiple components. One piece is the server, which does data processing, and the other is the client, which communicates with the user. A database server with front and back ends is a good example. The front end records user requests and displays formatted data to the user. Users can make queries, write reports, and create new **databases**. The back end manages data, concurrency control, and security. Basically, when a user submits a query for data, all search and **sorting** through the database is done by the server rather than the user's computer.

The back-end returns the specific record requested rather than the entire file, as in the case of network-aware applications, which expect the user's computer to then do the processing. With a database server, the question of multiple user traffic is addressed by concurrency control at the server back-end. The two programs, front- and back-end, work together to create one application. Network-intrinsic applications include distributed databases, compile servers, compute servers, and **multitasking** communications servers. Network operating systems today are seeking to provide more multitasking, more **memory**, faster processors, and **programming** interfaces in order to make network-intrinsic programs more powerful.

Cross-platform connectivity has become an increasingly important issue as dissimilar **hardware** and software platforms are distributed across networks. In the past organizations sought to standardize on one platform or another, an approach no longer followed, as platform innovation continues. Interoperability across diverse platforms is a vital goal for any architecture that claims to be suitable for network applications. On the Internet, TCP/IP offers a means to ensure cross-platform connectivity across **Windows**, Macintosh, and UNIX platforms.

# NETWORK SECURITY

Network security comprises the growing science of protecting **data** stored and transmitted across information networks. Security of data (and voice) transmissions has become an increasingly important issue as the **Internet** has expanded, and once-private corporate networks conduct a great deal of business in public cyberspace over the Internet and wide area networks. The danger of information being intercepted, corrupted, or misappropriated has escalated, as has the fear of hackers breaking into servers and altering source **code** published on Web sites or conducting Denial-of-Service attacks. As a result computer and network security procedures, practices, and technologies have developed into a science of their own. Today computer and network security take many forms and offer varying levels of protection, ranging from physical measures such as data-drive locks to access codes, user identification passwords, **authentication** devices, firewalls, data encryption, router access-control lists (ACLs), virtual LANS (VLANS), and Virtual Private Networks (**VPNs**). Methodologies to increase security are also proliferating and include the concept of layering defenses to engaging in intrusion detection to using a demilitarized zone (DMZ) for unprotected communications.

Physical measures to ensure network security include such precautions as confining network wiring to locked closets, restricting access to data and network **operation** centers (NOCs), installing electronic locks on doors, requiring visitor registration and badges, and installing security guard stations at key access points. These measures, long evident at all telephone companies and carrier headquarters—such as MCI WorldCOM, Sprint, Qwest, AT&T—are increasing in use at many companies using networks. Physical measures extend to using keyboard locks, data-drive locks, or desk locks, which become especially useful in places where workstations offer network access to wiring hubs, **LAN** servers, and bridge-routers.

Authentication measures on networks also offer a fairly standard means of network security. Basic authentication occurs on dial-up ports at networks when users using modems dial in and first transmit a user id and **password**. If this data corresponds with data stored on access control lists, then the user is permitted access to the network. Limits on access attempts also prevent unauthorized users from breaking in. Log-on security can be applied on any network, local or remote, and can be fine-tuned to identify users by workgroup or department. Complex and newer measures include the use of multilevel passwords, and biometric measures such as hand prints, voice patterns, or retinal prints.

Access levels offer another means of securing networks. Network administrators can delineate access levels for users as public, private, or shared. Public access would allow users to read but not alter data. Private access would allow read-write access, meaning users can both read and alter data. Shared access would allow all users to read and write to all files.

Data encryption is another means of ensuring privacy over networks. This has evolved in many ways over the last two decades and comprises an almost essential feature of data transmission these days on major networks. Encryption defines the conversion of data into a form unreadable by anyone without a secret decryption key. Its purpose is to ensure privacy by keeping the data hidden from all unintentional recipients, even those who can see the encrypted data. On networks, this measure requires that data and voice be scrambled first with an encryption algorithm before traversing the network. Pretty-Good Privacy (**PGP**) is an example of a highly effective encryption algorithm that uses a public key to protect **e-mail** and computer data. Public-key **cryptography** means that all recipients are supplied a public key with the **message**, while a corresponding private key resides already on the recipient's computer. The private key is then used to decode the message. Data encryption is often accompanied by digital authentication through a **digital signature**, which ensures that the receiver can be confident of the identity of the sender or the integrity of the message. Authentication **protocols** can be based on either conventional secret-key cryptosystems or on public-key systems; authentication in public-key systems uses digital signatures. The **signature** is an unforgeable piece of data asserting that a named person wrote or otherwise consented to the document to which the signature is attached.

Firewalls offer means of protecting a network from other, untrustable networks. A **firewall** can be thought of as a shield that blocks untrustworthy communications while simultaneously allowing reliable communications to enter and go through. Firewalls can take many forms, and like everything else on the Internet, are constantly evolving. Some firewalls specialize in blocking unsafe traffic while others emphasize permitting safe traffic. Firewalls can be set up around whole networks or on specific routers or servers. Packet filtering offers one kind of firewall protection; here, data packets received by a network are first screened through a firewall device. The screening limits access based on the packet's source or originating machine or site, time of day, date, or even day of week, number of sessions permitted or other such specification.

Transparent proxies are often used with firewalls to secure communications. In this case, firewalls act as deflectors, creating dynamic, transparent proxy routers to deflect and forward data. When packets looking for a router hit the firewall (set up as the default router), the firewall software immediately sets up a proxy that does not route the packets but connects to an intermediate host, which then forwards the data. Proxies are often used instead of routers as a means of traffic control, in order to ensure that traffic does not pass directly between trusted and untrusted networks. Proxies can implement protocol-specific security as well, since they necessarily understand application protocols. This means that they can be used, for instance, to allow outgoing FTPs and block incoming FTPs.

Virtual LANS (VLANS) offer another means of internal security. Virtual networking refers to the ability of switches and routers to configure logical topologies on top of the physical network infrastructure, allowing **variable** network elements to be configured to appear as a single LAN. Virtual LANs function by logically segmenting a network into different broadcast domains so that packets are only switched between ports designated for the same VLAN. Data traffic, whether internal or external, is then confined to a specific area within the company network, and can be further controlled internally by the network. This technology promotes highly targeted and secure communications and preserves bandwidth.

For both public communications over the Internet and for private corporate traffic, Virtual Private Networks (VPNs) are increasing in usage. VPNs allow companies to use public networks or the open, distributed infrastructure of the Internet, to privately transmit data between corporate sites. Companies using an Internet VPN would connect to their **Internet service provider (ISP)** and use their ISP's VPN to transmit data. Over the VPN, data is encrypted to increase security, since the Internet is a public network. VPNs can be used at corporate sites, branch offices, and by mobile workers. Because all workers can connect to their company's VPN by dialing into the local **POP** (Point of Presence) of their ISP, this greatly cuts down on long-distance charges and capital outlays while ensuring private and secure communications.

IPSEC, short for IP Security, is a set of protocols developed by the Internet Engineering Task Force (IETF) to support secure exchange of packets at the IP layer, and it has been deployed widely to implement VPNs. IPSEC requires that the sending and receiving devices must share a public key, and accomplishes this through a protocol that allows the receiver to obtain a public key and authenticate the sender using digital certificates.

SSL, short for Secure Sockets Layer, is another protocol that allows the transmission of private documents via the Internet. SSL uses a public key to encrypt data and is supported by both major browsers, Netscape Navigator and Internet Explorer. Many web sites use SSL to obtain confidential user information such as credit card numbers and bank account information. Web pages carrying confidential data

over an SSL connection start with https: instead of http:. Secure **HTTP** (S-HTTP) is a very similar secure transmission protocol. The difference between the two is that SSL allows any number of communiqués to be exchanged over a secure connection established between a client and a server, while S-HTTP is designed to transmit individual messages securely. SSL and S-HTTP, therefore, are complementary rather than competing technologies and have both been approved by the IETF as a standard.

# NETWORKED COMPUTING

Networked computing has evolved from networks connecting computers and distributed computing through thin-client network computing in the 1980s and 1990s to **Internet** computing today. Centralized computing—which started with mainframes at the outset of the computing evolution, evolved to PCs, and lasted up to the 1980s—focused mainly on automating existing processes. This approach gave way as **applications** and systems evolved to the client-server model and the distributed computing model. The client-server model allowed for the creation of server applications responsible for the storage, analysis, and **sorting** of large amounts of **data** on central data servers, with connected workstations responsible only for front-end client applications capable of running queries, producing reports, and adding new records. Distributed computing meant that dedicated file servers also could be used throughout an internal **Local-Area Network (LAN)**, each supporting a single application, such as **e-mail**, facsimile, **data storage**, **graphics** storage, or documentation storage. Computers, sometimes using different operating systems, could store different components of a single application, such as a spellchecker and thesaurus stored on different computers. Printers and other **peripherals** connected to the LAN offered users shared **access** over the network. Network monitoring and backups offered a high degree of **data security** and integrity. Personal computing entered a new era of productivity as spreadsheets, database programs, and word processors came increasingly into use at personal workstations.

The concept of network computing had its origins in 1995 with Oracle Corporation's concept of full-service client-server computing, where individual computers would rely on central servers on an internal network for all applications, **databases**, and information. Desktops would be minimally equipped with application-specific thin clients intended primarily to communicate with servers that would be responsible for all data processing. (In contrast, a fat client would comprise a stand-alone PC workstation fully equipped with all requisite applications.) This model of network computing allows for lower costs of installation, security, and maintenance, since databases and applications would need to be maintained only on the central server, not at every workstation. This model has been found particularly useful for task-oriented professionals in engineering, medicine, accounting, and real-estate focused on content rather than technology, as well as in back-office operations supported by clerical and sales staff. One disadvantage to this model is that as clients increase in number, servers need to be upgraded given the additional computing burden placed on them, thus raising infrastructure and maintenance costs.

Networked computing has evolved with the advent and progress of the Internet to mean Internet computing. This means that computers linked over the Internet would access large central servers outfitted with pre-packaged server software and Internet database applications for all processing purposes. Oracle8i, developed by Oracle Corporation to replace thin-client computing in 1998, offers such a platform; it functions as an Internet database that supports **Java**, and it can consolidate data, Java objects, and **Windows** files. Java is important because it is being used as a foundation to develop interactive, real-time exchange of information by allowing dynamic querying of databases and managing logical workflow processing. Java **applets** and **servlets**, which are compact Java programs supported and run by larger applications such as the major Internet browsers (e.g., Netscape and Explorer) are increasingly being used to streamline online banking, interactive trading, investment planning, and online purchasing. Through the use of Java applets and servlets Web users need not download whole workflow applications and can thereby save space, **memory**, and **hardware** wear-and-tear at their desktops. In this model, computing is focused on facilitating the search and dissemination of information. Applications are distributed across the network, which means that various functions can be accessed through the network as though they were stand-alone components, dynamically loaded and discarded when used.

Internet computing also means that business data is consolidated onto large servers for global Internet access, easy management, and speedier business application usage. Remote access computing is supported through remote access servers and concentrators. The Internet computing model is valuable to businesses because it can lower computing costs without the complexity of general-purpose operating systems. Computers with different operating systems would utilize Internet **protocols** as they accessed, computed, and communicated over the Internet. This model is thought to combine the best of the **mainframe** and client-server worlds by centralizing backups and offering users an intuitive graphical interface. In effect, client-server computing would expand to allow computing via **TCP/IP** over the Internet, allowing the use of different systems and platforms as long as a Web **browser** with a graphical interface provided a point of entry for a Web user. Additionally, mobile and remote computing becomes possible in this model, with all users required only to have access to the Internet and a Web browser installed on their machines.

In fact, the trend toward mobile and other computing devices is expected to change the profile of Internet computing in the next 10 years, with an increase in the usage of handhelds, wireless, and miniature "wearable" computers. Increased reliance on Internet computing will lead to data storage, synchronization, and scheduling being consolidated at centralized server farms that connect the corporate office and remote workers through broadband links. The concept of building hard-wired applications for functions such as inven-

tory and accounting will evolve into a more dynamic reliance on toolkits for a particular task, as is already evident in the proliferation of shareware, freeware, and discountware on the Internet. More than ever before, a menu of software tools is now available to complete any project. These tools, while occasionally downloaded to the desktop, are increasingly expected to reside on the network.

Futurists predict that PCs will soon be replaced by network computers, Internet appliances (from telephone-like devices to televisions), and non-desktop computers, such as enterprise servers and wearable computers. As business transactions increasingly take place online, issues such as security, **authentication**, and quality of service (QoS) are expected to be resolved. Constant wireless connectivity and virtual private networks will allow users to be connected anytime, anywhere to their corporate nets over the Internet. As wireless communications expands, the convergence of video, voice, and data will allow users to download books, movies, television, and radio signals to their portables over broadband wireless connections. Computers will not only be everywhere, they will be held centrally on a network and controlled remotely. You could go to work, connect to your home server and control devices such as security cameras, motion detectors, lights, alarm clocks, heating and cooling systems, refrigerators, microwaves, PCs, televisions, and VCRs remotely.

# NEURAL NETWORKS

A *neural network* is a biologically inspired form of computing device. Neural networks are parallel computing systems that hold the promise—according to their advocates—of being someday able to perform common cognitive tasks, such as pattern and speech recognition, that are hard for more common computational architectures yet are performed almost effortlessly by the human brain. The slight success seen by neural networks in these arenas so far is thanks to their parallel architecture, which mimics, albeit at a far lower level of complexity, certain aspects of our own brains.

In a human brain, the basic information-processing unit is a cell called the *neuron*. A neuron consists of a cell body where the nucleus resides. Networks of branching fibers called *dendrites* communicate with other neurons across synaptic gaps, across which chemical signals can travel. An action potential is carried from its cell body along a long fiber called an *axon* that, in turn, branches near its end. The transmission of signals from one neuron to another across the junction between axon and dendrite, the *synapse*, is a complex chemical process in which neurotransmitters (special chemicals floated like messages through the thin fluid layer between one cell and the next) lower the electrical potential (voltage) across the receiving cell's outer membrane. If a cell receives enough input from other neurons, its potential is lowered so far that it *fires*—sends an electrical signal down its axon, which can in turn help induce other neurons to fire. The human brain consists of about $10^{11}$ such neurons all acting in parallel (simultaneously), with synaptic connections between neurons numbering in the trillions. Even the most complex computers—conventional or neural—are thousands or millions of time times less complex than the human brain.

Artificial neural networks (ANNs) abstract a few simple ingredients from the huge complexity of the human brain. An ANN consists of a set of $N$ nodes $n_i$ ($0 < i < N$) corresponding to neurons, and a set of connection weights $w_{ij}$ ($0 < i < N, 0 < j < N$) representing the strength of the connection from **node** $j$ to node $i$. At any given time step each node $n_i$ has an output $o_i$. To determine its output **value** at the next time-step, node $n_i$ first computes a weighted sum of the outputs of all other nodes $n_j$ that are connected to it, where each output $o_j$ received by node $n_i$ is weighted by the connection weight $w_{ij}$. In other words, this weighted sum of outputs is the net input to node $n_i$. The resulting output of node $n_i$ is then some **function** $f$ of this input, where $f$ is an activation function characteristic of the node. There are many possible choices for the activation function, the simplest being a simple threshold function which yields 1 if the weighted sum input is positive and is 0 otherwise. Other possibilities are smoothed threshold functions or sigmoidal curves. This setup captures, though in a simplistic way, essential aspects of the workings of real neurons in the brain.

The next important ingredient in the **design** of an ANN is the topology or layout of connections between neurons (nodes) in the network. Usually most neurons in an ANN can be categorized into three classes: input neurons, output neurons, and hidden neurons. The inputs to input neurons are provided by an outside source, whereas the values of the output neurons represent the ANN's response to that source. For example, if the ANN is a pattern **classifier** then the input neurons would take on a set of values that would somehow encode the pattern to be classified, and the output would represent the ANN's answer to what **class** the pattern falls into. If the ANN were part of a control system then the input might be some stimulus (e.g., video image of approaching truck), while the output would encode some response or control **action** needed to influence the system as desired (e.g., get out of the way!). Hidden neurons, on the other hand have no connections to the outside world. They exist only as intermediate neurons on pathways from input to output neurons, and their output values may not have a clear interpretation. Sometimes in ANN pattern recognition systems the values of hidden neurons can denote the presence or absence of interesting features in the input pattern to be recognized.

In an abstract sense an ANN does nothing more than compute a mapping between its **input and output** neurons. Once the network topology and activation functions are chosen for the ANN, this mapping is fully determined solely by the connection weights $w_{ij}$. The knowledge implicit in a neural network's structure lies, then, in the connection weights and the topography of the net. A fundamental question is, how does one choose these weights to get the neural network to accomplish its desired goals, that is, its desired mapping between inputs and outputs?

The notion of modifying the weights in order to improve network performance is called training or learning. There are two major modes of learning: supervised and unsupervised. In supervised learning a teacher is present to provide a set of examples of good input-output mappings. The network uses these examples to learn what it should do in the more general case. Unsupervised learning is simpler, slower, and involves no teacher. The simplest example of unsupervised learning is Hebbian learning. The principle behind this approach is that if one neuron tends to persistently cause another neuron to fire, then this activity should be encouraged and the weight between these two neurons should be increased. There is biological evidence that Hebbian learning goes on in the human brain, that is, that the brain learns by reinforcing correlations between firing neurons. For pattern classifiers that are trained using Hebbian learning it is not always clear what exactly the outputs mean, but usually when a neural network is presented with a sequence of patterns that have some **redundancy** in them and its weights are modified in a Hebbian fashion, its outputs tend to categorize the input pattern. If the output neurons yield a set of distinct functions, for example, the neural network may be performing a clustering algorithm in which the network organizes the set of all input patterns into clusters of patterns that are more similar to each other than to those in other clusters. Hebbian learning can thus be a method of automatically identifying such regularities in input patterns. Another possible application of unsupervised learning is **data compression**, where the output represents a smaller, encoded version of the input that has done away with all redundancies.

In supervised learning one can make use of training **data**, namely a set of examples of inputs and what the corresponding outputs should be, in order to force the network to encode certain behaviors. For example in one military pattern recognition project, the examples consisted of pictures of tanks and pictures of trees. The desired outputs in such a case might be 1 for tanks and 0 for trees. In order to train the ANN to make this distinction one might use a simple "hill-climbing" procedure. We recall that the neural network's output is a function of both its weights and its inputs. One can create an error function that measures how poorly the network is doing simply by calculating for any training-set input the squared difference between the network's actual output and the desired output and summing this squared difference over all examples in the training set. This error function is then viewed as a function of the weights. The best possible network would minimize this function with respect to the weights. This minimization problem is then solved by gradient descent, namely by starting with a random set of weights, then moving in the weight space at every point in that direction that decreases the error function the most. This algorithm can be implemented quite efficiently in a feed-forward network, which consists of an input layer, a series of hidden layers, and finally an output layer, with connections only going forward from layer to layer in the direction of input to output. In this type of topology weights can be modified layer by layer, starting from the output layer, in such a way that the modifications are propagated backwards. This implementation of the gradient-descent training procedure is called backpropagation and was a breakthrough in the field of neural networks when it was discovered by P. Werbos in 1974. Mathematically, the whole procedure can be viewed as a least-squared-error fit of the neural network's input-to-output mapping function with respect to the weights. An interesting aspect of this approach is that it is not always clear what the neural network will learn from the training. For example, in the military application, it just so happened that all the pictures of tanks were taken on a sunny day whereas pictures of trees were taken on a cloudy day. When trained on this data set the neural network failed to perform adequately on new pictures of tanks and trees; it turned out that all the network had really learned to do was distinguish sunny weather from cloudy weather.

## NEWELL, ALLEN (1927-1992)
### American computer scientist

Allen Newell, an expert on how people think and a developer of complex **information processing** programs, was a pioneer in the field of **artificial intelligence**. From his development in the 1950s of Logic Theorist, one of the initial forays into artificial intelligence, to his presentation of the sophisticated problem-solving software system know as "SOAR" in the 1980s, Newell worked to link computer science and advances in understanding human cognition.

Newell was born in San Francisco on March 19, 1927, the son of Robert R. and Jeannette (LeValley) Newell. Robert Newell, a professor of radiology at Stanford Medical School, had a strong influence on his son. "[My father] was in many respects a complete man," Newell told Pamela McCorduck in an interview reported in *Machines Who Think*. "We used to go up and spend our summers on the High Sierra. He'd built a log cabin up in the mountains in the 1920s. And my father knew all about how to do things out in the woods—he could fish, pan for gold, the whole bit. At the same time, he was the complete intellectual.... My father knew literature, all the classics, and he also knew a lot of physics." Newell told McCorduck, however, that his own desire for scientific achievement had led him to focus his interests much more narrowly than had his father.

Newell served for two years on active duty in the Naval Reserve during World War II. In 1947, he married Noel Marie McKenna; they would have one son, **Paul Allen** Newell. After obtaining his B.S. in physics from Stanford University in 1949, Newell spent a year at Princeton University doing postgraduate work in mathematics, then went to work in 1950 as a research scientist for the RAND (Research and Development) Corporation in Santa Monica, California.

While at RAND, Newell worked with the Air Force to simulate an early warning monitoring station with radar screens and a crew. His need to simulate the crew's reactions led to his interest in determining how people think. Working together throughout the 1950s and into the 1960s, Newell and his colleagues Herbert A. Simon and Clifford Shaw were able to identify general reasoning techniques by observing the problem-solving behavior of human subjects. One of the best known of these techniques is means-ends analysis, a process that analyzes the gap between a current situation and a desired end and searches for the means to close that gap.

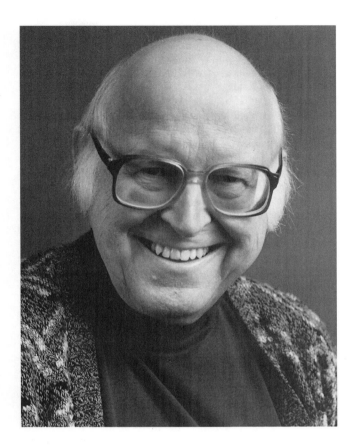

**Allen Newell**

In order to make use of computers in studying problem-solving behavior, Newell, Simon, and Shaw observed individuals as they worked through well-structured problems of logic. Subjects verbalized their reasoning as they worked through the problems. The three scientists were then able to **code** this reasoning in the form of a computer program. To make the program work, the scientists used a language called Information Processing Language (IPL) that they had developed previously for a computerized chess game. Their program, known as Logic Theorist, was not subject-matter specific; rather, it focused on the problem-solving process. Newell, Simon, and Shaw followed Logic Theorist with the development of General Problem Solver, a program that used means-end analysis to solve problems. Like Logic Theorist, General Problem Solver used the IPL language they had developed earlier.

During the summer of 1956, Newell and Simon were among a group of about a dozen scientists that gathered at Dartmouth College. The scientists came from a wide variety of fields, including mathematics, psychology, neurology, and electrical engineering. Though their backgrounds differed, they all had one thing in common: all were using computers in their research in an effort to simulate some aspect of human intelligence. With their Logic Theorist program, however, Newell and Simon were the only participants who could offer a working program in what would come to be known as "artificial intelligence." The Dartmouth Conference is generally viewed as the formal beginning of the field of artificial intelligence.

In 1957, Newell earned his Ph.D. in industrial administration from Carnegie Institute of Technology in Pittsburgh, Pennsylvania. In 1961 he left his position at RAND to join the faculty of Carnegie-Mellon University (formerly the Carnegie Institute of Technology), where he helped develop the School of Computer Science.

During the 1980s, Newell, along with his former students John Laird and Paul Rosenbloom, developed a more sophisticated software system that solved problems in a manner similar to the human mind. This system, called SOAR (State, **Operator**, and Result), was a general problem-solving program that learned from experience in that it was able to remember how it solved problems and to make use of that knowledge in subsequent problem-solving. SOAR, like humans, used working **memory** and long-term memory to solve problems. If SOAR was working toward a desired goal, it used working memory to keep track of the current situation, or "state," in the problem-solving process compared with the desired goal or "result." In order to make the decisions necessary to achieve a goal, people use information they have accumulated through experience. People use long-term memory to **access** information; SOAR also used long-term memory, programmed as a series of IF/THEN statements.

While the use of IF/THEN statements in a computer program wasn't a new idea, the way in which SOAR processed those statements was new. In the past, only one IF/THEN statement could **control** a computer program at any given time. If conflicting statements could apply to a problem, the problem-solving process would break down. SOAR, on the other hand, was designed to look at all of the programmed IF/THEN statements at once. After looking at all of the statements, SOAR would weigh them as suggestions, then decide which move, or "operator," would best advance it towards the desired result. If there were no IF/THEN statements stored in memory that applied specifically to the problem at hand, SOAR would use any available information that seemed potentially useful to try to resolve the problem. Whenever it solved one of these unexpected problems, SOAR would remember how it solved the problem, adding this information to its long-term memory. Like the human mind, SOAR was thus able both to generate original responses to new problems and to "learn" from its experiences.

In the late 1980s, Newell began an active campaign to promote the use of SOAR as the basis for a new effort to develop a unified theory of cognition. Whereas current research in artificial intelligence tended to focus on narrow and isolated aspects of cognition, Newell hoped SOAR would help cognitive psychologists devise broad theories of human cognition and advance towards an integrated understanding of all aspects of human thought.

Newell received the National Medal of Science from President George Bush just a month before his death from cancer on July 19, 1992. His work had already brought him a number of other honors, including the Harry Goode Memorial Award, which he received from the American Federation of

Information Processing Societies in 1971, and the A. M. Turing Award, presented jointly to Newell and Simon by the Association for Computing Machinery in 1975. Newell was founding president of the American Association for Artificial Intelligence and also served as head of the Cognitive Science Society. Along with his colleague **Herbert Simon** and computer scientists **Marvin Minsky** and John Mc Carthy, he is considered one of the fathers of artificial intelligence.

# NIELSEN, JAKOB (1957-    )
## *Danish web consultant*

Jakob Nielsen is a well-known Web **design** consultant and is considered to be the world's leading expert on Web usability. He calls himself a guru of Web usability in his promotional material and is regarded as one of the Web's most influential people.

Jakob Nielsen was born in Copenhagen, Denmark, in 1957 where he went to school. In 1973, at the age of 16, Nielsen owned his first computer. This computer was a Gier and it worked on a punch tape system and had four kilobytes of **memory**. This experience helped to reinforce the young Nielsen's interest in computers. When he went to university (Aarhus University, Denmark) it was to study computer science. Here he was awarded a B.Sc. and subsequently an M.Sc., both in computer science. He then moved to the Technical University of Denmark at Copenhagen where he studied for a Ph.D. in user interface design and computer science. In 1985 Nielsen worked at **IBM** as a visiting scientist—at their User Interface Institute at the T.J. Watson Research Center—where he studied users and how they interacted with various interfaces. This had been a recurring theme in Nielsen's studies since 1983 when he became interested in human interactions with computers. From 1986 to 1990 Nielsen worked as an assistant professor at the Technical University of Denmark, where he taught user interface design and other topics. He was awarded his Ph.D. in 1988. In 1990 Nielsen took up a position at Bell Communications Research (Bellcore) where he worked with **hypertext**, online systems, and telephony interfaces. He left Bell in 1994 to work for Sun Microsystems where, as a distinguished engineer, he worked on defining the next generation of **object** orientated interfaces. Nielsen was employed by SunSoft, which is the software arm of Sun Microsystems. His other work at Sun included designing the user interface for their next generation of online documentation and enhancing the maturity level of current usability engineering methodology. Nielsen also co-designed the Sun Microsystems internal **intranet** system—SunWeb—in 1994.

Since leaving Sun in 1998 Nielsen has worked as a consultant for businesses seeking a Web presence—he advises on human factors and their relationship with Web browsing. He carries this out through his position as a user advocate and principal of the Nielsen Norman Group, which he co-founded with Donald A. Norman (former vice president of research at **Apple** Computers) in 1998. As part of his consultancy business

Nielsen advocates a user-centered Web design approach, believes that a Web page should ease rather than hinder a user's interactions with the Web site, and discourages the use of unnecessary technology and gimmicks. As a logical extension of his core work Nielsen also regards himself as an e-commerce consultant—Nielsen makes Web sites easier to use, and the easier they are to use the more items they can sell. At a daily consulting rate of $20,000, only Web sites that sell a lot can afford to use him, although much useful information is available in his numerous publications. For those wondering whether Nielsen advocates total Web site designs (not just a tacking on of something that seems like a good idea at the time), he also preaches the avoidance of any technology that is less than two years old—he feels it needs this time to penetrate to the majority of users. Nielsen is also an advocate of the abolition of the Mac and **Windows** graphic user interfaces. The Nielsen Norman Group is based in California where Nielsen lives with his wife. For relaxation Nielsen indulges in his loves of science fiction, travel, and good food. In 2000 Nielsen was inducted into the Scandinavian Interactive Media Hall of Fame.

As of 2001 Nielsen holds nearly 60 U.S. patents, the majority concerned with ways to make the **Internet** easier to use. Nielsen founded the "discount usability engineering" movement to aid in rapid improvements of the user interface system, one output of which is heuristic evaluation. He writes several Web columns on the Internet, one of which regularly gets over nine million views per year. Nielsen also serves on the editorial boards of several noted technology journals including *The New Review of Hypermedia and Multimedia*, *Personal Technologies*, and a number of Association of Computer Machinery (ACM) publications. With nine popular books on Web usability to his name, including *Designing Web Usability: The Practice of Simplicity* and *Multimedia and Hypertext: The Internet and Beyond*, and over 130 separate publications in scientific journals, it is no exaggeration to say that Jakob Nielsen has had, and will continue to have, a profound affect on how we use and Interact with the Web.

*See also* Graphical user interface; Internet; Intranet; World Wide Web

# NODE

The term node has several meanings in computer science.

In the context of computer networks, a node is a location where processing of information occurs. A computer can be a node, as can a **printer**. Every node in a network has its own unique address, which is referred to as a **Data** Link Control (DLC address) or a Media Access Control (MAC) address.

In the context of the **tree** structure arrangement of hierarchical data, a node is a data point that is linked to other nodes of data. Each node represents a collection of information. The information in each node is retained in **memory** at a single location.

Trees are often constructed from a single node known as a root, or from a set of nodes—a forest of trees. The system of linked nodes generates a multilevel data network.

Nodes can also exist in **graphs**. Each data point in the graph represents a node. Similar to a tree, the data points in a graph are linked to other nodes.

*See also* Data; Tree

# NON-COMPUTABLE PROBLEMS

Computational **Complexity Theory** is the discipline of recognising solvable problems that are intractable in the sense that no efficient algorithm exists to solve them. Problems that computational processes are intended to solve can be divided into "decision problems," "functions," and "relations." It is possible to reformulate both decision problems and relations functions, which means that effectively **computability** can be reduced to solving **function** problems.

A function is considered "computable" if there exists an algorithm for calculating the function that for any given legal combination of input values produces the correct result within a finite time.

In 1936, English mathematician **Alan Turing** published a paper called "On computable numbers, with an application to the Entscheidungsproblem [decision problem]." Turing proposed a simple abstract computing machine, based on a notional mathematician with a pencil, an eraser, and a **stack** of paper. Turing stated that any function is computable if it is computable by one of these machines. He then investigated if there were any mathematical problems that such a machine would be unable to solve. These abstract machines are now called "Turing machines."

Turing's 1936 paper concluded that there is a set of well-defined problems that cannot be solved by any computational procedure. If these problems are formulated as functions, they are called "non-computable functions," and if they are formulated as predicates, which are problems that are presented as **assertions** with the only possible answers being "true" or "false," they are called "undecidable."

Turing said, effectively, that a function is non-computable if there exists no **Turing machine** that can compute it. Turing's assertion has been proven correct: there are in fact problems that cannot be answered by algorithmic means no matter for how long the algorithm is allowed to run.

Turing proved his thesis by demonstrating that the "halting problem" is undecidable. The **halting problem** is formally stated as: "Given a Turing machine M and an initial tape T, does M halt when started on tape T?" A more useful way of stating this for computer scientists is: "Given a program P and a **string** x, does P halt on input x?" Informally the question is: "Is it possible to predict whether a given computation will terminate?"

And in his paper, Turing proved that the answer is unequivocally "no." For computer programmers and computer scientists this means that it is impossible to write a computer program that can tell if any arbitrary program will ever terminate.

As many problems can be recast in terms of the halting problem, this means that computer scientists know there are a lot of problems that computers can never solve. Nevertheless, there are compromises in the form of partial solutions and heuristic **algorithms** that usually, but not always work and nearly always give the right answer.

## NON-TERMINAL

A non-terminal element operates in context-free grammar. This form of grammar is necessary to enable the translation of source **code** to **object** code in a meaningful way, so as to preserve all the information. Specifically, a non-terminal element, which can also be called a **variable**, is capable of being broken down into other elements, called tokens or **terminal** elements. A terminal element cannot be broken down into other symbols. Terminal elements of source code are typically passed on to the parser, which is a program that dissects the source code in order that the code can be translated into object code.

A second meaning for non-terminal relates to query languages such as the Abundantia Verborum, languages that are hierarchical, or tree-like, in their structure. The hierarchical approach to problem solving in this scheme is also referred to as a semantic **tree**. In this structure, the non-terminal nodes types the AND, OR, and NOT function to combine so-called atomic queries—that address a single issue and are not qualifiable—into more complex queries. The non-terminal **node** types are Boolean operators; that is, they produce an outcome that is true or false. The larger queries, which are qualifiable due to the AND, OR, and NOT nodes, enable a more all-encompassing query to be constructed.

*See also* Context-free grammar; Parser and parsing; Query language

## NORRIS, WILLIAM C. (1911-    )

*American electronic engineer and computer scientist*

William C. Norris is a computer pioneer who was instrumental in producing some of the early **supercomputers**. Norris is also a firm believer in education and technology to help the underprivileged and has set up many organizations aimed at addressing social issues.

William C. Norris was born in 1911 in Nebraska on his family's farm. His early education was carried out in a one-roomed schoolhouse until he moved to high school. At high school Norris developed a passion for physics and electronics. This interest took him to the University of Nebraska, and he graduated with a B.S. in electrical engineering in 1932. His academic career was halted by the death of his father—he had to return to run the family farm. During the Depression Norris was able to take a part-time position at the local Agricultural Adjustment Administration office, where he helped farmers hit by the hard times. These conditions affected Norris deeply and contributed to his life-long interest in helping others. In 1934

Norris was able to use his degree when he started to work for the Westinghouse Electric Company as a sales engineer. When the United States entered World War II Norris immediately joined the U.S. Naval Reserve. Norris was put to work intercepting and decoding enemy radio transmissions in order to locate submarines. To aid them in this endeavor Norris and his colleagues were attempting to make better and faster calculators that could crack the encryption codes. At the end of the war Norris and others set up a company called Engineering Research Associates (ERA) in St Paul, Minnesota, where they constructed electronic **hardware**. By 1947 Norris changed the **design** of the systems they were making so that they were general-purpose rather than single-task machines. The Navy received the first of these machines in 1950. In 1951 ERA was so attractive it was bought by the Remington-Rand Corporation for the **UNIVAC** project. In 1955 Remington-Rand was bought by the Sperry Corporation and Norris was made vice president and general manager for computing—this allowed more thorough coordination of the design and manufacturing work. In 1957, due to lack of support, Norris left to found the **Control Data Corporation (CDC)**. One of his employees, **Seymour Cray**, had a number of ideas that appealed to Norris, and he allowed Cray to build a team to pursue them. In 1960 the CDC 1604, then the world's most powerful computer, was delivered to the Navy. This heralded bitter rivalries between CDC and **IBM**, eventually leading Norris to file an antitrust suit in 1968 when the CDC 7600 was released. IBM could not match this supercomputer—and they dared not pretend they could—and the CDC became one of the most successful supercomputers ever. In 1973 the lawsuit was settled in favor of CDC. Norris continued to build CDC and eventually the company started producing software for its own machines.

During the 1960s Norris was able to help others—he gave machines to the University of Illinois for educational purposes and erected manufacturing plants in socially deprived areas. Between 1975 and 1977 Norris set up several database systems to allow searches for technological information; this was intended to help businesses make the most of modern developments. The system was subsequently extended to allow searches for employees with specific skills. Subsequent projects included setting up support systems for small businesses, advisory systems, training schemes, umbrella organizations for inner-city revitalization, rural equivalents, and prison training schemes. By 1980, at age 69, Norris became CEO at CDC and turned general management over to Robert Price and Norbert Berg. This change freed him to devote time to persuading other industrialists to follow in his social footsteps. Norris promoted social issues and continued manufacturing electronics. By 1985 CDC was in a decline and suffering closures—many thought Norris' unusual business practices and ideas were to blame. In 1986 Norris retired from CDC, allowing himself more time to help developing countries with education programs and run social schemes in the United States. In 1988 Norris formed the William C. Norris Institute to enhance education with computers, a task which took him into the 21st century.

*See also* Supercomputers; UNIVAC

# NOYCE, ROBERT (1927-1990)

*American physicist and inventor*

Robert Noyce coinvented the **integrated circuit**, an electronic component which is considered to be among the twentieth century's most significant technological developments. The laptop computer, the ignition control in a modern automobile, the "brain" of a VCR that allows for its **programming**, and thousands of other computing devices all depend for their **operation** on the integrated circuit. Noyce was not only a brilliant inventor, credited with more than a dozen patents for **semiconductor** devices and processes, but a forceful businessman who founded the Fairchild Semiconductor Corporation and the **Intel** Corporation and who, at the time of his death, was president and CEO of Sematech.

Robert Norton Noyce was born December 12, 1927, in Burlington, Iowa, the third of four boys in the family. His parents were Ralph Noyce, a minister who worked for the Iowa Conference of Congregational Churches, and Harriet Norton Noyce. Growing up in a two-story church-owned house in Grinnell, a small town in central Iowa, Noyce was gifted in many areas, excelling in sports, music, and acting as well as academic work. He exhibited a talent for math and science while in high school and took the Grinnell college freshman physics course in his senior year. Noyce went on to receive his baccalaureate degree in physics from Grinnell, graduating Phi Beta Kappa in 1949. It was at Grinnell that he was introduced to the **transistor** (an electronic device that allows a small current to control a larger one in another location) by his mentor Grant Gale, head of Grinnell's physics department. Noyce was excited by the invention, seeing it as freeing electronics from the constraints of the bulky and inefficient vacuum tube. After he received his Ph.D. in physics from the Massachusetts Institute of Technology in 1954, Noyce—who had no interest in pure research—started working for Philco in Philadelphia, Pennsylvania, where the company was making semiconductors (materials whose conductivity of an electrical current puts them midway between conductors and insulators).

After three years, Noyce became convinced Philco did not have as much interest in transistors as he did. By chance in 1956 he was asked by **William Shockley**, Nobel laureate and coinventor of the transistor, to come work for him in California. Excited by the opportunity to develop state-of-the-art transistor technology, Noyce moved to Palo Alto, which is located in an area that came to be known as Silicon Valley (named for the silicon compounds used in the manufacture of computer chips). But Noyce was no happier with Shockley than he had been with Philco; both Shockley's management style and the direction of his work—which ignored transistors—were disappointing. In 1957 Noyce left with seven other Shockley engineers to form a new company, financed by Fairchild Camera and Instrument, to be called Fairchild Semiconductor. At age twenty-nine, Noyce was chosen as the new corporation's leader.

The first important development during the early years at Fairchild was the 1958 invention, by Jean Hoerni (an ex-Shockley scientist), of a process to protect the elements on a

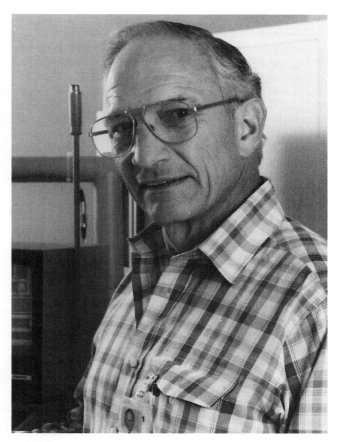

**Robert Noyce**

transistor from contaminants during manufacturing. This was called the planar process, and involved laying down a layer of silicon oxide over the transistor's elements. In 1959, after prodding from one of his patent attorneys to find more applications for the planar process, Noyce took the next step of putting several electronic components, such as resistors and transistors, on the same chip and layering them over with silicon oxide. Combining components in this fashion eliminated the need to wire individual transistors to each other and made possible tremendous reductions in the size of circuit components with a corresponding increase in the speed of their operation. The integrated circuit, or microchip as it became commonly known, had been born. More than one person, however, was working toward this invention at the same time. **Jack Kilby** of **Texas Instruments** had devised an integrated circuit the year before, but it had no commercial application. Nevertheless, both Kilby and Noyce are considered coinventors of the integrated circuit. In 1959 Noyce applied for a semiconductor integrated circuit patent using his process, which was awarded in 1961.

Both technological advances and competition in the new microchip industry increased rapidly. The number of transistors that could be put on a microchip grew from ten in 1964 to one thousand in 1969 to thirty-two thousand in 1975. (By

1993 up to 3.1 million transistors could be put on a 2.15-inch-square **microprocessor** chip.) The number of manufacturers eventually grew from two (Fairchild and Shockley) to dozens. During the 1960s Noyce's company was the leading producer of microchips, and by 1968 he was a millionaire. However, Noyce still felt constricted at Fairchild; he wanted more control and so—along with Gordon Moore (also a former Shockley employee)—he formed Intel in Santa Clara, California. Intel went to work making semiconductor **memory**, or **data storage**. Subsequently, Ted Hoff, an Intel scientist, invented the microprocessor and propelled Intel into the forefront of the industry. By 1982 Intel could claim to have pioneered three-quarters of the previous decade's advances in microtechnology.

Noyce's management style could be called "roll up your sleeves." He shunned fancy corporate cars, offices, and furnishings in favor of a less-structured, relaxed working environment in which everyone contributed and no one benefited from lavish perquisites. Becoming chairman of the board of Intel in 1974, he left the work of daily operations behind him, founding and later becoming chairman of the Semiconductor Industry Association. In 1980 Noyce was honored with the National Medal of Science and in 1983, the same year that Intel's sales reached one billion dollars, he was made a member of the National Inventor's Hall of Fame. He was dubbed the Mayor of Silicon Valley during the 1980s, not only for his scientific contributions but also for his role as a spokesperson for the industry. Noyce spent much of his later career working to improve the international competitiveness of American industry. Early on he recognized the strengths of foreign competitors in the electronics market and the corresponding weaknesses of domestic companies. In 1988 Noyce took charge of Sematech, a consortium of semiconductor manufacturers working together and with the United States government to increase U.S. competitiveness in the world marketplace.

Noyce was married twice. His first marriage to Elizabeth Bottomley ended in divorce (which he attributed to his intense involvement in his work); the couple had four children together. In 1975 he married Ann Bowers, who was then Intel's personnel director. Noyce enjoyed reading Hemingway, flying his own airplane, hang gliding, and scuba diving. He believed that microelectronics would continue to advance in complexity and sophistication well beyond its current state, and that the question would finally lead to what use society would make of the technology. Noyce died on June 3, 1990, of a sudden heart attack.

# NP-COMPLETE

The term NP-Complete refers to a complexity class of decision problems. A "complexity class" is simply a collection of computational problems that all have the same bounds on time and space, and a "decision problem" is a problem for which the answer is "yes" or "no." This is equivalent to a computational **function** that has a range comprising just two discrete values, such as 0 and 1.

NP-Complete is a subset of NP or "Non-deterministic Polynomial time," which is a set of problems for which answers can be checked by an algorithm whose run time is polynomial in the size of the input. The **complexity of algorithms** is generally measured using "Big-O" notation, which is a theoretical measure of how quickly an algorithm will run in terms of the time or computer **memory** required given the size of the problem itself. The number of items in the problem typically defines the size of the problem.

An algorithm that runs in "polynomial time" has an average running time that is no more than a polynomial function of the size of the input. Polynomial **algorithms** have running times formally expressed as:

$$t(n) = O(n^k)$$

where "k" is a constant. Problems that have a solution that runs in polynomial time are in the class P. Problems that are in NP have algorithms that run in exponential or factorial time.

However, the fact that a purported solution can be quickly verified or refuted does not require or imply that an answer can be found swiftly. An example of this is the factoring problem. Factoring a number involves finding which other numbers when multiplied together form the original. The factors of ten, for instance are {1,10} and {2,5} because both 1x10 and 2x5 equal 10. Even the best known factoring algorithms have exponential running times, where as the checking algorithm, plain ordinary multiplication, has polynomial running time. Factoring is in the class of NP-Complete problems.

NP-Complete problems are NP problems that have the added qualification that no other NP problem is more than a polynomial factor harder. Informally, a problem is NP-Complete if answers can be verified quickly, and a fast algorithm to solve this problem can be used to solve all other NP problems quickly. There is also much argument among mathematicians as to whether NP=NP-Complete; that is, does the subset NP-Complete comprise all NP problems. If it does and anyone ever finds a polynomial algorithm to solve an NP problem, then it will effectively prove that NP=P.

Although it may seem a bit esoteric and possibly irrelevant, this is extremely important to computer scientists, even if they don't know it. This is because the algorithms that provide most of the world's computer security are based on NP-Complete problems. Therefore, if NP is ever shown to be equal to P, it means that there exist fast algorithms to break this security. And all that remains then is to find them

# NUMERICAL LIMITS

Numerical limits are part of **object-oriented programming** languages such as **C** and **Unix**. Numerical limits define the sizes and characteristics for numerical **data**.

There are two types of numerical data, integral (whole number) or floating-point (including decimals). The criteria for these numerical types are specified in the limits.h and float.h header files. The files contain specifications for the length, in bits, of numerical types. These specifications include signed and unsigned numbers; that is "+" and "−" values.

Some examples of numerical limits in the limits.h and float.h header files are given below:

- Each character of type "char" is represented in 8 bits.
- Each character of type "wchar_t" is represented in 32 bits.
- Open VMS system values for the "int", "signed int", and "unsigned long int" types are the same.
- Open VMS system values for 'unsigned int' and 'unsigned long int' types are the same.

The limits.h header file also defines many resources that are used in various applications, in terms of the minimum and maximum limits that pertain to their content. The following are examples of numerical limits within the limits.h file:

- maximum length of a login name
- maximum number of files that one process can have open at any one time
- size in bytes of a page
- maximum number of significant bytes in a password
- maximum number of links to a single file

The adoption and use of numerical limits is one of the steps that has standardized the writing and performance of **programming** languages such as C and Unix.

*See also* C; Unix

# O

## OBJECT

An object is "anything with a boundary." This can be extended in computer science to be "anything with a boundary that represents a uniquely identifiable entity; unit; or item, real or abstract; that represents some element in the problem domain."

What this means is that an object represents a "thing" or an idea in the real world. Although programmers talk of objects in non-object orientated languages like **C**, this is a bit misleading because in Object Orientated **Design** objects typically have both **data**, sometimes called "state" or "identity," and they have behavior, things that they can do, either on their own data or data given to them by other objects. The behaviour of objects is defined by the methods it supports. A **method** is basically a **function**, or self-contained block of **code** that performs some **action** and returns a **value**. The semantic difference between methods and functions is merely that a method always belongs to an object, whereas a function can be "global" in the sense that it belongs to the program as a whole or to a code module. **C++** supports conventional functions and methods, but in **Java**, every function is a method.

Typically, an object will be of a certain type or "class." If an object is a thing, then a **class** is a description or blueprint for what that thing looks like, what is in it, and what it can do. Special methods declared for the class construct instances of the class - objects - from the raw bits and bytes of computer **memory**. These special methods are called "constructors," for obvious reasons.

It is this distinction that draws the line between genuine objects as instance of classes and loose collections of data like C and C++ structures and **Pascal** records. Objects are living, breathing entities in a program that can do things of their own accord in response to stimuli; structures and records are dull, lifeless things that are manipulated by external functions and procedures. Objects do; structures are done to.

Objects are strongly tied up with the idea of **encapsulation**, which, in computer science is broadly the practice of bringing together elements to produce a new entity. In the more specific case of object-orientated **programming**, encapsulation implies data hiding and the **abstraction** of behaviour from implementation: if the internal data and workings of the object are encapsulated, then objects have to interact through a set of clearly defined interfaces. These interfaces are represented by the class methods or member functions. By invoking a method on an object, the programmer sends the object a **message** that tells it to do something or send back some data. Object-oriented programs are defined as sequences of interactions between objects. Objects maintain their own state and identity and have clearly defined responsibilities in terms of the behavioural contract they make with other objects in the program.

Object-orientated languages like C++ and Java rely heavily on encapsulation to create classes and objects as instances of those classes. Both of these languages contain keywords like "public," "private" and "protected" that force the **compiler** to enforce rigidly the encapsulation of both data and functionality; encapsulating data in this way is called "data hiding."

Classes have "visibility modifiers" that the compiler enforces to say what external entities can see in an object. A "public" item, whether it is a member **variable** or method, is in C++ and Java is visible to anyone and everyone. A "protected" item in C++ is visible only to objects of that specific type or objects of classes derived from that type; in Java a "protected" member is visible only to objects of its own class, objects of subclasses, or within classes in the same package, where a package is a logical collection of classes that have some (possibly) arbitrary common attributes. In both C++ and Java, "private" member items are visible only to the class they are defined in. These visibility modifiers enforce encapsulation and facilitate data hiding.

Data hiding is where the details of an object or function are invisible to the outside world. The data can be accessed via methods that are privileged to see them, the "accessor methods," but they are not immediately visible in themselves. If the data are to be changed in some way, say because of external events, the program sends a message to the object by invoking a method, or function owned by the object, and that makes the change to the encapsulated data. Functions that change the internal state of an object are called "mutators." Methods can themselves be encapsulated, which means they may be accessible only from within the object itself. Methods that are encapsulated are typically those that would reveal details of the object's implementation to the outside world.

It is also possible to use a class as the basis for deriving another class. This is called "subclassing" and the **derived class** is called a "subclass" or a "derived class." The class the subclass is based on is called the "base class," or the "superclass," or, in some circles, the "parent class." The **base class** is related to the subclass in a "kind of" relationship where the subclass is a "kind of" the base class. For example, a PlymouthFury might be derived from a Car class, and it is clear that a Plymouth Fury is a "kind of" car, and not the other way around.

Properly designed and implemented object oriented programs tend to be less complex and hence more easily written and maintained than their non-object orientated counterparts. Specifying program behaviour in terms of object interfaces and hiding the details of implementation from the users of the objects means that the effects of code changes is minimised, thus reinforcing the principle of less complex and hence more reliable code.

# OBJECT-BASED DEVELOPMENT

Object-based development is the **programming** thrust that determines **object-oriented programming** languages such as **Java**. As its name implies, object-based development focuses on an **object**. An object is defined as something that has the capacity to store information, manipulate its own information, and carry out some task when requested by another object to do so.

In object-based development, blocks of a program **code**, the objects, can be recognized and used based on their names, without the necessity of understanding how exactly the object works. Also, this development technique encourages code to be re-used, as long as it works in the context to which it is applied. In other words, an object of constant structure can participate in different functions.

Objects can be data-storing entities, such as a line of text or a database. Also, objects can be components of a software system, such as a user interface. The latter are known as processing objects. The power of object-based development is that such objects can be programmed to one another relatively easily to create functions. An object can be called for different functions at the same time. Thus, parallel programming, where programs can be running at the same time, is possible.

Object-based development also enables personalized responses to be tailored to user requests "on-the-fly". In fact, multi-user requests can be accommodated. This aspect of object-based development is attractive to businesses, who can **design** their web pages, particularly the catalog section, to be flexible to user order requests.

Another use of object-based development based software has been in the area of architectural design. Software programs, such as AutoCAD, have made it possible to obtain three-dimensional like, interactive, "walk-through" images of the modeled program (such as a house). The increased realism that can be achieved enhances the creative energies of the architect.

Object-based development, while currently popular, has been a programming tool since the early 1980s. Then, the dBASE **data** management system was created. The dBASE format for storing data has since become the de facto standard, and is supported by most database management and spreadsheet systems. Examples of software based on the object-based development approach have included WebObjects (NeXT), Oracle8 (Oracle), ActiveX and Visual Basic (**Microsoft**), and Java Sun Microsystems).

*See also* Object-oriented programming

# OBJECT-ORIENTED PROGRAMMING

Software **applications** tend to be very large, expensive, and complex to create. There also tend to be changing requirements encountered during their creation (due to changes in marketplace conditions, new offerings from competitors, and additional demands from customers) and new problems that were not foreseen in the **design** stage. Even after software has been created, the "debugging" of **code** tends to take more time than the original coding itself, and need for revisions and improvements may also be expected. Typical software systems are so large and complex that no single individual has a holistic view that takes in every detail. To build such systems, it is essential that there be some way to break down the task into manageable parts that allow there to be a cooperative effort by a team of developers. Practices and tools that work well for a solo programmer often do not work well for large teams.

The goal of software development is to produce software that is useful, delivered in a timely fashion, reliable, maintainable, reusable, user-friendly, and efficient. The practice of software development requires two parts: the model, which is an **abstraction** of some problem or aspect of a part of the real world, and the algorithm, which describes a well-defined process for solving the problem that has been encapsulated in the model.

In the early days of software development, the main focus was on development of **algorithms** that were efficient, and the models received less attention. Early software development efforts chose to focus on computation, and were based on control flow. Later on, other efforts tried the opposite perspective, choosing to focus primarily on the **data** flow, while computation was relegated to a secondary place. All these efforts were handicapped by the lack of a viable model.

As developers realized that more attention needed to be given to the model, different efforts began to be made that took on a balanced perspective of the data and computation aspects, and also helped provide techniques to optimize software development. The most important achievement in this regard was the development of the object-oriented model, which consists of objects, each having data and making computations. Exceedingly large software systems which have complex interactions among their constituent parts can be described in the object-oriented model, based on the structure of the objects, classes, and the relationships between them.

Objects and classes are fundamental to object-oriented **programming**. Each has a representation in the model, and an interpretation in describing something in the real world. An **object** represents something in the real world that has a distinct nature and function. In the model, the object is entity with a unique identity, a distinct set of possible states, and well-defined behaviors. A **class** is a set of objects that are similar in nature; all objects belonging to a certain class are called instances of that class. In the model, a class is characteristic of the states and behaviors that all its instances share.

The state of an object is given by its fields (also called attributes), and their existing values. The behavior of an object is defined by its methods, which may read or change the state. The state and behavior of an object are together called its features.

A class serves as a **template** to allow creation of instances, i.e., objects (the terms "object' and "instance' are often taken to be interchangeable in this context). Instead of defining individual objects, programmers define the feature of the classes of these objects

The principle of **modularity** is central to object-oriented programming. Modularity is simply the style of analysis which requires that any complex system be broken down into a set of cohesive but independent modules which can each be analyzed and developed independently of the others. In order to achieve modularity, two aims are sought after: abstraction and **encapsulation**.

Abstraction is simply the characterization of the essential functional aspects of a module, leaving out any details that don't have to be known to users of the module. A precise description, commonly called the contractual interface for the module, has to be generated. A contractual interface is merely a means of capturing the behavior of the module while leaving its inner workings implicit and undescribed. For instance, such an interface for a telephone would simply say that if one lifts the handset of a functional phone instrument and dials a number on the keypad, a call will take place, which can be terminated by hanging up. This is the only level of detail that common phone users need to know, and inner workings of phone instruments or the phone system do not have to be part of their understanding.

Encapsulation is a closely related principle that says that the implementation of a module should be kept completely distinct from its contractual interface, and should be hidden from clients of the module. In our example, we could say that the workings of the phone should be kept separate from the instructions for using the phone. This principle is also called **information hiding**, and is important in helping software developers from becoming overloaded with irrelevant detail.

In object-oriented development, the practice is to split the task of building a complex software system into many modules that interact in a specific way. The design of these modules says nothing about how the modules are to be implemented, but just specifies how they are to behave. Each developer (or team of developers) works on a certain module that has to perform exactly as per the requirements specified of its contractual interface. Developers know nothing of others' modules save what is stated in their contractual interfaces; this information suffices even if they have to use other people's modules in their own work. The inner workings of each module are thus known only to the people working on that particular module. Finally, when all the modules are ready, it is possible to put them together to obtain the final system.

Other important concepts in object-oriented programming that may be mentioned include:

- Inheritance—This defines a relationship among classes, so that a class may "inherit' from another class, in which case it is called a subclass and uses the implementation of its superclass.

- Association—This represents general binary relationships among classes, such as relationships among classes titled "Employee' and "Pay'.

- Sequence Diagrams—These are used to show object interaction by showing the time order of method invocations.

- Unified Modeling Language(UML)—This is a graphical notation for describing object-oriented systems, developed jointly by the "three amigos" of software engineering: Grady Booch, Ivar Jacobsen, and James Rumbaugh.

*See also* Applications; Software; Verification

# OCL (OBJECT CONSTRAINT LANGUAGE)

The **Object** Constraint Language (OCL) is not a **programming** language; it is a formal **expression** language used to express constraints and conditions on object-oriented models. The evaluation of an OCL expression always delivers a **value**. It does not change anything in the system model. As an expression language OCL is also neutral about implementation decisions. This means that the usage of OCL is not tied to any specific platform or programming language.

The OCL is a subset of the **UML (Unified Modeling Language)**, which is mainly used for documentation. Based on the Syntropy object-oriented analysis and **design** method, the OCL was originally developed within **IBM** as a language for business modeling. One of the guidelines of the OCL was that an easy-to-use standard was needed to document constraints. It was incorporated into the UML 1.1 specification in 1997 and is considered the standard notation for constraints on object-oriented systems.

A constraint is a restriction or set of rules that governs an object. The context of the constraint is the **attribute**, method, **class**, or other object that is being constrained. These constraints may be noted within the UML diagram or documented separately.

Constraints and conditions provide an additional level of detail not provided by standard UML diagrams. This additional detail helps formalize system requirements. Without the OCL, additional information to clarify models could be written in natural language. However, as natural language varies between modelers, it is prone to ambiguity and misinterpretation. The OCL provides a textual description of constraints on attributes, methods, and classes within object-oriented models. As a formal language for constraint notation, the OCL reduces ambiguity and increases **precision** of the system descriptions.

Specific types of constraints include invariants, preconditions, postconditions, and guards. An invariant is a condition that must be met at all times by all instances of the class or type. A precondition is a condition that must be true at the moment of execution of an **operation**. A postcondition is a condition that must be true at the moment after execution of an operation. A guard is a constraint that must be true before a state **transition** occurs.

OCL is a typed language, meaning that part of the definition of the OCL includes value types. The basic predefined types are Boolean, integer, **string**, and real. Additionally there are more advanced types, including collection types, meta types, and user-defined types. Various operations can be performed on each value types as part of evaluating an OCL expression. For example, operations for the integer and real types include mathematical functions.

*See also* Constraint; UML (Unified Modeling Language)

# OCTAL NOTATION

Octal notation is a method of representing octal (base 8) numbers using the eight numerals 0–7. Octal notation uses *positional notation* and *powers of 8* to express to express numbers in a manner similar to that of the familiar decimal system. In the decimal number system, the *positions* of the digits 0–9 determine their values. Consider the decimal number 375; the digits 5, 7, and 3 are understood to be multiplied by increasing powers of 10. Explicitly, $375_{10} = (3 \times 10^2) + (7 \times 10^1) + (5 \times 10^0) = 300 + 70 + 5$. Octal 567 is the same number as decimal 375: $567_8 = (5 \times 8^2) + (6 \times 8^1) + (7 \times 8^0) = 5 \times 64 + 6 \times 8 + 7 \times 1 = 320 + 48 + 7 = 375$.

Each octal digit is the equivalent **value** of three binary digits. For example, octal 235 can be converted to a binary number by transforming each of its three digits to a binary triple. The leading 2 is 010 in binary notation, that is, $(0 \times 2^2) + (1 \times 2^1) + (0 \times 2^0) = 0 + 2 + 0 = 2$; the 3 is 011 by $(0 \times 2^2) + (1 \times 2^1) + (1 \times 2^0) = 0 + 2 + 1 = 3$; and the 5, similarly, is equivalent to binary101. Thus octal 235 equals binary 010010101. **Hexadecimal notation** is more commonly used in contemporary computer work than octal notation.

*See also* Binary number system; Hexadecimal notation

# OCTET

An octet is a storage unit that is always composed of a sequence of exactly eight bits. A *bit* (a contraction of *bi*nary dig*it*) is the smallest piece of information (or unit of **data**) used by a computer. A **bit** possesses a binary **value**, either zero (0) or one (1). By general definition of the binary numbering system, an octet ranges in mathematical value from zero (00000000) to 255 (11111111) because 2 to the power of 8 ($2^8$) produces 256 different combinations (or possibilities). Nearly all computers are designed to store data and execute instructions in multiples (or strings) of bits. A *byte* (from *bi*nary *te*rm) is formed from strings of bits, and is a unit of data that can represent information such as single characters, numerals, etc. An octet is a **byte** of eight bits. The smallest value of an octet is "00000000" (zero), and the largest value is "11111111" (255 in decimal notation). Although bytes are most often eight-bit strings, they are not required to be of that particular size. For instance, a byte may be a sequence of 9 bits on some 36-bit computers. Octet, on the other hand, is always designated as an eight-bit unit. For instance, four eight-bit octets form a 32-bit *word*.

The term octet is normally used in networking, in preference to the term byte, because, as said earlier, some systems use the term byte for units that are not eight bits long. Historically, the octet was applied to eight bits when some computer systems began to represent a byte as a size other than eight bits. Today bytes usually range in size from four to ten bits, but octets always consist of eight bits. The term octet is derived from the Latin word "octo" that means "eight."

*See also* Bit; Boolean algebra; Byte

# ON-LINE EDUCATION

On-line education refers to the use of the **Internet** for the delivery of long distance education. Electronic education allows people to study without having to be physically on a campus.

As educational costs have increased over the past several decades, the ability to train and educate students without the necessity to house them and provide classroom facilities has become a greater incentive to establish on-line education services. Aside from issues such as expense and access, Internet based education offers collaborative benefits that are not easily attained in a traditional classroom setting. For example, real-time chat room software permits students from diverse locations and cultures to communicate. This almost instantaneous interchange can be incorporated into a course, to provide both a practical learning experience (such as language study) and an exposure to another culture. Hundreds of institutions dedicated to on-line learning have been established. An example is The Virtual On-line University. As well, traditional academic institutions are incorporating on-line education into their educational delivery repertoire. Examples of the latter include Diversity University (DU MOO), the University of Missouri (Zoo MOO), and the University of Phoenix (Pueblo MOO).

The interactive and multimedia nature of on-line education attempts to provide an enhanced educational experience. The Internet can take the best of the classroom experience— plus the use of textbooks, videos, CD-ROMs, and the presence of a dedicated leader to facilitate a fruitful and stimulating interchange of opinions—and extend its reach to the world. The Internet facilitates outside communication and collaboration, and provides access to diverse external sources (and so diverse points of view) of information. On-line education is student-centered, rather than being teacher-centered, as is often the case in the traditional classroom setting.

Typically, a student enrolled in an on-line education program will pay tuition for a set length of study. Lessons, assignments or chat room interactions occur at designated Internet addresses. Some institutions also provide on-site facilities for students. Others conduct all business electronically and remotely. Some institutions provide their students with computers and the necessary electronic connections during their period of study. This ensures that everyone has the same software and **hardware** to provide equal access. Other institutions require the student to provide the needed technologies.

The delivery of education, and interaction between teacher, students, and other students occur asynchronously or synchronously with on-line education. Asynchronous delivery is typically done using technologies like **e-mail**, multimedia Web pages and **USENET**. Synchronous, or real-time, instruction can be done using MOOs or MUDs and **IRC** (**Internet Relay Chat**, a system that enables multiple users to engage in real-time communications). In contrast to some public chat rooms, the educational chat rooms are in general well organized and strictly moderated.

To date, on-line education has been largely the domain of those who have the financial means to invest in the computer technology, and is most prevalent in the United States. Other areas of the world, particularly developing regions, stand to benefit enormously from on-line education. While these opportunities have not yet been realized, efforts are underway to assess the feasibility of limited on-line education in several developing countries.

*See also* Computer-Assisted Instruction; IRC (Internet Relay Chat); MOOs and MUDs

## OPEN-SOURCE SOFTWARE

Open-source software is software in which the source **code**, or the code that permits the software to function, the executable program, and the software license are available free of charge to the general public. Typically, because the license is supplied, open-source software can be freely modified and redistributed by public users as well as the software originators. Examples of open-source software are **UNIX**, **Perl**, **Linux** and FreeBSD (Berkeley Source Distribution).

In contrast too open-source software, proprietary software must be purchased, and is not subject to modification and redistribution by users. The license for a proprietary software ensures that only the company or original software developer has the legal right to see and modify the software's source code.

Open-source software is often an evolving process. Users identify shortcomings, modify, and redistribute the software, primarily on the **Internet**. Proprietary software, on the other hand, is developed with the aim of identifying and correcting shortcomings prior to its issue. The process of eliminating problems and improving the software happens at a much quicker rate in an open-source environment, as the information is shared throughout the open-source community, and does not pass through the developmental hierarchies of a company.

In the 1960's, when computers were far less easy to operate, users tended to be software developers, and software tended to be supplied with the source code included. Beginning in the 1970's, however, a proprietary atmosphere began to dominate, and source codes became the domain of the commercial software developer.

A cadre of software developers, such as **Richard Stallman**, continued to advocate for an open software development community. Under Stallman's direction, the Free Software Foundation was created in 1983. Stallman was also the driving force behind The GNU Project (GNU is a recursive acronym for "GNU's not Unix"). The GNU Project was one of the first initiatives to challenge the emerging trend of proprietary software.

Another major impetus for open-source software came in 1991, when **Linus Torvalds** publicly released his first version of an open-source version of the Unix operating system (now called Linux). Finally, the Open-Source Initiative (OSI) was formed in1998, stimulated by the announced public distribution of the formerly proprietary Netscape Internet **browser**.

Open-source software is closely allied to open communications **protocols**, which allows many different types of computer equipment to run the software and communicate with one another. Although the development of open-source software is communal and virtually unrestricted, often there is some sort of central authority that collects and combines the changes made by users. For example, Linus Tovalds still fulfills this role for Linux software.

A number of companies, such as Red Hat and Corel, supply functional add-ons to open-source software. Despite its freely available nature, such opportunities have made open-source software economically viable. Open-source software such as Linux can be packaged into a convenient and easy to install package, with **programming** support available. This tact has proven so attractive that consumers will often pay to acquire the convenience surrounding a free piece of software.

*See also* Architecture; Linux

## OPEN ARCHITECTURE

A computer's *architecture* can refer to the components of the computer (i.e., its **hardware**); to the software that is executed by the computer; or both. An *open architecture* is an architecture whose specifications are in the public domain. These specifications can be approved and sanctioned by regulatory bodies, or they can be developed commercially (i.e., by a company, corporation, etc.) and then published for general distribution. The public access to a particular **design** allows any designer or manufacturer to produce products to those specifications. Open architecture is a great boon to the consumer because, in general, more manufacturers mean more competition, which leads to lower prices and greater choice in the choice of a particular product.

Open architecture has found its greatest application in the **personal computer** (PC) industry. When microcomputers were introduced in the early 1970s, most manufacturers produced computers whose software and hardware were mostly incompatible with their competitor's computers and **peripherals** (peripherals are auxiliary components attached to, and directed by, a computer). A sort of de-facto open architecture for microcomputers developed in the mid-1970s after the introduction of the **Intel** 8080 processor (in 1974), the Zilog Z80 **microprocessor** (in 1976), and the **CP/M operating system** (in 1972). Different manufacturers began making microcomputers that often had major components in common with one another. In 1981 **International Business Machines** (**IBM**) Corporation introduced the IBM PC, and for several years IBM became the dominant personal computer manufacturer. IBM management chose an open architecture for their PC, which meant that any company could produce similar computers or computer components in direct competition with them. Companies large and small produced an entire range of "IBM-compatible" products, such as motherboards, expansion boards (including sound cards, video cards, modems, etc.), disk drives, monitors, printers, keyboards, mice, and other components used to produce or enhance a computer. Not long after the introduction of the IBM PC, dozens of "IBM clones"—PCs similar in appearance and performance to the IBM PC—were being produced by a variety of manufacturers. Because of open architecture, parts from one "IBM-compatible" PC would work in any other. Inter-compatibility between IBM-compatible computer brands did not stop with hardware: different operating systems could be installed in the same PC, such as MS **DOS** (**Microsoft** Disk Operating System), IBM DOS, Norton DOS, and versions of the **Unix** operating system.

One might rightly wonder if IBM made an error in choosing an open architecture instead of a proprietary (or closed) architecture. After all, a proprietary architecture means that a company can control the numbers and types of clones (i.e., architecturally-similar products) that other manufacturers can make and sell. While open architecture was undoubtedly of great benefit to the consumer, it nonetheless meant unbridled competition from IBM's competitors. However, companies that went the "proprietary route" when it came to personal computers and related equipment found themselves with a niche market at best. Two such companies were **Apple** Computer and its line of Macintosh personal computers, and Commodore Business Machines with its Amiga personal computer line. (Interestingly, the Amiga and Macintosh computer lines used the same type of microprocessor, namely the Motorola 680x0 series of microprocessors; however, because the Amiga and Macintosh used different (proprietary) operating systems, the two computer systems were incompatible with one another, as well as with the dominant IBM-compatible PCs.) Apple, Commodore, and several other "closed architecture" computer makers eventually accounted for only a small minority of the total personal computer market, and most went out of business (e.g., Commodore).

There are many important open architecture hardware **protocols** that are followed by equipment manufacturers. A couple of examples are Ethernet, which is a Local Area Network (**LAN**) protocol used for **data** communication; and Small Computer System Interface (SCSI), a high-speed parallel interface for connecting PCs to peripherals, to other computers, and to LANs, and defined by **ANSI** (**American National Standards Institute**).

As stated previously, open architecture can apply to software as well as hardware. On the one hand, a software vendor can choose to produce a proprietary product; an important example is the Microsoft operating system software, which dominated the PC market starting in the 1980s and continuing throughout the 1990s. However, open architecture software is increasingly being employed by a variety of computer users. In recent times so-called *component software* has garnered attention from a variety of software buyers. The goal of component software is to allow individual software programs, or components, to be interlaced and run with other components as part of a larger application. Standards such as "OLE" and "OpenDoc" have been published to ensure that different software components, even if purchased from different vendors, will run seamlessly with other software components that follow the same standard. Just as a consumer can purchase a **modem, mouse**, keyboard, etc. from any of a number of PC manufacturers with the confidence that they will function properly on his open-architecture PC, so too can a consumer purchase various software components and have the confidence that they will operate together properly.

*See also* Apple; Architecture (hardware); Architecture (software); International Business Machines (IBM); Protocols

# OPERATING SYSTEMS (THEORY)

An operating system is, simply speaking, the software that operates the **hardware** on behalf of the user(s). It is that software which makes the hardware usable to the humans. Among the important functions of an operating system are that it:

- defines the user interface;
- allows sharing of resources among users, while preserving privacy;
- schedules resources;
- facilitates I/O functions;
- provides routines for **applications** to use **peripherals**;

One of the oldest views of the operating system is to consider it as a resource manager that doles out rations of scarce resources to competing processes. Although many resources, such as **memory** sizes and **CPU** speeds, have grown exponentially since this view was first developed, it remains current because the demands on these resources have more than kept pace with their growth.

It is common practice to speak of an operating system kernel, which is the smallest core of the operating system. Typically, the kernel of an operating system does not include fancy features for memory management, plug-and-play for peripherals, or so on. It really is the most basic amount of software required to define the immediate working environment of the CPU. Further features of an operating system are acquired by adding artifacts to the kernel. The kernel itself takes only a miniscule amount of resources compared with the add-ons; for example, the original **Unix** kernel from about 1970 could run on a machine with just 4 KB of RAM! More advanced kernels exist today, of course, but it is still typical for kernels, especially for Unix variants, to be quite small in their demands.

An operating system must exercise control in order to allocate input-output **access** to contending requests. This is typically done using a method called I/O interlock, wherein it is ensured that mutual exclusion is maintained among various processes that need to use an I/O resource. Operating systems also have to allocate I/O to processes keeping in mind the limited bandwidth of the channels used; the **code** used for this can be as complex as the code that is used to schedule CPU time among processes.

The secondary memory is the most important resource that is overseen by the operating system, at least from the perspective of the user. In the traditional shell environment such as on Unix or DOS, the operating system is seen as little more than a command-line interface that is used to launch programs and execute specific commands for printing or accessing secondary storage. In a more advanced sense, the function of an operating system is the allocation of space on disk drives and such media among competing files. Since the physical structure of memory units on disk drives is very different from that in main memory, the **algorithms** used tend to be very different. Another problem in this context is that read and write times to secondary memory tend to be much slower (by several orders of magnitude) that those to main memory. For example, a hard drive can be read from or written to at about 10 MB a second, while a floppy drive can be read or written at just about 30 KB a second. These numbers compare very poorly with the speeds for main memory, which are of the order of 1 GB a second.

Security and reliability are two other functions provided by operating systems. Security is the feature of the operating system that makes it impervious to malicious attack. On small systems, security is not bothered with to any great degree, and anyone with physical access to the computer has access to all its workings. On larger systems which nowadays are constantly connected to the Internet and are used by many users, security is a serious issue. Reliability is similarly the feature of the system to be protected against accidental damage. In general, though the relationship between security and reliability is often debated and the terminology is not fixed, it is accepted that whatever a malicious user can do on purpose, a careless user can do by accident. Since there are more careless people in the world than malicious ones, the risks from carelessness

and malice are both equally significant, even granting that a catastrophe is more likely to result from malice than from carelessness.

Sharing of resources and information is a challenging issue in operating systems. Sharing is trivial when there is no protection or privacy, and protection is trivial when there is no sharing. In practice, a balance must be struck between these incompatible extremes. Operating systems use features such as access control lists (ACLs) that provide safe sharing, whether on disk or on main memory. Every user has some regions of memory that are private, and some that are shared with others, but not with all. On Unix and other operating systems, the 'superuser', also called root, has access to all user resources. A process has the priority associated with the user who created it; thus a user process cannot mess up the system because the system files are not write-accessible to users. A user process cannot interfere with another user process, but the root can kill any user process, a useful feature for system administration in case of a careless or malicious user.

***See also*** Applications; Central processing unit; Hardware; Mutual exclusion; Operating systems types

# OPERATING SYSTEM (TYPES)

An operating system is a specialized software package that operates something on behalf of someone. The **object** it operates is clearly the computer itself—the operating system operates the computer. The entity it operates on behalf of is a human user, or a community of human users. Functions of an operating system include providing a uniform interface across differing **hardware**, providing abstractions such as files, **windows**, clocks, etc., that humans prefer, and providing mechanisms for enforcing security policies. Every general-purpose computer requires some type of operating system that tells the computer how to operate and how to utilize software **applications** and hardware that are installed. This frees the user from the tedium of having to worry about the minute details of file reads, writes, scheduling of process threads, and the like.

Operating systems can be classified in various ways, depending for example on whether they allow only a single user or more than one user at a time; or depending on whether they allow one **thread** or many; or depending on whether they allow multiprocessing (the use of more than one processor) or **multitasking** (the running of more than one task on a processor).

The earliest operating systems were rudimentary and only allowed for text input. This kind of operating system is now said to be text-based, or to have a text shell. Examples of this kind include MS-DOS (the precursor to **Microsoft** Windows), and **Unix**, which was first released in 1969 from Bell Labs. It became obvious, after a time, that a mere text interface was not adequate, and efforts began to be made to develop a **Graphical User Interface** (**GUI**) which would allow for **graphics**, icons, drag-and-drop, and so on. The first successful GUI for personal computing devices was the system used on the **Apple** Macintosh, which grew partly from research done at Xerox's Palo Alto Research Center. GUI interfaces were also developed for Unix (X-Windows), and for MS-DOS (Windows 3.1). The Macintosh system was a real operating system with a GUI interface, rather than being a GUI interface running on top of a text shell. However, early X-Windows and Microsoft Windows 3.1 were both GUIs running on text shells, where **mouse** movements and operations on icons, etc., would be translated into text **commands** and executed by the underlying shell operating system that was hidden from the user. Later, with the coming of Windows 95, this shortcoming was fixed.

Early operating systems did not allow for multiprocessing or multitasking, but nearly every one of recent date does, for obvious reasons, as computers and software have continued to increase in complexity and user demands continue to increase likewise.

In the 1960s, there was a project called MULTICS, which aimed to create a "computing utility." This was back in the day when computers were owned soley by corporate owners and were housed in separate large rooms and were expensive to purchase and operate. Few envisioned that it would ever be possible for individuals and families to purchase and use their own computers, and the idea of MULTICS was to form a computing utility that would enable people to purchase computing services, much as they might purchase electricity, water, or heating gas for home use. After several years and much money spent, MULTICS failed and the sponsors withdrew. A few of the researchers who had worked on MULTICS decided to work on a more modest effort that nonetheless preserved some of the worthwhile aims of the failed grand effort, and Unix was born. (The name "Unix" is merely a pun on MULTICS, and does not stand for anything.)

Unix is, and has always been, a multi-user operating system. In fact, it is partly for this reason that Unix continues to be a popular choice for college and university computing networks with hundreds or thousands of users. By contrast, many other operating systems, including Windows 95 and the MacOS versions, are meant for a single user at a time. Microsoft has its own Windows variant called Windows NT which is supposed to be a competitor to Unix in the multi-user area, but it has not succeeded in dislodging Unix as the predominant choice. One of the important concerns in a multi-user system is obviously security—it is important for multiple independent users to be able to use the system in a meaningful way without being able to intrude upon each other, and without having to fear loss of privacy. On Unix, this is done by providing a method for file security, and a way to create individual accounts that are protected by passwords. These features are missing on most operating systems for personal computers, but **Linux**, a freeware Unix variant developed in the 1990s, has them.

Unix is also preferred for scientific computing where robustness, i.e., the lack of operating system crashes, is an issue. In personal computing where the applications used might be just for personal use or amusement, such as for electronic mail, **Internet** access, **word processing**, and the like, robustness is not as serious an issue since most people don't use a computer continuously for very many hours at once.

However, anyone who has used Windows or other PC operating system has experienced crash failures (in fact, Windows 98, the successor to Windows 95, crashed during its demonstration to the world by **Bill Gates**, chairman of Microsoft). In technical terms, it would be said that the "mean time between failures" of an OS such as Windows is rather small perhaps just a day or less. This may just cause a little irritation to a lay user, but is a very serious matter in scientific computing, where for instance a **simulation** or a long-running program may have to be run continuously for weeks or months. Such a program obviously has no chance of being run to completion on Windows 95, and needs to be on Unix, which is a stable operating system that can go years without crashing.

On the other hand, it is true that Unix is a less user-friendly operating system than modern Windows and other releases. This is largely because it was originally conceived in a different era, and still retains some of the distinctive features of its humble beginnings. Lay users who have little training or interest in a deep study of computers and are thus keen to use them with minimal training, often find it easier to use Windows, which is thus the predominant operating system in the personal computing market.

*See also* Applications; Hardware; Software

# OPERATION

An operation is an **action** or instruction that is performed on or by an **object**. A program consists of set of operations. A program can be compared to a process. A process consists of many steps. Let's use a laundry example. Mary is going to program her robot maid, Robbie to do the laundry. She would have to create operations or steps for Robbie.

These steps are:

- Open the laundry hamper.
- Place clothes in laundry basket
- Taking the clothes to the washing machine.
- Open the lid.
- Place clothes in the washing machine.
- Adding the laundry detergent to the washing machine.
- Closing the lid.
- Set the dial to the appropriate cycle.
- Turn the washing machine on.
- Remove clothes after washing cycle.
- Place clothes in dryer.
- Remove clothes after drying cycle.
- Fold clothes.
- Place clothes in closet.

In this example all of then operations are being performed on the clothes (the object). However, Robbie, the washing machine and dryer, which are also objects are performing actions.

Other names used for operations are **method**, **message**, functions or events. Examples of operations are jump, load, store, open and close. Functions are different because they do not change the object's state. Examples of functions would be add, subtract, multiply, divide and count.

*See also* Action; Function; Message; Method; Object-oriented programming; Object; Variable

# OPERATOR

In the context of computer science the term operator has two different meanings. The first, and relatively trivial meaning, refers to the person whose responsibility it is to ensure that a computer or computer system is running properly. Tasks associated with the operator's position include preparing storage media and making backup copies of files.

The second meaning of operator is a symbol representative of a specific **action**. Many operators exist in the myriad of available programs and **programming** languages. For example, a plus sign is an operator, which represents addition. The other basic mathematical operators are the subtraction sign and the multiplication and division signs. For example, in the **expression** $5 + x$, the + is the operator. The 5 and the $x$, the objects that are being manipulated, are called operands.

Mathematical operators are relatively simple in their actions. Other operators allow the manipulation of numbers and text in more complicated ways. A Boolean operator is one example. Boolean operators allow for a TRUE or FALSE determination of information. One type of Boolean operator is known as an OR operator. It can also be called an inclusive OR. This operator returns a **value** of TRUE if either or both of its operands is TRUE. Another type of operator, the exclusive OR, returns a TRUE value only when one of the operands is TRUE. If both operands have the same value, an exclusive OR does not return a TRUE value. Put another way, an inclusive OR can be "this, that, or both", while an exclusive OR means "this or that, but not both."

Another operator is called a relational operator. This type of operator allows one value to be compared to another. Hence, this operator is also known as a comparison operator. An example of a relational operator is the expression $x > 10$ ($x$ is greater than 10). This expression will have a value of TRUE if the **variable** $x$ is greater than 10. If $x$ is less than 10, the expression will be FALSE.

Operators are essential for the construction of expressions, and so are a vital component of programs and programming languages.

*See also* Computer language; Programming languages, types

# OPTICAL CHARACTER RECOGNITION (OCR)

Although computers have made tremendous strides over the last few decades in terms of their **hardware**, especially the processor speeds and sophistication, some things have not

changed nearly as much. The most important thing that is still the same now as twenty years ago is the constraint of the **WIMP** interface used in **human-computer interaction**. WIMP is an acronym denoting window, **icon**, menu, and pointing device, and is used to describe the sort of interface that has been common for quite some time now. A human user typically interacts with the computer through a screen, a keyboard, and a **mouse**. The screen is the most important, or often the only, means for the computer to communicate its output. The screen typically consists of one or more **windows**, each of which may be used for separate files or other environments; the screen also shows icons for various objects, and menus from which the human user may choose options. The human uses a pointing device (typically a mouse) to choose icons, menus, or windows.

The WIMP menu certainly has its good points, but the fact that it has changed so little over such a long period of time, while other aspects of computing have become a lot better, is certainly troublesome. It is undoubtedly true in many contexts that if only one were able to take regular notes in longhand and have a computer interpret them, one would find life so much easier than having to use a keyboard and format text. Although handwriting recognition systems that can serve limited purposes do exist, such systems are not widespread at present for several reasons: human handwriting is very varied, and it is difficult to create a system that will handle the diverse range of possible styles; a single individual's handwriting can also change with age, illness, injury, moods, and the like. Lastly, certain specialized subjects like medicine or mathematics have their own very involved styles and notations that are sufficiently different from common language that the computer would almost need to be a physician or a mathematician to understand the writings of professionals in those subject.

Although full-scale computer comprehension of human writing is impossible at this time, systems that can, to a limited extent, translate writing into computer files do exist. Such systems are also useful in the context of reading off printed text (either computer printouts where the software and files are unavailable, or printed text not generated by a computer) and creating a computer file that can be edited or used for other purposes. The common feature of such systems is optical character recognition (OCR). The term stands for general character recognition by a machine, including the transformation of anything humanly readable to a machine manipulable representation. As noted, character recognition may involve either recognition of machine-printed characters, or of human handwriting. At this time, there have been significant advances only in the field of machine-printed character recognition, and most software that is available in the market is geared toward that function. For this reason, some pople like to use a separate term ICR, or intelligent character recognition, for systems that explicitly are also meant to recognize handwritten characters. ICR is very much an active research area at this time, and a conclusion does not seem to be imminent. Most working models are based on the constraints of using only limited vocabularies and "clean" handwriting. Some may also involve "training" the software with large, known samples of a person's writing before it can recognize characters produced by her hand.

With OCR software, converting printed text on paper into electronic files can be almost as easy as feeding the pages to a scanner. An OCR package takes an image (actually, a bitmap graphic) from the scanner, analyzes it, and tries to translate it into a text file. Each character is recognized by its shape, and a corresponding character is generated and placed in the file. It is possible to edit and format this file using a **word processing** package, just as you would any other text file. This is a significant advantage in cases where large quantities of printed text have to be converted into electronic **data**. However, though the characters are recognized in a way that allows most words and even sentences to appear correctly in the generated file, a significant limitation is that most OCR software today does not correctly recognize footnotes, page numbers, marginal comments, headers, italicized text, and the like. Strange fonts, drop caps, and the like may produce incorrect results also. Contemporary OCR also does not format the text into a replica that of the original document; all that it achieves is the creation of a computer file containing all the text on the original page. A fair amount of post-processing by hand is thus called for in order to achieve a version that is actually close or identical to that of the original text.

The success of an OCR effort depends on several factors, among them the quality of the original text and the quality of the scanned image—if the original page is smudged, or if the image is not scanned to an adequate resolution, the results may not be satisfactory. Having a higher quality image is often useful, but may not necessarily be so.

Another major research area in OCR is the recognition of text in foreign languages that do not use the Roman script (common to modern English, French, German, etc.). Certain scripts that have characters based on phonetic syllables or pictographs are especially difficult even with printed text, and much work needs to be done in their respect. Such work also has the potential of one day allowing for automatic machine translation of printed text in foreign languages into English.

*See also* Computer architecture; Graphics

# OPTICAL COMPUTING

For over forty years—ever since the invention of the laser in 1960—researchers have sought avidly for a way to compute with light. Why have they done so, and why are computers still electronic, not optical?

In conventional, electronic computing, the elementary carrier of information is the electron. Most computational actions—transmitting signals from one chip to another, storing a **bit** of information in **random access memory**, changing the state of a **memory** circuit, and so on—involve the shifting of electrons in space by the application of electric fields. An electron is charged, so an electric field causes it to accelerate; nearby atoms tend to impede this motion.

In optical computing, the elementary carrier of information is the photon. Depending on the physical context, light can behave either as very small particles (photons) or as a self-propelled wave comprised of an electric field and a magnetic field working in tandem. Both aspects of light, wave and particle, are essential to optical computing techniques.

The lure of optical computing depends on the difference between photons and electrons. The same property of electrons that makes them so useful—their charge, which is responsive to electric and magnetic fields—is also their most inconvenient property, for several reasons. First, like charges repel. It is therefore not practical for two electronic devices, say two chips on a printed circuit board, to communicate by simply shooting electrons back and forth; an electron beam, squirted into free space, quickly spreads as the electrons push each other apart. As a result, flows of electrons must be confined by conductive wires. When these wires are closely spaced, as the conductive paths on a printed circuit board are, the electrons in one wire may be affected by those in the others: electric and magnetic fields generated by the electrons in one wire tend to influence those flowing in others, a form of interference called "crosstalk." If crosstalk is too strong, errors will result. Therefore there are physical limits on how closely spaced the conducting paths by which signals are transmitted inside chips and between them can be. Second, any stray electromagnetic fields that may occur inside the system ("noise") can corrupt electronic signals. Third, in order to send an electrical signal down a wire the wire must be charged, which requires time and energy. The ability to store charge is called *capacitance*; all electronic transmission lines exhibit capacitance. The longer the line, the greater its capacitance and the poorer its performance.

Photons, in contrast, interact weakly with each other. Any number of beams of light can pass through the same volume of space without affecting each other. (Something like this property can be observed by throwing two stones into still water a few yards apart and watching the ripples from each splash pass through each other without being changed.) Photons also pass freely through many common materials, and so can be beamed directly from one device to another through the air (in the technique called "free-space optics") or steered through glass (in the form of optical fibers) over long distances. At the distances relevant to computer engineering, both kinds of transmission are essentially lossless.

The *speed* of light, surprisingly, turns out not to be one of its great advantages. "Electronic signals in wires and optical signals in fibers have roughly identical upper speed limits," states H. John Caulfield, director of the Center for Applied Optics at the University of Alabama at Huntsville. This caveat does not apply to free-space optics, for the speed of light in air is significantly greater than the speed of light in glass, but free-space optics suffer from the disadvantage of being able to transmit information only in straight lines.

Photons are no cure-all. While electrons require confinement in a material medium, they *can* be confined, and thus accumulated as charges in (say) a small volume of crystalline silicon. The crystal medium even does double duty by supplying positive charges in the form of atomic nuclei, which are just as important to device **design** as electrons. Photons, on the other hand, cannot be hoarded; when they cease to move at the speed of light they cease to exist. Optical logic devices must therefore shift from one state to another ("0" to "1" or vice versa) by altering their optical properties, a trick that turns out to be somewhat more difficult than that of confining charges. A variety of bistable optical logic devices have been built in laboratories, but all have fallen far short of their electronic rivals in terms of size, speed, and cost.

A natural division of labor suggests itself: sticky electrons for logic, lightfooted photons for messengers. This is, in fact, the trend of most current research. *Optically interconnected computers* exploit photons for communication and electrons for computation. Supercomputer designers are already using ribbons of 10 or more optical fibers to link cabinet-sized sub-units, each fiber carrying up to 2 billion bits per second. Future designs may utilize integrated optical waveguides to interconnect individual transistors; free-space optics to interconnect chips and modules; and optical fibers for interconnecting modules, shelves, and other larger units.

In addition to communications there are two major roles for optical computing. The first is storage. Optical **data storage** devices (CD-ROMs, etc.) are already standard in desktop computers, while **holographic storage** in solid metallic crystals or on the surface of disks is a strong candidate technology for the next generation of cheap, archival **data** storage.

The second role is image processing. Images are not only a common source of large quantities of data, they are *inherently* optical and thus amenable to optical computing techniques. Consider, for example, the common task of obtaining the two-dimensional Fourier transform of an image. To create a numerical representation of the image and to crunch those numbers in order to determine the Fourier transform of the original is very computation-intensive, requiring at approximately $N \log_2 N$ calculations for an image containing N pixels. In contrast, a raw optical image can be Fourier transformed in a single step and regardless of its size by passing it through an appropriately designed lens. A computer that needs to obtain many image transforms—a targeting system or video indexer, for example—may therefore benefit by handing off this task to a dedicated optical unit. Indeed, this form of analog computing has proved useful in military and other applications since the 1960s, and remains commercially viable.

Several decades ago, optical computing enthusiasts believed that electronic computing was about to run up against performance limits set by the laws of physics, and that optical computing would pick up where electronics left off. However, the physical limits on electronic computing turned out to be less confining than was thought and the optical revolution has never occurred. All-optical computers have been built, but only as one-of-a-kind demonstrations, not as working tools. However, optical-computing technologies have proved their worth as helper devices that accelerate electronic computing and cheapen data storage, and computer designs will probable incorporate them more and more intimately as time goes on.

# OPTIMIZATION PROBLEMS

Some important problems in the computing sciences or in engineering require that a certain performance metric or func-

tion be optimized while under conflicting constraints. An practical example of an optimization problem would be the **design** of an automobile engine to deliver maximum possible fuel efficiency while staying within size, weight, and cost constraints. Optimization problems are analyzed and solved by stripping away the inessential details of the problem domain to obtain an abstract specification of the problem. This requires a clear understanding of just what features of the problem domain are relevant and what are not—that is part of the challenge of meaningful abstraction.

The oldest and best-known technique used in optimization is linear **programming**. The word "programming" is in some respects an unfortunate choice here, since it does not connote programming in the sense of creating software programs or **applications**. It really means "planning," and the "linear" means that the system of equations to be solved for is linear in a mathematical sense.

A Linear Program (LP) is a problem that can be expressed as follows (the so-called Standard Form):

minimize cx

subject to Ax = b

$x \geq 0$

—where x is the vector of variables to be solved for, A is a matrix of known coefficients, and c and b are vectors of known coefficients. The expression "cx" is called the objective function, and the equations "Ax=b" are called the constraints. All these entities must have consistent dimensions, of course, and you can add "transpose" symbols to taste. The matrix A is generally not square, hence you don't solve an LP by just inverting A. Usually A has more columns than rows, and Ax=b is therefore quite likely to be under-determined, leaving great latitude in the choice of x with which to minimize cx.

Although all LPs can be converted to the Standard Form if required, in most cases it is not essential to make such an effort, and a solution may be attempted while the problem specification is in a different form.

Two major types of solutions are in widespread use today—each approach creates a series of trial solutions of increasing accuracy, until a candidate achieves conditions necessary for it to satisfy the optimality requirements. The simplex method, introduced in the 1940s by George B. Dantzig (then working for the U.S. Air Force, later a professor at Stanford) tries to fix enough of the variables at their bounds to reduce the constraints Ax = b to a square system, which can be solved for unique values of the remaining variables. Barrier or interior-point methods, made possible by Narendra Karmarkar in 1984, visit points within the interior of the feasible region.

A more difficult type of optimization problem is the one involved in Nonlinear Programming (NLP). A non-linear objective function is sought to be maximized while subject to constraints. Nonlinear programming is, in general, extremely complicated, and methods used typically do not apply except to special cases. One such well-studied special case in NLP is Quadratic Programming (QP), where the objective function is quadratic (has at most degree two).

The reasons why NLP is so much harder than LP may be briefly given as follows.

In geometry, linearity refers to Euclidean objects: lines, planes, (flat) three-dimensional space, etc.—these appear the same no matter how we examine them. On the other hand, a nonlinear object, such as a sphere for example, looks different on different scales—when looked at closely enough it looks like a plane, and from a far enough distance it looks like a point.

In elementary algebra, we define linearity in terms of functions that have the property $f(x+y) = f(x)+f(y)$ and $f(ax) = af(x)$. Nonlinear is defined as the negation of linear. This means that the result f may be out of proportion to the input x or y. The result may be more than linear, as when a diode begins to pass current when it reaches a threshold; or less than linear, as when finite resources limit Malthusian population growth. Thus the fundamental simplifying tools of linear analysis are no longer available: for example, for a linear system, if we have two zeros, $f(x) = 0$ and $f(y) = 0$, then we automatically have a third zero $f(x+y) = 0$ (in fact there are infinitely many zeros as well, since linearity implies that $f(ax+by) = 0$ for any a and b). This is called the principle of superposition—it gives many solutions from a few. For nonlinear systems, each solution must be achieved separately.

One computational tool particularly relevant to optimization in nonlinear problem domains is **Genetic Algorithms** (GA). A genetic algorithm has the advantage that it can often search the solution space much more thoroughly and efficiently than other methods—a well-created GA is often also able to find the right global optimum rather than local optima that other methods might converge on.

*See also* Abstraction; Computer science and mathematics; Genetic algorithms

# OUTPUT FILE STREAM

Output is anything, meaningful or otherwise, that comes out of a computer. In a number of **programming** languages, including **C++** and **Java**, a type of output is termed the output **file stream**. The output file **stream** refers to the stream of information that flows between two objects. In this case, one of the objects is information entered via a keyboard or from a file (the sender) and the other **object** is a file to which the information is to be routed (the receiver).

The file stream is in the form of bytes, such as **ASCII** characters. The output file stream can be used to place the output from a program directly into a file. When a file is opened, an object is created and a stream is associated with that object. The object that is opened is referred to as an ofstream object. The ofstream can write the **data** to an output file.

Generally, the output file stream ofstream is written as

&lt;stream **variable** name&gt;

&lt;stream variable name&gt;.open(&lt;file name&gt;)

The variable name can be any **identifier** that is recognizable in the programming language; out_file, for example.

The output file stream is closed when a particular task is completed (when the data has been placed in a file). To continue the above example, if the variable name selected was out_file, then the command to close would be:

out_file.close()

*See also* Data flow

# OVERFLOW

Overflow is the general condition that occurs when input or output **data** within a computer requires more bits than have been reserved in **hardware** or software in order to store that data. In a digital computer overflow is synonymous with *arithmetic overflow*, the overflow condition that occurs with mathematical calculations. An example of overflow can be something as simple as the **central processing unit** (**CPU**) not accommodating a negative number. Suppose a financial spreadsheet program calculates a checking account balance. Normally all numbers will be in the form of currency (such as $15.46), which are positive. But if the balance should fall below zero, and the program does not allow negative numbers that normally require an additional **bit** (the smallest piece of information used by the computer) to accommodate the negative sign (e.g., -$3.45) or bracket (e.g., ($3.45)), then an overflow condition occurs. Other examples of overflow include (1) a floating-point **operation** whose result is too large for the number of bits allowed to be stored in a particular location (that is, if the operation only allows 3 units to the right of the decimal point, then numbers containing fractional (e.g., 3/7) or irrational (e.g., 1.3645...) parts may lie outside the allowed range when being operated upon); and (2) a **string** that exceeds the bounds of the **array** allocated for it (that is, if a person's name is allowed a maximum of 10 characters, then a name with over 10 characters will cause an overflow in storage capacity).

When an overflow occurs an overflow error often results. An *overflow error* is an error that occurs when the computer attempts to handle data that is too large to be contained in the **data structure** that a program provides for it. If during the execution of a program the CPU locates data outside a predetermined range, it will experience an overflow error. Overflow errors, sometimes called overflow conditions, often result when mathematical calculations produce erroneous results. For instance the addition of the 3-bit binary sequence 111 (7 in decimal notation) and the 3-bit binary sequence 001 (1 in decimal notation) will produce an overflow error if the maximum number of places for digits is three, because the result is 1000 (8 in decimal notation), a 4-bit binary sequence.

Overflow can be contrasted with *underflow*, which occurs when a mathematical calculation produces a result too near to zero to be represented by the range of binary digits available to the computer for holding that **value** in the specified **precision**.

*See also* Bit

# OVERLOADING

"Overloading" in computer **programming** is a form of "polymorphism" which itself means "can take many forms." What it "overloading" in practice is that the **compiler** of a language that supports it can distinguish between two or more functions or operators that are different but that are represented by the same name or symbol.

In computer programming, a "function" is a self-contained sequence of **code** statements that perform a set of actions and return a **value** of a known type, and an "operator" is a symbol that represents a specific **action**. For example, a **function** called timeEgg() might contain code that times the boiling of an egg, and the "+" symbol is an **operator** that represents addition. Most programming languages also support other operators that allow the code to manipulate numbers and character strings in more complicated ways.

Every function in the same program must have a unique "signature" so the compiler can tell which one is being called at any point of the code. When there are two or more functions in the same program that have the same name but have different "signatures," the function is said to be "overloaded".

The compiler creates the function's "signature" by combining information about the name of the function; the type or order, or both, of the parameters passed when the function is called; it's "visibility qualifiers," or information about what else in the program is allowed to "see" the function; and its return type. So long as each function has a **signature** that is different from every other function's signature in the program, it will be able to treat them as different functions even if their names are the same.

It is useful to understand that operators themselves can be considered to be functions in the same way as timeEgg() is a function, but the way they are presented to the compiler is different in order to make computer programs easier to read.

For example, the **C++** programming language allows operators to be "overloaded" for derived classes, or classes that are a "kind of" another **class**. What this means is that it is possible to give different semantics or meaning to the **expression** "b + c" in the following code, depending on what type of **data** b and c represent.

    myClass a, b, c;

    a = b + c;

The interesting thing is that the programmer can arbitrarily decide what the "b+c" means by adding code to the "operator+()" function in the definition of the class myClass. The declaration might look something like this:

    class myClass {

    myClass& operator+(const myClass& obj);

    }

And the programmer can **call** it like the conventional function it is:

    a = b.operator +(c);

or using the syntactic shortcut the compiler allows:

    a = b+c;

Thus operator overloading and function overloading can be seen to boil down to much the same thing at the language level. **Java** does not allow operator overloading although it breaks its own rule in the single case of the "String" class, where the language definition means that the "+" operator is overloaded and it is legal to write Java code like this:

    String a = "hello, ";

    String b = "world!";

    String c = a + b; // c contains "hello, world!";

Overloading tends to be characteristic of languages where every item of data is strictly defined in terms of what it is and what it can do. Languages of this kind are called "strongly typed" languages. C++ and Java are both strongly typed languages.

Weakly typed languages allow programmers to be more relaxed in how they use data objects in the program. The **C** programming language is not very strongly typed, and scripting languages like **Perl** are practically untyped. In C the **function signature** is based on the name of the function alone, which makes it impossible for the C compiler to distinguish between functions that have the same name so it is impossible to have two functions with the same name in the same C program.

Function overloading is a useful addition to programming languages that helps programmers write more easily understood, and thus more easily and cheaply maintained programs.

# OVERRIDING

Overriding in computer **programming** is a form of polymorphism which itself means "can take many forms." In Object-Oriented terminology, an overridden **method** or **function** is one that is redefined in subclass derived from a superclass.

What it means in practice is that the **compiler** of a language that supports overriding can distinguish between two or more functions or operators that are both represented by the same name or symbol, and have the same **function signature**.

In computer programming, a "function" is a self-contained sequence of **code** statements that perform a set of actions and return a **value** of a known type, and an "operator" is a symbol that represents a specific **action**. A function's **signature** is a combination of the function's name; the number, order, and **types** of its parameters; as well as any qualifiers that can be applied to the function. Operators and functions are implemented in much the same way in the details of the compiler, so from a technical point of view, there is little difference between them. In **C++**, for example, it is possible to assign functionality to operators like "+" and "-" by declaring them as functions like this:

    **class** myClass {

    myClass& operator+(const myClass& obj);

    myClass& operator-(const myClass& obj);

    }

and then **call** them in either one of two ways:

myClass a, b, c;

a = b.operator +(c);

or by using the syntactic shortcut the compiler allows:

myClass a, b, c;

a = b+c;

Conceptually, overriding is very much like **overloading**, which is where the compiler can distinguish between identically named functions as long as they have different function signatures. Overriding goes one step further and allows the compiler to distinguish between identically named functions that also have identical function signatures but belong to different objects in the same class hierarchy i.e., where the class of one of the objects is derived from the class of the other.

As an example, given a **base class** Mammal, **polymorphism** enables the programmer to define different methods for calculating the volume of the shape for any number of classes derived from Mammal. So, derived objects such as "Sloth," "Gibbon," "Dolphin," and "Platypus" will probably all support the "CountLegs()" method, but "overriding" means that the compiler will ensure that the right version of the method is called for any given **object**.

In C++ the classes could be declared like this:

class Mammal {

public:

virtual int CountLegs () const;

};


class Gibbon : public Mammal {

public:

int CountLegs () const;

};

class Platypus : public Mammal {

public:

int CountLegs () const;

};

The "virtual" keyword tells the compiler it can override the function "CountLegs()" in any derived classes. If the programmer now creates a Gibbon and a Platypus, she will be able to get the number of legs the animal has by calling the CountLegs() method.

Gibbon* myGibbon = new Gibbon();

Platypus* myPlatypus = new Platypus();

int gibbonLegs = myGibbon→CountLegs();

int platypusLegs = myPlatypus→CountLegs();

However, it is also legal and possible to do this:

Mammal* myMammalPtr = myGibbon;

gibbonLegs = myMammalPtr →CountLegs ();

myMammalPtr = myPlatypus;

platypusLegs = myMammalPtr →CountLegs ();

And the compiler will still call the correct method. This is because the compiler chooses which method to call depending on the type of the underlying object and not the type of the pointer. It can do this because it builds a table in its own internal **memory** at run time, when the program is actually executed.

It then knows that although myMammalPtr is a basic Mammal pointer, the object it represents is actually first a Gibbon and then a Platypus. By using its internal tables it can select the correct code to run when the call is made. In C++, this table is called the "v-table" or "virtual table."

One advantage of this that is not immediately obvious, is that it is possible to write code that will call functions on classes that do not even exist yet. This makes overriding and polymorphism an extremely powerful feature of object orientated languages.

# P

## PACKET SWITCHING

Packet switching is the process by which **data** is broken into smaller chunks, or packets, for transmission over a network. Packet switching divides a **message** into smaller units, sends each unit individually via the best route possible at the time, and reassembles the units into the complete message at the destination. Most **wide-area network** (WAN) **protocols** are based on packet-switching technologies.

Until the late 1960s computers could only talk to one other computer at a time, using dedicated, circuit-switched communication lines. This was inefficient, as it resulted in brief, intermittent data communications. In 1968 packet switching was first implemented in a government laboratory in England. The idea behind packet switching was that it was a more efficient use of communication time.

Upon hearing about the use of this technology in England, the Department of Defense issued a Request for Proposal (RFP) to implement packet switching for the **ARPAnet**. Faculty members and graduate students from UCLA responded with a proposal to determine the feasibility and reliability of using packet switching on the ARPAnet. This team designed communication protocols and interfaces to send and receive messages from other computers. By 1969 four university computers were connected via a WAN and exchanging packet switched messages.

The implementation of packet switching requires communications protocols, a router, and network software. **TCP/IP**, X.25, and frame relay are WAN communications protocols that use packet switching.

Every host connected to a WAN needs a router. A router is a specialized piece of **hardware** that connects a **local-area network** (**LAN**) to a WAN. A router sends packets to other destinations, monitors packets on the WAN for any that are addressed to computers on its LAN, and captures packets addressed to computers on its LAN.

Network software breaks up outgoing messages into packets. Each packet is about one kilobyte in length. The beginning of each packet is called a packet header. The packet header contains the IP address of the source computer sending the packet, the IP address of the destination computer, the length of the packet (measured in bytes), the total number of packets in the complete message, and the sequence number of this packet compared to the other packets comprising the message. Packet header information allows individual packets to be correlated with other packets when they reach the destination computer.

The order of transmission of individual packets is not important, nor is the route that each packet takes to get to its destination. As long as one packet of a message reaches its destination, the receiving computer can determine from the packet header how many packets there were supposed to be and request retransmission of the packets that are missing. When a connection is broken or a computer is down, packets are rerouted across other connections. Also, routers dynamically adjust their internal routing tables according to network conditions to bypass downed or unreliable connections.

*See also* ARPAnet; Local-area network (LAN); Message; TCP/IP protocol; Wide-area network (WAN)

## PAGING

Starting in the late 1960s and early 1970s, there arose the problem that software programs and their **data** would take up more memory space than was available in the primary storage (RAM). It became necessary to think of ways to break up such a larger program and its data into parts, with less-relevant parts being held in some auxiliary storage. If such additional **memory** is available, such as in the form of secondary storage on disk, then there are three major ways of doing this:

- Overlays—sections of the application **code** or data are stored on secondary storage (typically hard drives), and the application has to load them whenever required. This was a common method in personal computers under **DOS** right up to the early 1990s, but has the disadvantage that **applications** are slowed down by drive access speeds.

- Swapping—this is slightly similar to the use of overlays, but involves the process scheduler; a whole process, along with its data, is swapped on to disk (or other medium) when necessary, and is swapped back, with the required context-switching by the **CPU**, when it needs to be run again. Swapping has been there since the 1960s, and is still used in many systems.

- Virtual memory—this is a technique where the apparent memory available to the process or application is expanded seamlessly, without it being made aware of the dirty details involved. Hence, a "virtual memory" is created which is all that the process sees; this virtual memory may be thought of as a magnified memory made available to the process through the action of other components.

The last technique, that of **virtual memory**, is most pertinent in modern-day architectures and operating systems. It works as follows. A "page" is a small fixed-size block of memory; a "segment" is a variable-size block of memory, usually larger in size. Architectures are commonly either "paged" or "segmented" depending on which they use, but it is not unknown for there to be architectures where a segment is further subdivided into pages. On paged systems, there is a "virtual address" for each page in memory, which is the only address that the process needs to know about. The hardware (specifically, the memory management unit or MMU) takes care of locating the page physically given the virtual address.

If a page requested by the process currently running is already in main memory, well and good. If it is not in main memory, then a "page fault" is said to occur, and it needs to be brought into memory—this is done by use of a special piece of system software called a "page fault trap service routine." Of course, the process will not be given the page as quickly as it would be if the page were already in main memory, but this is of little consequence as the process never has to bother with the details of how the pages it asks for are obtained, and it only sees a virtual memory of more pages than the main memory itself can intrinsically support.

If the pages are only copied on to main memory when they are needed by a process, then we have "demand paging." Pages are then moved into main memory only by the occurrence of page faults. This is a very basic technique, but in many cases, it is possible to do better. For that we use "anticipatory paging," where a page is brought into main memory in anticipation of its possible use. For example, when a certain page has been loaded into main memory because of a page fault, other pages which contain related blocks of data or application code, may be needed shortly. Hence, some software systems even allow user programs to explicitly ask for certain pages to be brought into main memory even before they are referenced.

A question now arises—how does one know which page that is already in memory to replace, when a new one is brought in? Some of the common page replacement techniques are:

- Belady's optimal replacement policy—this is the optimal page replacement policy, unimplementable in practice, which requires precise knowledge of when a page will be needed in future; under this method, one has to know which page will not be required for the longest time in future, and replace it with the one being moved in. Lacking a crystal ball for always knowing which pages will be needed in future, we have to come up with various reasonable guesses, so this method cannot be used in its stated form.

- Random—just pick whichever page in main memory, with no regard, and replace it with the one that is being moved. This is obviously the least sophisticated page-replacement method there could be, and it would be really hard for any method to do worse!

- FIFO (first in, first out)—pick the page that has been in main memory the longest, and replace it. This method sounds reasonable, but empirical studies have shown that it is nearly as bad as random replacement—the mere fact that a page has been in main memory a long time does not mean it is useless and can be swapped; in fact, it is possible it should there a long time because it is very useful.

- LRU (least recently used)—pick the page in main memory that has not been used for the longest time, and remove it. This is a sensible policy, but unfortunately it requires that the MMU do a fairly complex job of bookkeeping in order to keep track of times of accesses to pages. Various approximations to LRU replacement are found to be good in practice, and empirical studies have shown that it is the policy that comes the closest to realizing the performance of the impossible Belady policy. That is, the fact that a page has not been used for the longest time is a good indicator generally that it is not going to be used for the longest time to come.

***See also*** Central processing unit; Computer architecture; Operating systems (theory)

# PARALLEL ALGORITHMS

With the advent of **parallel processing**, the raw computing power available to solve many problems is now immense, well beyond what was available using conventional uniprocessor computing techniques. This is especially significant in solving the so-called Grand Challenge problems of computing. A Grand Challenge problem (such as accurate weather forecasting) is a fundamental problem of science or engineering, having a broad social or economic impact, whose solution requires the use of very high-end computing power.

Many problem domains are also naturally suited to parallel processing. For instance, applications such as weather prediction, biosphere modeling, population analyses, and the like are modeled by assuming a grid on the domain being modeled. The segments (squares or cubes) of the grid are analyzed for their influences on surrounding segments, and vice versa. This often requires solutions to large systems of differential equations, with the **granularity** of the grid chosen determining the accuracy of the model. Such a problem often cannot be solved using sequential **algorithms** running on a uniprocessor.

As an example of such a problem, consider the task of modeling the weather over the lower 48 states of the United States. We may say that the area being modeled is approximately 3000 miles $\times$ 3000 miles, and that the atmosphere up to a height of 10 miles is significant in determining the weather. Assume that the $3000 \times 3000 \times 10$ cubic mile weather domain is partitioned into segments of size $0.1 \times 0.1 \times 0.1$ cubic miles. There are thus about $10^{11}$ different segments.

In a weather modeling system, time is an additional dimension in the computations, since the model has to show the changes of weather over time. Let us say that in our model we need to model the weather over a two-day (48 hour) period, and that the variables must be updated every half hour—these are very conservative assumptions, likely to be highly inaccurate in practice (practical weather forecasting models require much faster updates, often within minutes). The computation of variables (temperature, pressure, wind speed, humidity, cloud cover, etc.) in each segment may be taken to require the previous values of the variables in that segment, as well as the values from neighboring segments. Assume that this computation requires 100 instructions to be executed (again, a very conservative estimate). Thus, a single half-hourly update of the variables for the whole system requires $10^{11} \times 100$, or $10^{13}$ instructions. As there are about 100 such updates over two days, the total number of instructions to be executed is about $10^{15}$. On a high-end serial computer capable of computing one billion instructions a second, this computation would require about 280 hours, or almost twelve days.

This illustrates one important problem with serial computing even using fast computers—a weather forecasting system that takes twelve days to forecast the weather over the next two days is obviously useless. Parallel algorithms running on many machines thus are required—by partitioning the large problem among many processors (such as by allocating large chunks of the three-dimensional segment space to them for individual processing), problems such as weather forecasting may be solved.

A basic approach to the study of parallel algorithms is to assume that the size of the input space is equal to the number of available processors that can be used in parallel. This is obviously not always accurate—it is unrealistic to grant that one could have $10^{11}$ processors to solve the weather forecasting problem described above. However, the assumption is useful to the extent that it illustrates which problems are capable of being solved in parallel. In general, it is good for the size of the input space to be divisible by the number of processors available, but this too may be an over-simplistic assumption. Most processors in real life are also not dedicated to just one task such as weather modeling, and may have other **variable**

loads that change from time to time. The number of processors available may also change periodically due to crashes or maintenance, or as new ones are added to the system. Randomization and other techniques are often applied to distribute the load among processors running in parallel.

In running a parallel algorithm, the ideal case would be where with $n$ processors each of which takes time T to solve the problem, one would be able to solve the problem in T divided by $n$ time. However, there are communication overheads (time and processor cycles taken for communication between processors), network delays, and the like—the problem itself may also not be easily parallelizable. For such reasons, this is usually more than the gain actually achieved with $n$ processors. The "Principle of Unitary Speedup" says that the gain from using $n$ each of which takes time T, is at most equal to that of using a single processor which takes time T/$n$.

In randomized parallel algorithms, sometimes the principle given above may not hold true, and super-linear gain may be observed occasionally due to the unpredictable performance of **randomized algorithms**. In deterministic algorithms, however, the principle is always true.

*See also* Parallel processing; Randomization

# PARALLEL PROCESSING

For the last three decades or more, computer processor speeds have grown at the rapid pace expected by Moore's Law. This tremendous increase has allowed for there to be great advances in the range and sophistication of **applications** supported, and tasks that some years ago could not even be performed on specialized scientific supercomputers costing millions of dollars are now routine affairs even on personal desktop machines. However, it has been observed that sequential uniprocessor computing is approaching a fundamental restriction on its performance—the speed of light. Since processor speeds are already up to the gigahertz level and **transistor** sizes on chips are already in the micron range, it is felt that the current technology is unlikely to sustain the rate of progress for much longer before coming up against the laws of physics. Of course, it can always be hoped that a different type of processor architecture will come forward and allow for advances even beyond the point where the current technology hits its ultimate bottleneck, but that is uncertain at best.

One definite way in which performance improvement is likely is by the use of multiprocessor architectures. The idea that by using multiple processors running in parallel it is possible to obtain a higher performance than any one processor running by itself is basically sound, though it comes with its own special set of challenges. Some that may be mentioned are that parallel processing is a large and diverse field, with much study still in its infancy. Advances in parallel processing are also likely to require advances in compiler **design** and construction, in the understanding and use of parallel **algorithms**, and in distributed computing.

The notion that one can use a parallel architecture to enhance performance beyond that achievable with a single processor is of course not new. The basic taxonomy for classifying processor architectures was proposed in the 1960s, and is as follows:

- Single instruction **stream**, single **data** stream (SISD)—this is your regular uniprocessor.

- Single instruction stream, multiple data streams (SIMD)—in this architecture, the same instruction is executed by more than one processor using different data streams. Every processor has a distinct data memory (hence multiple data streams) but there is a single instruction memory, and a control processor whose function is to fetch and dispatch instructions. This is most often used with special-purpose processors where full generality is not required.

- Multiple instruction streams, single data stream (MISD)—this is a somewhat counter-intuitive style of architecture, and no such machine has ever been built, though one could be in future.

- Multiple instruction streams, multiple data streams (MIMD)—every processor gets its own instructions separately, and uses its own data. The processors are usually generic, off-the-shelf.

In early years, multiprocessor architectures were generally of the SIMD type, but MIMD has gained favor in the last few years. Two reasons may be mentioned for this. The first is that MIMDs offer flexibility, functioning either as single-user machines running one specialized application, or as multi-user machines running many different tasks at one time, or some combination of these extremes. The second is that MIMDs use regular off-the-shelf chips that are also used in uniprocessors, rather than requiring special chips to be custom-built for them. This allows MIMDs to be constructed cheaply.

Processors in MIMD machines can share a single centralized memory with the processors and **memory** being connected by a common bus. This is most practical on systems of a small number of processors. For architectures with a larger number of processors, it is a better idea to use a physically distributed memory, where each processor has a cache and a local memory, and is connected to the other processors by an interconnection network. Distributing the memory this way has two major benefits: lowered cost, and reduced **access** latency.

With physically distributed memory, there are two ways in which the memory may be addressed by the processors. The first is to treat the entire memory cumulus spread over all processors as one logical address space, so that any processor may, if it has access privileges, address any logical unit of memory without concern for where the relevant memory component is actually located in the system. Such systems are called distributed shared memory (DSM) architectures, or just shared memory systems. Alternatively, if the memory is partitioned into disjoint private address spaces, processors cannot address memory units they do not own; each processor-memory unit may be considered a distinct computer. In fact, this architecture can be implemented simply by having desktop machines connected by a local area network (**LAN**). For applications where little or no communication is required among the processors and the separate memory units are sufficient,

this architecture is used. All communication among the separate computing units is by passing of messages over the connecting network, hence these systems are called **message-passing** machines.

Parallel processing systems are distinguished by their memory models and their communication mechanisms, as outlined above. Older attempts at parallel processing typically used the message-passing model, since it was easier to understand and shared memory was hard to implement in **hardware**. In recent years, however, shared memory has made strides and is finding favor with the computing community.

Ideally, any parallel processing architecture should achieve linear speedup, that is, the advantage gained should be proportional to the number of processors used. For example, if it took ten hours to run a computation on a uniprocessor machine, it should take just one for a multiprocessor system with ten chips of the same kind as before. In practice, however, linear speedup is infrequent, and in rare degenerate cases, the speedup may actually be completely absent, i.e., it may take as much or more time to run a program on a multiprocessor system as it does on a uniprocessor. Two important reasons for the lack of optimal speedup are software or algorithmic limitations in parallelism, and large latencies for remote memory access or **message** passing, as compared to local access. The first has to do with some computing tasks and problems not being efficiently partible into arbitrary numbers of smaller subtasks—if one has a large problem that cannot be efficiently broken up into multiple subproblems, then having multiple processors working on it would not help much. Much research in parallel processing therefore focuses on the development of algorithms to allow for the parallelizing of larger problems into parts that can be run on parallel architectures. The problem of latency has received much attention also.

*See also* Computer architecture

# PARAMETER

A parameter is an entity that represents a **value** supplied by one **function** that desires to render the services of another function. It is sometimes referred to as an **argument** or "arg" rather than a parameter. Parameters can be a value, a constant or a **variable** but in any case they are values that facilitate the evaluation of a function, procedure or **subroutine**. Constant parameters, or actual parameters, cannot be altered by the function whereas variable parameters, or formal parameters, represent values that can be changed within the function or procedure. All the parameters used in a function or procedure must be listed in the header of that function or procedure or the function must include a directive to where the parameters are listed, as is the case when using global parameters. There are certain functions that can be designed to operate well without the need of parameters listed outside of the function. It is also possible to **design** a function that can **access** global parameters from a subroutine, function or procedure. Although both of these designs are possible designing a program where parameters are passed in and out of subroutines is sometimes the best solution when the programmer wants the function to be independent from the calling function. If parameters can be passed back and forth, between the subroutines of the program the **code** for a particular function can be used in other projects, **debugging** this code will be greatly simplified, therefore less time consuming, and any subsequent versions of the function will not affect the entire program. Also, this transfer allows the values or entities represented as parameters to be transferred back and forth and utilized by these functions without having to redefine them within each piece. This saves programmers much time and effort.

Parameters are usually listed in the header of a subroutine or of the main program as parameter **declarations**. The **parameter declaration** contains one or a comma-delimited series of parameters, as the identifying name(s), followed by a colon and a type **identifier** specific to that parameter. Occasionally a parameter is given a default value and so the type identifier is followed by an equals-sign and a value. The identifying name of a parameter must be a valid identifier. A parameter is an entity used by the **compiler** to identify a piece of a function or procedure.

It is the parameter declaration that determines where the parameter is evaluated, either by the called function or the caller function. If the parameter declaration defines the parameter as a variable then the specific **method** used to pass the parameter is important in affecting whether the value of the parameter is computed by the caller or the called function and whether the called function can modify the value of the parameter as seen by the caller. Three popular methods of passing parameters between called functions and function that **call** are call-by-value, call-by-name, and call-by-need. Employing the call-by-value method results in a parameter that is evaluated before it is passed to the called function so only the value is transferred. The caller sees the value of the parameter is unaffected by called function. Call-by-name passes the parameter as an unevaluated **expression**. The call-by-need method delays evaluation of function parameters until they are needed.

# PARAMETER DECLARATION

A **parameter** declaration tells the **compiler** the name of the **function** and the number, type and order of parameters utilized in that function. It is a composed of a series of parameters, contained in parenthesis, delimited by commas, with the other identifying information such as type and order. It is sometimes called an **argument** declaration. The parameter declaration can be contained in either the same source **code** file along with the function or procedure or it can be contained in a separate file and included in the source code file for the function using some sort of include directive. Parameter **declarations** are sometimes incorporated into lists such as parameter lists. In these lists parameter declarations are separated by a semicolon.

There are several **types** of parameter declarations. Two types are constant or **value parameter** declaration, and **variable** or a **reference parameter** declaration. A constant parameter

declaration is evaluated at **runtime** and its actual **value** is transferred from the caller function to the called module. Unlike a constant parameter declaration a variable parameter declaration is not transferred to the called function but instead only its address is transferred.

Although it is the type of parameter declaration by definition that determines where the parameter is evaluated there are many different conventions for passing parameters to functions and procedures including call-by-value, call-by-name, and call-by-need. The specific method used to transfer the parameter will affect whether the value of the parameter is computed by the caller or the called function and whether the called function can modify the value of the parameter as seen by the caller, assuming it is a variable. The call-by-value method is an evaluation method where parameters are evaluated before the function or procedure is entered. In this way only the value of the parameter is transferred and so any changes that occur to the parameter in the called function are not seen to affect the parameter by the caller. Although this method is efficient it is less likely to terminate in the presence of infinite **data** structures and recursive functions. The call-by-name method utilizes a method that passes the parameter as an unevaluated **expression**. It is the opposite of the call-by-value method. Parameters to macros are usually passed using call-by-name. In order to implement **functional programming languages**, call-by-name is often combined with graph reduction, a technique that represents an expression as a directed graph, to avoid repeated evaluation of the same expression. This combination is then known as the call-by-need method, the third method mentioned above. This is a method that delays evaluation of function parameters until they are needed because they are parameters to a primitive function or a conditional.

# PARAMETER LIST

A **parameter** list, sometimes called an **argument** list, is a sequence of parameter **declarations** found in the header of a **function**, procedure, program or **subroutine**. All the parameters used in such types of **code** must be listed in the header of that function or procedure or the function must include a directive to where the parameters are listed, as is the case when using global parameters. The parameter list is basically just a list of the parameters and their characteristics, the parameter declarations. In some **programming** languages the entire parameter list is enclosed in parenthesis and each **parameter declaration** is separated from the next by a semicolon. Further each parameter declaration is composed of the parameter **identifier**, followed by a colon and the type identifier, and in some cases this is followed by symbols that assign the parameter a default **value**. The different parameter declarations are ordered in the parameter list. That is that there is a **constraint** or limiting **attribute** attached to an **association** to signify that the objects at one end are specified in some explicit order.

Parameters that can be transferred from one function or procedure to another have a transfer or passing protocol specified by its parameter list. Also the number and types of parameters that a function accepts and the number and types of values it returns are described in the parameter list. For a generic function all methods for that function must have congruent parameter lists.

## PARAMETER PASSING

**Parameter** passing is a type of technique used to transfer parameters from a **function** or procedure to another function or procedure. There are certain functions that can operate well without needing outside parameters. It is also possible to **access** global parameters from a **subroutine**, function or procedure. Although these designs are possible parameter passing is sometimes the best solution when the programmer wants the function to be independent from the calling function. If parameter passing is employed the **code** for a particular function can be used in other projects, **debugging** this code will be greatly simplified, therefore less time consuming, and any subsequent versions of the function will not affect the entire program. This is a very useful technique since many complex programs are written in special pieces or functions where each has a defined task. Parameter passing allows the values or entities represented as parameters to be transferred back and forth and utilized by these functions without having to redefine them within each piece. This saves programmers much time and effort. There are many types of parameter passing techniques with call-by-value, call-by-name, and call-by-need being three of the most widely utilized. The specific parameter passing technique employed in a situation where a parameter is declared as a **variable** affects whether the **value** of the parameter is computed by the caller or the called function and whether the called function can modify the value of the parameter as seen by the caller.

Call-by-value is a parameter passing technique that utilizes parameters that are evaluated or defined before the called function is entered. Only the value of the parameter is transferred to the called function and so the caller function does not see the value of the parameter being affected by the called function. This parameter passing **method** is efficient but less likely to terminate when dealing with infinite **data** structures and recursive functions.

Call-by-name is the opposite of call-by-value in that it is a parameter passing technique that does not pre-evaluate the parameter before passing it. This parameter passing technique was first established by Algorithmic Language 1960, a portable language for scientific computations. Usually when dealing with macros a parameter is passed using call-by-name. Instead of passing the evaluated parameter a pointer to some code that will return the value of the parameter and an environment giving the values of its free variables are passed. Using this technique a normal form, the state of a term that contains no reducible expressions, is guaranteed to be achieved if one exists. In order to avoid repeated evaluation of the same **expression** over and over when implementing **functional programming languages** the call-by-name parameter passing is often combined with graph reduction. Graph reduc-

tion is a technique that represents and expression as a directed graph. The combination of graph reduction and call-by-name is called call-by-need parameter passing.

Call-by-need parameter passing is a technique that delays evaluation of a function parameter until it is needed by that function. This is done because the parameter is part of a conditional or primitive function. This term first appeared in 1971 in a thesis written by Chris Wadsworth, a student from Oxford.

## PARENT

The parent, or mother or predecessor as it is often called, is a term that refers to the more general element in a relationship that is formulated in a generalization-type architecture or hierarchical structure. In this type of architecture things associated with child, a more specialized element, are substitutable for a parent of that child. Often times it is common to say "the child is a kind of the parent." The parent is the **object** or element that is immediately above another object in a hierarchical structure. It can also be an object or element that contains other objects or elements.

This kind of generalization architecture is often found in organizational trees of classes of elements, **databases**, and directory file structure in some **computer languages**. In **Unix** files are organized into directories that contain files and other directories. This type of file structure looks similar to a **tree** with its different branches. It is a directed acyclic graph, that is a graph that has only a single route between any pair of nodes. The top of a tree file structure is called the root **node**. Each entry on a different branch is a node and considered a **child node**, or daughter node, of the parent branch. Each parent branch is, in turn, considered a child node of the next higher parent branch closer to the root node to which it falls under. No node can have more than one parent. If a node has no parents but does have child nodes then it is called a root node. A superclass is a parent of another **class** within that generalization, and a supertype is a patent of another class within a generalization.

## PARITY

Parity is a technique for determining whether **data** has been lost or overwritten during a move. It can be used within a single computer when moving bits of data between storage locations, and it can be used between computers when data is transmitted. Parity checking is the most basic form of error detection in communications.

When data is moved, it is moved in groups of bits. An extra binary **bit**, called a parity bit, is added to each group of bits that is moved. This bit does not become part of the data; it is used only for the purpose of identifying whether the bits being moved arrived successfully. Parity bits can be either odd or even, depending on the systems involved. When data is transmitted between computers, the sending system and receiving system must agree to use parity checking and whether to use even parity or odd parity. Even parity is more commonly used.

When even parity is used, each group of bits must total an even number. To accomplish this, the parity bit is set to zero or one, depending on the total of the bits in the group (before the parity bit is added). If the total number of bits is odd, the parity bit is set to one; if the total number of bits is even, the parity bit is set to zero. This results in each group of bits totaling an even number.

Parity checking is the calculation at the receiving end of the transmission to ensure that the total number of bits in the group totals an even number. If the number is odd, there has been a transmission error. The receiving system can either request a retransmission or generate an error **message**.

*See also* Bit

# PARSER AND PARSING

A parser is a program that enables the translation of source **code**, which is the original form of program instruction, into **object** code, or language that the computer is able to understand. As such, parsing is part of the compilation process. The mechanics of dividing the source code into it component parts and identifying those components, so that translation into object code can occur, constitutes parsing. Parsers are available for all standard **programming** languages, such as **XML**, **Perl** and **Java**.

The parse function has and input series to which specific rules of analysis are applied. The input series may be a group of characters (**string**) or numerical **data** (block). If it is a sting, it will be parsed by character. If it is a block, it will be parsed by **value**. The rules supply the parameters that determine how the information will be parsed. The parse function can be modified in two ways. The function "/all refinement" forces a parsing of all the characters in a string, including aspects usually ignored by the parser—spaces, tabs, new lines, and other nonprintable characters. The "/case refinement" specifies that the string to be parsed be done so in a case sensitive manner. Normally, upper and lower cases are not distinguished.

Parsing is vital to the **operation** of many computer science disciplines. The **compiler**, the program that actually accomplishes the source code to object code translation, does so by examining the entire source code and then reorganizing the information. While the parser is the program that dissects the information, the compiler is essentially the language that specifies the way parsing is accomplished. Without the compiler and the ability to parse the information, the reorganization of the information could not occur. Parsing also is important for many **applications**, which require the processing of **commands**.

Parsing constitutes lexical analysis and semantic analysis. Lexical analysis divides strings, which are a series of characters grouped together, into their components, which are called tokens. For example, a sentence could be divided into several tokens corresponding to a noun phrase, verb phrase, and prepositional phrase. Semantic parsing then functions to try and determine the meaning of the string. In the above example, semantic parsing would establish the nouns, verb, preposition, and article constituents. A drawing of the process, with the string at the top and the completely parsed string components at the bottom, is reminiscent of an evergreen **tree**, with its broad base tapering upwards to a tip. The visual image inspired the name treebank, which refers to the arrangement of the parsing process.

The parsing process utilizes a form of grammar known as **constraint** grammar. In constraint grammar, the grammatical functions of words in a sentence and the relationships between these words are codified. Not all parsing systems are the same. There are two main differences: the number of constituent types, or tools used to dissect the grouped information, that a system uses, and the way in which the constituent types are allowed to combine with each other. Despite these differences, most parsing schemes are based on a form that is known as context-free structure grammar. Within this form are two distinctly different forms of parsing; full parsing and skeleton parsing.

Full parsing aims to provide the highest level of detail possible of the structure of the grouped information. Skeleton parsing is less detailed. For example, in full parsing there are several types of noun phrases, which are distinguished by features such as their singular or plural nature. Several constituent labels are also used for adjective phrases, prepositional phrases, adverbial phrases, and verb phrases. Each label has a character code. Skeleton parsing, on the other hand, labels all noun phrases the same, with the letter N. There are fewer codes in skeleton parsing than in full parsing (relative clause, noun phrase, prepositional phrase, compound sentence, verb phrase).

Parsing is a term applied to other, computer-dependent tasks. The medium of digital video also involved parsing. Digital video needs to be properly processed before it can be inserted into a video server. One processing need is parsing. Video parsing is the process of detecting scene changes or the **transition** from one camera shot to another in a video montage, which is often in a compressed state in a JPEG or MPEG file. Another aspect of parsing is found in biology, specifically in the emerging field of proteomics—the mapping of the identity and activities of all the proteins in a cell. Parsing comes in at the level of the genetic material. Deciphering the sequences of DNA that code for the thousands of functional proteins that operate in humans requires vast computational power.

*See also* Compiler; Data structure; Information processing

# PARTICIPATORY DESIGN

Participatory **design** is a method of giving the end user of a product a part in the construction and implementation of the design. It aims to bring together all the stakeholders in a project (users, designers, managers, etc.) at the earliest possible stage of development, before anything is set in stone. Often the method involves game-playing exercises, using pen and paper mock-ups, to help define how a product will be used. Using paper allows for many different designs to be imagined and for any number of changes to be made immediately and at minimal cost. In software design, one person usually plays the role of the computer by holding up a drawn version of the screen, and adding to it paste-on menus and function boxes. Users say what they want to click on, or write down what they want to type, and the paper screen is changed to represent what the software would show. These design sessions may be videotaped, so a record exists of what designs were rejected, and why modifications were made. Only when all those concerned are satisfied with the design concept is it actually programmed into a computer.

Participatory design methods originated in Europe in the 1970s, primarily in Scandinavia. The concept of involving workers in the design of their workplace was an offspring of the trend to democratize business, and was seen as a method of empowering employees. While the concept had some notable successes, it was initially not widely adopted outside of Scandinavia. The growth of the information technology industry, however, and the increasing frustration many companies have with expensive software products that do not perform as desired, has lead to a revival of interest in participatory design.

Participatory design aims to reduce the need for fixes to a product once it has been implemented, and, therefore, also reduce costs. Some estimates suggest that up to eighty percent of software development costs occur after a product is implemented, often due to unforeseen or unmet user requirements. By involving users in the earliest design process, many such problems can be avoided. Product development and testing times are often shortened, and a friendlier design can also lead to greater worker satisfaction and increased productivity.

The use of low-tech materials during participatory design, such as pen and paper, makes it possible for anyone, no matter what their computer skill, to contribute to the design. The process can make better users, as they are more informed about the products they are using, and can recognise the intentions and limitations of the system. The life span of the product may be increased, as a design better suited to the user will not become obsolete as quickly.

While software design remains the most common application of participatory design, is has also been used in areas such as urban planning, where community residents help determine their environment, and in architectural projects, where buyers consult with the developer and architect on the specifications for their project.

Perhaps the biggest limitation of participatory design is that users do not always know what they need, nor will they necessarily have an initial clear idea of exactly they want from a product. The method of participatory design is best used in situations where it is easy to simulate the end product by paper prototyping. The simplicity of pen and paper designing does not allow fine detail to be fully explored, however, nor can it reveal technical aspects, such as system response times for software. There are also a bewildering number of participatory design methods that can be used. For example, PANDA (Participatory Analysis, Design, & Assessment), CARD (Collaborative Analysis of Requirements and Design) and PICTIVE (Plastic Interface for Collaborative Technology Initiative through Video Exploration), are all participatory design models whose methods slightly differ.

Despite these limitations, participatory design has the potential to change the nature of design. Participatory design assumes that everyone can be a designer, and that design should be a social process. It can reduce development costs and time, and redefine the role technology and software plays in the workplace. While it has many limitations, and is not suitable for all projects, it does offer a refreshing alternative to traditional design methods.

***See also*** Computer science and corporations; Design; Software, design, engineering, and testing

# PASCAL, BLAISE (1623-1662)
*French geometer, probabilist, physicist, inventor, and philosopher*

Although Blaise **Pascal** can be seen in retrospect as an important scientist in his time, he was a controversial figure to his contemporaries. There is no doubt that Pascal was of a superior intelligence, but he was a modest man, embarrassed by his own genius. The reason for his contemporaries' doubt was perhaps in part due to the fact that much of his work was not published in his lifetime, which limited how his accomplishments could be viewed. Still, Pascal gave the world, mathematical and otherwise, many things: he opened up new forms of calculus, projective geometry, probability theory, and he designed and manufactured the first calculating machine run by cogs and wheels.

Pascal was born in Clermont (now known as Clermont–Ferrand), Auvergne, France, on June 19, 1623. He was the son of a mathematician and civil servant Ètienne and Antoinette (nee Bégon) Pascal. His mother died when Pascal was three. With his two sisters, Gilberte (Madame Périer after marrying Florin Périer in 1641) and Jacqueline, Pascal was educated at home, primarily by his father. Pascal was part of a very tightly knit family, and he was especially close to his sisters. Pascal's sister Jacqueline was a child literary prodigy, and, despite being sickly all his life, Pascal was also a gifted child. In 1631, the family moved to Paris, where Pascal began his mathematical education when he was 10 or 11. His father insisted that his education start with the study of ancient languages, before learning geometry.

At age 13, Pascal and his father began attending discussions in Paris with a group of scientists and mathematicians, such as René Descartes, called the Académie Parisienne. By the time he was 16 years old, Pascal had already done a significant amount of his mathematical ground work. He continued his studies in Rouen where the family moved in 1639, when his father was appointed to the tax office there. Pascal continued to go to Paris occasionally while living in Rouen, and it was on one of these trips that he presented one of his important mathematical discoveries.

Published in 1640 as a pamphlet, *Essai sur les coniques* was a vital step in the development of projective geometry and it contained what came to be known as Pascal's mystic hexagram. Pascal began writing this treatise on conic sections to clarify the 1639 publication of Gérard Desargues' *Brouillon project d'une atteinte aux evenements des rencontres du cone avec un plan* ("Experimental project aiming to describe what happens when the cone comes into contact with a plane"). Desargues had written his book in a manner that was very difficult to understand, even for other mathematicians.

But as Pascal began to work with the propositions that Desargues made, he went beyond what Desargues accomplished. Pascal developed his own theorem which he used to deduce some 400 propositions as corollaries. His theorem, describing a figure known as Pascal's mystic hexagram, states that the three points of intersection of the pairs of opposite sides of a hexagon inscribed in a conic are collinear. When he presented his findings to the Académie Parisienne, Descartes could not believe a 16–year–old boy had written this work. Only part of the manuscript was published in the 1640 essay, but a whole manuscript did exist at one time.

Soon after this pamphlet was published, in 1641, Pascal's health began to decline. He suffered from headaches (perhaps caused by a deformed skull), insomnia, and indigestion but he continued his work. To help with his father's lengthy tax work in Rouen, Pascal worked on what became the first manufactured **calculator** from 1642 to 1644. This machine could automatically add and subtract, using cogged wheels to do the calculations. The invention was patented and Pascal received a monopoly by a royal decree dated May 22, 1649. He wanted to manufacture these machines as a full scale business enterprise but it proved too costly. The basic principle behind Pascal's calculator was still used in this century before the electronic age.

The year 1646 was key in Pascal's life. He became part of an anti–Jesuit Catholic sect called Jansenism, which believed in predestination and that divine grace was the only way to achieve salvation. He persuaded his family to join him, and the influence of Jansenism played a dominant role in the rest of the life.

Pascal also began doing work in physics, conducting experiments in atmospheric and barometric pressure, and vacuums. Pascal used the theories of Evangelista Torricelli as a starting point for his work. In Pascal's experiments, he had his brothers–in–law climb Puy de Dôme with tubes filled with different liquids to test his theories. The results were not just more information about atmospheric pressure, for Pascal invented the syringe and the hydraulic press based on them. More importantly, he delineated what came to be known as Pascal's principle, which says that pressure will be transmitted equally throughout a confined fluid at rest, regardless of where the pressure is applied.

Pascal published his some of his results in 1647 under the title *Experiences nouvelles touchant le vide*, and in 1648 as *Récit de la grande experience sur l'equilibre des liqueurs*. He completed the work already done on hydrostatics theory,

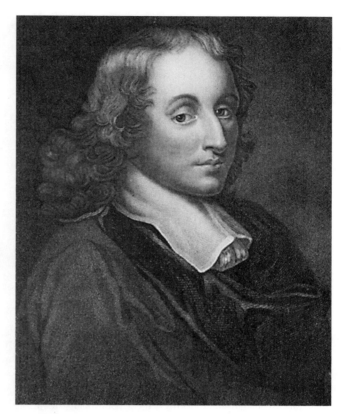

**Blaise Pascal**

bringing together the mechanics of both fluids and rigid bodies. His whole treatise on this subject was not published until a year after his death.

The Pascal family returned to Paris in 1647. His father died there in 1650, and his sister Jacqueline entered the Jansenism Convent at Port–Royale. Pascal himself had a profound religious experience four years later on the night of November 23, 1654. That night, Pascal was nearly killed in a riding accident. A few months later, Pascal left the secular world to live in the Port–Royal Convent. He did a little more work in mathematics and science, but primarily published religious philosophy.

Before Pascal's religious experience, earlier in 1654, he and Pierre de Fermat began writing each other about problems on dice and other games of chance. This correspondence laid the foundation for the mathematical theory of probability.

During his work on probability, Pascal made a comprehensive study of the arithmetic triangle. Although this triangle of numbers was more than 600 years old, Pascal used it so ingeniously in his probability studies that it became known as Pascal's triangle. His work on the binomial coefficients that make up the triangle helped to lead Isaac Newton to his discovery of the general binomial theorem.

Pascal's last mathematical work was on the cycloid, the curve traced by the motion of a fixed point on the circumference of a circle rolling along a straight line. This curve was known as far back as the early 16th century, but in 1658, over the course of eight intensive days of effort, Pascal solved many of the remaining problems about the geometry of the cycloid. The "theory of indivisibles," a forerunner of integral calculus, allowed him to find the area and center of gravity of any segment of the cycloid. He also computed the volume and surface area of the solid of revolution formed by rotating the curve around a straight line. As was customary in those days, once having found these solutions, Pascal proposed a challenge to other mathematicians to solve a set of problems about the cycloid and offered two prizes. Neither prize was ever awarded and Pascal eventually published his own solutions.

The fruition of Pascal's correspondence with Fermat came in 1658, when he was trying to forget the pain of a toothache. Pascal came up with solutions to problems related to the curve cycloid, also known as roulette. He solved the problems using what became known as Pascal's arithmetic triangle (also known as the triangle of numbers) to calculate probability. His results were published in 1658 as *Lettre circulaire relative a la cycloïde*. This work played a major role in the development of calculus, both differential and integral. With this framework, areas and volumes could be calculated, and infinitesimal problems could be solved.

Though Pascal had been sickly all his life, his health became much worse later in 1658. His last project was developing a public transportation system of carriages in Paris in the first part of 1662. He did not live to see the system running. He died in his sister Gilberte's home on August 19, 1662, probably of a malignant stomach ulcer. Before his death, he may have parted company with his Jansenist friends.

Pascal was often underestimated in his time, and the bulk of his work was published posthumously. For example, *Traité de la pesanteur de la masse de l'air* was published in 1663, and *Traité du triangle arithmétique* in 1665, although these are only two of many.

# PASCAL

Pascal is a high-level **programming** language, which is named after **Blaise Pascal**, a seventeenth century French mathematician who constructed one of the first mechanical adding machines. The language was developed by **Niklaus Wirth** in 1971. It resembles ALGOL, a now little used language devised for scientific computing

The person for whom Pascal is named, Blaise Pascal, lived from 1623 to 1662. He was a child prodigy and accomplished mathematician. In 1642, at 21 years of age, he invented a calculation machine. Pascal is credited with the discovery of the mathematical theory of probability. He also made fundamentally important contributions to number theory, geometry, and the advancement of scientific theory in the face of religious criticism.

A programming language contains a vocabulary, certain keywords and set of grammatical rules for instructing a computer to perform specific tasks. A high level programming language like Pascal is more or less independent of any particular type of computer. Also, the language uses English type state-

ments that are converted to machine statements, which provide the computer with the instructions for a particular **action**.

Since 1971 many versions of Pascal have emerged, including versions by Borland, Inc. (Turbo Pascal), **Microsoft** (Quick Pascal), and **Apple**, Inc. (Macintosh Pascal). Pascal is a general purpose programming language, which enjoyed great popularity throughout the 1970s and the 1980s. Today, it remains a popular teaching tool.

The popularity of Pascal can be attributed in large measure to two things. First, in the early 1980's, the Educational Testing Service, the company that creates the primary college entrance exam in the United States, added a Computer Service exam to the placement exams taken by high school students. The computer language chosen was Pascal (it remained the choice until 1999). Thus, many students were of necessity exposed to Pascal programming. Secondly, the Borland International company marketed the Turbo Pascal **compiler**. The compiler was revolutionary because of its speed—a compilation rate of several thousand lines per minute. The benefit of speed made many users gravitate to the use of Pascal.

Pascal is best known for its high performance with **structured programming** techniques. Because the language is very data-oriented, the structure is imposed to prevent the mix up of **data types**. Even though Pascal reads very much like a natural language, the rigid structure of the language forces programmers to write programs that are methodically and carefully designed. This rigidity is one feature that has made it a popular teaching language. Another feature of Pascal is that it highlights concepts that are similar to all **computer languages**. So, learning Pascal makes the learning of other languages easier. Also, Pascal uses standardized language, which makes the writing of programs less arduous.

However, Pascal success in other spheres, such as a business tool, was not as pervasive due to the inflexibility of the language and the dearth of application development tools. In other applications too, Pascal has been supplanted by other languages, such a **C**, **C++** and **Java**. To address some of the criticisms against Pascal, Wirth designed a new language called Modula-2. Modula-2 is similar to Pascal, but contains additional features enabling the separate compilation of program routines and **multitasking**.

In order to create a functional Pascal program, an editor, compiler and linker are needed. The editor create the Pascal source **code**. The compiler converts this source code to a machine readable form known as the **object** code. A number of compilers are marketed, such as Turbo Pascal. Finally, the linker functions to link the object code to create the executable code.

Pascal is comprised of simple text files, just like regular ASCI files, that contain so-called program statements. They are created using a text editor—a program, such as EMACA, that enables the user to create and edit text files. These files are also called the source program, and are denoted with the file extension ".pas" or ".p.". The text must then be compiled to turn it into a file capable of generating an action. Pascal programs can be compiled using the compiler called pc.

The basic format of every Pascal program is the same. The "PROGRAM" is always the first word of a Pascal program and is a keyword. The designation "TITLE" refers to the

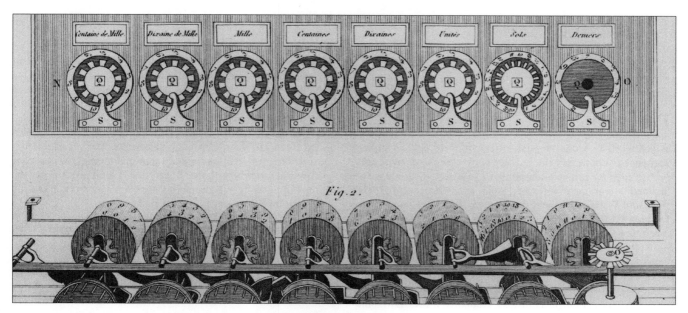

**Illustration of Blaise Pascal's calculating machine, made in 1642, called La Pascaline**

name that the programmer gives to the program. It is an **identifier**. There are rules concerning the format and length of the identifier. The "INPUT/OUTPUT" statement states what the program will do. Data is inputted from the keyboard and outputted to the screen. The begin statement defines the starting point of the program and provides a means of grouping statements together. All statements that are between the begin and end **commands** are considered part of the same group or block. The end statement must always be the final statement

A recent Pascal innovation is a revitalized system for the **Windows** operating environment. Called Delphi, the system's graphical **design** tools permit a much more rapid assembly of graphical interfaces than is possible using the C and C++ programming languages.

*See also* C; C++; Java; Modula

# PASCALINE

The *Pascaline*was a mechanical adding machine, or rather a family of such machines, designed by **Blaise Pascal** (1623–1662). Only one true mechanical **calculator**, Schickard's "calculating clock," had been created before **Pascal** invented the Pascaline, and Pascal almost certainly never saw Schickard's device or even heard how it worked. Thus Pascal and Schickard must both be credited with independent invention of the "first" true calculator. However, Pascal has the distinction that a large number—about 50—of his adding machines were actually produced and used.

Pascal's father was a tax collector, and put his son to work adding columns of tax figures. The tedium of this job moved Pascal to conceive the basic **design** of his adding machine when he was 19 years old. By today's standards the

Pascaline was crude: a shoebox-size device that could add base-10 (ordinary decimal) numbers anywhere from 6 to 8 digits long, depending on the individual Pascaline. The mechanism inside the box used gear positions to represent numbers. Addends were entered by hand, and carries from one column to the next were propagated internally by falling weights lifted and dropped by pins attached to the gears. The device did work, but somewhat unreliably; a slight knock could generate unwanted carries by causing the weights to fall prematurely.

Subtraction was accomplished by adding the nine's-complement version of the number to be subtracted. (See the article on **Two's Complement Arithmetic** in this volume for an explanation of how subtraction can by accomplished by adding complements.) Multiplication was performed by repeated additions, and division by repeated subtractions. Although these techniques may seem crude, they correspond rather closely to those employed inside the **central processing unit (CPU)** of a modern computer. In a modern CPU, the adder is the device on which all arithmetic operations are based: subtraction is often achieved by adding numbers in two's-complement format, multiplication by repeated additions, and division by repeated subtractions. In the case of the Pascaline, the human **operator** had to perform all those manipulations of the adder which in a CPU are performed electronically by microcode, control lines, registers, and the like. Indeed, the fact that everything the Pascaline did was the result of direct manual intervention by the human operator is what made it an adding machine rather than a true computer: it was not programmable. Still, it was a great achievement.

Unlike Schickard's "clock," knowledge of which was lost in the European wars of the period, the Pascaline directly inspired further work on calculating machines by Leibniz, Samuel Morland, and others. Pascal is also known for his work in pure mathematics, especially geometry and early probability theory, and for his religious and philosophical writings, including the classic Penseées (1670).

*See also* Adder; Leibniz's mechanical multiplier; Schickard's calculating clock; Two's complement

# PASSWORD

A password is a confidential, often arbitrary, and unspaced sequence of characters entered by a computer user to verify his or her identity when attempting to log onto restrictive (or "locked") computer software, such as systems, programs, files, and Web browsers. It is similar to the secret **code** that a banking customer uses to gain **access** to an automatic teller machine (ATM).

Passwords are instituted as a security device in order to restrict access to only authorized users of private and/or sensitive software. Within these secured pieces of computer software, the prospective user first encounters some type of a *password protection* program that compares a user ID (some unique identification) and a password with a stored list of authorized codes for that particular user. (A password protection program employs the use of passwords as a means of allowing only authorized users access to computer software.) If the user ID and password are legitimate, the system authenticates the user's entry and allows the now authorized user access to only that particular software at a pre-approved security level. To prevent unauthorized users from gaining access to software by random luck, most password protection systems restrict the number of attempts that a user has to input a correct password. The password is normally a combination of alphabetic, numeric, and punctuation (or other similar characters). A possible password is to use a mnemonic device (something that is easy to remember but has no significance to the general population) followed by a series of numbers that has some relevance to the user. For example, a computer user might combine the first letter from each word of the sentence ("My cat is named Tinker Bell") with the user's birthday ("May 14th, 1953") to produce "McinTB531405" as the user's password.

A password is typically between four and 16 characters, depending on how the computer system is set up. Most users create passwords that are difficult to guess in order to maintain a level of security against computer "hackers" who try to gain access to restricted information. Unfortunately, many people choose a password that is easy to remember, such as their name or their initials. This is one reason why it is sometimes easy to break into computer software. It is, therefore, recommended not to use words that are: (1) easily guessed (i.e., social security number, birthday, or maiden name), (2) found in the dictionary, (3) currently newsworthy or historically relevant, (4) similar to a previous password, (5) only letters, and (6) difficult to remember. In fact, some people, called "crackers," write programs in order to discover passwords by using lists of commonly chosen passwords such as last names spelled forwards and backwards. To protect against such dishonest practices passwords should optimally be a mixture of upper and lower case letters or digits that avoid proper names and real words.

Four major threats to computer information are countered with the help of passwords: (1) theft of **data**, such as military secrets from government computers; (2) vandalism, including the destruction of data from computer **viruses**; (3) fraud, such as employees at financial institutions switching monies into special accounts; and (4) invasion of privacy, such as the illegal accessing of protected personal (e.g., medical and financial) data from large **databases**. The primary use of passwords for computer system administrators is to electronically track and record the access to, and activities of, the various users of their computer system in order to maintain the highest level of security within that software.

*See also* Computers and privacy; Computer spying; Data security; Hacking

# PATTERN MATCHING

Pattern matching is a basic search mechanism. The term pattern matching refers to the process of locating a specific pattern inside **data**.

When the pattern of data is a collection of groups of data known as a **string** (a series of characters that are manipulated as a unit), the pattern matching is called string matching. The location of a certain string having a certain length in a text of much longer length is an example of string matching.

A variety of search formulas, or **algorithms**, has been devised for string matching. These algorithms make use of a process known as hashing. In hashing, a number, also called a hash, is generated from a string via one of the devised formulas. The mathematical derivation process renders it unlikely that some other string will produce the same **value**. The number and its corresponding string form an index, called a **hash table**, to which a search formula can be applied to quickly yield the **record** of interest.

Pattern matching extends beyond text. In recent years, a flow of high-quality research on pattern matching has opened up this area to new applications. Pattern recognition is an important field of computer science, concerned with the recognition of visual and audio patterns. Such pattern matching is vital to **optical character recognition**, **voice recognition**, **holographic storage** of data, and handwriting recognition. In the disciplines of molecular biology and bioinformatics, it is important to search out similar sequences of the bases that comprise genetic material along with the amino acids that comprise proteins, in order to elucidate the structure and the function of the macromolecules.

Other areas that benefit from pattern matching techniques are **information retrieval**, **data compression**, and security. Quality control of on-line **databases** is important, especially as it concerns the retrieval of information. Variations in spelling of a word and misspellings decrease the fidelity of retrieval. The technique of approximate string matching can help increase the efficiency and accuracy of information retrieval. Data compression relies upon the recognition of repeated patterns of text, digital or audio information. Two compression techniques that use pattern matching are run-length encoding and Huffman encoding.

Run-length encoding uses pattern matching to identify sequences where the same information is repeated, and then replaces each sequence by an interpretable **code**. For example, sequences of zeros could be identified and replaced in the run-length code by a single zero followed by a number indicating the number of zeros in the original string—an original sequence of "0 0 0 0" would be run-length encoded as "0 4". When done for an entire file, the file is significantly compressed. An example of a run-length scheme is PackBits, which was created for Macintosh users.

Huffman encoding is named after D.A. Huffman, who developed the procedure in the 1950's. The Huffman scheme is based on the frequency of occurrence of characters in **ASCII** text. For example, in a typical section of text, the most common characters are lower case letters, the space, and the carriage return. The Huffman scheme assigns a probability of occurrence to each character and then arranges equal probabilities into common groups. The information is recovered from these probability groups in order to restore the original text. While efficient, the algorithms involved are complex and are not within the domain of the typical user.

Pattern matching is important in **data security**, particularly in the encryption of data. Recognition of data patterns and the assigning of interpretable codes to these patterns enable data conversion into a code that is unrecognizable to a human. The recipient is, however, able to program the conversion of the compressed patterns to the original and recognizable text.

Visual pattern matching represents a particular challenge. A computer image consists of pixels instead of continuous functions, such as a string, or a waveform, such as in an audio spectrum. The gray-scale image typically used for visual pattern matching is a difficult medium from which to discern a pattern of similar intensity. Typically, two matices of pixel values are collected. One matrix contains the gray-scale values of the image. The other matrix contains the gray-scale values from a test image—a background level of values. Gray-scale correlation algorithms, which focus on the differing intensities, or shades of gray, of the pixels, are adversely affected by processing steps in image analysis, such as the normalization of light intensity over the entire image. Geometric pattern matching, which acquires information from the edge of a pattern in an image, eases the detection and matching of image information.

As the quantity of data on databases increases and the electronic transmission of data continues to grow, the ability to recognize data patterns will also continue to increase in importance.

*See also* Hash table; Holographic storage technology; Optical character recognition; Pretty good privacy; Voice recognition

# PERCEPTRONS

The perceptron is a special type of neural network that is especially useful for recognizing and classifiying various types of patterns. The simplest perceptron is the single layer perceptron, developed by Rosenblatt in 1958, which is capable of classifying linearly separable patterns as explained below. More complicated perceptrons involve hidden layers and additional nonlinearities introduced into neuronal output functions. In the 1970's, after the breakthrough discovery of the back propagation algorithm used to train these multilayer perceptrons, this particular class of **neural networks** gained popularity and were successfully used in many pattern classification problems.

Like any neural network, a perceptron consists of a set of nodes, or neurons. Each neuron N has a set of inputs $x_i$ and one output which can subsequently serve as the input to another neuron. Each input is multiplied by a weight $w_i$. The neuron N computes the weighted sum of its inputs and yields as output some **function** of this weighted sum. Usually this function is a step function centered around zero, or a more smooth sigmoidal threshold function. In a multilayer perceptron, the nodes are ordered in layers, with the first layer being the input layer, and the last layer being the output layer. There may be many intervening hidden layers of neurons inbetween. For any given input, the network propagates signals through the hidden layers forward to the output layer, whose neuron values give the result of the computation. For example a neural network trained to recognize enemy tanks could have as its set of possible inputs a small bitmap image. This network could then have two outputs, one which will yield a large output **value** if it recognizes its input image to be a tank, whereas the other one will have a large value if the network's input is some other, less threatening image.

Again, the simplest perceptron is the single layer perceptron, whose behavior can be understood quantitatively. Such a neural network consists of a single neuron with p inputs $x_1,...,x_p$ and a single output O. Here O is simply the sum over i of the product $w_i x_i$ where the weights $w_i$ characterize the properties of the perceptron. One should think of the set of inputs $X = (x_1,...,x_p)$ as a p-dimensional vector space. Then it can be seen that the perceptron can classify this set of inputs into two classes $C_1$ or $C_2$, where the perceptron yields a positive output for inputs in $C_1$ and a negative output for inputs in $C_2$. Futhermore, from a geometric viewpoint, the class $C_1$ is simply the set of inputs that lie on the positive side of the hyperplane defined by $W^TX = 0$. Here $W = (w_1,...,w_p)$ are the weights thought of as a vector and $W^TX$ is the dot product of W and X. Similarly $C_2$ is the set of inputs that lie on the negative side of the same hyperplane. Two classes of inputs that lie on separate sides of a hyperplane are said to be linearly separable. Thus the set of classes that a single layer perceptron can distinguish are exactly those that are linearly separable. Indeed given any two linearly separable classes, there exists an algorithm to train the perceptron to classify these patterns. The result of the training is to find the correct set of weights that define the separating hyperplane $W^TX=0$. The perceptron convergence theorem guarantees that this algorithm will work as long as the two classes are linearly separable. Otherwise the single layer perceptron cannot classify non-linearly separable patterns and one must resort to the more involved case of multilayer perceptrons and backpropagation.

*See also* Neural networks

# PERIPHERALS

A computer as a whole consists of both **hardware** and software. The hardware includes such items as the **central processing unit** (**CPU**), the computer's primary storage (RAM), and other hardware devices such as disk drives, monitor, keyboard, **printer**, and the like. Of these, all hardware devices other than the CPU and the RAM are generically referred to as peripherals. The use of this term reflects a great bias in **computer architecture** and hardware **design**, where the CPU and its immediate environment are considered to be central to computing, and everything else is merely an **object** in the periphery. To some extent it is sensible to give importance to the CPU, of course, but there also a case to be made for why the excessive fixation on the CPU is unhealthy. It is certainly true that peripherals have improved little over the years compared with the tremendous advances made by CPUs over the same time, so much so that a quantum leap in computer performance would probably occur more by improving the performance of peripherals than anything else.

A computer is traditionally held to perform four functions that are characteristic of it—any device that performs these functions is a computer, and any that does not, is not. These functions are input, processing, output, and storage. Of these, processing is the province of the CPU, aided by the RAM, and the others are the province of the peripherals.

**Input and output** are generally done by peripherals that interact with humans, and must either convert **data** given by humans into computer-accessible form, or else must present the results of computation in a form that humans find useful. The most common peripherals used for input are devices such as keyboard, **mouse**, joystick, microphone, touch-screen, and so on. In special circumstances, such as computers that are designed to work with physically challenged people, or computers that are designed to work with industrial equipment, we may have other kinds of peripherals that are used for input.

Peripherals that produce output for humans are most commonly of two kinds, those that produce screen output, or those that produce paper output. Screen output is most commonly preferred in case of non-final results, where the results of change must be continually updated on an ongoing basis. Screen output devices are commonly called monitors, and are of two major kinds: cathode ray tube (CRT) and liquid crystal display (LCD). CRT monitors use largely the same technology as household television sets, although they have a much higher resolution. They are generally much heavier, use more power, and are part of non-portable desktop machines. LCD monitors are lighter, and are similar to displays used on digital wristwatches or portable calculators. They are lighter and are hence used in portable handheld and laptop devices, use much less

power and hence can be supplied by battery, and are more expensive.

Paper output via peripherals comes largely from printers, which themselves are of two major kinds: impact and non-impact. In case of impact printers, there is a physical impact of a print head or some such device against the sheet of paper on which the printed impression is to be conveyed. Examples of impact printers include dot-matrix printers, current into the early 1990s but now mostly gone, and line printers, which were used in the 1960s and later but are nowhere used now. Impact printers were standard technology upto the 1970s, but have lost favor since. Part of the reason for this is that owing to their large numbers of moving parts, they suffer greater wear and tear and have greater need for maintenance. The print quality is also often not very good, and is restricted besides to certain font styles or sizes, which is an inconvenient restriction for **desktop publishing**, high quality **typesetting**, or when working with images, **graphics**, or foreign language material. Impact printers can also be quite noisy, which restricts their use in environments where noise is undesirable. Non-impact printers, such as laser printers, have become the standard technology, as they remedy all these ills.

Peripherals for storage are the secondary (persistent) storage devices on which it is possible to store data that survives even after the computer is turned off. Storage devices in common use can be classified in either of two ways: as using magnetic storage versus optical storage, or as offering sequential **access** versus random access. Magnetic storage devices, such as hard drives, disk drives, and tape drives record the information to be stored in the form of magnetic fields generated in a suitably designed stable artifact such as a diskette or a cassette tape, and by reading these magnetic fields when the diskette or cassette is played back, it is possible to recover the data that was encoded. Optical storage typically is in the form of using laser beams to record and read bits (0s and 1s) of information. Magnetic storage media are susceptible to distortion or loss by exposure to strong electric or magnetic fields, but have the advantage that they can be erased and re-written relatively easily. Optical storage is generally more reliable, but optical media may be harder to write to, and may not allow for as many erasures and re-writes as magnetic media do.

Sequential access is the restriction that data can only be read in the exact sequence in which they were recorded; an example of this is cassette tape drives, where the tape has to be forwarded or rewound to access non-contiguous data. Cassette players for music have largely given way to CD players because people have found that it is a hassle to have to rewind or fast-forward the tape when one wants to listen to songs in some arbitrary order of personal choice. For like reason, tape drives are no longer the mainstay of secondary storage, and are used only for limited purposes like creating system backups that do not have to be accessed at random. Random access devices such as hard drives and CD drives are suitable for most uses where individual items stored need to be read.

*See also* Central Processing Unit (CPU); Computer architecture; Computer science and electrical engineering; Hardware

# PERL

Perl is an acronym for Practical Extraction and Report Language. The language, which was authored by Larry Wall in 1987, is designed to scan text files, extract information from those files, and print out reports based on the extracted information.

Following its 1987 release, new versions appeared almost yearly, culminating in the 1995 release of a Perl version for the Macintosh computer. Versions also exist for **DOS** and **Linux** based operating systems. Because of its strong text processing capabilities, Perl has become one of the most popular languages for writing so-called **CGI** scripts. CGI, or **Common Gateway Interface**, enables Web servers to react with users in a dynamic and responsive way. Other scripting languages are Python and Eiffel.

Perl is an interpretive language—it executes instructions by translating the instructions into an intermediate form, rather the conversion directly into **machine language** (called compiling). An interpreted language can be beneficial to the programmer, as it allows the modification and testing of small sections of the program. Another benefit of an interpretive language like Perl is its educational **value**, because of its interactive capability.

Although optimized for scanning text, Perl can also deal with binary **data**. Sophisticate **pattern matching** techniques enable the rapid scanning of large amounts of data. Unlike most **Unix** utilities, Perl does not arbitrarily limit the size of the data. The amount of data that can be accommodated is limited only by the **memory** available. Version 5 of Perl represented a nearly complete rewrite of the earlier versions, and included features that enhanced its utility, such as simplified grammar, which allows the user to learn the language progressively as experience builds. Also, the program can resolve local ambiguities, so that rigid **programming** definition of every character is not required. The overarching theme of Perl is that the language is designed to be useable and efficient, rather than to produce a program that is technically elegant to the programmer.

Perl was conceived as a language designed for change. The latest version contains an extension system that, much like the module system of Linux, allows the continued development of the language without the necessity to change the core language. The user is able to tailor the language to their particular use, while not changing the core that is more global in its use.

The applications for Perl include financial analysis, analysis of population statistics, and, in the biological world, the Human Genome Project. In the latter, Perl enabled sequencing data from various laboratories to be scanned, patterns recognized, and a cohesive entire sequence assembled.

*See also* Open source software; Shareware and freeware

# PERLIS, ALAN J. (1922-1990)

*American computer scientist*

Alan J. Perlis is best known for his innovative work in computer **programming** languages and compilers. Perlis was a keen educator and helped set up several computer departments at universities throughout the United States.

Alan J. Perlis was born in Pittsburgh, Pennsylvania, in 1922. After a local education Perlis received a B.S. in chemistry from the Carnegie Institute of Technology (now the Carnegie Melon University) in 1943. Immediately upon completing his studies Perlis joined the war effort, serving in the United States Army Air Force until 1945. Upon cessation of hostilities Perlis continued his studies and he was awarded an M.S. in 1949 and a Ph.D. in 1950. Both of these degrees were in mathematics from the Massachusetts Institute of Technology (MIT). Between 1948 and 1949, while at MIT, Perlis was employed as an adviser on Project Whirlwind between. (Project Whirlwind was originally conceived as an analog computer flight simulator, but with the advent of **ENIAC** and **EDVAC** it was changed to be a digital device.) Perlis returned to it in 1952 after a period at the Ballistic Research Laboratories, Aberdeen Proving Ground, where he worked at the Multi Machine Computing Laboratory. At the end of 1952 Perlis became an assistant professor of mathematics at Purdue University as well as the director of the Digital Computer Center Laboratory, which he founded. During this time Perlis worked extensively on the development of the Internal Translator (IT) **compiler**. In 1956 Perlis moved to become an assistant professor of mathematics at the Carnegie Institute of Technology (now Carnegie Melon University), and while there he founded the Computation Center of which he was made the first director. Perlis became chair of the Department of Mathematics in 1960. During his time at Carnegie Perlis completed his development of the IT compiler. In 1957 Perlis became the chair of the Association for Computing Machinery (ACM) committee for developing a common universal programming language. As part of this work the team developed Algol58 in 1958. This was subsequently modified to produce Algol60, and Perlis was involved in this and subsequent versions of the Algol language. The development of both Algol58 and Algol60 led to other languages, as well as establishing standards in the development of programming languages. In 1965 Perlis was given a chair in the computer science department at the Carnegie Institute of Technology, a department which he had proposed. Perlis retained this position until 1971. At the same time he was also the chairman of the department. In 1966 Perlis received the ACM's first Turing Award. In 1971 Perlis was made Eugene Higgins Professor of Computer Science at Yale and was chair of the computer science department between 1976 and 1980. During this period he spent a year, 1977 to 1978, at the California Institute of Technology as the Gordon and Betty Moore Professor of Computer Science. Throughout his time at Yale Perlis devoted part of his research studies to the programming language **APL** (A Programming Language). When Perlis died in 1990 he was still a professor of computer science at Yale.

Perlis had a long association with the ACM. In 1958 he founded their journal *Communications of the ACM*, of which he was also the first editor until 1962. From 1962 to 1964 he was president of the ACM and in 1966 he received the society's first Turing Award, for which his citation reads, "For his influence in the area of advanced programming techniques and compiler construction." In 1973 Perlis was elected as a fellow of the American Academy of Arts and Sciences and in 1976 he became a member of the National Academy of Engineering. Throughout his life Perlis published widely. He believed strongly in the educational thrust of his role and felt that publications would help in the spread of his work. As well as articles for numerous research journals Perlis published several text books on programming, compilers, and **computer languages**. In 1984 Perlis received the AFIPS Education Award. In 1985 Perlis was given the IEEE Computer Pioneer Award for significant contributions to concepts and developments in the electronic computer field, which have clearly advanced the state of the art in computing. Alan J. Perlis died in 1990 aged 67. In his **memory** Yale now holds an annual Alan J. Perlis Symposium, and Carnegie Melon University established the Alan J. Perlis Chair of Computer Science in 1991.

*See also* Algol60; Algol68; APL; Compiler; Simulation

## PERMISSION, ACCESS

Permission, in the context of **access**, refers to the privilege to use some computer information. The use can be restricted to the viewing of information for some users, while, for other users, the ability to manipulate or alter the information may be granted.

Many operating systems, particularly those serving multiple users, have several different types of access privileges—a hierarchical scheme of permissions—that can be granted or denied to certain individual users or to groups of users.

Permission can be granted by means of a **password**. A password is a series of characters, selected by the user and known to them and a system administrator if one exists. If the user supplies the correct password, access is granted to the particular file, program or computer. Passwords are very useful in computer systems where there are many users, ensuring that unauthorized entry does not occur.

*See also* Data security; Password

## PERSONAL AREA NETWORK (PAN)

A personal area network (PAN) is a technological concept that would enable information to be passed from person to person or from a person to a machine, by touch. Technology being developed principally at the Alamaden Research Center of the International Business Machine Corporation would, in effect, turn the human body into a copper cable. A PAN would enable someone to identify themselves to a device they own, such as a car or telephone, and eliminate the need for keys or coins.

The genesis of the PAN was the development of the **data** glove in 1982 by Thomas Zimmerman. Although initially used more for game purposes, the data glove spawned the idea that the body could be used as a conduit for the transmission of electronic information. This idea gained credence when the **IBM** researchers worked with the renowned cellist Yo Yo Ma

to expand the capabilities of his instrument. In the course of their work, the researchers found that interference with the electrical circuitry was due to passage of some of the signal through Ma's body.

By establishing a PAN, a person might become capable of being the conduit that will enable cross-talk with the information and communication devices he or she carries—pagers, cell phones, personal digital assistants and watches. The contact number of an incoming page could be automatically identified in the digital assistant and the number dialed on the cell phone.

Another form of a PAN can link one portable device to another device without the necessity of a human as the connecting bridge. The standards and specifications for the technology goes by the name of Bluetooth. Its origins date back to 1994 when the Swedish mobile phone maker, Ericsson, was joined by Nokia, Toshiba, **Intel** and IBM to develop the technology

The technology relies on radio waves with a frequency of 2.4 GHz. The radio waves allow the interconnection of devices positioned close together—within a radius of 10 meters. A network, known as a Piconet, can accommodate eight devices. In turn, up to 10 Piconets can overlap to form a Scatternet. In a Scatternet, up to 80 appliances could be linked.

Bluetooth's limited broadcast range is not suited for the establishment of wireless local area networks. However, the technology is well positioned as the hub of a PAN, where a single user could establish linkages with devices in close proximity, such as in a home office.

With still largely in the development stage, a Bluetooth-enabled cellular phone has been marketed by Ericsson. The phone uses Bluetooth to communicate with a headset. A user wearing the headset can use the phone, even if the phone is, for example, in a briefcase. The market for such technology may be very vast, with some predictions forecasting 1.4 billion users by 2005.

*See also* Computers and privacy; Computers and music; Cybernetics; Wireless networks

## PERSONAL COMPUTER

The personal computer (abbreviated PC) is a computer that does not need to be connected to a larger computer in order to operate, and is capable of repetitively and efficiently performing calculations and instructions while being operated by an individual. It is smaller, less expensive, and easier to use than other types of computers such as minicomputers, mainframes, and **supercomputers**. The PC traces its ancestry to the mainframes and minicomputers of the 1950s and 1960s, which were all based on **microprocessor** technology that enabled manufacturers to place an entire central-processing-unit (**CPU**) on one **semiconductor** chip in order to perform all arithmetic, logic, and control functions.

In the 1960s, when microcomputers (they were not yet called personal computers) were evolving, they were distinguished from other computers by their size—they were smaller than minicomputers, which in turn were smaller than mainframes. While early mainframes needed the floor space of a house, minicomputers were the size of that home's refrigerator; microcomputers could fit on a desk inside that house. At that time the term microcomputer referred to any machine with the characteristics of being: (1) digital (rather than analog), (2) user programmable, (3) mostly automatic, (4) transportable, (5) sold either as a commercially manufactured product, an unassembled kit, or a published kit plan, and (6) did not require a programmer or technician to operate.

The following is a brief outline of microcomputer development, which eventually lead to the personal computer. Conceived in 1949 by Edmund Berkeley and built in 1950, the Simon was called a "mechanical brain." Although not considered the first personal computer, it did satisfy the microcomputer requirements mentioned above. Built in 1965, Digital Equipment Corporation's PDP-8 inspired Steven Gray to found the Amateur Computer Society (ACS) in 1966. The birth of the ACS is often thought to mark the dawn of personal computing. Even so, the PDP-8 is still not usually considered the first personal computer.

Up until the early 1970s most people thought of a computer only as a large, sluggish "number cruncher"; a mammoth device, contained in a glass-enclosed, climate-controlled room, that consumed vast amounts of electricity processing the **data** on punch cards, storing information on magnetic tape spools, and then printing the results on green-and-white-striped paper. Most people never imagined that a computer could be small enough to sit on a desk. But in 1969 **Intel** Corporation developed a CPU chip that could receive data and perform simple functions; by 1971 the chip had became a microprocessor, the first single-chip CPU that performed complex calculations. The Intel chip owed its existence to the miniaturization of integrated electronic circuits, which allowed computer manufacturers to increase computer performance and decrease expense. The Hewlett Packard HP 9830, introduced in 1972, was the first desktop "all-in-one" computer, but few people knew about it because HP marketed it exclusively to the scientific sector. The Xerox Alto, designed in 1973, was never commercially produced because Xerox's Palo Alto Research Center development team could not convince management of its usefulness. The Alto is often considered that era's most innovative **design** because it possessed a **mouse**, a point-and-click graphic user interface (**GUI**), an object-oriented operating system, and fast networking with the first ethernet cards.

None of the largest computer corporations of that time would introduce the world to the modern PC. Those behemoths did not see financial **value** in manufacturing an inexpensive product that might replace the mainframes that they were successfully selling. Fortunately, idealistic individuals succeeded where corporate leaders failed, eventually introducing the first personal computer.

In 1975 Micro Instrumentation and Telemetry Systems (MITS) introduced the **Altair** 8800, enabling hobbyists to assemble their own computers. It had no monitor, no keyboard, no **printer**, and couldn't store data, but it created enormous demand. Although not the first available microcomputer, it is often considered the computer that began the personal computer industry. MITS went out of business, but its existence helped two young software programmers, **Bill Gates** and **Paul Allen** (whose version of **BASIC** was used for the Altair), in the creation of **Microsoft** Corporation.

In 1977 American entrepreneur **Steven Jobs** and computer designer **Stephen Wozniak** created the **Apple** II, a fairly inexpensive computer with a keyboard, monitor, and **modem**. It was the first personal computer mass-produced and preassembled in a factory and the first capable of color **graphics**. Apple Computer incorporated the Visicalc spreadsheet program on the Apple II, enabling users for the first time to change one number and watch the effect it had on the entire budget. This combination made the Apple II a standard business device, and today it is considered the first "true" personal computer, largely because it proved that computers were more than just "expensive calculators."

Even with all of the successes of the early PC manufacturers, the PC was not seen as a serious business tool until, in 1981, **International Business Machines** (**IBM**) introduced the IBM PC. It was the first computer to stamp "personal computer" on its name and is often called "the computer that launched an industry". The IBM PC was designed with an **open architecture**, meaning that other manufacturers could create similar machines, or clones, that would also run IBM PC-designed software. The IBM PC and its clones soon became the PC standard. Because old-time **mainframe** computer maker IBM sold this product, the PC became a legitimate business tool. The Apple Lisa (1982) and Macintosh (1984) featured the first **graphical user interface** (GUI), which enabled a "point-and-click" mouse to select **commands**, point to icons, call up files, start programs, and perform other routine tasks; this eliminated the need to memorize the often arcane and complex commands required by the IBM PC's operating system, **DOS**.

Today PCs generally consist of (1) a microprocessor, the CPU that directs logical and arithmetical functions and runs computer programs through electronic circuits; (2) **memory** to temporarily store programs and data, and mass storage devices (such as hard-, floppy-, and **CD-ROM** drives) to permanently store information; (3) a keyboard and mouse; 4) a video monitor; (5) a printer; (6) a sound-adapter and speakers; and (7) a modem to connect to the **Internet**. But its parts do not define the personal computer because many of these same components are common across the spectrum of computers, from calculators to supercomputers.

## PÉTER, RÓZSA (1905-1977)
*Hungarian mathematician*

Rózsa Péter was one of the early investigators in the field of recursive functions, a branch of mathematical logic. Recursive functions are those mathematical functions whose values can be established at every point, for whole numbers one and above. These functions are used to study the structure of number classes or functions in terms of the complexity of the calculations required to determine them, and have useful applications to computers and other automatic systems. Péter wrote two books and numerous papers on recursive functions, which are related to **Alan Turing** 's theory of **algorithms** and machines and to **Kurt Gödel** 's **undecidability** theorem of self-referential equations. Péter also wrote a popular treatment of mathematics, *Playing with Infinity,* which was translated into fourteen languages. A teacher and teacher-training instructor before her appointment to a university post, Péter won national awards for her contributions to mathematics education and to mathematics.

Péter was born in Budapest on February 17, 1905. She received her high school diploma from Mária Terézia Girls' School in 1922, then entered the university in Budapest to study chemistry. Although her father, an attorney, wanted her to stay in that field, Péter changed to the study of mathematics. One of her classmates was László Kalmár, her future teacher and colleague. Péter graduated from the university in 1927, and for two years after graduation she had no permanent job, but tutored privately and took temporary teaching assignments.

In 1932, Péter attended the International Mathematics Conference in Zurich, where she presented a lecture on mathematical logic. She published papers on recursive functions in the period 1934 to 1936, and received her Ph.D. summa cum laude in 1935. In 1937, Péter became a contributing editor of the *Journal of Symbolic Logic.* Péter lost her teaching position in 1939 due to the Fascist laws of that year; Hungary was an ally of Nazi Germany and held similar purges of academics. Nevertheless, she published papers in Hungarian journals in 1940 and 1941.

In 1943, Péter published her book, *Playing with Infinity,* which described ideas in number theory, geometry, calculus and logic, including Gödel's undecidability theory, for the layman. The book, many copies of which were destroyed by bombing during World War II, could not be distributed until 1945. The war claimed the life of Péter's brother, Dr. Nicholas Politzer, in 1945, as well as the lives of her friend and fellow mathematician, Pál Csillag, and her young pupil, Káto Fuchs, who had assisted Péter with *Playing with Infinity.*

In the late 1940s, Péter taught high school and then became Head of the Mathematics Department of the Pedological College in Budapest. She also wrote textbooks for high school mathematics. In the fifties, Péter published further studies of recursive functions; her 1951 book, *Recursive Functions,* was the first treatment of the subject in book form and reinforced her status as "the leading contributor to the special theory of recursive functions," as S. C. Kleene observed in the *Bulletin of the American Mathematical Society.*

Péter was appointed Professor of Mathematics at Eötvös Loránd University in Budapest in 1955, where she taught mathematical logic and set theory. The official publication of *Playing with Infinity* occurred in 1957. In this book, she wrote in the preface, she tried "to present concepts with complete clarity and purity so that some new light may have been thrown on the subject even for mathematicians and certainly for teachers."

In the sixties and seventies, Péter studied the relationship between recursive functions and computer **programming**, in particular, the relationship of recursive functions to the pro-

gramming languages Algol and Lisp. Péter retired in 1975. She continued her research, however, publishing *Recursive Functions in Computer Theory* in 1976.

Péter's awards included the Kossuth Prize in 1951 for her scientific and pedological work, and the State Award, Silver Degree in 1970 and Gold Degree in 1973. Péter was a member of the Hungarian Academy of Sciences and was made honorary President of the János Bolyai Mathematical Association in 1975. Interested in literature, film and art as well as mathematics, Péter translated poetry from German and corresponded with the literary critic Marcel Benedek. She noted in *Playing with Infinity* that her mathematical studies were not so different from the arts: "I love mathematics not only for its technical applications, but principally because it is beautiful; because man has breathed his spirit of play into it, and because it has given him his greatest game—the encompassing of the infinite." Péter died on February 17, 1977.

# PETRI NET

A Petri net, also called a place-transition net, is a mathematical representation of concurrent systems—systems in which an activity of one component of the system can occur simultaneously with other component activities. Modeling of a system based on a Petri net can reveal information about the structure and behavior of that system.

Examples of concurrent systems are the dynamic structure of an atom, high-speed computers, air traffic control systems, chemical reactions, and economic systems. In a computer system, for example, peripheral devices, such as printers and tape drives may operate concurrently under the master control of the computer. In an economic system, manufacturers may be producing some products while retailers are selling other products, and customers are using still other products, all at the same time. In such concurrent systems, each component can be described independently of the other components, although interaction of the components is necessary for the functioning of the system as a whole. Each component also has its state of being, which can change with time.

This concurrent nature of activity makes modeling a challenge. The transfer of information or materials from one of the system components to another means that all component activities need to be synchronized while the transfer is occurring, although not necessarily before or after the time of transfer. Thus, one component may wait for the other. Other activities may occur in a random fashion. Describing such actions can be complex.

Petri nets were conceived by Carl Adam Petri in the 1960s to describe the complex activities of concurrent systems. Part of Petri's doctoral dissertation concerned the communication between components of computer systems. From his work came the basic concepts on which Petri net have developed.

In mathematical terms, a Petri net is a so-called four-tuple, consisting of a number of places (P, also the state of being of a component), an equal number of transitions (T, the change from one component state to another), an input **function** (IN) that defines the movement from one place to a **transition** (the beginning of a change of state of being), and an output function (OUT) that defines the movement from a transition to a place (the completion of a change in state). In a Petri net model, a place is denoted by a circle and a transition is denoted by a line.

Different arrangements of circles and lines are used to model various component activities, such as:

- sequential execution, where one transition requires the completion of a first transition
- conflict, where two component transitions are trying to occur but only one is acceptable
- concurrency, where component activities are occurring at the same time in a independent way
- synchronization, where component activities are occurring at the same time in a related way
- merging, where several transitions lead to the same place
- priorities, a sorting-out of transition event order so as to permit the overall system functioning to continue.

The power of Petri nets as an analytical modeling system has increased since the development of high-level Petri nets. Also known as Colored Petri nets, these permit very large models to be constructed, which can have separate but interconnected sub-models. Currently, an XML-based language called Petri net Markup Language is being developed to provide an information interchange format between Petri nets.

*See also* Automata theory; Concurrency; Transition

# PHOTONIC NETWORKS

Photonic networks, currently at the research stage, hold the potential of being able to utilize optical signals to transmit information. As with electrical signals, photonic signals would be capable of amplifying, switching, and processing signals. Photonics can, however, manipulate signals of very high bandwidth—far beyond the bandwidth achievable using electronics—resulting in a potential for exceptionally high information content.

Optical fiber cables enable great amounts of information to be transported over long distances at a much cheaper cost than using electrical cable or radio. The limitation to the amount of information carried in a photonic network currently is the **information processing** ability of the electronically driven computers at either end of the optical fibers. In the future, this electronic bottleneck would be removed by using photonic devices.

The development in early 2001 of an ultra-fast photonic switch is bringing the era of photonic devices closer to reality.

*See also* Dataflow

# PHYSICAL AND VIRTUAL MEMORY

Physical and **virtual memory** are forms of **memory** (internal storage of **data**). Physical memory exists on chips (RAM memory) and on storage devices such as hard disks. Before a process can be executed, it must first load into RAM physical memory (also termed main memory). Virtual memory is a process whereby data (e.g., **programming** code,) can be rapidly exchanged between physical memory storage locations and RAM memory. The rapid interchanges of data are seamless and transparent to the user. The use of virtual memory allows the use of larger programs and enables those programs to run faster.

In modern operating systems, data can be constantly exchanged between the hard disk and RAM memory via virtual memory. A process termed swapping is used to exchange data via virtual memory. The use of virtual memory makes it appear that a computer has a greater RAM capacity because virtual memory allows the **emulation** of the transfer of whole blocks of data, enabling programs to run smoothly and efficiently. Instead of trying to put data into often-limited volatile RAM memory, data is actually written onto the hard disk. Accordingly, the size of virtual memory is limited only by the size of the hard disk, or the space allocated to virtual memory on the hard disk. When information is needed in RAM, the exchanges system rapidly swaps blocks of memory (also often termed pages of memory) between RAM and the hard disk.

Modern virtual-memory systems replace earlier forms of physical file swapping and fragmentation of programs.

In a sense, virtual memory is a specialized secondary type of **data storage**, and a portion of the **hard drive** is dedicated to the storage of specialized virtual-memory files (also termed pages). The area of the hard drive dedicated to storing blocks of data to be swapped via virtual memory interface is termed the page file. In most operating systems, there is a preset size for the page file area of the hard disk, and page files can exist on multiple disk drives. Users of most modern operating systems can, however, vary the size of the page file to meet specific performance requirements. As with the page file size, although the actual size of the pages is preset, modern operating systems usually allow the user to vary the size of the page. Virtual memory pages range in size from a thousand bites to many megabytes.

The use of virtual memory allows an entire block of data or programming (e.g., an application process) to reside in virtual memory, while only the part of the **code** being executed is in physical memory. Accordingly, the use of virtual memory allows operating systems to run many programs and thus, increase the degree of multiprogramming within an operating system.

Virtual memory integration is accomplished through either a process termed demand-segmentation or through another process termed demand-paging. Demand-paging is more common because it is simpler in **design**. Demand-paging virtual-memory processes do not transfer data from disk to RAM until the program calls for the page. There are also anticipatory **paging** processes utilized by operating systems that attempt to read ahead and execute the transfer of data before the data is actually required to be in RAM. After data is paged, paging processes track memory usage and constantly **call** data back and forth between RAM and the hard disk. Page states (valid or invalid, available or unavailable to the **CPU**) are registered in the virtual page table. When **applications** attempt to **access** invalid pages, a virtual-memory manager that initiates memory swapping intercepts the page fault **message**. Rapid translation of virtual addresses into a real physical address is via a process termed mapping. Mapping is a critical concept to the virtual-memory process. Virtual-memory mapping works by linking real **hardware** addresses (a physical storage address) for a block or page of stored data to a virtual address maintained by the virtual-memory process. The registry of virtual address allows for the selective and randomized translation of data from otherwise serial reading drives. In essence, virtual-memory processes supply alternate memory addresses for data, and programs can rapidly utilize data by using these virtual addresses instead of the physical address of the data page.

Virtual memory is a part of many operating systems, including **Windows**, but is not a feature of **DOS**. In addition to increasing the speed of execution and operational size of programs (lines of code), the use of virtual memory systems provide a valuable economic benefit. Hard-disk memory is currently far less expensive than RAM memory. Accordingly, the use of virtual memory allows the design of high-capacity computing systems at a relatively low cost.

Although swaps of pages of data (specific lengths of data or clocks of data) via virtual-memory swaps between the hard drive and RAM memory are very fast,an over-reliance upon virtual-memory swaps can slow overall system performance. If the amount of the hard drive dedicated to storing page files is insufficient to meet the demands of a system that relies heavily on the exchange of data via virtual memory, it is possible for users to receive "OUT OF MEMORY" messages and faults, even though they have large amounts of unused hard disk space.

*See also* Multitasking; Software management; Thrashing

# PIPELINING

Pipelining is a technique used by advanced microprocessors where the **microprocessor** begins executing a second instruction before the first has been completed. In other words, several instructions are in the "pipeline" simultaneously, but each at a different processing stage within the microprocessor (also called the **central processing unit** (**CPU**)) or a **functional unit** of the CPU, such as the arithmetic logic unit (**ALU**). By performing this function, pipelining (or "pipeline processing" as it is sometimes called) is able to efficiently coordinate execution times of a microprocessor so that optimal use of the microprocessor is achieved. Pipelining can be compared to an automobile assembly line in which a car is assembled one step at a time throughout a line that may contain hundreds of stages. When a particular car is at a certain stage in the process, other cars are at various stages further on in the assembly process while others are being assembled at earlier

points along the line. In each case, all of the cars are going through the same assembly process but at different times relative to other cars. The salient point of this analogy is that just as it would be highly inefficient to have only one car on the entire assembly line at any one time, it is also inefficient to have only one instruction at any time being processed by the CPU, and hence the need for pipelining.

The method of pipelining assures that a second instruction begins to execute before the first instruction has completed. In this way, several instructions are in the "pipeline" simultaneously, each at a different processing stage. In order to perform these simultaneous functions, the pipeline is divided into instructional segments (or "stages"), where each stage can execute its **operation** concurrently with other stages. When a stage completes an operation, the result is passed on to the next stage in the pipeline and the next operation is fetched from the preceding stage. The final results of each instruction emerge at the end of the pipeline in rapid succession. The **control** unit of the computer's CPU directs this entire process of fetching and forwarding instructions (or **data**).

As an example of not taking advantage of pipelining, consider groups of unprocessed data taken out of storage. Instructions performed on each group might first "add" numbers together, and then secondly "multiply" these results by some constant. After the ALU performs these two distinct instructions on the first group, the processed data is placed back into storage. The addition operation could be called stage 1, and the multiplication operation could be called stage 2. The ALU would perform the two operations on the first group, store the result in **memory**, and only then pass the second group through the two operations. For small groups of numbers this would be adequate, but when performing calculations on huge groups of numbers this technique would be inefficient, because only one group of data is being processed at any one time.

Pipelining overcomes the source of inefficiency associated with the microprocessor by performing a "sequence" of operations. Going back to the previous example, the pipeline method would take the first group out of storage, perform a specific operation on it during stage 1, and move it to stage 2. As the result of the first group moving to stage 2, a second group is moved from storage into stage 1. The operations unique to stage 1 and stage 2 are then performed simultaneously on their respective groups. Now, a third group is taken from storage and placed into stage 1 while the results of the previous operations are moved ahead in the pipeline; the second group goes to stage 2, and the first group is returned to storage. All calculations are performed in this pipelining manner, with the specific stages within the ALU always operating on some group. Since the time within the ALU is a critical part of processing, it is essential that this time is made as efficient as possible. Pipelining coordinates this efficient "sequential" use of the microprocessor.

Pipelining is often combined with *instruction prefetch* (a technique to minimize the time a microprocessor spends waiting for instructions in an attempt to keep the pipeline busy). Pipelining is also sometimes divided into an instruction pipeline and an arithmetic pipeline. The *instruction pipeline* represents the stages in which an instruction is moved through the microprocessor, including its being fetched, perhaps buffered, and then executed. The *arithmetic pipeline* represents the parts of an arithmetic operation that can be broken down and overlapped as they are performed.

**Supercomputers** were some of the first computers that used pipelining. This was because supercomputers were specifically designed to perform many complex mathematical calculations as quickly as possible. Although at one time pipelining was a near-exclusive feature of supercomputers, it is now common in smaller computers, such as personal computers (PCs). For instance, Intel's line of Pentium® microprocessors that operates inside many PCs incorporate pipeline processing.

*See also* Central processing unit (CPU); Integrated circuit; Microprocessor; Supercomputers

# PL1 PROGRAMMING LANGUAGE

The PL1 **programming** language is a third-generation, procedural programming language that bears some resemblance to **FORTRAN** and **BASIC**. It is a general-purpose programming language that is versatile enough to be used in commercial, scientific, and technical applications.

PL1 was developed by **IBM** in the early 1960s in an attempt to combine the best features of Algol, FORTRAN, and **COBOL** into a new, all-purpose language. It was originally named New Programming Language (NPL) but was soon changed to PL1 to avoid confusion with the National Physical Laboratory in England.

PL1 is a comprehensive language that includes a number of common programming concepts. It is block-oriented, which helps programmers modularize their applications. PL1 supports standard control structures such as SELECT-WHEN-OTHERWISE and DO-WHILE. There is also built-in support for many common functions, including arithmetic computation, mathematical computation, **string** manipulation, **precision** handling, input/output (I/O), storage control, and date/time manipulation.

In addition to containing many of the best features of other programming languages, PL1 also has some unique features. The language is freeform text and has no reserved keywords. There are some words with specific meanings in specific instances, but PL1 determines the meaning of words from the context of their use. In addition PL1 defines the precision of its **data types** without regard to the operating system or **hardware**. These precision data types include real, complex, floating-point, fixed-point, signed, unsigned, binary, decimal, character, **bit**, graphic, and string.

Another one of PL1's novel features is the definition of four different storage classes. The data type of an **object** usually determines whether to use automatic, **static**, controlled, or based storage. The default storage **class** is automatic, which is allocated on entry to a block and freed upon exit. Static storage exists throughout the life of the program. Controlled storage must be explicitly allocated by the program. Based storage

provides a mapping for storage otherwise allocated or referenced, or may also be explicitly allocated and freed.

One of PL1's strongest areas is **exception handling** of error conditions detected by hardware, PL1 itself, or the operating system. PL1 allows exceptions to be intercepted and handled without interrupting execution of the program.

In order to serve a variety of programming purposes, PL1 evolved into a complex language. The complexity of the language as well as the supporting tools and diagnostics made writing and **debugging** PL1 programs somewhat burdensome. As newer programming languages have arrived, the popularity of PL1 has declined.

*See also* Programming languages, types

# POLYMORPHISM

The word "polymorphism" quite literally means "ability to take more than one form." Polymorphism in **object-oriented programming** specifically refers to the ability of a **programming** language deal with objects differently, depending on their **data** type or **class**.

More important, it is the ability of the programming language to redefine or override methods in base classes with new methods in derived classes. This means that methods in derived classes have identical names, input parameters, and return values as methods in the **base class** but the program can figure out which one to **call** in any given situation, depending on the exact type of the **object**.

As an example, given a base class ThreeDimensionalObject, polymorphism enables the programmer to define different methods for calculating the volume of the shape for any number of classes derived from ThreeDimensionalObject. So, derived objects such as "Cube," "Sphere," "Cone," and "Dodecahedron" will all support the "CalculateVolume()" **method**, but polymorphism means that the **compiler** will ensure that the right version of the method is called for any given object.

In **C++** the classes could be declared like this:

```
class ThreeDimensionalObject {
 public:
 virtual int CalculateVolume() const;
};

class Cube : public ThreeDimensionalObject {
 public:
 int CalculateVolume() const;
};

class Sphere : public ThreeDimensionalObject {
 public:
 int CalculateVolume() const;
};
```

The "virtual" keyword tells the compiler it can override the **function** "CalculateVolume()" in any derived classes. If the programmer now creates a Cube and a Sphere, she will be able to get the volume by calling the CalculateVolume() method.

Cube* myCube = new Cube();

Sphere* mySphere = new Sphere();

int cubeVol = myCube→CalculateVolume();

int sphereVol = mySphere→CalculateVolume();

However, it is also legal and possible to do this:

ThreeDimensionalObject* myObjPtr = myCube;

cubeVol = myCube→CalculateVolume();

myObjPtr = mySphere;

sphereVol = mySphere→CalculateVolume();

And the compiler will still call the correct method. This is because the compiler chooses which method to call depending on the type of the underlying object and not the type of the pointer.

Polymorphism is a requirement of any real object-oriented programming language. The polymorphism described above is often called "parametric polymorphism" to distinguish it from a second kind of polymorphism called "overloading," which allows the compiler to treat identical symbols ("operator overloading"), and functions ("function overloading") differently depending on the context in which they are being used.

# POP (POST OFFICE PROTOCOL)

Post Office Protocol (POP) is a client/server protocol that allows client **e-mail** software to retrieve e-mail from a server that receives and stores it. The first version of the protocol was issued in October 1984, and the most recent version, POP3, was introduced in November 1988.

A POP3 server provides e-mail services to e-mail client software. When an e-mail client needs to use the services of a POP3 server, it opens a connection over the **Internet** and waits for a greeting from the server. The sequence of a POP3 session progresses through three states—the Authorization state, the Transaction state, and the Update state.

In the Authorization state, the client receives a greeting from the server and sends the user name and **password** to **access** a specific mailbox. If the user name and password match the server's records, the server authorizes the client to access the e-mail messages.

In the Transaction state, the client requests to read the messages. The server opens the mailbox with an exclusive lock and transfers the messages to the computer running the e-mail client software. These messages can be read immediately or stored for future, offline reading.

The Update state begins when the client software terminates the POP3 session. The server removes e-mail messages marked as "deleted" by the client software and releases the lock on the mailbox. This completes the POP3 session.

*See also* E-mail; Protocols

# PORT

In general, a port is an interface on a computer through which the computer, or more precisely the computer's **central processing unit,** may be connected to a device. One type of port is termed an I/O port. I/O refers to Input/Output, the communications **channel** between the computer and the world. It is via the I/O port that **peripherals** such as printers, external floppy disk drives and monitors can be attached to the computer's processor.

The I/O port is a so-called parallel port. A parallel port is a port through which more than one **bit** of information can be transferred at a time. On personal computers, the I/O port is a Centronics interface that utilizes a 25-pin connector. Some I/O connections enable up to seven devices to be connected to a computer through the same port.

*See also* Input and output; Peripherals

# PORTAL

A portal is a web site that serves as an all-purpose entry point to the **Internet.** Designed with rich navigation structures, portals provide easy-to-use interfaces to access resources on the web and the content contained on the site itself. Portal designers seek to make the portal site the central place for users to find what they need on the web. Portals usually display ads to generate income and pay for the services they provide. Popular portals include Yahoo, CNET, and America Online's AOL.com.

### Services

Portals offer a broad array of resources and services, such as search engines, **e-mail,** news, discussion groups, classified ads, online shopping, stock quotes, weather, sports scores, white and yellow pages, and links to other useful or popular sites. Portals attempt to offer as many services as possible to retain large audiences, hoping that users will make the site their default home page or at least visit it often. The number and types of services portals provide are the defining difference between portals and other web sites.

### Special Types of Portals

Specialty portals have developed for specific audiences and industries. One such type is a corporate portal. Corporate portals are contained in intranets, or internal sites. They are used to help company employees access internal information as well as useful public web sites. Corporate portals also possess search engines and can be customized for various company divisions or groups. Corporate portals are usually restricted to information relevant to the company.

A vortal is a vertical industry portal. A vortal targets a specific industry, such as banking, medicine, computers, or pets. It offers services, information, research, and other resources particular to the industry to which it is catering. Vortals can be considered a hybrid cross between web portals and **intranet** portals. Vortals can also be business-to-business sites that provide a common site for buyers and sellers in a specific industry to interact.

### The Future of Portals

Some Internet analysts considered portals the future of the web and particularly intranets. The nature of portals as a central location for accessing information on the Internet reduces, what some may consider, unnecessary web surfing. Portals allow for the aggregation of a variety of content, such as documents and database queries, and can provide a front-end to software **applications** companies use. Portals also allow for scaling. As the amount of information available continues to grow, the ability to categorize and group information that portals provide may become essential.

# PORT, MEMORY

A **port memory**, also known as memory mapped I/O, is, along with port mapped I/O, a means to connect external devices to a computer's **central processing unit**.

In memory mapped I/O, each device has a separate address that is mapped into the system memory, along with **Random Access Memory** (RAM) and Read Only Memory (**ROM**). The machine's normal memory **access** instructions enables a device to be activated and used.

An advantage of memory mapped I/O is that every instruction that can convey information to memory can be used to manipulate an I/O device, such as a **printer** or a monitor. A disadvantage to this mode of **operation** is that the entire identifying address must be fully decoded for every device. For extensive addresses, this can add to **hardware** costs.

*See also* Peripheral devices; Port, I/O

# POS SYSTEM (POINT-OF-SALE)

The point-of-sale (POS) system is a computerized retail transaction system, such as the one commonly seen at supermarket checkout counters. POS is also sometimes called EPOS for "electronic point-of-sale" in order to emphasize the computerized character of the current point-of-sale system. This system may use personal computers (PCs) or other specialized terminals that are combined with electronic cash registers, **bar code** readers, optical scanners, magnetic strip readers, among others, for accurately and instantly recording transactions at the time and place of the sale, hence the term "point-of-sale."

A POS system may be connected to an **intranet** (a private network within a company or organization) via a centralized computer for such activities as inventory updating and credit checking, or it may be a stand-alone machine that stores transactions until they can be delivered or transmitted to the main computer for processing. Some of the point-of-sale operations performed by the POS system are reading product tags, updating inventory, and checking customer credit. It often also

includes such retail activities as merchandising techniques and aids, advertising displays, and the methods used to enable transactions. The total system generally includes the **hardware** and software that runs both the front counter and the back office **operation** of the business.

The following are important advantages of the POS system: (1) fully tested pre-installed hardware and software configurations, (2) same vendor/representative support for all system aspects such as training and technical maintenance and service, (3) more reliable than other systems, (4) few software conflicts because all terminals support the fully integrated POS software, (5) restricted **access** to the operating system so unauthorized modifications cannot be performed, (6) software accessible "keycode" to allow customized coding of the keyboard (with "keylock" to prevent unauthorized changes), (7) labeled function keyboard to increase **throughput** and reduce training (e.g., to input employee discounts), (8) lockable journal tape and diskette drive in order to prevent removal of sensitive information, (9) control totals kept in protected area of main **memory** (normally random-assess memory (RAM)), and (10) hardware and software error detection.

A POS system provides control over transactions, with access to a large amount of historic **data** for comparisons over periods of years, months, and weeks with regards to such thing as profitability on different retail lines, stock comparisons, and other important financial and marketing indicators. The system can also track inventory, provide efficient computer stock control and reordering, and automatically create order lists as needed (even adjusting quantities for seasonal demand).

*See also* Bar code

# POSTSCRIPT

Postscript is a **programming** language that describes the appearance of a printed page. Postscript describes the text and graphic elements on a page using mathematical shapes and curves. This results in higher resolution on the printed page than is achieved using the **ASCII** characters and bit-mapped images.

Adobe Systems developed Postscript and first released it with the **Apple** LaserWriter **printer** in 1985. It has since become a printing and imaging standard and has been designated by the **International Organization for Standardization** (**ISO**) as the standard page-description language.

Postscript is used by many desktop and midrange printers as well as commercial printing presses. It is device-independent, meaning that a single specification can take advantage of the resolution of multiple devices. For a printer or other output device to support Postscript, it must have a specialized interpreter with sufficient **memory** to support the execution of Postscript instructions. To print a page, a Postscript file is sent to the output device and executed within the Postscript interpreter. The Postscript interpreter creates the requested page image, and the drawing engine prints the image.

# PRECISION

Precision is the extent of detail (or "exactness") used in expressing a number. Precision is specified as the number of significant digits (or the number of decimal places) with which a quantity is reliably expressed and can be repeatedly expressed. For example, the **value** of pi ($\pi$, the circumference of a circle divided by that circle's diameter) is expressed with more precision when pi's value is stated as 3.14159285, rather than when pi is expressed as 3.14. Precision is related to, but different from, *accuracy*. Precision indicates "degree" of detail, while accuracy indicates "correctness" of detail. That is, accuracy involves how close to the real value a measurement is, or the degree to which the result of a calculation or measurement approximates the true value. Therefore, a value of pi stated as 3.14159285 has both more precision and more accuracy than a value of pi stated as 3.14 because it has more digits to the right of the decimal point and is closer to pi's actual value, respectively.

Precision is often used within computer **programming** when referring to values of floating-point numbers as being *single-precision* or *double-precision*. Used in this format, precision specifically refers to the number of bits used to hold the fractional part of the floating-point number. A **bit**, short for *bi*nary digi*t*, is the smallest unit of information used in a computer, where a single bit can represent only one of two values: zero (0) or one (1). The more precision a computer system uses, the more exactly it can represent fractional quantities. Normally, programming languages use one of the two options of single- or double-precision numbers for coding. The difference between the two is in the amount of storage space allowed for the value of a particular floating-point number. A double-precision number uses twice as many bits (to store that number) as a single-precision value, so it can represent fractional quantities much more precisely. Commonly, double-precision numbers are stored with 8 bytes (equivalent to two words) of computer **memory**, while single-precision numbers are stored with 4 bytes (equivalent to one word) of computer memory. The extra bits increase not only the precision but also the range of magnitudes that can be represented. The exact amount by which the precision and range of magnitudes are increased depends on what format the computer is using to represent floating-point values. Most computers use a standard format known as the "IEEE (Institute of Electrical and Electronics Engineers) floating-point format."

*See also* Bytes; Double-precision variable; Floating-point representation

# PREPROCESSOR

A preprocessor is a program that transforms **data** or a computer language into suitable input for another program or a **compiler**. A preprocessor performs preliminary operations on data, such as organization, formatting, and computation, before that data is passed on for further processing. For example, in the **C programming** language the line #define PI 3.14159 instructs the preprocessor to replace every occurrence of PI with the numerical **value** 3.14159. In the case of a computer program, a preprocessor may be used to transform a program into a simpler or less complete computer language, for example, transforming **C++** into C. This processing **operation** can detect and correct problems in **code** before the compiler can reject them.

Preprocessor operations can be similar to **macro** expansions. Macro expansion replaces an instruction with a sequence of instructions prior to assembly or compiling. However, preprocessors differ from compilers. A compiler translates a **high-level language** into assembly or **machine language**. A preprocessor does not translate code into machine language, but transforms into suitable language for the compiler.

Preprocessing may require data or computer programs to be translated twice. The source data or program is inputted into the preprocessor. The preprocessor then passes the modified code to the compiler, which then translates it into **machine code**.

*See also* Compiler; Macro

# PRETTY GOOD PRIVACY (PGP)

PGP, or Pretty Good Privacy, is a security software application used for the encryption and decryption of **data**. In 1991, Philip R. Zimmermann wrote PGP for the purpose of sending secured data across an insecure network, such as the **Internet**. Individuals, businesses, and governments use strong **cryptography** programs such as PGP to secure networks, e-mails, documents, and stored data.

PGP was originally designed as a combination of RSA encryption and a symmetric key cipher known as Bass-O-Matic. RSA is a public key cryptographic algorithm named after its designers **Ronald Rivest**, **Adi Shamir**, and **Leonard Adleman**. The RSA algorithm developed in 1977 (earlier versions of which were partially developed by intelligence agencies) quickly became a major advancement in cryptology. The RSA algorithm depends upon the difficulty in factoring very large composite numbers and is currently the most commonly used encryption and **authentication** algorithm in the world. The RSA algorithm forms were used in the development of modern Internet web browsers, spreadsheets, **e-mail**, and **word processing** programs.

Bass-O-Matic is a conventional (often referred to as symmetric) key algorithm designed by Zimmermann. Bass-O-Matic was later replaced by another conventional key algorithm known as IDEA, which enabled more powerful encryption technology.

Conventional cryptology is based on the concept that one key is used in both the encryption and decryption process. The major benefit of conventional cryptology is the speed in which the encryption process takes place. Conventional encryption can be up to one thousand times faster than public key encryption. However, secure key distribution is a major problem in this form of cryptology.

In 1975, **Whitfield Diffie** and **Martin Hellman** developed public key cryptology to increase the security of exchanging keys. Each user of a public key–based system has a public and private key. First, the user publishes the public key to a server or contact. Next, the contact encrypts the **message** to the user's public key. Finally, the user employs the private key to decrypt the cipher text (encoded message) received. The combination of both public and conventional key cryptology makes PGP a hybrid cryptosystem. This allows for users of PGP to be able to securely exchange keys and still have a speedy transaction of secured data.

PGP follows a simple process when encrypting plaintext (data easily understandable) into cipher text. PGP first compresses the document desired for encryption. This saves **modem** transmission time and strengthens the cryptographic security of the plaintext. Next, PGP creates a session key. The key is a number correlating to the random movements of the user's **mouse** and the keys that are typed. The key then works with a cryptographic algorithm to encrypt the plaintext. A cryptographic algorithm is a mathematical **function** in which a computable set of steps must be followed to achieve a desired result. The strength of this encryption is dependent on the strength of the algorithm.

After the data has been encrypted into cipher text, PGP encrypts the session key. The session key is encrypted to the recipient's public key. PGP uses digital certificates to prove the identity of a public key. The cipher text and encrypted session key are then transmitted to the recipient. When the recipient receives the data, PGP uses the user's private key to decrypt the session key. When PGP has recovered the session key, it can be used to decrypt the cipher text.

Though the plaintext has been recovered, there is still a question of authentication. PGP uses digital signatures to provide the recipient of an encryption with an origin and identification. Digital signatures are created in the opposite way a public cryptography system works. The sender encrypts a **digital signature** with their private key and attaches it to the rest of the data transmitted. When the digital **signature** is received, PGP decrypts it with the sender's public key. Through this process, PGP is able to determine the authenticity of the signature.

Digital signatures produce large amounts of data, slowing transmission and processing speeds. PGP uses a hash function to regulate the amount of data sent. The hash function takes **variable** amounts of data (the size of the plaintext) and produces a fixed amount called a message digest. PGP then creates a digital signature with the message digest and the user's private key. The hash function also helps to prove the authenticity of the encryption. If the encryption is changed after this process takes place, an entirely new message digest is created. This allows for PGP to detect encryption tampering.

Although PGP encryption has been available to the general public for several years, debate regarding encryption technologies and national security issues, especially in the United States, has ensued. Many government officials argue that strong cryptography programs should not be exported outside the United States. Due to these concerns, there are presently two available PGP **applications**: PGP and PGPi (interna-

tional). Any user outside of the United States is currently required to utilize PGPi.

***See also*** Authentication; Cryptography; Data security

# PRIMARY AND SECONDARY MEMORY

Modern electronic computers generally possess several distinct types of **memory**, each of which "holds" or stores information for subsequent use. The vast majority of computer memory can be placed into one of two categories: *primary memory* and *secondary memory*.

Primary memory, often called *main memory*, constitutes that device, or group of devices, that holds instructions and **data** for rapid and direct **access** by the computer's **central processing unit** (**CPU**). Primary memory is synonymous with **random access memory** (RAM). As a computer performs its calculations, it is continuously reading and writing (i.e., storing and retrieving) information to and from RAM. For instance, instructions and data are retrieved from RAM for processing by the CPU, and the results are returned to RAM. Modern RAM is made of **semiconductor** circuitry, which replaced the magnetic core memory widely used in computers in the 1960s. RAM is a volatile form of information storage, meaning that when electrical power is terminated any data that it contains is lost. There are other semiconductor memory devices accessed by the CPU that are generally considered as being distinct from primary memory (i.e., different from RAM). These memory units include cache memory, **ROM** (Read Only Memory), and PROM (Programmable Read Only Memory).

Secondary memory, also called *auxiliary memory* or *mass storage*, consists of devices not directly accessible by the CPU. Hard drives, floppy disks, tapes, and optical disks are widely used for secondary storage. The **input and output** of these devices is much slower than for the semiconductor devices that provide the computer's primary memory. Although access times (i.e., the time to read or write information) are slow as compared to that of primary memory, secondary memory devices have important features that are unmatched by primary memory. First, most secondary storage devices are capable of containing much more information than is feasible for primary memory (hence the use of the term "mass storage" as a synonym for secondary memory). A second, and essential, feature of secondary memory is that it is non-volatile. This means that data is stored with or without electrical power being supplied to the device, as opposed to RAM, which can retain its data only so long as electrical power is present.

Like primary memory, many secondary memory devices are capable of storing information, as well as retrieving it. Magnetic technology devices (such as hard drives, floppy disks, and tape) have this read-write capability, as do magneto-optical drives. However, some mass storage devices can only read data, as in the case of **CD-ROM** (Compact Disk-Read Only Memory) drives. CD-ROMs utilize optical technology; however, newer optical technologies, such as CD-RW (compact disk-rewriteable), can both read and write information like magnetic storage devices.

*See also* Central processing unit (CPU); Disk storage; Hard drive; Memory; Random-access memory (RAM); Semiconductor

# PRINTER

A *printer* is a device that converts computer output into printed text or images on paper or some other medium. A printer is considered a *peripheral* device, as is any part of a computer other than the **central processing unit** or its working **memory**: monitors, printers, disk drives, digital cameras, scanners, and so on.

In 1953, the Remington-Rand company developed the first high-speed printer for use with the **UNIVAC** computer. Today, laser and inkjet printers are two popular types of printers. The original laser printer was developed in 1978 at the Xerox Palo Alto Research Center when Xerox engineer Gary Starkweather added a laser beam to Xerox copier technology. The **Hewlett-Packard** Company introduced the first desktop laser printer in 1984, basing their device on technology developed by Canon, Inc. Laser printers quickly became popular due to their high-quality printouts and their relatively low operating expenses. Though the inkjet printer was invented in 1976, it wasn't until 1988, when Hewlett-Packard released its DeskJet inkjet printer, that it become a popular consumer item.

Printers are categorized in several ways. The primary distinction is whether a printer prints by *impact* or *non-impact* means.

*Impact printers* are older, noisier, and generally produce lower-quality output than non-impact printers. In this method of printing, the printing mechanism physically comes into contact with the paper. Examples include the dot-matrix, line, and daisywheel printers.

A *dot-matrix printer* places ink on paper using a matrix of small, closely packed needles or pins, like a miniature bed of nails. As this print head repeatedly tracks across the page, different pins are activated at each point and hit an ink ribbon, striking a small portion of the ribbon against the paper. Typically, the dot-matrix print head consists of 24 pins in a 4 × 6 arrangement. Dot-matrix printers are noisy and cannot produce high-quality printout, but they are inexpensive and have many uses. Dot-matrix printers were once a relatively low-cost printing option for many people and businesses, but they have been largely replaced by inkjet printers (described in more detail below).

A *line printer* is, in most cases, a dot matrix printer. However, instead of printing one character at a time, the line printer prints an entire line at a time using a long, narrow matrix of pins. Line printers are very fast, but still produce low-quality print. They are commonly used in **data** centers and industrial complexes where large amounts of printed material are required. They tend to be large, fast, expensive, and noisy.

A *daisywheel printer*, similar to a ball-head typewriter, has characters arranged on the ends of the spokes of a plastic or metal wheel (shaped somewhat like a daisy). The wheel is rotated to select the character to print and then an electrically operated hammer mechanism knocks the selected spoke forward, pressing an ink ribbon against the paper. A daisywheel printer can produce letter-quality print but cannot print **graphics**. Daisywheel printers were common in the 1980s, but declined in use when laser and inkjet printers became affordable. Of similar construction, specially designed electronic typewriter keyboards, such as the line of **IBM** Selectric Typewriters, were connected to computer logic and memory circuits in order to perform automatic functions such as printing multiple copies of a given letter. These devices, too, have fallen out of general use.

*Non-impact printers* print without striking the paper. They are much quieter than impact printers, are faster due to the absence of moving parts in the print head, and generally produce higher-quality print. Examples include laser, inkjet, LED/LCD, and thermal printers. A *laser printer* uses a laser beam to form an electrostatic image on a drum (i.e., a pattern of electric charge that corresponds to the image to be printed). This attracts electrically charged dry ink powder (toner) which is then transferred to paper and heat-fused (melted on). Laser printer resolution ranges from 300 to 600 dots per inch (dpi), allowing for increased flexibility of character shapes, which in turn allows the use of TrueType font formats. The highest-quality laser printers, which use chemical photoduplication techniques, can produce resolutions of 2,400 dpi (fine photographic quality). All laser printers produce high-quality text and graphics. An *inkjet printer* sprays very small ink droplets electrostatically from a nozzle onto a sheet of paper. Charged plates in the ink's path direct the ink **stream** (broken up into thousands of discrete droplets per second) onto the paper in the desired pattern. Inkjet printers produce high-quality text and graphics, and have become the most popular personal printer technology. An *LED printer* is one that is similar in **operation** to a laser printer, but instead of a laser an arrangement of light-emitting diodes (LEDs) are used to produce a charge image on the drum. A *thermal printer* is an inexpensive printer that works by pushing heated pins against heat-sensitive paper. Thermal printers are widely used in printing calculators and in barcode and fax machines.

Methods of categorizing printers include: (1) *print technology* used (dot-matrix, inkjet, laser, etc.); (2) *character formation* technique used, which may involve either (a) completely formed, solid characters (e.g., laser, daisywheel) or (b) characters composed of patterns of dots (e.g., dot-matrix and inkjet); (3) *method of transmission* from computer to printer, such as (a) byte-by-byte transmission with parallel ports or (b) bit-by-bit transmission with serial ports; (4) *method of printing*, namely (a) character-by-character (e.g., dot-matrix, inkjet), (b) line-by-line (line printers), or (c) page-by-page (laser); (5) *quality*, namely photo quality, letter quality, or draft quality; and (6) *speed*, namely output speed measured in either characters per second (cps) or pages per minute (ppm). Daisywheel printers are usually the slowest, printing about 30 cps (less than a page per minute), while dot-matrix printers can print up to 500 cps. Laser printers range from about 4 to 20 ppm.

**Word processing** programs have transformed the processes of typing and editing, contributing dramatic new flexibility to the writing process. Computer printers tracked this process as they moved through several stages of innovation, from the first impact printers (daisywheel and dot-matrix) to the current generation of affordable, high-quality non-impact printers (inkjet and laser).

*See also* Word processing

# PRIVILEGED INSTRUCTION

Privileged instruction is an instruction (usually in **machine code**) that can be executed only by the operating system in a specific mode. (An *instruction* is a statement that is acted upon by any computer language.) Examples of where privileged instructions are used include operations involving input/output and **memory** management (the coordinated effort to provide sufficient memory to all processes of a computer system). The existence of privileged instructions is to specifically allow the operating system to perform certain operations that **applications** should not be allowed to perform. To allow for privileged instructions a "mode bit" is added into the computer's software to indicate one of two dual modes: monitor mode or user mode. The privileged instruction can only be executed when the **microprocessor** is running in *monitor* (or supervisor) mode, a mode that enables execution of all instructions. Thus, the operating system contains routines that execute these particular (privileged) instructions. The monitor mode is the normal operating state of computers. If an attempt is made to execute a privileged instruction in the user state, then the microprocessor does not execute the instruction. The *user* mode is the least privileged of the states, being the state from which all application programs run.

*See also* Application; Instruction set; Machine code

# PROCEDURAL ABSTRACTION

Procedural **abstraction** is the process of converting a specific procedure into a general procedure by ignoring certain details. This is used during the **design** process to allow the programmer to focus on the structure of the program instead of the detail of the individual functions.

A procedural abstraction specifies everything the users require from the procedure but nothing more. All other details are left up to the programmer to determine during the implementation. Procedural abstractions are sometimes referred to as "black boxes" since they describe what a procedure does without describing how it does it.

Defining a procedural abstraction requires two steps. The first step names the **input and output** parameters as well as their **types**. The second step defines the conditions (called the *requires* clause), any side effects (the *modifies* clause) and what the abstraction achieves (the *effects* clause).

When a procedural abstraction is defined completely, it has the properties of locality and modifiability. Locality means that the details of the implementation are local to the individual procedure and only need to be known by the programmer dealing with the implementation. Modifiability means that replacing the implementation of the procedure does not affect the rest of the program.

*See also* Abstraction; Parameter; Side effect

# PROGRAM DESIGN

The **design** of large computer programs and the software systems they implement is a complex task. An old saw in **programming** goes, "Software is harder than hardware," and it means that new computer **hardware** is developed faster and more easily than new computer software. There is certainly a degree of truth to this statement, though computer architects are unlikely to be pleased by the seeming trivialization of their domain!

Program design is not a totally unique discipline, and cannot be practiced on a stand-alone basis. To give some idea of what program design is in relation to other aspects of program development, we may say that program design is to programming what building architecture is to masonry. A good architect can, if he chooses, take off his jacket and do a mason's job, but his comprehension has to be greater, encompassing more than the mason's point of view. Likewise, the designer of a program has to be a proficient programmer himself, and has to be alive to the concerns of programmers, but his function is more refined.

Many outsiders have difficulty understanding why the design of good large programs is difficult. To see why, we should distinguish between two types of complexity, physical and logical. Physical complexity has to do with how hard it is to implement a given system, i.e., the logistics of translating a plausible design into a successful product. Logical complexity has to do with comprehending the **operation** of a system, i.e., understanding how many states the system has, and the transitions between them. Physical artifacts such as buildings have enormous physical complexity but relatively little logical complexity. Software, on the other hand, has enormous logical complexity but little physical complexity.

For many people, however, physical complexity is all that is apparent, so there is a dangerous fallacy that because software has low physical complexity, it must be "easy," and that program design is "just a matter of programming." These misconceptions have resulted in the history of software development being replete with horror stories, with many high-profile development efforts costing millions having ended in dismal failures that finished careers and companies. Even today, it is not uncommon for large software projects to miss deadlines and schedules and deliver unsatisfactory products.

The current state of **the software industry** in which a program designer may expect to work, is one of intense competition which increasingly calls for short and cost-effective development cycles. So much so that sometimes, if a product cannot be fully debugged before it is shipped out, innovative marketing tries to pass off persistent bugs as "features" of the software. Products have low shelf-lives and require frequent upgrades. Customers require or expect greater reliability and the ability to use the software with minimal or no special training.

A program designer has to have the ability to understand the customer's (or user's) requirements and expectations. In some cases, the customer may be unfamiliar with the workings of computers and thus may not be able to clarify what his expectations are, and the designer must help out. Early communication is essential to avoid later misunderstandings. The designer must then translate the customer's vaguely-formulated wishes into precise specifications for the proposed system, and must then perform conceptual modeling and high-level design, to allow the planning of a development effort with meaningful estimates for timelines and resources required.

In designing a large program, it is often also necessary to be able to evaluate competing alternatives and make trade-offs between incompatible objectives. For example, as the apparent simplicity of the software from the perspective of the user increases, making for an easier-to-use product, so does the complexity for the programmer developing the software. Since the program design has to make sense both to the user as well as to the programmer, it is essential that a balance be struck in this regard.

In the formal models of software development such as the **Waterfall Model**, design proceeds in two distinct phases. The first phase occurs once the specification has been fixed—an overall system design is then attempted. At this time, the **macro** system structure must be determined, key elements and their major interactions must be identified, and the larger system functions must be allocated. The second stage, occurring next, involves the identification of system modules (objects) and the allocation of functionality to these. The modules or objects have to be defined at the functional or algorithmic level, with detailed consideration of the specific **data** structures involved.

Nearly all modern program design is by application of object-oriented principles. This ensures, among other things, that **code** and experience gained from previous efforts can be reused in later designs, and that the development effort that follows the design is efficient and productive.

*See also* Computer architecture; Correctness; Object-oriented programming; Programming; Software

# PROGRAMMING

Computers have one big problem—they do not comprehend English, nor in fact any other human language. Strictly speaking, the **CPU** of a computer only understands its own **machine language**, the vocabulary of which is given by its **instruction set**. The machine language of a CPU is extremely rudimentary, of perhaps the same level of sophistication as the limited language of **commands** used to order a trained dog to perform certain actions like bark, run, fetch, etc. Such a language is simply incapable of expressing the vast majority of concepts,

ideas, and abstractions that the human mind in all its ingenuity comes up with.

Therefore, it is not difficult to see why it is necessary for there to be some way in which the concepts and procedures created in the human mind and expressed in human language can be reduced in level to the extremely limited vocabulary of the CPU, so that a machine may carry out the actions the human wishes it to. However, the gulf between human language and machine language is so great that there is no sensible way of bridging it in just one step—it is far more reasonable to try to bridge it in two (or more).

Thus, for the first step, the humans who wish the computer to carry out some task specify, in a clearly phrased and well-defined subset of the human language, what it is exactly that they want it to do. The description thus created should be completely free of ambiguities, errors, and inaccuracies. The description of the task should also state, in a step-wise fashion, a sequence of actions, each of which the computer is capable of performing. Such a well-specified procedure by which the computer is to carry out the desired task is called an algorithm. The word "algorithm' is given in honor of the name of the ancient Arab mathematician Al-Khowarezmi, who, around the year 825 CE, wrote a treatise in Arabic titled *Hisab al-jabr w'al muqa-balah*, or "The Science of the Union and the Opposition."

This specification in simplified and clear human language of the task to be performed is an important first step. After an algorithm is thus created, it is used by humans (perhaps the same ones, perhaps not) to create a translation into a weaker language called a programming language. There are literally hundreds of programming languages; some that are well known and in current use would be **C**, **C++**, **Java**, Fortran, **COBOL**, and **Pascal**. The process of translating an algorithm into programming language is called programming. A programming language is much weaker in its expressive power than mature human language, and has the sophistication of the language used by a very young child. Just as it is not always easy for adults to communicate their ideas clearly to young children, it is not always easy for programmers to translate **algorithms** into programs. This often makes for many anxious moments and frustrations for programmers and their clients, who may be facing deadlines and other difficulties, or may be be facing competition to bring their software to market ahead of rival products.

After the program is created, it is then necessary to take the final step and convert from the programming language **code** to the machine langauge code that the computer can directly understand. This final step is typically (in modern programming languages) carried out by specialized software programs called compilers. There are special compilers that convert code from a certain language to machine code for a particular CPU. Compilers are thus specific to the CPU they produce the code for, and it is important for a **compiler** to be available for a certain CPU, before one can use any programs on it.

Of course, the previous discussion is to some extent an oversimplification, because a programmer does not produce final working code and then compile it all at once: what happens almost always is that some code is produced, then compiled to see if it has any errors (called bugs), and then those bugs are fixed and the code is compiled again—programming is very much a process of incremental improvement rather than huge leaps. Compilers thus also have the role of helping the programmer produce bug-free code; this they do by issuing error messages during compilation that announce that the code has syntactical errors in it (for example, a missed semicolon after an executable statement is an error in the C language); they may also issue warnings, which may mean that while the code may be correct, it may not function exactly the way it was intended to. While it is desirable that the compiler's error and warning messages convey in exact detail what the problem is with the code, in practice it often takes some skill and ingenuity on the part of the programmer to find the exact nature of the problem that is causing a particular error to be returned. For example, a compiler may complain of an error at a certain location in the program while the real problem is elsewhere, hundreds of lines away.

For serious programming, there are other specialized software packages called debuggers, whose sole function is to help the programmer trace errors in the code. Sometimes, such **debugging** and constant revisions can also help the programmer find and rectify any logic errors in the code as well. A logic error is a statement in programming language that is correct syntactically but conveys an incorrect meaning, or else does not fit in with the purpose it is meant for.

A good programmer should also document the code carefully, i.e., should add suitable comments and explanations throughout the program to clarify for human readers what is being done and why—it is likely as not that the program will have to be updated, corrected, or otherwise modified by others in times to come. Even if the author of the code comes back to it after some months or years, the ideas that were clear in the beginning will no longer be so, and programming language code is typically very hard to read and understand if one doesn't already have a good idea of what's in it. Other than documenting, other concepts like **structured programming** are often mentioned as good programming practices. The great computer scientist Don Knuth, Professor Emeritus of The Art of Computer Programming at Stanford University, wrote a famous book called The Art of Computer Programming in three volumes totally over 2000 pages, and is presently working on more volumes, and is also revising existing ones.

*See also* Computer language; CPU; Object-Oriented programming; Program design; Software; Verification

# PROGRAMMING LANGUAGES, THEORY

Although **programming** languages are many in number and diverse in nature, nearly all of them rely on an essential set of a small number of basic concepts. Knowledge of these concepts is essential to programmers, **compiler** writers, and others.

A programming language, like any formal language, must have a specific alphabet associated with it. As almost all programming languages have been designed in the U.S. and

other English-speaking countries, the 7-bit **ASCII** character set that encompasses the Roman characters used in English is the most common alphabet, used with older programming languages such as **C**. However, this does not allow for the use of umlauts and other singular features—these are found with characters in European languages (such as Ç, ä, etc.) Nor does the 7-bit ASCII allow characters from other scripts such as Chinese to be used. Hence, newer languages often allow a larger character set—for instance, **Java** allows the 16-bit **Unicode** character set to be used. Even if 7-bit ASCII is used, as is most common, the strings are converted internally into the equivalent 16-bit Unicode.

It is possible for a programmer to define either variables, which can take different values, or constants, which are assigned a value which is never changed. These variables are given names, which are strings in the program's alphabet. However, every programming language has some "reserved words" which are already used as "identifiers,", i.e., are assigned special meanings, and are used in assignments, **declarations**, and so on; these are not available to the programmer for use in naming variables.

A program works with two kinds of **data**: problem data and control data. Problem data are associated with the computations performed, and may include numerical data, logical data, and descriptive data, obtained from the program's input. The control data, such as labels, addresses, and offsets, is internal to the program and is fixed by the creator of the program.

The numerical data used by the program and assigned to its variables and constants can be of several types—fixed-point, floating-point, signed integer, unsigned integer, character, and so on. In modern programming languages, it is essential for a variable to be "declared" as being of a certain type, before it is used. Some languages such as C are "weakly typed" and allow variables to be used in a manner different from their declaration (for example, a character **variable** may be dealt with as an integer), but other languages such as Java are "strongly typed" and do not allow this practice. It is not a good idea for a variable to be used in a manner inconsistent with its definition, even if the language allows it. Strongly-typed languages are considered to have greater security than weakly-typed ones.

A programming language allows a variety of functions to be performed on mathematical data. Some of these are: arithmetic functions (such as addition); logical functions (such as comparison); data movement; sequence and control functions; and input and output. These functions are available to the programmer through the use of "operators" such as the addition **operator** + or the multiplication operator ×. Older programming languages such as **COBOL** allowed the use of English-like statements such as "ADD A TO B", but this is rare in newer languages, and an algebraic notation such as "A + B" is preferred.

Operators such as the addition operator are called infix operators, because they come in between their operands. Other operators, such as the negation operator, are called prefix operators, because they come prior to their operands. The actual representation of some operators may vary—the logical "and" operator is denoted by .AND. in **FORTRAN**, by just AND in COBOL, by & in PL/I, and by & in C and **C++**. However, most programming languages have nearly the same set of operators, with the same meanings. Some advanced languages such as C++ and Java allow programmers to define their own operators, which are usually proprietory or special operators acting on data structures used within the program. For example, it is possible to define an addition operator that acts on sets instead of numbers, with the result of adding two sets being a larger set with the elements of both sets. Some languages such as C++ specifically allow "operator overloading," that is the use of a standard operator representation to stand for a newly defined operator as well. For example, it is possible to write a C++ program in which the set-addition operator given above is also invoked by +, the same symbol used for regular arithmetic addition. The language compiler is able to know which operator is meant, based on the context. However, operator **overloading** should be used with care.

Statements in programming languages that involve multiple operators are evaluated according to standard mathematical operator precedence—for example, A + 3 × B is evaluated as A + (3 × B). However, the programmer should use parentheses to force the precedence in complex expressions. The expressions are internally converted to **Reverse Polish Notation**, during compilation.

***See also*** ASCII; C; C++; Computer languages, types; Data Structures; Java; Programming; Reverse Polish notation; Unicode

# PROGRAMMING LANGUAGES, TYPES

A **programming** language is the communication bridge between a programmer and computer. A programming language allows a programmer to create sets of executable instructions, or a program, that the computer can understand. This communication bridge is needed because computers process (or "understand") only **machine language**, which is an instruction language in which **data** are represented by binary digits ("bits"). For example, the binary digits 1000 represent the instruction ADD.

Writing instructions in machine language is a long, tedious process; for this reason it is prone to errors. Additionally, humans speaking natural languages (e.g., English) may find it very difficult to grasp, understand, and use machine language. Programming languages represent a middle ground between the binary machine language computers understand and our own natural languages.

A programming language assists a programmer in using a computer to solve a problem. Computers solve problems by storing and manipulating data that represent things in the real world. For example, a person can be represented by name, address, social security number, gender, etc. A computer can perform operations on this data to make, for example, a person an employee of a company by assigning an employee number to all the data associated with that person. To perform operations on data and solve problems, such as creating a list of employees, programming languages are used.

Like our own natural languages, programming languages have their own vocabulary and rules governing how the vocabulary can be used. Languages whose vocabulary and rules are closer to that of the computer's machine language are called low-level languages. Languages that are closer to how humans write and speak are called high-level languages. Whether low or high, the programming language must be translated into machine language. This is done by a **compiler** or interpreter.

A compiler translates an entire program into machine language and then executes the instructions. An interpreter reads and executes a program one statement at a time. A compiled program executes faster, but the user must wait for it to be compiled in entirety. In contrast, if a program is interpreted, the user does not have to wait while the entire program is read, but execution is slower. The method of translation, compilation or interpretation, is one **variable** that affects the type of programming language chosen to solve a particular problem.

### A Brief History

As discussed earlier, programming in machine language has several drawbacks. In addition to being tedious, it requires the programmer to keep track of where individual bits of data are stored in the computer's **memory**. Changing the address of one **bit** of data could affect the memory addresses used in the rest of the program. To combat these and other difficulties, other languages were developed.

**Assembly language** is a low-level language that allows names to represent instructions and data. Instead of writing the binary digits 1000, an assembly language programmer can write ADD. Although an improvement, assembly language fails to ease the burden on programmers.

In short, assembly language:

- is machine dependent, meaning it cannot be easily moved from one machine to another
- has to manage size and location of data in memory addresses similar to machine language
- cannot be easily shared between programmers
- does not produce a significant enough improvement in shortening program length
- does not resemble natural languages

Higher-level programming languages were developed to overcome these limitations. High-level languages leave the problem of tracking memory addresses up to the computer. This allows the programmer to focus on the instructions for solving the problem.

High-level languages are:

- less error prone and easier to debug
- machine independent
- more like natural languages
- easily shared between programmers

Currently there are over 1,000 programming languages. Many are designed for specific **applications**, such as **simulation**, business processes, mathematical or scientific applications, and systems software.

## Procedural Languages

There are two categories of programming languages: procedural (imperative) and non-procedural (declarative). In a procedural programming language, the programmer defines the set of executable instructions and the exact sequence in which those instructions are to be executed. The computer simply obeys the instructions in the sequence it is told. For example, to sort a list, a programmer would have to give the computer step-by-step instructions on how to sort. The sequential instructions would compare each item to the next item on the list, determine if its **value** is greater than or less than the value of the next item, and repeat this procedure until each item has been compared to all other items in the list.

Procedural languages execute faster than other types of languages but tend to be harder to write. Usually designed for compilation rather than interpretation, procedural languages sacrifice programming convenience for speed of execution. One reason for the higher execution speed is a procedural language's reliance on the **von Neumann architecture**. In the von Neumann architecture, the ability to manipulate the sequential flow of **control** is a defining characteristic. With sequential flow of control, the programmer can define the order in which instructions are executed. In other computer architectures, flow of control does not exist, thereby causing slower execution. Procedural languages include **FORTRAN**, Ada, and **Pascal**.

Within the procedural category, object-oriented languages are a major **class**. Object-oriented languages use **abstract data types**, which are structures in which the data and its operations are defined together in a single unit, in this case an **object**. These objects are instances of a class. A class defines the properties of its objects. A major characteristic of object-oriented languages is **inheritance**. Inheritance allows the abstract data types to "inherit" data and functionality from **parent**, or hierarchically higher, classes. For example, you can have a class called "Employee" with instances of the class called "Manager" and "Cashier." Both Manager and Cashier inherit all the characteristics of the parent Employee class, such as employee number, department, etc. However, the operations of the Manager object are different from the operations of an Employee object.

Object-oriented languages differ from other procedural languages in that the objects contain a description of the operations that can act upon them. Objects are sent messages stating which operations to execute. In other procedural languages, the operations are defined in procedures that are separate from the data on which they act. Object-oriented languages, though requiring more initial analysis, can reduce development, be more accurately coded, provide greater **data security**, and be easily reused. **C++** is an example of an object-oriented language.

ADVANTAGES AND DISADVANTAGES OF PROCEDURAL LANGUAGES Programming in procedural languages can be very efficient. Since the programmer is giving an explicit set of instructions to the computer, the computer does not have to determine how to solve a problem. The programmer has done all the work; the computer simply has to execute the steps. A drawback to this is that the burden is put on the programmer to not only under-stand the problem, but **design** the best way to solve the problem. Some question whether procedural languages will continue to be able to handle the increasing complexity of large programs and the ability to support concurrent execution of programs.

## Non-procedural Languages

In non-procedural languages the computer is not limited to a set of precise instructions. Instead, the programmer defines only the problem—*not* the instructions—to solve the problem. The computer determines the necessary steps to solve the problem. In essence, non-procedural languages emphasize the result (or *what*) is to be achieved rather than the methods (or *how*) a result is achieved. For example, to sort a list, the programmer instructs the computer to output a list in which adjacent items are in increasing or decreasing order.

The term non-procedural is relative in that it changes as languages continue to evolve. What may have been considered non-procedural 40 years ago may be procedural today because computer **hardware** and programming capabilities have improved. Additionally, most non-procedural programming languages cannot be defined purely as such; many have features of both procedural languages as well.

There are two major classes of non-procedural languages: functional and logic languages. Functional languages apply functions to given parameters. Functions are statements that return a single value based on the arguments, or inputs, it is passed. Functional programs attempt to act like mathematical functions. They are harder to implement efficiently than procedural languages. Until computers are designed on which functional languages can execute more efficiently, they will not replace procedural languages. Examples of functional languages are **LISP** and Miranda.

In logic languages, the programmer defines the problems through **declarations** or facts. Declarations are propositions that can be written in symbolic logic or as "if-then" statements. For example, if X is the mother of Y then X is a parent of Y. Given inputs, the computer determines if the declarations are true. Logic languages have the potential to be powerful and flexible. However, they are not as efficient as other languages, and methods for solving large problems this way still need to be developed. Prolog is the best known logic language.

ADVANTAGES AND DISADVANTAGES OF NON-PROCEDURAL LANGUAGES Much of the onus for designing a step-by-step procedure for solving a problem is taken on by the computer. Programming in a non-procedural language allows the programmer to concentrate on understanding and describing the problem, while the computer does the work of figuring out how to solve the problem. A disadvantage of this type of language is that efficiency can suffer. The computer may not select the "best" method for solving the problem, resulting in the computer taking longer to solve it then if the programmer had provided it with a set of explicit instructions. Good methods that allow non-procedural languages to solve large problems efficiently are yet to be developed.

### Re-Entrant Program

A capability of some procedural and non-procedural programs is the coding of a re-entrant program. A re-entrant program allows multiple users (a user can be a program or person) to share the same program at the same time, such as an operating system or network protocol. Users can be interrupted by another user and then re-enter the program. This interruption is possible because the program's instructions are not modifiable and each user's data is stored separately from any other users. When a user re-enters the program, the saved data is recovered.

*See also* Assembly language; Compiler; Functional Programming Language; Interpreter; Machine language; Object-oriented programming; Von Neumann Architecture

# PROPOSITIONAL LOGIC

Propositional logic explains how to work with the most basic elements of logic, propositions. A proposition is any statement that is either true or false but not both. Declarative sentences such as "The sky is blue," "I have one arm," and "1 + 1 = 3" are all propositions. **Commands** ("Close the door!"), interrogatives ("What are you doing?"), and sentences that include variables ("Someone is watching me.") are not propositions.

The truth or falsity of a proposition might change depending on the speaker and the time it is uttered. The proposition "I have one arm" is true only when spoken by a person with one arm and false when spoken by those with two or no arms. A proposition that is always true, for example, "Either it is raining or it is not raining," is called a tautology; a proposition that is always false, as with "1 + 1 = 3," is called a contradiction. The truth **value** of a proposition is T if it is true and F if it is false.

Compound propositions can be created through the use of logical operators. For example, if $p$ is any proposition, the negation of $p$ can be written, "It is not the case that $p$." Other logical operators include "and," "or," "if, then," and "if and only if." The truth or falsity of a compound proposition is determined by examining the truth or falsity of each of its component propositions. The truth of the compound proposition "$p$ and $q$," for example, is true only when both $p$ is true and $q$ is true.

A statement that contains a **variable**, such as "$x$ is divisible by 6," can be turned into a proposition through the use of a quantifier and a universe of discourse. The quantifiers come in two forms: universal ("For all $x$,...") and existential ("There exists an $x$ such that..."). The universe of discourse tells us what values $x$ can possibly be. Through quantifiers the statement above can become the (false) proposition, "For all $x$ such that $x$ is a whole number, $x$ is divisible by 6." Using the existential quantifier on the above statement produces a true proposition since there does exist at least one whole number that is divisible by six, six itself being one example.

*See also* First-order logic; Theorem proving

# PROTOCOLS

Protocols are conventions that facilitate intercomputer communications. Simply put, protocols are agreed-on formats for transmitting **data** at the **bit** and **byte** level between two computing devices. Protocols determine how data will be compressed and sent, what kind of error checking will be used, how the sending device will indicate completion of send, and how the receiving device will indicate reception of the **message**. Protocols are an intrinsic aspect of data communications across networks. A range of standard protocols varying from highly reliable, to highly efficient, to speedy, currently exist and offer a diversity of communications options. Choosing protocols for data communications is greatly facilitated these days by the range available. An essential aspect of this choice is that both computing devices seeking to be in communication must support the protocols used, which can be implemented either in **hardware** or in software.

The Open Systems Interconnect (OSI) Reference Model developed by the **International Organization for Standardization (ISO)** is commonly used to describe the structure and function of data communication protocols. This model contains seven layers, each defining a separate communications function performed (possibly by a number of protocols) when data is transferred between **applications** across a network. Each layer can contain multiple protocols. The seven layers of the OSI model are:

- Layer 7—Application layer
- Layer 6—Presentation layer
- Layer 5—Session layer
- Layer 4—Transport layer
- Layer 3—Network layer
- Layer 2—Data Link layer
- Layer 1—Physical layer

Every protocol communicates exclusively with its "peer," which is an implementation of the same protocol in the corresponding layer on a remote system. However, the layers also pass data between each other on a single computer.

Network protocols are layered on top of each other, with each layer using functionalities provided by the lower layer while adding new functionality. The term "protocol stack" describes a set of network protocol layers that work together. The OSI Reference Model is often called a **stack**, as is the slightly different set of Transmission Control Protocol/Internet Protocol (**TCP/IP**) protocols that define communication over the **Internet**. The actual software used to process the protocols is also described by the term "stack."

The term "layered protocols" also indicates that the protocols are stacked on top of each other. Data received by a computer is passed up from the lowest-level protocol to the highest, while data being sent to other computers moves down the protocol stack within the host. Each layer at the sender's end communicates with the corresponding layer at the receiver's end. When a device prepares to transmit data to the network, each protocol layer processes the data in turn. For instance, at the network layer (layer 3), data to be transmitted is received from the higher transport layer (layer 4). Network-layer information on routing is appended in the form of a header to the front of the data. Control information for a layer along with data from the higher layer is described by the term Protocol Data Unit (PDU). Each layer appends a header to the PDU, except the physical layer, which manages data in bit form. The physical and the data link layers, layers 1 and 2, together define a machine's physical network interface. Typically network-interface software defines how the Ethernet **device driver** gets data from or to the network. Ethernet is the most common implementation of the physical- and data-link layers, and it can be run over a variety of media, including thinnet, thicknet, and unshielded twisted-pair cables.

The layered model is useful because it allows network services to be defined by their functions. This means that new protocols can be substituted at lower levels without affecting the higher-level protocols, as long as they perform the requisite layer function. Communication in a network is successful only if the functions in each layer are executed successfully. Essentially each layer needs only to carry out its task and deliver the data to the next layer in the process. Protocols in layers can also be mixed and matched to fulfill different requirements.

Most modern **Wide-Area Network** (WAN) protocols, including TCP/IP, X.25, and Frame Relay, are based on packet-switching technologies. "Packets" refer to protocols in which data messages are divided into parts that are transmitted individually and can follow different routes to their destination. When all packets comprising a message arrive at their destination, they are recompiled into the original message. **Packet switching** is an efficient and robust method for transmitting data that is amenable to delays in transmission, such as **e-mail** messages and Web pages. (In contrast, normal telephone service—in which delays are unacceptable—is based on a circuit-switching technology, where a dedicated line is allocated for transmission between two parties.)

Because errors can occur at any of the layers in a protocol stack, error-controlling and detecting mechanisms need to be in place to correct errors or notify the sender. To ensure the reliable transmission of data, error-control **algorithms** are used to detect those errors and in some cases correct them so upper layers will see an error-free link. Two error control strategies have been popular in practice. They are the FEC (Forward Error Correction) strategy, which uses error correction alone, and the more popular ARQ (Automatic Repeat Request) strategy, which detects errors as well as retransmits corrupted data. The FEC strategy is mainly used in links where retransmission is impossible or impractical.

Two other error-detection techniques are called checksum and CRC. Checksum is a simple error-detection scheme in which each transmitted message also carries the numeric sum of set bits in the message. The receiving station checks to ensure the numeric sum **value** when received is the same. If not, the message has been garbled. CRC refers to Cyclic **Redundancy** Check, a common technique for detecting data transmission errors, in use by a number of file transfer protocols.

# PROTONIC MEMORY

Protonic **memory** uses embedded protons as a memory storage medium. The embedded protons remain in place even when the power has been turned off. The information embedded in the protons is not lost. In devices such as dynamic **random access memory** (DRAM), which are based on the flow of electrons, the cessation of power results in the loss of the information.

Development of the process occurred at the Sandia National Labs, in Albuquerque, New Mexico in the mid to late 1990s. The researchers created a protonic memory-retentive chip by incorporating a few steps to the hundreds of steps used to make microchips. The key was putting the hot microchip in an atmosphere of hydrogen gas. Protons become trapped in the central layer of silicone dioxide in the chip. In this condition, the protons respond to positive or negative charges. A positive low voltage sends the protons to the far side of the central layer, which represents a binary "1". Negative low voltage has the opposite effect, attracting the protons to the near side of the silicone dioxide layer, which represents a binary "0". The protons remain in their respective positions when the power is turned off, retaining the information in the chip.

The simplicity, economy, and memory preserving ability of the protonic chip may allow them to replace a computer's main memory. Exploration of the commercial potential of protonic memory has begun.

*See also* Memory

# PSEUDOCODE

In the specification of **algorithms**, as well as in consideration of the **design** and **verification** of completed programs, it is common practice to use a notational technique called pseudocode. Pseudocode is simply a convention for specifying a procedure or algorithm fragment in a semi-rigorous way that can be followed by programmers. Well-written pseudocode can often be translated line-by-line into program **code**.

As with program code itself, pseudocode should be well commented so that it can be easily understood. If the pseudocode conventions (the notation used, which is not rigorous and can vary by author's choice and application domain) are somewhat relaxed, then additional comments may not have to be extensive since a fair amount of English-like comments and phrases can be built into the pseudocode fragment itself.

As an example of a pseudocode specification, consider the following. A person is entitled to vote if she is 18 years of age or older, if she is registered to vote in the relevant jurisdiction, and if she has not lost her right to vote on account of a felony conviction. This voter-validation protocol may be specified in the following format, which could be easily converted to a program for asking questions of a prospective voter to determine eligibility. Comments are included after the double slash marks (//).

```
// Variable declaration—
LEGAL is 18 // Global variable for age restriction
// Query for age, felony convictions, registration
input (age) // Query the person's age
input (conviction) // Boolean for felony conviction; 0
means not, 1 means yes.
input (is_registered) // Boolean for voter registration; 1
means registered, 0 means not.
if (age ≥ LEGAL) then // If it is true that the person is
of legal age
if (is_registered) then // If she is registered
if (!conviction) then // If it is not true that she has been
convicted
else
print ("Sorry, felons are not allowed to vote")
endif
print("You can vote")
else
print ("Sorry, you aren't registered to vote")
endif
else
print ("Sorry, you must wait a little longer to vote")
endif
```

*See also* Programming

# PSP (PERSONAL SOFTWARE PACKAGE)

**PSP**, or Personal Software Package, is the supporting resource package for the Personal Software Program. The latter, which can also be called PSP, is a software engineering methodology that is designed to promote improvement in the work efficiency and software **design** skills of programmers.

PSP will refer from now on to the software package.

The software tools that form the PSP are varied and are intended to enhance a software designers abilities in accurately predicting the time required to produce a product of stellar quality, to seek ways to improve the quality of the software being designed, and to improve their ability to evaluate technologies and methods.

Part of the PSP consists of files. While some differences exist between vendors, the following summary of the intent of the files is fairly inclusive:

- Logging of worktime (time log), defects (defect log) and interruptions. Work events can be logged in as they commence and end. Premature termination of work due to an interruption or a mistake can be recorded. This provides a diary of work patterns, which can be useful in revealing areas where efficiencies can be gained.
- Logging of individual work events.
- Statistical analysis of time and defect logs.
- Summary reports of log information.

- Tracking work time on various aspects of a development project.
- Accounting. These files have been written for a variety of operating languages, including **DOS**, **Perl**, Turbo **Pascal** and **Unix**.

Another component of a PSP is termed the defect type standard. The standard, which is meant to be refined for the particular use it is being applied to, is a means of categorizing defects into classes. One scheme that is in use has three categories. The first category is termed the injection phase, and groups defects based on when they were produced. The second category is termed defect type. This category is product related, and groups defects based on their structure or the repairs needed to correct them. The last category is termed defect reason. This is process related and groups defects based on the reason for their introduction (mistake or otherwise).

The PSP is designed to address improved software quality by improving the performance of the human engineers. Seventy per cent of the cost of developing software is attributable to personnel costs. Thus, the skills, experience and work habits of the engineers involved in software design are crucial to the success of development. In order to address the human component of software design, the PSP has been made as easy to navigate and use as possible. A complete PSP should include tools to track the efficiency of the engineer in various ways and tools to allow the engineer to discover ways of improving their performance. The use of plans and procedures that are part of a PSP brings order and efficiency to a job and allows the engineer to concentrate on producing a product of excellence. The enhanced discipline that can result from application of the PSP tools can lessen error, waste and inefficiency, which frees financial resources for better uses.

*See also* Programming; Software design, engineering and testing

# PSP (PERSONAL SOFTWARE PROCESS)

The Personal Software Process (PSP) is a structured approach for improving the process of software development. The PSP assists engineers and other such professionals in improving their performance by bringing discipline to the way they develop software. Based on the principles found in the Capability Maturity Model® (CMM) for Software, the PSP is applied by engineers as a guide to a disciplined approach to consistently develop high quality software products in a timely manner. Because much of the research and development cost of software is directly related to personnel costs, the experience, skills, and work habits of engineers mainly determine the results of the software development process. This relationship of the engineer to the results of the development process is the foundation on which PSP is based.

Competent work in most professions requires the disciplined use of established practices. PSP principles assert that creativity and performance are rarely compromised when discipline is introduced into the work place. In fact, PSP experts maintain that bringing discipline to the work place actually improves creativity and performance. The use of plans and procedures can bring order and efficiency to any job and can allow workers to concentrate on producing a superior product and/or service. Disciplined work minimizes wastes, errors, and inefficiencies, and, as a result, frees resources for more and better uses. Because software engineers are generally not taught to plan and track processes, and to measure quality, they usually do not record their work, and rarely measure software quality.

PSP training involves about 150 hours per engineer to complete the course. The extensive course goes beyond just "telling" engineers what to do, but rather "shows" them the appropriate principles to use and how to efficiently collect and analyze the resulting **data**. The PSP teacher explains to engineers how to manage the quality of their products and how to make reasonable commitments. The teacher also provides them with the data to justify their plans. The PSP can be applied to different pieces of the software development process, including small program development, rules and requirements definitions, document writing and editing, systems test procedures, and maintenance and enhancement of large software systems. The PSP has been verified to substantially improve the estimating and planning ability of engineers while strongly reducing product defects. While PSP training teaches a specific personal process, the real point of the training is to teach "process improvement" concepts and to emphasize to the engineer the **value** of a defined process. PSP-trained engineers are expected to assertively control and optimize their work processes by deciding what works for them and what does not work for them.

Because the PSP improves the way the engineer does his or her work, a new way of working in teams is also required. PSP training is most beneficial when followed up by the Team Software Process® (TSP). The TSP emphasizes the new skills and knowledge of the PSP-trained engineer in order to form an effective software development team. Team members use TSP at the beginning of each phase of a project and throughout the project in order to keep it under control.

*See also* Software design, engineering, and testing; Software management

## PUNCH-CARD TECHNOLOGY

Punch-card (or "punched card") technology involves an essentially outdated computer **input and output** storage medium consisting of stiff, thin paper that stores **data** as a series of punched holes arranged in columns. The method for creating the punch-card patterns is called Hollerith coding, where the punch-card was sometimes called the "Hollerith card." From 1890 until the 1970s—at the apex of its popularity—punch-card technology was synonymous with data processing. During this time it was the most popular storage control system for the input and output of data and programs for com-

puters or other data processing machines. Traditionally, a punch-card was a manila card about 3 inches high by 7 inches long, on which 80 columns of data could be entered in the form of holes punched with a keypunch machine or card-punch device. The punched holes corresponded to letters, numbers, and other characters that could be read by a computer connected to a punched-card reader.

Some of the early mechanical information storage devices, the precursors to modern day data processing, were 18th century music boxes that encoded sequences of musical notes as pins on such mechanisms as a revolving drum. The use of punched cards is considered to have originated with the **Jacquard loom** that was invented in 1801 by French silk-weaver and inventor **Joseph-Marie Jacquard** (1752–1834). Jacquard used paper cards with information recorded as holes punched in them to control weaving looms. The Jacquard loom was the first automatic loom able to weave complex patterns with the use of punched cards that controlled its **operation** (however, it did no computations based on the cards). As a result of using punched cards, the Jacquard loom transformed the 19th century textile industry and became the idea for using punched cards in future calculating and tabulating machines. British mathematician and inventor **Charles Babbage** (1791–1871) later used Jacquard's idea of punched-card storage in his mechanical calculating machine, the **Analytical Engine**. The holes on each card allowed an arm to pass through and activate a mechanism on the other side. In the United States census of 1890, American inventor **Herman Hollerith** (1860–1929) used punched cards to hold data within his statistical Hollerith's tabulator. Intrigued with the idea of tabulating large amounts of data, Hollerith developed over the next several years a number of machines for punching and tabulating cards. These punch-cards were later read by various machines in which rows of electrical contacts sensed when a hole was present. In the 1940s the first electronic computers used punched cards and rolls of paper tape with punched holes for storing both programs and data.

In 1896 Hollerith founded the Tabulating Machine Company that later expanded into the **International Business Machines** (**IBM**) Corporation. IBM, originally a producer of punch-card tabulating-machines in 1911, eventually combined the punch-card technology with computers by encoding binary information as patterns of small rectangular holes, one character per column, 80 columns per card. Other coding schemes, card sizes, and hole shapes were tried at different times, but the 80-column width of most character terminals became the foundation of the IBM punched card. Even today, the size of quick-reference cards distributed with many computers follows the size of the 80-column punched cards. The punched card is all but obsolete today, being replaced with such input devices as the keyboard and **mouse** used in conjunction with the computer monitor.

*See also* Analytic engine

# PUSH TECHNOLOGY

Push technology, also called netcasting, is a **World Wide Web** (WWW or Web) applied **data** distribution technology designed to provide end users with personalized Web **access**. The owner of a Web site actively sends, or "pushes" information to registered **Internet** users, either automatically or at specified intervals. Generally, the application of push technology is usually initiated by the user or pre-selected by a Web site administrator, and arrives only as the result of client requests. Push was developed by information services companies (i.e., the broadcast media) as a means of (1) promoting ("pushing") products or services onto potential customers and (2) relieving users from the task of manually retrieving ("pulling") requested information from the Web.

In the past and even today, the Web is mostly based on *pull technologies*, where the user must actively request a Web page before it is delivered. The broadcast media, on the other hand, is an active promoter of push technologies because companies within that industry are able to send information through Webcast servers (the technology to either push or pull selected information from a server to a client) regardless of whether the user is actually at their web site or not. The software that supports push technology can be internal to a Web **browser**, such as **Microsoft** Internet Explorer and Netscape Navigator, or in a stand-along program, such as PointCast and BackWeb.

An important example of a Web-based company using early push technology is PointCast. The now-defunct company, PointCast, founded in 1992 was one of the first companies to deploy push technology when in 1996 it become very popular on the Internet by "pushing" (delivering) customized news, stock quotes, and other selected information through their PointCast Network. Supported by advertisement revenues the PointCast Network used the Internet to transmit its information to registered users at specified intervals. PointCast Network was free, but in order to use it computer users were required to download the PointCast "push client" program. In 1999, LaunchPad Technologies acquired the product, and turned it into EntryPoint, which later became Infogate, often called a "personalized online newspaper."

Companies are more and more frequently using the Internet to deliver information with "assertive" push technology, rather than relying on "passive" pull technology. Probably the oldest and most widely used push technology that is currently on the Internet is electronic mail (**e-mail**). This is a push technology because the user receives mail in a mailbox at their Internet service provide from senders whether it is asked for or not; that is, the sender "pushes" the **message** to the receiver.

The two leaders in Internet browsing software delivered new versions of their browser in 1997 that aimed to make computing less passive and more active. Netscape introduced Navigator 4.0, while Microsoft introduced Explorer 4.0. Both new browsers incorporated "push" technology for the first time, which allowed subscribers to receive Internet data automatically through what some Internet companies called "channels," rather than having to go out and search for it.

*See also* Internet; World Wide Web (WWW)

# Q

## QUANTUM COMPUTING

Quantum computing refers to the current theoretical use of quantum physics in the processing and **memory** functions of computing. Certain properties of atoms or nuclei could allow the processing and memory functions to cooperatively function. These quantum bits, or qubits, would be the computer's processor and memory. The operating speed of qubits is much faster than current technologies permit. Quantum computing is well suited for tasks like **cryptography**, modeling of **data**, and the indexing of very large **databases**. It is, however, not suitable for tasks like **word processing** and **e-mail**.

Qubits operate differently from the current binary system of computing. Now, computers encode information into so-called bits using binary numbers, 0 or 1, and can only do calculations on one set of numbers at a time. In contrast, quantum computers encode information according to quantum mechanical states of the involved atomic constituents, such as spin directions of electrons or the orientation of photons. The various possibilities could also represent 0 or 1, or could represent a combination of the two, or could represent a combination between 0 and 1, and finally, could simultaneously represent many different numbers. All these possibilities could be addressed at the same time—a phenomenon called super-position— something a binary system cannot do.

By doing a computation on many different numbers at once, then using these results to arrive at a single answer, a quantum computer is potentially much faster and more powerful than a classical computer of equivalent size. For example, in cryptography, factoring a number having 400 digits—which could be necessary to break a security code— would take a fast modern day supercomputer millions of years. But a quantum computer could complete the process in about a year. And, while the supercomputer is a bulky instrument that is typically housed in a dedicated space, the quantum computer could theoretically be no larger, and might actually resemble, an average coffee cup.

The orientation of the photons in a qubit also may serve another function. Scientists, including Albert Einstein, noticed that if the polarization of one photon (the pattern of its light emission) is measured, then the state of the polarization of another photon becomes oriented too, no matter how far away the second photon is from the first. The phenomenon, called entanglement, effectively wires qubits together, and makes the electric transfer of information transfer from one qubit to another. While not practically useable as yet, quantum teleportation has been demonstrated in the laboratory setting.

A major hurdle to quantum computing is how to isolate the qubits from the environment, since even a stray interaction of an external atom would produce a measurement. The inner working of a quantum computer must somehow be separated from its surroundings, while at the same time being accessible to operations like loading of information, execution of information and reading-out of information. Currently, the best approach involves the exposure of liquids to magnetic fields, much like the technique of nuclear magnetic resonance. Atoms in the liquid can orient themselves in the field, producing the entanglement behavior.

If successful, the use of liquids as computing devices will eliminate the need for extremely small **hardware** components. The discipline of **nanotechnology** would not be applicable to a quantum computer.

*See also* Nanotechnology

## QUERY LANGUAGE

Query language is crucial to the construction and manipulation of the repositories of computerized **data**. The **design** of query languages allows the user to, in effect, ask a question of the data, and then to examine only a selected data point or larger portions of the data to attempt to answer the question. An important feature of query languages is the utility with multiple **databases** that have been constructed using the same platform. In the age of the **Internet**, with the multitude of databases, the ability to retrieve and compare data from a wide variety of sources is extremely useful and productive.

One of the most important of these database building blocks is the Structured Query Language, or SQL. It is used to navigate through the so-called **relational databases**, where data can be spread across multiple tables. It is a flexible query language, and so enjoys great popularity and use.

SQL has several variations, which enable it to function with variously designed databases, such as the versions offered by Oracle or **Microsoft**. All of these variations, however, are based upon the industry standard **American National Standards Institute** SQL. The **commands** used in SQL can be divided into two main sublanguages. These are the Data Definition Language and the Data Manipulaton Language. The Data Definition Language contains all the commands necessary to make or destroy databases and the objects within these databases. Once a database has been made, those who use the database utilize the Data Manipulation Language to insert new data, retrieve existing data, and work with the data.

The Data Definition Language as four basic commands to create or destroy databases. The "CREATE" command establishes a database. For example, "CREATE DATABASE PAYROLL" creates an empty database named "payroll." A variant of the "CREATE" command, "CREATE TABLE", will create the tables within the database that will house the data. The second core command of SQL is called "USE". This command selects the target database from among those in the computer. The third command is "ALTER". As its name implies, "ALTER" allows the user to modify how the information is presented in the selected table in the database. Finally, the "DROP" command facilitates the removal of an entire database. The "DROP" command should be used with prudence, given its ability to remove large amounts of information. A variant of the "DROP" command, called "DELETE", is used to remove individual records, instead of globally deleting all the data. "DELETE" is used more often in everyday database manipulations than is "DROP".

The Data Manipulation Language has its own commands to facilitate other manipulations of data. The "INSERT" command is used to add records to an existing table. The "SELECT" command is the most commonly used command in SQL. It permits specific information to be retrieved, ranging from the information in an entire table ("SELECT*") to only selected information contained in that table ("SELECT" or "SELECT*" followed by "FROM" or "FROM WHERE"). The "UPDATE" command can be used to modify the information in a table. The modification can be on all the data in the table or on selected data within the table. A variant of this command, "INSERT", permits the addition of new rows to a table, so that new data can be entered. Finally, as its name implies, "DELETE" is used to remove data. Use of "DELETE FROM" followed by "WHERE" allows the user to target and delete specific information.

Another SQL language that exists is called Data Control Language. This language can be used to specify various security features of a database, and so its **access** is typically restricted to those users who are authorized to perform security-related functions. Typical commands include permission "GRANT" and "REVOKE" commands, "SELECT" and "INSERT".

In addition to the commands listed above, other subcommands exist, permitting a fine-tuning of the use of data by the user.

Other query languages exist, with more specialized intents. The Object-Protocol Model (OPM) Query Language supports scientific, particularly molecular biology, databases, in terms of objects and **protocols** and attributes. A protocol can be a lab experiment, for example. A query language has been developed for the **Extensible Markup Language** (**XML**), a language that permits the interchange of electronic data between multiple sources on the Internet. XML data is proliferating on the Internet. The design of a query language specifically for XML makes the retrieval, manipulation and comparison of data from multiple sources possible.

***See also*** American National Standards Institute; Architecture (software); Data

# QUEUE

In England, lining up to get on a bus is called queuing. In computer language, a queue means to line up a job for the computer's **Central Processing Unit** (**CPU**) or a peripheral device. A job is any task that a computer system does. One type of queue is called a **memory** queue, which is a storage space in memory or on a disk that holds incoming transmissions until the computer can process them. Another example of a queue occurs when printing a file. When the user enters a PRINT command, the document is first copied into a special area called the print **buffer** or print queue, which is a temporary storage area, usually in RAM. This allows the **printer** to print the characters at its own much slower pace and frees up the central processing unit to perform other tasks while the printer is running in the background. Another name for this process is print spooling. SPOOL stands for simultaneous peripheral operations online. SPOOL is a holdover term that originated with mainframes in order to optimize such slow operations as reading cards and printing.

The order in which a system completes a task in the queue depends on the priority system being used. A normal queue would elicit the computer to complete first the first task entered. However, certain devices automatically jump ahead in the queue. For example, **mouse commands** are given a higher priority queue, so that a user would not wait around for the mouse to respond to a click while the CPU is completing some other task. Another example of a higher priority command would be those of the keyboard **driver**. It might be disconcerting to wait for a character to appear on the screen minutes after typing it, the same with making corrections in the text of a document. A priority queue, therefore, is one where the elements of the queue are removed according to their priority, as opposed to a normal queue in which the elements are removed according to their arrival. Thus, a mouse click, having a higher priority than a normal program **operation** will be removed and processed sooner then other program elements, even though it arrived later. Likewise, something with an even higher priority would be removed sooner than a mouse click-data coming in over a serial **port**, for example.

A queue has a similar meaning when referring to **programming**. In this instance, a queue is considered a **data structure**. In this way elements of the queue are removed in the same order as they were entered. Another way to refer to this structure type is first in first out (FIFO). Another type of **data** structure is referred to as a **STACK**. Elements in this type of structure are removed in the reverse order from which they are entered or last in, first out (LIFO). A double-ended queue is one where the elements can be added to or deleted from, either end (input or output). In a normal queue, the elements can only be added to the tail (input) and removed (deleted) only from the head. A double-ended queue is also referred to as a deque. This should not be confused with a dequeue. To dequeue means to remove an element from the queue./

*See also* Buffered file input; Control structure; Physical and virtual memory

# R

## RABIN, MICHAEL O. (1931- )

*German computer scientist*

Michael Rabin is particularly known for his work on the theory and application of computer **algorithms**. He is especially interested in computer security and the application of randomization in computers.

Michael Rabin was born in Breslau, Germany (known as Wrocav, Poland, since the end of the Second World War), in 1931. His father was from Russia and was a Rabbi, as were many of his forefathers. Recognizing the threat of remaining in Germany at this time the family moved to Palestine in 1935. Rabin went to a religious elementary school where he was initially interested in microbiology, though his interests soon changed to mathematics. Against his fathers wishes Rabin went to the Reali School, a school that specialized in the sciences (his father wanted him to attend a religious school prior to becoming a Rabbi). Rabin eventually entered the Hebrew University where he studied mathematics and was awarded an M.Sc. in algebra in 1953. During his studies Rabin became interested in computers (after reading of the work of **Alan Turing** in *Metamathematics* by S. C. Kleene). At this time Israel had no computers so to pursue this interest Rabin had to move to the United States. Initial studies at the State University of Pennsylvania soon gave way to Ph.D. studies in logic at Princeton University under **Alonzo Church**. Rabin's doctoral thesis showed that many problems concerning the mathematical field of groups could not be solved by computers. In 1957, while writing his thesis, Rabin was offered a summer job with **IBM** research (along with Dana S. Scott). Given free reign to research anything they wanted, the pair proposed a computer that could "guess" solutions using **finite-state machines**. The paper relating to this work was not published until 1959 and it had many ramifications for nondeterministic machines. After completing his thesis Rabin returned to IBM Research for another summer job and worked with **John McCarthy**. During this period Rabin came up with the idea of the one-way **function** (a function that is easy to compute in one direction but not the other). In 1974, Rabin returned to the use of randomness in computing to achieve results more quickly; randomness results in a small degree of error, but Rabin found that the increase in speed more than outweighs this problem. Work on **cryptography**, such as the RSA public key system, is built on the randomization process that Rabin discovered. In 1975, Rabin (while on sabbatical to MIT) discovered the work of Gary Miller on the Riemann Hypothesis, which lead Rabin to come up with the fastest known method of finding if a number is a prime.

As of 2001, Rabin is the Thomas J. Watson Professor of Computer Science at Harvard. In his quest for increased computer security Rabin uses sophisticated algorithms to prevent **access**. Rabin and his graduate student D. Tygar invented ITOSS (Integrated Toolkit for Operating System Security), a new model for computer security along with a set of tools that can be incorporated into operating systems to increase levels of security. Rabin is also the developer of IDA—the Information Dispersal Algorithm that is used to spread information within parallel computer arrays and networks as well as the storage of information in arrays of disks (RAIDs). Rabin is also working on the MCB system—a software environment to allow large processing to be carried out on multiple, connected workstations. MCB allows the usage of several computers as if they were one—this has the advantage of increased computing power and a high fault tolerance. This latter aspect of the MCB system is a direct result of the presence of the IDA software as an integral part of MCB. Rabin is also Albert Einstein Professor of Mathematics and Computer Science at the Hebrew University in Jerusalem. He was awarded the ACM Turing award in 1976 (jointly with Dana S. Scott) for "their joint paper *Finite Automata and Their Decision Problem,* which introduced the idea of nondeterministic machines. Their (Scott & Rabin) classic paper has been a continuous source of inspiration for subsequent work in this field."

Rabin spends half of the year living in the United States working at Harvard and the rest of the year working in

Jerusalem at the Hebrew University. His family lives in Jerusalem full time.

*See also* Cryptography; Parallel computing; RAID

# RAID (REDUNDANT ARRAY OF INDEPENDENT DISKS)

RAID is an acronym that stands for Redundant Array of Independent Disks. It is a method of spreading information across several disks. Information can be duplicated on several disks, hence the word **redundancy** in the technique's name. By spreading stored **data** across several hard disks instead of one, users can get both faster performance and much greater **data security**. Depending upon the RAID system being used, a failed drive can be replaced without having to shut down the **host system**.

In 1987, a group at University of California, Berkley published a paper proposing a form of **data storage** they called RAID. The technology was designed to increase the speed of secondary **memory**, so as to keep pace with the increasing speed of central processing units.

There are several levels of RAID configurations. RAID 0 writes data across the different drives, one segment of a drive at a time. Also called striping, it is a linear means of writing the data, where writing begins at a segment of the first drive and then works progressively through the drives.

RAID 1 writes data to two drives at the same time. If one drive fails, the data is not lost, since it resides on the other drive. This process is called mirroring, and it provides total redundancy. Besides providing the protection associated with two copies of the data, mirroring speeds up the reading of data. Different blocks of data can be read simultaneously from the two drives, and then compiled together in the original order. There are several disadvantages to RAID 1. Redundancy is inefficient with respect to space, and the need for more data storage space affects the cost. Also, RAID 1 is often implemented in software rather than **hardware** (also called host based RAID). Software performance demands much from the **CPU**, and so can lower the overall performance of the system. The reliability it offers can be worth the expense, however, in **applications** where data loss could be disastrous, such as accounting or payroll settings.

The original RAID configurations included RAID 2. Instead of creating a backup of all the data, RAID 2 uses a so-called error correction **code**. The code detects and corrects single errors during their input, so that mirroring of data is not necessary. The storage requirements for the code are considerable, however. Due to the inefficiency for small data transfers and the high cost of the additional drives required for the code, RAID 2 as not been commercially available.

RAID 3, also called RAID 0+1, is a combination of striping and a technique called **parity** checking. Parity checking involves determining whether each given block of each drive has an odd or even **value**. When all the values across a stripe are added up, the parity value is obtained. Once a drive's parity value is known, then the failed area of a failed drive can be determined and the information rebuilt on another drive. Parity checking provides redundancy without having to double drive capacity. Because of its efficiency in large data transfers, RAID 3 is used where large files are being stored and where quickness is necessary. Video production and live streaming of images utilize RAID 3 technology.

RAID 4 is similar to RAID 3 except that the size of the stripe written across the drives is larger. This means that the information is spread out across the drives more, and that each drive will not contain exactly the same information. The drives are more independent of one another. The parity information about all the drives is stored only on one of the drives. While this spreads the writing of the information to the drives, recovery of data in the event of a drive failure is more complex and time consuming.

Finally, RAID5 is a combination of striping and a form of parity checking where the parity information is distributed across all the drives. This improves the speed at which data can be read and makes for the most efficient storage of data. Rebuilding a failed drive can still be onerous. Nonetheless, RAID 5 is widely used in servers for **databases**, email, newsgroups, and intranets.

Of all the implementations of RAID, the most commonly used are RAID 1, 3, and 5. Each has their niche with respect to application. Technological advances have created newer forms of RAID (6, 7, 10, 53). Each offers variations on the partitioning of data based on striping or mirroring. Some of the improvements in speed and security of data storage come with greatly increased price tags. The choice of a RAID system becomes one of a balanced consideration of the data storage needs and budget.

*See also* Data storage; Redundancy

# RANDOM ACCESS MEMORY

A computer has two kinds of **memory**. The first is called primary storage, and is used to hold program instructions and **data** while the computer is running. The other kind, called secondary storage, is used for storage of data even while the computer is not running. The primary storage is memory of a kind called Random Access Memory, RAM for short. It is volatile, i.e., susceptible to loss easily upon power outage. The secondary storage can be of many kinds—hard drives, disk drives, tape drives, and so on. The secondary storage is persistent, i.e., retains its contents even when the power is switched off.

RAM is said to be "random access" because any memory cell in RAM can be accessed directly, if the physical address of that cell is known. The counterpart of RAM is SAM, Sequential Access Memory. This kind of memory requires sequential access, i.e., access to items in the order in which they are stored. One example of a sequential-access device from common experience is a cassette tape and its recorder/player—if one wishes to listen to the fifth song on a music cassette, for instance, one has no choice but to go past the first four (either by playing or fast-forwarding). A random-access device from common experience is a music CD player, which by contrast allows for the fifth song on a CD to be played directly.

For obvious reasons, random access is preferable to sequential access—witness the fact that CD players have largely supplanted cassette players in the music business. However, there are some cases where SAM works well enough to be used—such as in memory buffers, where data are normally accessed only in the order in which they were written. One example of such a SAM **buffer** is the texture buffer memory in a video card.

RAM is implemented in a manner very similar to microprocessors, using an **integrated circuit** consisting of transistors and capacitors. The common form of RAM device is called a Dynamic Random Access Memory (DRAM), and uses a pair consisting of a **transistor** and a capacitor, to create a cell that can store a single **bit** of data. The function of the capacitor is to maintain an electric potential difference as appropriate to store a 0 or a 1; the transistor acts as a tiny switch to allow read and write access to the capacitor. Usually, the default **value** of a capacitor when there is no potential difference is considered a 0, while an appropriate potential counts as a 1.

There is a significant problem to be faced—the capacitor in a DRAM memory cell cannot hold its state for long. Within a few thousandths of a second, any potential difference that may have been imposed on it is lost due to leakage, thus erasing any bit information that may have been stored. Thus, for DRAMs to work, it is necessary for either the **CPU** or a dedicated memory controller device to come along every so often and refresh the values stored in the memory cells. This refresh must be done by first reading the value that exists in each cell, and then writing it right back on to it, thus prolonging its life. This process has to carry on automatically thousands of times a second—hence the name, Dynamic RAM. It takes a very small amount of time, usually a few dozen nanoseconds (billionths of a second) to read and recharge a memory cell.

DRAM memory cells are created by a **VLSI** etching process in an **array**, whose columns are called bitlines, and whose rows are called wordlines. The address of an individual memory cell is completely specified by its bitline and wordline. In order to access the memory cells, a set of specialized circuitry exists as part of the DRAM device to perform support functions.

The other major kind of RAM is **static** RAM (SRAM), which does not need refreshing. Bits are stored in memory using logic gates known as flip-flops, with one flip-flop required to store each bit. To implement a flip-flop requires about a half-dozen transistors along with appropriate wiring. Because no time is taken for refreshing, static RAM is significantly faster than DRAM. However, because more **hardware** is required per bit of storage, static RAM is more expensive for a given storage size, as well.

In CPU caches, speed is of the essence—a 1 gigahertz CPU has a **cycle time** of one nanosecond, and waiting for a DRAM to be read in 50 or so nanoseconds is very inefficient because many cycles have to be wasted in the wait. The size of the cache is also quite small (rarely exceeding a few hundred

kilobytes, and often significantly less). For these reasons, static RAM is preferred in CPU caches. Dynamic RAM is used for the computer's main primary storage, where the speed requirement is less severe but storage has to be a lot larger.

***See also*** Central processing unit; Computer architecture; Peripherals

# RANDOM NUMBERS, GENERATION OF

At first it might seem odd to want *random* numbers: that is, numbers in which no patterns can be found, which do not "say" anything. Yet it would be difficult to name a branch of science that does not rely, heavily or occasionally, on random numbers.

The most common scientific use for random numbers is in Monte Carlo simulations. A Monte Carlo **simulation** is any calculation that feeds random numbers into a set of deterministic rules (such as Newton's laws of motion) to model the outcome of a physical process. (Monte Carlo simulations are named after the city of Monte Carlo, famous for its gambling casinos.) Most real-world processes involve a random element, such as the arrival times of photons or of phone calls, the decay times of atomic nuclei, or the thermal jigglings of particles. In Monte Carlo simulations, therefore, the purpose of randomness is realism. Another feature of randomness is secrecy; if someone picks a number purely at random, there is no systematic way for someone else to guess what that number is. Random numbers are thus important in **cryptography**, the study of secret codes.

There are two basic ways to make random numbers. One is to perform physical experiments that produce apparently random outcomes: coin-flipping, sampling electronic noise, or the like. To the outcome of each experiment one assigns a number, thus obtaining a random series. The second approach is arithmetical. One may perform calculations that produce sequences of digits that behave for certain purposes as if they were random, even though they are known not to be. Such numbers are called *pseudo-random numbers*, and the recipes or **algorithms** for producing them are called *pseudo-random number generators* (PRNGs).

Both ways of making "random" numbers have their advantages, but PRNGs are much favored today over physical methods for several reasons. First, the speed with which a physical process produces random numbers depends on the process itself, whereas the speed of a PRNG increases with computer speed. Second, physical random number generators tend to be fussy devices requiring regular readjustment. Third, the non-randomness of pseudo-random numbers is really an advantage; a PRNG, being merely a series of calculations, can reproduce the same series of pseudo-random numbers on demand. This property is important in **debugging** Monte Carlo simulations, because it requires a defective simulation to go wrong exactly the same way every time. It is also important in spread-spectrum digital communications systems, which use pseudo-random numbers to smear out transmitted information signals into noise-like signals that are resistant to interference and interception. This technique is made possible by the repeatability of pseudo-random numbers, for the receiver of a spread-spectrum signal can only reassemble the scrambled signal if it is set to generate the same pseudo-random sequence as the transmitter. Only in **applications** where unpredictability is more important than repeatability, such as cryptography, are physical devices still used to produce random numbers.

Many PRNGs are variations on a single, simple algorithm. Consider a series generated by the following rule:

$$x_i = Kx_{i-1} \text{ (modulo } M\text{)}, i = \{1, 2, 3, \ldots \}.$$

That is, each new number in the series ($x_i$) is found by multiplying the previous number in the series ($x_{i-1}$) by some constant $K$, then taking the result modulo $M$. "Taking the result modulo $M$" means that the result of the multiplication $Kx_{i-1}$ is divided by $M$ and only the remainder kept. Thus if $K = 4$, $x_{i-1} = 5$, and $M = 7$, then $Kx_{i-1} = 5 \times 4 = 20$, and $x_i$ is given by 20 modulo 7, which is by definition the remainder of 20/7 (2 6/7). This remainder is 6/7 or approximately .857142—an apparently random number. The first number in the series, $x_0$, is called the "seed" and may take on any chosen **value**, some choices being better than others; 0, for instance, would make a terrible $x_0$, resulting in $x_i = 0$ for all $i$. Every distinct seed produces a distinct, repeating sequence of pseudo-random numbers.

*Pseudo*-random, however, means not truly random. There are several ways in which the numbers generated by a PRNG (such as the one just described) fail to behave like truly random numbers. Their first and most basic failing is repetition or *periodicity*. Periodicity follows from the fact that a binary computer using N-bit words can only name $2^N$ different numbers. Any possible PRNG running on any real computer is therefore doomed to eventually run out of numbers and start repeating itself. The reality is even worse, for no PRNG produces anywhere near the theoretical limit of $2^N$ pseudo-random numbers before starting to repeat itself. Furthermore, other, more subtle failures of randomness can also be detected in the output of any PRNG, and these non-random qualities can (depending on many factors) be disastrous for practical Monte Carlo simulations.

In an effort to overcome these limitations, many PRNGs have been invented over the last 50 or so years. Most are variations on the theme described above: each new number in the series is calculated by subjecting an earlier number in the series to some simple set of arithmetic operations. For example, the PRNG described above is a special case of a slightly more complex group of PRNGs in common use, *linear congruential generators* (LCGs). LCG algorithms have the form

$$x_i = Ax_{i-1} + B \text{ (modulo } M\text{)}, i = \{1, 2, 3, \ldots \}.$$

where $A$ and $B$ are mutually prime numbers. (It can easily be seen that setting $B = 0$ recovers the basic PRNG given earlier.) The PRNG built into the **ANSI C programming** language, for example, is an LCG algorithm with $M = 2^{31}$, $A = 1103515245$, $B = 12345$, and seed $x_0 = 12345$.

Other PRNGs in widespread use are multiple recursive generators, lagged Fibonnaci generators, inversive congruential generators, and explicit-inversive congruential generators. Much effort goes into testing these algorithms to characterize

the statistical qualities of the numbers they generate. A cautious researcher using Monte Carlo simulation will sometimes run her or his simulation several times, using a different PRNG for each run to see how this affects the results.

The field of PRNG **design** and evaluation continues to be an active one, driven by the ever-increasing use of computer simulation as a scientific tool.

***See also*** Cryptography; Floating-point arithmetic; Long-distance communication; Simulation

# RANDOMIZED ALGORITHMS

A randomized algorithm is one which is able to take one or more steps in a non-deterministic fashion, on purpose. Such **algorithms** are used in many cases. The **correctness**, or the worst-case or average performance of many deterministic algorithms is often derived from an "adversary argument" which posits the existence of a hypothetical "adversary" who is able to arrange things so as to make things as difficult as possible for the algorithm. In this context, it is often assumed that the adversary has full knowledge of the expected behavior of the algorithm. A randomized algorithm which may behave in several ways at one or more steps may be thought of as a probability distribution on a set of deterministic algorithms (one for each possible choice the randomized algorithm may make). An adversary in such a situation may not be able to devise a single input strategy that defeats any randomly chosen algorithm from this set. This is the paradigm that lies behind the success of randomized algorithms.

Randomized algorithms are used for many reasons, some of which we look at below.

- Random sampling—if a population space of items to be evaluated is very large so that not every member of the space can be measured, then a randomization procedure is applied to draw a sample whose characteristics are likely to be close to that of the whole population itself. A real-life example of random sampling is in political polls and the like (where instead of asking the whole electorate whom they will vote for in the next election, a sample of a few thousand or so is asked, and the results extrapolated for the whole community), but in computer science the technique is used most notably in selection algorithms, geometric and **graph algorithms**, and approximate counting.

- Abundance of witnesses—if it is required for an algorithm to determine whether a given input has a certain property (such as whether a number given is prime), then the problem is often solved by finding a "witness" which can attest to the property in the input, or conversely, by showing that no witness exists. In many problems, the search space in which to look for such a witness is very large, and an exhaustive search cannot be made. However, if one is able to establish that there are many witnesses in the search space, it is possible to draw candidates from that space at random and test whether they are witnesses. If the randomization is done well, then after a limited number of trials it can be said with a high degree of assurance that if no witness is found, then the input does not have the required property.

- Fingerprinting—a long input such as a **string** can often be represented by a short "fingerprint" using a random algorithm. If two inputs are to be compared, for example, it may suffice to show that their fingerprints are identical, rather than having to compare the complete inputs in every detail.

- Random reordering—in card games, it is almost always the practice to shuffle the deck well before the cards are dealt. The reason for this is that shuffling removes any patterns there may be in the deck (from previous games, etc.), and makes the game fair. Likewise, in many **sorting algorithms** and the like, it is a good idea to use a pre-processing step and randomly reorder the input before the main algorithm is applied. The chances that the reordered input will be a pathological worst-case for the algorithm is then reduced considerably.

- Load balancing—in parallel or distributed computing applications where it is desirable for processors to share the computing burden evenly, randomization is often a good technique to spread the load around. Deterministic load-balancing is usually not possible because real-time global information concerning all processors is not available at any one location in the system.

Randomized algorithms are of two basic types, called Las Vegas and Monte Carlo algorithms. A Las Vegas algorithm will always give a correct result, but its performance with respect to running time and use of other resources may vary. A Monte Carlo algorithm, by contrast, is one that may fail. Monte Carlo algorithms that compute decision problems—those for which the answer is always YES or NO, such as, "Can this non-planar graph be colored with five or fewer colors?"—may be of two types, having either one-sided error or two-sided error. A Monte Carlo algorithm with one-sided error can only be wrong one way; for instance, it may be wrong when it says NO, but it will always be right if it says YES. One with two-sided error can be wrong both ways.

**Genetic algorithms** are a special kind of randomized algorithms which scour a large search space using randomization.

One important issue in all randomization procedures used in algorithms—or even in the real world—is how one obtains a random value for use. In the real world, it is common to toss a coin or roll a die; if there are no structural deformities that bias the coin or the die to land a particular way, we are able to say that the result is a random **value**. However, within computers, the problem is more difficult. It has been shown mathematically that no deterministic algorithm can be used to generate truly random numbers. However, a sufficiently complex and well-designed program or routine may generate "pseudo-random numbers" that look sufficiently random unless one understands the workings of the program used to create them. Such a routine is usually begun by taking as input a specific value, called a "seed," and then generates a fixed but random-looking sequence. Every sequence of invocations of the routine starting with a particular seed is the same, which can be useful in some cases. If such repetitive behavior is not desirable, it is common practice to seed a pseudo-random generator using an unpredictable **variable**, such as the process id or the time of day. (Every process on **Unix** and other operating systems has a unique process id, one that cannot easily be predicted because on a larger system, many processes are created and killed constantly and the complete process history since the most recent start of the system is not known. Likewise, the time-of-day with an accuracy of microseconds is almost impossible to fix with any accuracy by an adversary.)

*See also* Genetic algorithms

# RASKIN, JEFFREY (1943- )
*American artist, musician, computer scientist, writer*

Jef Raskin has held a wide variety of positions in computing and other spheres, but he is fated to be forever associated with the development of the **Apple** Macintosh computer, as he was the manager of advanced systems at Apple for this particular project.

In 1943 Jef (Jeffrey) Raskin was born in Brentwood, New York, on Long Island. After local schooling Raskin was awarded a B.S. in mathematics and physics from the State University of New York at Stony Brook in 1964. Following this Raskin was awarded a B.A. in 1965 in the philosophy of science with a minor in music—this was also from the State University of New York at Stony Brook (the two courses had been taken part concurrently). Raskin moved to Pennsylvania State University to study for a Ph.D. in philosophy, but decided he wanted to switch to computer science. Unfortunately Pennsylvania State did not offer a Ph.D. in computer science, so Raskin had to transfer to an M.S. course. He was awarded this degree in 1967 with a thesis on *"A Hardware Independent Computer Graphics System"*. From here Raskin decided to continue in computers and moved to the University of California at San Diego where from 1967 to 1969 he undertook graduate studies in electronic and computer music. These studies were halted when Raskin joined the faculty. During all of his time at various universities Raskin took a number of different jobs to support himself, the majority of these involved computer projects of some sort. From 1970 to 1974 Raskin was an assistant professor at the University of California at San Diego, he taught chiefly in the computing department although he did also teach a small number of courses within the music faculty. From 1974 to 1979 Raskin was a faculty member at the San Francisco Community Music Center, and from 1976 to 1978 he was also working as a computer consultant and writer. At the Music Center Raskin taught recorder, harpsichord, chamber ensemble, and music theory. Another side job at this time for Raskin was Jef's Friends Model Aircraft Company, which he and several partners ran from 1974 to 1979. Raskin is on record as saying that this particular experience taught him more about business than he ever earned in money from it. One reason he may have had difficulty in making money from running his own business was that at various times during the period from 1974 to 1979 he was also involved in Bannister and Crun (a software consulting and documentation service). He also spent two years working as an advertising and portfolio photographer and as a recreation leader for the city of Brisbane recreation department.

From 1978 to 1982 Raskin had what must surely be his most famous position—at Apple Computers Incorporated. From 1978 to 1979 Raskin was the Manager of New Publications and New Product Review. He then moved to become manager of Applications Software from 1979 to 1980. From 1980 to 1982 Raskin was the manager of advanced systems for the Macintosh project. In 1982 Raskin took a position in Denmark, working as an instructor in operating systems and documentation for the Dansk Datamatic Institute of Lyngby. From 1982 to 1989 Raskin was chairman and CEO of Information Appliance Incorporated. Since 1989 Jef Raskin has worked full-time as a user-interface and system-design consultant, based in California. Here his contracts include many world famous names such as **Intel**, Xerox, and **IBM**, as well as many smaller, less well-known companies. His position as a consultant has not stopped Raskin from holding positions with other companies at the same time. From 1999 to 2000 Raskin was the VP for Interaction **Design** in California. A prolific writer, Raskin has authored several books, including *The Humane Interface*, published in 2000, and he has also had over 500 articles published. In 1982 Raskin married Linda Blum and together they live in California where they have two daughters and a son. There are many other positions that Raskin has held, usually in parallel with the ones here listed; many were short-term projects or part-time positions. For all of the different fields he has worked in, it is still his position as part of the design team for Apple Computers in the late 1970s and early 1980s that Raskin will be remembered for.

*See also* Apple

## READ-ONLY MEMORY (ROM)

Read-only **memory** (ROM) is a **semiconductor integrated circuit** that functions as a computer device for the permanent storage of **data** and **programming** instructions. Once it is pre-recorded at the time of manufacture the ROM can be read randomly but cannot be modified. A ROM memory device is made when a **design** company provides a semiconductor manufacturer with the instructions or data that is to be stored, and then the manufacturer makes the specified devices according to those specifications. Since making memory devices is an expensive procedure, ROM devices are almost always made in very large quantities. Before making ROM devices, experimental designs are created in small quantities using PROM (programmable read-only memory) or EPROM (erasable programmable read-only memory). The evolved definition of ROM has expanded to also include forms of memory that can be modified, but generally only under particular circum-

stances, so that, in general usage, ROM means any read-only device, including PROM and EPROM.

ROM is often compared to random-access memory (RAM), also called main memory. ROM is called non-volatile storage because it retains its contents even when the power is switched off. RAM, on the other hand, is called volatile because it (generally) does lose its contents under the same conditions.

ROM, informally called nonerasable storage, is often a small amount of memory used inside computers to hold programs for embedded systems (components of computers systems used without human intervention) since they usually have a fixed purpose. On computer motherboards, ROM is normally present in the form of an integrated circuit (commonly called a "chip") such as the computer **BIOS** chip. The BIOS (basic input/output system) is the set of software control routines that tests **hardware** at startup, starts the operating system, and supports the transfer of data among hardware devices. This information is stored in ROM so that it can be executed when the computer is turned on. It is critical that the data within the BIOS remains fixed so that the computer starts ("boots up") exactly the same way each time it is turned on. For this reason, the ROM is used to maintain a consistency in the operating system of the computer. In addition, ROMs are used extensively as controllers in peripheral devices (such as printers, whose fonts are usually stored in ROMs) and other electronic devices. ROM is also used in many other **applications**. A major purpose of this technology is within video games where a cartridge uses many ROM chips in order to store all the information that is necessary for the running of the game. ROM does not only exist in the form of chips. Compact disks (CDs) are ROM, too. When computers are used in hand-held instruments, household appliances, automobiles, and other such products, the program instructions for their routines are generally stored in ROM chips or some other non-volatile chip such as a PROM or EPROM.

*See also* Integrated circuit; Memory; Microprocessors; Random-access memory (RAM)

## REAL MODE

Real mode is an operating mode of x86 **microprocessor** chips that emulates the **memory** management used by the 8086 or 8088 microprocessor chips manufactured by **Intel**. The real mode of execution is supported by Intel 80286 processors ad those developed subsequently.

Real mode limits the processor to 1MB of memory and does not provide any memory management or memory protection. In real mode, adding a so-called address offset to an existing segment **register** creates addresses. This generates an address that is 20 bits long. In another mode, called protected mode, memory protection and management features are available, as the segment register can link to a table of descriptors. The descriptors contain the memory protection information. The protected mode also supports **multitasking**, while real mode does not.

Examples of real mode of **operation** include the drivers that support various devices and MS-DOS. The 80386 and later microprocessors also support a third mode called virtual 8086 mode. In virtual mode, the microprocessors can run several real mode programs simultaneously.

*See also* DOS (Disk Operating System; Intel microprocessors; Memory

# REAL-TIME COMPUTING

In some **applications**, it is not sufficient for a computation to be merely carried out successfully at some time or the other. It is also necessary for it to be carried out within a specified time period, not sooner or later. One example of this is the computer systems that help control a space shuttle during takeoff. It is necessary for the computer to receive sensory **data** about thrust, tilt, altitude, velocity, air resistance, and the like, and make suitable changes at exactly the right time. Either too soon or too late could be disastrous. Another example is an automated assembly line where a robotic arm has to pick up an **object** off a moving conveyor belt. If the arm moves too soon, the object will not be there yet, and if the arm moves too late, then it will no longer be there. In either case, the task would be considered not to have been performed correctly.

The canonical definition of a real-time system is by Donald Gillies, and says, "A real-time system is one in which the [overall] correctness of the computation not only depends upon the logical correctness of the computation, but also upon the time at which the result is produced. If the timing constraints of the system are not met, system failure is said to have occurred."

The discipline or practice of real-time computing is often confounded with fast or **interactive computing**, especially as a result of marketing hype or uninformed usage. Real-time computing can be fast or interactive, but it is not necessarily either. A robotic device working on a factory floor may be working in real time and yet may be quite slow, performing actions in seconds or minutes. It may also not allow for much interactive control beyond initialization, starting, and stoppage. Conversely, not all fast computing is necessarily real-time, and interactive systems that are often fast but have no specific bounds on response times are not real-time either. The point to be noted in this context is that in the correct sense, a real-time system is merely one which offers a specific performance guarantee on the temporal latency of a solution generated by it. Such a guarantee is almost always required for the specific application which the system is to be used for.

A distinction is sometimes sought to be made between "soft' and "hard' real-time. This is not standardized, and vigorous disputes exist about the meanings of these terms. In general, however, it is perhaps safe to say that hard real-time often refers to systems with rigorous constraints, while soft real-time is used to refer to systems with some temporal constraints but less rigorous ones.

Much interest in real-time systems arises from a perceived need for a single purpose—streaming audio/video feeds (often live and interactive as well) for teleconferencing and similar applications. A moving video sequence is generated as a sequence of still frames, typically thirty or so a second. The human eye, upon being shown the sequence of frames, is unable to distinguish individual frames and observes fluid motion. Unfortunately, video frames also typically require huge amounts of **memory** and bandwidth, though audio takes much less bandwidth and can be comfortably transmitted in real time. Thus, at the present time, bandwidths on the **Internet** and most public networks are still too small to permit such applications. If there is insufficient bandwidth to transmit the video frames at the required rate, what happens is that several frames are generated at the source in the time it takes to transmit a single frame. The only meaningful way to handle this situation is to drop all the frames that have been generated in the time it has taken to transmit a frame, and only transmit the latest frame. At the receiving end, this results in non-contiguous frames updating at a slow enough rate for the human eye to distinguish them, thus causing the appearance of jerky or irregular motion.

Thus, real-time video transmission is closely linked to the problems of high-bandwidth systems, and also to data compression, especially image and video compression. However, even if high bandwidths or **data compression** techniques are available, it may be necessary to process the received video feed prior to display, and this entails the need to be able to process each frame in less time than it is generated, with the latency requirement that the processed output should be made available soon enough for the human user not to notice any difference. This is a serious challenge in real-time computing, and is a major area of contemporary research.

Real-time computing often requires fast **hardware**, of course, but that is not typically enough. It is essential that the operating system running on the hardware be able to deliver the goods as well. A special kind of operating system, called Real-Time Operating System (RTOS) is considered desirable for real-time computing. An RTOS has to be multi-threaded and pre-emptible, and should have some manner of enforcing **thread** priority. It should have proper mechanisms for synchronizing threads, and its behavior should be well known. An RTOS also should have a small and known **interrupt** latency (the time it takes for an interrupt to take effect) and system **call** latency (the time it takes for a system call to complete). The RTOS should also specify whether it, or device drivers, **mask** the interrupts, and if so for what maximum duration.

Real-time systems often are extremely difficult to **design** and verify. **Temporal logic** is often used in analyzing them.

*See also* System reliability; Temporal logic; Verification

# RECORD

A record is an ordered set of fields in a database or spreadsheet file. In database and spreadsheet files, the record commonly refers to the row of the sheet or page contained within the database or spreadsheet. The rows are further divided into cells that may contain text, numbers, formula, or program instructions. When used in connection with files, a record refers to the line of the file.

The record field may be preset to a fixed width in terms of bits or characters. The use of delimiting characters such as a comma or tabs can also be used to separate fields of **variable** length within a field. Fields delimited by commas are, for example, denoted as CSV (comma separated **value**) fields.

In contrast to the usually horizontal orientation of records, columns are usually vertically oriented collections of all records in a particular field. If records are denoted by numbers (1, 2, 3...) and columns by numbers (A, B, C...), then a spreadsheet record or row would be composed of cells A1, A2, A3...etc. In contrast, column B would be composed of all the **data** in cells denoted by B1, B2, B3...etc.

Accordingly, fields are areas or cells of a record (the columns in a particular row of a spreadsheet).

A **linked list** is a **programming** element that contains a pointer to the next element in order to compose a directional list. Some lists, termed doubly linked lists, contain pointers to the next element in the list and the previous element used. Lists offer reliable sequential **access** to data.

When data access may be random rather than sequential, an **array** is often used to store the data. Records differ from arrays because arrays are grouped and identified by their particular indices (the dimensions identified by bracketed identifiers or subscripts). Arrays are usually stored next to each other, but the particular programming language in use determines whether the storage is by rows or columns.

*See also* Data structure; Spreadsheet programs

# RECURSION

When a computed **function** (or procedure) calls itself, it is called "recursive." If the **call** is via one or more other functions then this group of functions are collectively called "mutually recursive." If a function were to always call itself whenever it is called, then it would never terminate. Since each call of the function requires an activation frame in the computer's **memory**, it would soon use up all of the computer's resources and bring it to a complete halt as well. Therefore, a recursive function first performs some test on its arguments to check for a "base case"—a condition under which it can return a **value** without calling itself. When it is called with higher values, then it calls itself with a lower value, and so on, until a base case is reached and values can be returned to the higher-level calling routines.

The canonical example for a recursive function or computation is the factorial function, defined as the product of the first *n* natural numbers. The factorial of 0 and 1 are defined to be 1, and the factorial of any larger number is defined to be the product of that number and the factorial of its predecessor. Therefore, a factorial can be recursively computed. For example, let us compute the factorial of 4 in this way:

- The factorial of 4 is, by definition, 4 times the factorial of 3.
- The factorial of 4 therefore is, by extension, 4 times 3 times the factorial of 2.
- That in turn similarly is 4 times 3 times 2 times the factorial of 1.
- Since the factorial of 1 is already known to be 1, the computation need be carried no further, and it suffices to simply derive the answer, which is 24.

Recursion is in some ways analogous to mathematical induction, and a problem that can be solved recursively can also be solved inductively. The application of recursion is also often called tail recursion, because the recursion step where the original function is called with new, usually smaller parameters occurs near the end or the "tail" of the function definition, with previous parts accounting for base cases where the function can yield a value without invoking itself.

It is relatively simple to write program **code** for a recursive function. Many classes of problems, especially those that lend themselves to solutions by divide-and-conquer techniques, are natural candidates for application of recursion. The credit for realizing the importance of recursion goes to Professor **John McCarthy** (formerly of the Massachusetts Institute of Technology, now at Stanford University). McCarthy strongly advocated the use of recursion in the **design** of Algol60, a precursor of modern **programming** languages such as **Pascal** and **C**. Later on, he developed the language Lisp, which introduced recursive **data** structures, as well as recursive procedures and functions.

In considering the use of resources by recursive procedures, it is natural to use a mathematical construct known as a recurrence equation. A recurrence equation over the natural numbers defines the value of a mathematical function at a given integer in terms of the value of that very function for a smaller integer. As with induction or recursion, the base case has to be stated separately, and the recurrence only applies for input values larger than the base case. Recurrence equations are important in other areas of **discrete mathematics** as well, such as in forming discrete analogues of differential equations.

The concept of recursion plays a central role in **computability** theory as well. In considering the question of computability, i.e., just what mathematical functions that map the natural numbers to the natural numbers are computable, a special class of functions called primitive recursive functions are defined. The primitive recursive functions are just those that can be derived by composing the constant function, the successor function, and the projection functions. The work of the great 20th-century mathematician Stephen Kleene showed that a computable set is just one which can be expressed as the range of a primitive recursive function. Because of Kleene's work and influence, the branch of learning known as recursion theory was developed, and is now also known as computability theory.

Recursion theory is very closely tied to the work of **Alan Turing** and Kurt Gödel, and the **Halting Problem** on Turing machines, and the incompleteness theorems of Gödel are most commonly expressed in recursion-theoretic terms as set forth by Kleene. The Halting Problem, for instance, can be expressed by saying that there is a set of natural numbers that is recursively enumerable but not recursive. Therefore, the concept of recursion plays a central role in questions of **undecidability** also.

*See also* Abstract data types; Divide-and-conquer; Programming

# RECURSIVE DESCENT PARSER

A recursive descent parser is a computer program designed to take input as a language, such as a list of tokens generated by the lexer, interactive online **commands**, markup tags, sequential source program instructions, or some other form of defined interface, and convert it into an abstract **data structure** that can be handled by other programs, such as other parts of a **compiler**. Usually this conversion involves breaking the input up into usable parts that is done using **recursion**. It is basically a translator and is usually part of a compiler. This particular type of parser, a recursive descent parser, uses recursive procedures to model the parse **tree** that is to be constructed that is it is an algorithm that calls itself within some part of executing its own task. It can be as simple as taking a **string** of input and cutting off the first part of the string and loading it into a string list. Turbo **Pascal** is an example of a recursive descent parser.

There are typically three subsections to a recursive descent parser. The first part of the algorithm divides the problem into one or more simpler or smaller parts of the overall problem. In particular for each nonterminal in the grammar, a procedure that parses a nonterminal is constructed that processes the right-hand side of the production. Each of these constructed procedures can accept input, match **terminal** symbols, or **call** other procedures to accept input and match terminals in the right-hand side of a production. Because the right-hand side of the production itself is a nonterminal, the body of the procedure will consist of a call to itself. The second subsection invokes the **function** to be performed over and over on each part. The third subsection combines the solutions of the individual parts into a solution for the overall problem. In recursive descent parsing the grammar is thought of as a program with each production as a recursion or recursive procedure. So there would be a procedure corresponding to the nonterminal program.

LL(1) parsing is often described as table-driven recursive descent parsing. This is a top-down parsing method that proceeds by expansion of productions, beginning with a start symbol. Recursive descent parsing has the same restrictions as the general LL(1)-grammar type parsing method. This particular type of parsing is most effective and appealing when the language is LL(1), when a quick compiler is called for, and where there is no tool available.

# REDDY, RAJ (1937- )
*Indian American computer scientist*

Raj Reddy is one of the world's leading experts on **robotics** and **artificial intelligence**. The director from 1979 to 1992 of the Robotics Institute at Carnegie Mellon University in Pittsburgh, Pennsylvania, Reddy was responsible for the **operation** of thirteen laboratories and three program centers, and oversaw the research performed at the institute on numerous topics related to computer-integrated manufacturing and robotics **design**. He is currently the dean of computer science at Carnegie Mellon University.

Dabblal Rajagopal Reddy was born on June 13, 1937, in Katoor, India, near Madras. His father, Srdenivasulu Reddy, was an agricultural landlord and his mother, Pitchamma, was a homemaker. His interest in civil engineering led him to study at the University of Madras College of Engineering, where he received his bachelor's degree in 1958. Soon after finishing his undergraduate work in India, Reddy moved to Australia, calling it home for a number of years. While in Australia, Reddy worked as an applied science representative for the **International Business Machines** Corporation (**IBM**) in Sydney. His primary job used computers for structural analysis. Although his formal education was in civil engineering, his first employment and early practical experience were with computers, which prepared him for future work in the computer field. Reddy studied for and received a master's degree in computer science from the University of New South Wales in 1961. During his post-baccalaureate education his interest and course of study changed from the civil to the computer engineering disciplines.

Reddy moved to the United States in 1966 and received his doctorate from Stanford in the same year. He became a naturalized citizen and joined the faculty of Stanford University as an assistant professor of computer science. His time at Stanford only lasted three years; in 1969 he moved to Pittsburgh and joined the faculty of Carnegie Mellon University as a professor. It was here that Reddy began his study of the rapidly expanding fields of robotics and artificial intelligence. He was named director of the Robotics Institute in 1979.

Reddy has focused on two areas within the field of robotics: automatons capable of performing manufacturing and assembly-line tasks, and fully functional robots that can perform, understand, and use more complex functions like speech, hearing, and sight. Although the later part of the twentieth century has seen a tremendous growth in the use of robots for assembly-line manufacturing chores, Reddy feels that researchers are still thirty to one hundred years away from creating machines capable of speech and sight. Aiming to make this goal a reality, Reddy developed an interdisciplinary program at the Institute that trains students in mechanical engineering, computer science, and management in order to give them the background they need to design the complex robotics manufacturing systems of the future.

Reddy remains at the forefront of studies in **human-computer interaction**. His research projects include building robots capable of speech recognition and comprehension systems, and the Automated Machine Shop, a full manufacturing facility using robotics technology. Reddy is also exploring an area he calls "white-collar robotics," that is, robots programmed to perform such white-collar tasks as production scheduling and other management functions. Reddy and his colleagues at Carnegie Mellon also investigate the possibilities for **programming** robots to make subjective decisions (artificial intelligence), for building robots that can learn from observation, and for designing robots that can work in environments that are hazardous for humans, such as waste disposal sites and nuclear reactors.

A lecturer in his field and contributor to scholarly journals, Reddy was presented the Legion of Honor by President Mitterrand of France in 1984 for his service at the World Center for Personal Computation and Human Resources in Paris. He was awarded the IBM Research Ralph Gomory Visiting Scholar Award in 1991. He is a member of the National Academy of Engineering, and a fellow of the Institute of Electrical and Electronics Engineers, the Acoustical Society of America, and the American Association for Artificial Intelligence, which he also served as president from 1987 to 1989. Reddy married his wife Anu in 1966 and has two children, Shyamala and Geetha. He looks forward to the day when advances in computer and communication technology will allow every person to use computers in their daily lives.

# REDUNDANCY

Network systems, **Internet** Service providers, utilities and the military are all examples of systems that need to be failsafe. This is accomplished by having backup or redundant systems ready to take over in case the main system breaks down. Redundancy refers to any **peripherals**, computer system and network devices that take on the processing or transmission load when other units fail. This is also called a fault tolerant system. Reliability is achieved by having multiple backups of critical components such as central processing units, memories, disks and power supplies. If one unit fails, another is there to immediately take over. A true fault-tolerant system is expensive to maintain, as the redundant **hardware** is wasted if no system failure occurs. On the other hand, a fault tolerant system provides the same processing capability after a failure as before a system breakdown. This is not true in the case of the high availability systems that could be considered a low-end redundancy structure. These systems do not provide the seamless processing provided by more expensive models, as the software is required to resubmit the job to the second system once the first one fails.

Backing up **data** and files can be considered a form of redundancy, and is a necessary part of a fault-tolerant system. This process is referred to as disk mirroring or duplexing. Data is written on two partitions of the same disk, or on two different disks within the same system. Disk mirroring uses the same controller. Disk duplexing uses a controller for each disk. A controller is an electronic circuit board or system that

expands the computer's ability to handle peripheral devices. **Redundant Array of Independent Disks (RAID)** is a disk subsystem that increases performance and can also provide data backup for a fault-tolerant system. RAID is a set of two or more disks and a specialized disk controller that contains the RAID processing information. RAID also increases performance by disk striping. This allows more than one disk to read and write simultaneously by interleaving bytes or groups of bytes across multiple drives. When used to describe disk drives, interleaving refers to the way sectors on a disk are organized. One-to-one means the sectors are placed sequentially around each track. In two-to-one interleaving, the sectors are arranged so that consecutively numbered sectors are separated by an intervening sector.

Redundancy can also refer to error-checking data transmissions. Redundancy may be used as an abbreviation of cyclic redundancy check, a common technique for detecting data transmission errors. Data reliability is also obtained by checksum and error-Correcting **Code memory**.

*See also* Fault-tolerant computing

# REFERENCE PARAMETER

A reference **parameter** is a parameter, also called an **argument**, which defines the characteristics of a **function**. It is used when the function conveys a **value** to, or changes the value of, a **variable** from the calling block, without an **assignment statement** (such as D = A + B+ C, where D is the variable and the equation is the **expression**) in the calling block. In other words, a reference parameter specifies the location of the particular parameter, rather than containing the actual parameter information that defines the function.

When a function is called for, the reference parameter passes the **memory** address of the function parameter to a routine. The routine, in turn, executes the function.

A reference parameter is usually not information that is widely disseminated, since its use can alter functions that the user has installed.

*See also* Action; Argument; Assignment statement; Call

# REGENERATIVE MEMORY

*Regenerative memory* is any form of **data storage** which requires its contents to be refreshed or regenerated periodically. The first such device ever to be incorporated in a digital computer was the drum capacitor **memory** of the **Atanasoff-Berry Computer** (ABC), built 1942 and widely regarded as the first true electronic computer. The ABC's regenerative memory consisted of two small drums (about the size of coffee cans) spun by an electric motor and studded over their outer surfaces with capacitors. The charge (or lack thereof) on each capacitor represented a **bit** of information. As the drums rotated, charge leaked naturally from their capacitors (all capacitors lose charge over time). Lest the information stored on the drums disappear, a special circuit checked each capacitor once per revolution to see if it was charged: if it was, the circuit recharged the capacitor, preserving the information for another revolution of the drum.

The inconvenience of having to regenerate the contents of the drum memory was compensated by the speed with which **data** could be accessed from the drum, the relative cheapness of the solution, and the relatively high density of the storage system (bits per cubic inch) compared to other methods available at the time (e.g., vacuum tubes).

Despite numerous revolutions in computing technology since 1942, memories comprised of leaky capacitors continue to be a feature of virtually all computers. The CMOS (complementary metal-oxide **semiconductor**) DRAM (dynamic random-access memory) chips that populate most computers today function very much like the spinning drums of the ABC: each bit of information in a CMOS memory chip is stored as a charge on a microscopic capacitor. The charge tends to dissipate, so a special circuit must periodically (many times a second) read the contents of the memory and recharge its capacitors as needed. The frequency with which a DRAM chip's contents must be regenerated (or *refreshed*) is called its *refresh rate*. The reasons for using regenerative capacitive memory are essentially the same today as in 1942: high speed of **operation** and high device density. Some things *have* changed since 1942, however: the ABC regenerative memory stored a grand total of 300 bits, whereas a modern 256 MB DRAM chip stores about two billion bits. Optical regenerative memories are also a topic of research interest at this time.

*See also* Atanasoff-Berry Computer

# REGISTER

Registers are localized component cells of the **central processing unit** (**CPU**). Registers are designed to offer fast **memory** retrieval. There are two principal forms of registers. General-purpose registers are cells that allow the temporary storage of **data** actually being manipulated or utilized by the CPU. The general-purpose registers maintain data to be used as input for the operations performed by the arithmetic/logic unit (**ALU**), and also maintain the output or results from those operations.

Registers serve an important memory function that differs from other **random access memory** (RAM). Register sets comprise only a small area of Ram (typically, modern systems carry an allocation of 32 to 144 registers). The principal difference in register memory is that it may be addressed with only a few bits (e.g., a 4-**bit** or eight-bit register). Other RAM components usually require 20 bits to specify a location. In addition, registers contain actual memory addresses while other RAM memory is indirectly addressed. The use of registers vastly improves computational speed. Although several cycles may be required to **access** other memory components, multiple registers can be addressed, read and written within a single cycle.

Register allocation and register assignments are compiler functions used to designate the values to be placed in registers.

Computer performance and computation ability can suffer from shortage of registers. Without suitable register allocation, it can be difficult to save and store intermediate computational values and, especially in early generation computing systems, register dancing was a serious problem. Register dancing required the highly coordinated of saving and dumping of intermediate values in registers as operational proceeded. Even in modern systems, if there is insufficient register allocation, the system must spill data (register spillage) from the registers into other memory.

There are several forms of physical and functional register configurations. Data registers (DR) are usually 16-bit registers. Address registers (AR) are usually 12-bit registers designed to hold a memory address. **Accumulator** registers (AC) are usually 16-bit registers that function as processor registers. Program counter registers (PC) are usually 12-bit registers that can hold the address of an instruction. Instruction registers (IR) are usually 16-bit registers designed to hold instruction **code**. Input (INPR) and output (OUTR) registers are usually 8-bit registers that function to hold **input and output** characters.

Increment and decrement registers hold **increment and decrement operators** that function to increase or decrease the **value** of a **variable**. Temporary registers (TR) usually 16-bits are utilized to hold temporary data.

*See also* Bus; Compiler; Random-access memory RAM)

# RELATIONAL DATABASES

There are several kinds of **databases**, the common types being:
- Hierarchical;
- Network;
- Relational;
- **Object**;
- Object-Relational.

Among these, the hierarchical and network database types are of older **design** than relational databases, but the others are newer.

An hierarchical database is built upon **record** types and a parent-child relationship among record types. All accesses to child records must go through **parent** records. Relationships are strictly hierarchical, and every record type must be a child only to a single parent. This makes it difficult to represent **data** where loops or other cross-links exist in relationships. Information storage and retrieval are fast, but querying is not, and it is not possible to build a decision support system, using this database model.

Under the network model, a more realistic relationship is assumed between data elements—a record type can be linked to more than one other record type. The paths needed to be followed to **access** data are still predetermined, but they are less restricted than in the hierarchical database model. Overall, this makes the network model more capable than the hierarchical model.

The relational database model, of interest to us here, makes no assumptions about the kinds of relationships existing among the data elements. Data in many files are related through the use of a key field. The use of the key as an index enables the computer to locate records without having to read all the records in the file. Relations are dynamic and determined as needed. An object database, or an object-relational database, is a special case of a relational database, where storage of complex data types called objects is supported. Concepts such as inheritance, **polymorphism**, and **encapsulation** are allowed for the object model.

Historically, the development of relational databases may be traced to a paper titled "A Relational Model of Data for Large Shared Data Banks," written by E.F. Codd of **IBM** and published in the *Communications of the ACM* in 1970. This paper laid out the theoretical or mathematical principles upon which relational databases are founded. Later on, Dr. Codd presented a paper titled "The Relational Approach to Data Base Management: An Overview" at the Third Annual Texas Conference on Computing Systems in 1974; this was his presentation of the famous 12 principles of relational databases.

Software, called a relational database management system (RDBMS) is used to create, update, and manage relational databases. Common examples of RDBMS software in widespread use includes Oracle, Sybase, Informix, and Xbase. Billions of dollars are spent every year in research and development of newer systems as well.

A major thrust in recent times has been in the development of databases that are distributed across many nodes; this is, in a sense, a natural consequence of the growth of **distributed systems**. A distributed database is one where data elements are stored on different nodes, sometimes on geographically widespread systems. This kind of database is also referred to as a replicated database. Data elements may be read simply by accessing a local or nearby replica, but all replicas of the data must be changed when updating. CORBA is an example of a distributed database system.

Special issues that arise in case of relational databases that are distributed, are consistency, availability, and partitions.

- Consistency is the property that all replicas are identical in their contents.

- Availability is the property that the database, or certain parts thereof, are always available. A database cannot be always available, but good designs allow for a high degree (often expressed as a percentage) of availability, such as a design assurance that it will be available 95% of the time.

- Partitions are the splits of databases on account of faults in the underlying distributed system that cause communication failures. This can cause difficulties with updates, among other things.

A well-known result in distributed databases called the CAP theorem says that one may achieve only two of the three objectives above. That is, a database may be consistent and available, but it will not tolerate partitions; else, it may be consistent and tolerate partitions, but it will not always be available; else, it may be available and tolerant to partitions, but it will not always be consistent.

*See also* CORBA; Databases; Distributed systems

# RELATIONAL OPERATORS

Relational operators, sometimes called comparison operators, are operators (symbols that represent a specific **action**) that allow computer programmers to compare two or more values. Typical relational operators are: greater than ($>$), equal to ($=$), less than ($<$), not equal to ($<>$, #, !, or $\neq$), greater than or equal to ($\geq$), and less than or equal to ($\leq$).

A *relational expression* is an **expression** that uses a relational **operator** such as "less than" to compare two or more values (called "operands"). Every expression consists of at least two operands and can have one or more relational operators. Operands are values (usually alphanumeric constants or variables), whereas operators represent particular pre-specified actions. The general form of a relational expression is *a (rel-op) b* where *a* and *b* are operands and *rel-op* (from *relational-operator*) generically refers to the various possible relational operators. With respect to the relational operators listed above: (1) a $>$ b is true if a is greater than b, (2) a $=$ b is true if a and b have the same **value**, (3) a $<$ b is true if a is less than b, (4) a $<>$ b is true if a and b do not have the same value, (5) a $\geq$ b is true if a is greater than b or if a is equal to b, and (6) a $\leq$ b is true if a is less than b or if a is equal to b. For example, the relational expression x $>$ 6 states that the **variable** x is greater than the constant 6. The expression is TRUE if x is greater than 6, and is FALSE if x is less than or equal to 6.

The result of a relational expression becomes a Boolean value when used inside a computer. Boolean values are binary in nature, meaning that there are only two possibilities; for example, TRUE or FALSE, or 1 or 0). This mathematical method used within virtually all of today's digital computers, is called **digital logic**, and is generally used interchangeably with Boolean logic. The Boolean value is always a two-valued form (either 1 or 0) when used to represent all interactions and relationships among words, numbers, symbols, and other **data** entered and stored in the computer's **memory**. That is, the result of a relational operator is a zero (0) if the test that the operator implements fails in its conclusion, but is a one (1) if the test succeeds in its conclusion. In the previous example (x $>$ 6), the Boolean value is "zero" if x *is not* greater than 6, while the Boolean value is "one" if x *is* greater than 6 (where zero represents FALSE, and one represents TRUE).

Relational expressions (which always include relational operators) are used in such computer software as **programming** languages, database systems, and spreadsheet **applications**. Each programming language and application has its own rules for what constitutes an appropriate relational operator and how it is used. For example, database systems use relational expressions to specify which information is to be viewed. These types of expressions are called queries.

*See also* Bit; Boolean algebra; Expression; Digital logic; Operator; Logical operations; Value

# REMOTE PROCEDURE CALL (RPC)

One of the staples of modern computing systems is the concept of remote **method** invocation, where a client program calls a procedure or routine in another program running in a server process. This usually is confined to a single physical device, however. An extension of the same basic concept, called remote procedure **call** (RPC for short) allows a client to call a procedure or routine on a server that is running on a distant machine.

A server may itself be a client of another server, so RPCs can be chained. A server process has to have a defined format, called a service interface, that specifies the procedures that are available for remote calling. The service interface should specify which processes are eligible to be called remotely, what the format of a call should be, and what the range or type of acceptable parameters is. The invocation semantics for the service also should specify what should be done in case of failures or abnormal behavior.

Fault-tolerance or fault-masking are important concerns in all distributed computing environments, and certainly so in using RPCs. If the RPC invocation was lost, then the server will not have acted upon the client's request. However, if it was received but the result message it sent has been lost, then the client will not get what it expects. In asynchronous systems, the client often cannot tell the difference between these situations, yet they are often totally different.

Generally, it is possible to classify invocations made of servers into two types—idempotent and non-idempotent. Idempotent is something in possession of the quality referred to by mathematicians as "self-adjoint," and means "repeatable" in plain English. For instance, a command of the form: "Set the temperature of the boiler to 220 Celsius" is idempotent, because it can be repeated safely (if the first command was lost, then the second one takes effect; if the first was acted upon, then the second does nothing). However, a command: "Saw 12 centimeters off the end of this block of wood" is not idempotent; if the first **message** was lost, then the second will do the same thing as the first would have done if it had been received. If the first message was in fact received and acted upon, then the second will cause a problem. There are many examples of idempotent and non-idempotent requests that can be found in daily life; an ATM request to a bank: "Query my checking account balance" is idempotent, but: "Withdraw $100 from my checking account" is not.

Therefore, in deciding the invocation semantics to be used with RPC, it is necessary to know what kinds of procedures are involved, and the likelihood of failures. It may be necessary in some cases to warn the client of an earlier invocation it does not know was successful.

The software that implements or supports RPC can be quite complex, and there is no one universal standard. Generally, however, most RPC software is not concerned with objects or **object** references.

A client accessing a remote service includes one "stub procedure" for each remotely callable procedure in the service interface. The **stub** procedure functions as a proxy—it appears as a local procedure to the rest of the client, which does not know that a call to a remote procedure is going to be involved. When the stub procedure is called, it does not itself execute the call, but marshals the procedure **identifier** and the arguments into a request message, which it then sends to the server via the standard communication module or system. When the server's reply arrives, it unpacks the results contained therein, and passes them on to the other part of the client that called it. The calling part of the client is, as noted, completely unaware of the actual semantics of processing its request.

The server also, like the client, has a stub procedure which acts as a proxy. It receives the request from the client, unpacks it, and calls the corresponding service procedure; when it receives the results from this call, it marshals the values received into a reply message to be sent to the client. Once again, the other parts of the server beside the server stub procedure are not even aware that an external call is being serviced.

The advantage of the non-stub parts of the client and server not being aware of the call semantics is that it permits programmers to use RPC just as they would any other procedure call—the less the designer of software has to know and account for, the easier it is to create the software.

The definition of RPC should include an interface definition that allows one to generate the client and the server stub procedures and the dispatcher which forwards the messages back and forth. In order to do this, a specialized formal language called an interface definition language is used. However, there is no universal or standard interface definition language at this time, and different hardware or systems manufacturers have varying standards.

*See also* Client-server interaction; Butler Lampson; Object-oriented programming

# RESERVED WORD

A reserved word is a word or symbol that has a special meaning, specific to or part of a particular **programming** language or a specific program. Reserved or restricted keywords are used to control how that program is defined. Programs are simply a set of instructions for manipulating **data** within the computer environment. These instructions are written in a particular programming language. There are many different programming languages. **Java**, **C**, **C++**, **BASIC**, COBAL and **Pascal** are just a few of the high-level languages used by programmers. Some examples of reserved words in the Java programming language are "break," "while," "catch," and "try."

Instead of the term GOTO, Java uses the term "break." The goto term in other programming languages is a way to arbitrarily branch, i.e., a way to control flow. The term break refers to the process of breaking out of a block of **code**. Code is a colloquial term for written computer instructions and can appear in a variety of different forms. To illustrate, the code that a programmer writes is called source code. However, computers can only execute instructions that have been written in **machine language**. To get from a high level language that programmers use to one that the computer can understand it must first be transformed by a **compiler**. The compiler reorganizes the source code. Once it has been compiled, it is called **object** code. Executable code is code that is ready to run. When a user buys software, he is buying an executable version of that program. In the Java language, break is also used to break out of LOOPS and SWITCH statements.

"While" is Java's most basic and powerful looping statement. Simply put, looping executes a single statement over and over again until a certain condition has been met; for example, until a Boolean (true or false) statement continues to be true. Each pass through a **loop** is called an **iteration**. A SWITCH is just another word for an option or a **parameter**, i.e., something added to a command to somehow change or refine that instruction. Options, as the term implies, are not required. For example, within the **DOS** operating system, an option has a slash (/) in front of it. If you ask the computer to display it's directories with the DIR command, the /P option instructs the computer to pause between screens. Every application or operating system has different rules for identifying options.

"Catch" and "try" are two reserved words that handle exceptions in the Java programming language. An exception is any unusual or abnormal condition encountered during the running of a code sequence. Previously, other programming languages forced programmers to use return codes, but these are subject to many failures. This is because it is often necessary to understand, at many levels, the intimate details of possible error conditions. The try keyword can be used to specify a block of code that should be guarded against all exceptions. Immediately following a try statement, a catch clause is inserted, which specifies the exception type the user desires to catch.

Words and symbols that are reserved within each program have specific meanings to that program's compiler.

*See also* Programming linguistics

# REVERSE POLISH NOTATION

In school, while learning basic arithmetic, students are also taught precedence rules for the various arithmetic operators. This is often done using a mnemonic such as "My Dear Aunt Sally" (denoting the order as Multiplication, Division, Addition, and Subtraction). Therefore, given an **expression** 2 + 3 × 4 - 1, we know that the multiplication should be evaluated first, followed by the addition and finally the subtraction—the answer thus is 12 + 2 - 1, or 13.

This order of **operator** precedence is also important in **programming**, because expressions should be evaluated by the **compiler** in the same way that the programmer intended them to be. This happens only when the programmer who writes the

code, and the compiler writer who determines how program statements are translated into **machine code**, have the same notation in mind. In most programming languages in use today, the notation in use is as described above, and both compiler writers and programmers define their statements accordingly. However, in some early electronic calculators, the notation was not fixed or else was hard-wired incorrectly into the device, hence for example the expression given above would evaluate to 19.

In many cases, it is desirable to remove all ambiguity by using brackets. If the programmer specified the statement as (2 + (3 × 4)) - 1, even the most dense compiler would be rightly expected to interpret his intentions correctly.

In the early days of electronic calculators, these precedence rules proved to be very difficult to implement in the **hardware** of the time. **Calculator** designers, especially at Hewlett Packard, came to realize that another notation could be used. The Polish notation, named after its creator Polish mathematician Jan Lukasiewicz (1878-1956), was created in the 1920s for use in evaluating expressions in symbolic logic. A variant of this notation, called the Reverse Polish Notation, was what the engineers at **Hewlett-Packard** decided to use.

Reverse Polish Notation is a way of expressing arithmetic expressions fully and unambiguously while avoiding the use of brackets to define operator precedence. In ordinary notation, one might write an expression as (1 + 4) × (8 - 5)—the brackets just specify that first we have to add 1 to 4, then subtract 5 from 8, and lastly multiply the two results together.

In the Reverse Polish Notation, numbers and operators are listed one after the other, and an operator always acts on the closest numbers on the list. The whole situation can be thought of in terms of stacks—the most recent number goes on top of the **stack**; the operator takes the appropriate number of arguments from the top of the stack, and replaces them by the result of its **operation** on them. The expression has been evaluated completely once the stack contains just a single number and no arithmetic operator.

In this notation, the above expression would be: 1 <enter> 4 <enter> + 8 <enter> 5 - × (we need the <enter> key to separate the numbers, else the calculator would not know that 1 and 4 were separate numbers rather than the two digits of 14).

Read from left to right, this is interpreted as follows:

- Push 1 onto the stack.
- Push 4 onto the stack. The stack now contains (1, 4).
- Apply the + operation—take the top two numbers off the stack, add them together, and put the result back on the stack. The stack now contains just the number 5.
- Push 8 onto the stack.
- Push 5 onto the stack. It now contains (5, 8, 5).
- Apply the - operation—take the top two numbers off the stack, subtract the top one from the one below, and put the result back on the stack. The stack now contains (3, 5).
- Apply the × operation—take the top two numbers off the stack, multiply them together, and put the result back on the stack. The stack now contains just the num-

ber 15—the answer.

In the Polish notation, the one originally used by Lukasiewicz, the operators preceded their arguments, so that the expression above would be written as $\times$ + 1 <enter> 4 <enter> - 8 <enter> 5 <enter>. The "reversed" form, which is similar to German (all verbs at the end of the sentence!) has however been found more convenient in computation.

Calculators using conventional algebraic input semantics also work using the Reverse Polish Notation, but they convert the input expression into that form internally before evaluating it. Early calculators by Hewlett-Packard and other manufacturers were unable to do this, so they relied on the human user to correctly supply the expression in RPN format. This made for some effort on the part of the users initially, but most people got used to it when they needed to. Some hardware manufacturers, including Hewlett-Packard, still manufacture RPN devices for those who are used to the **syntax**. Some modern calculators also offer the choice between the Reverse Polish Notation and the conventional one, as a user-configurable option.

*See also* Stack

# RIFKIN, STANLEY MARK (1946-    )

*American computer programmer and hacker*

Stanley Rifkin, a mild-mannered computer wizard, used his skills to pull off the largest bank robbery in the history of the United States. Adding insult to injury, the bank was unaware that it had been victimized until federal officials informed them of Rifkin's scam.

In 1978, Stanley Rifkin operated a computer consulting firm out of his apartment in the San Fernando Valley in southern California. The balding thirty-two-year-old had numerous clients, including a company that serviced the computers of the Security Pacific National Bank, headquartered in Los Angeles, California. Located in a room on the bank's D level was Operations Unit One—a wire transfer room. A nationwide electronic wire network allows banks—including Security Pacific—to transfer money from one bank to another. Operated by the Federal Reserve Board, a government agency, the network allows banks to transfer funds throughout the United States and abroad. Like other banks, Security Pacific guarded against wire theft by using a numerical **code** to authorize transactions. The code changed on a daily basis.

Rifkin used his position as a consultant at the bank—and his knowledge of computers and bank practices—to rob the institution. In October 1978, he visited Security Pacific, where bank employees easily recognized him as a computer worker. He took an elevator to the D level, where the bank's wire transfer room was located. A pleasant and friendly young man, he managed to talk his way into the room where the bank's secret code-of-the-day was posted on the wall. Rifkin memorized the code and left without arousing suspicion.

Soon, bank employees in the transfer room received a phone call from a man who identified himself as Mike Hansen, an employee of the bank's international division. The

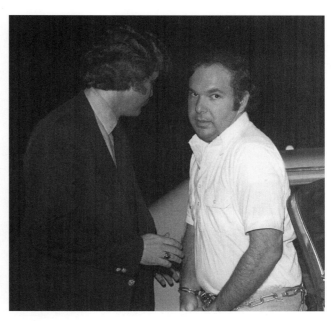

**Stanley Rifkin**

man ordered a routine transfer of funds into an account at the Irving Trust Company in New York—and he provided the secret code numbers to authorize the transaction. Nothing about the transfer appeared to be out of the ordinary, and Security Pacific transferred the money to the New York bank. What bank officials did not know was that the man who called himself Mike Hansen was in fact Stanley Rifkin, and he had used the bank's security code to rob the bank of $10.2 million.

Officials at Security Pacific were not aware of the theft until Federal Bureau of Investigation (FBI) agents informed them of the robbery. The heist went through without a problem—until the second part of Rifkin's plan came into play. Rifkin had actually begun preparations for the robbery in the summer of 1978, when he asked attorney Gary Goodgame for advice in finding an untraceable commodity. Goodgame suggested that Rifkin should speak to Lon Stein, a wellrespected diamond dealer in Los Angeles.

In early October, Rifkin laid the groundwork to convert stolen funds into diamonds. Claiming to be a representative of a reputable firm—Coast Diamond Distributors—he contacted Stein. He claimed to be interested in placing a multimillion dollar order for diamonds. Suspecting nothing, Stein ordered diamonds through a Soviet government trading firm called Russalmaz.

On October 14, the Russalmaz office in Geneva, Switzerland, received a phone call from a man who claimed to be an employee of the Security Pacific National Bank. The man, who called himself Mr. Nelson, informed the Russalmaz firm that Stein was acting as a representative of Coast Diamond Distributors. Further, he confirmed that Security Pacific had the funds to finance the multimillion dollar transaction. The man who called himself Mr. Nelson called again, to say that Stein would stop by Russalmaz's Geneva office on October 26 in order to look over the diamonds.

On October 26, Stein arrived at the Geneva office of Russalmaz. He spent that day inspecting diamonds and returned the following day with another man. (The identity of the second man is unknown. According to physical descriptions of the man, he did not resemble Rifkin.) Stein agreed to pay the Soviet firm $8.145 million in exchange for 43,200 carats of diamonds. (Diamonds are weighed by a basic unit called a carat, which is 200 milligrams. A wellcut round diamond of one carat measures almost exactly.25 inch in diameter.)

Somehow Rifkin managed to smuggle the diamonds into the United States. Five days after he robbed Security Pacific, he began to sell the Soviet diamonds. First, he sold twelve diamonds to a jeweler in Beverly Hills—an exclusive suburb of Los Angeles, California—for $12,000. Next, he traveled to Rochester, New York, where he attempted to sell more of the diamonds. There Rifkin's plot hit a snag.

On November 1, he visited Paul O'Brien, a former business associate. He informed O'Brien that he had received diamonds as payment for a West German real estate deal—and that he wanted to exchange the diamonds for cash. Before he had a chance to act on Rifkin's request, O'Brien saw a news item on television describing a multimilliondollar bank heist in Los Angeles. The story named Rifkin as the thief. O'Brien wasted no time in contacting the FBI.

Rifkin flew to San Diego, California, to spend a weekend with Daniel Wolfson, an old friend. He informed Wolfson that he planned to surrender. But he never had the opportunity to give himself up. O'Brien had given the FBI permission to record calls from Rifkin. On November 5, Rifkin called O'Brien. The conversation contained information that allowed FBI agents to track Rifkin to Wolfson's Carslbad, California, address.

Around midnight on Sunday, November 5, FBI agents Robin Brown and Norman Wight appeared at Wolfson's apartment. At first, Wolfson barred their entry with outstretched arms. When the agents informed him that they would force their way inside if necessary, he allowed them to enter. Rifkin surrendered without a struggle. He also turned over evidence to the federal agents: a suitcase containing the $12,000 from the Beverly Hills diamond sale and several dozen packets of diamonds that had been hidden in a plastic shirt cover.

Rifkin was taken to the Metropolitan Correctional Center in San Diego. Soon after he was released on bail, he got into more trouble with the FBI. He had begun to target the Union Bank of Los Angeles—using the same scheme that had worked at the Security Pacific National Bank. What he did not know was that someone involved in the scheme was a government informant who had set him up. Rifkin was arrested again on February 13, 1979. Federal agents also arrested Patricia Ferguson, who was helping Rifkin setup the bank. Tried on two counts of wire fraud, Rifkin faced the possibility of ten years imprisonment. He pleaded guilty, and on March 26, 1979, was sentenced to eight years in federal prison. In June 1979, Ferguson was convicted of three counts of conspiracy.

# RISC (REDUCED INSTRUCTION SET COMPUTER)

Microprocessors that are designed to perform fewer types of computer instructions but at higher speeds (millions of instructions per second, or MIPS) are known as *reduced instruction set computers*, or RISC.

The RISC concept has led to a more thoughtful **design** of the **microprocessor**, one that includes the following key architectural considerations:

- how well an instruction can be mapped to the clock speed of the microprocessor (ideally, an instruction can be performed in one clock cycle)
- how "simple" an architecture is required
- how much work can be done by the microchip itself without resorting to software help

Because each instruction type that a computer must perform requires additional transistors and circuitry, RISC-based processors offer several advantages over *complex instruction set computers*, or CISC-based processors:

- Smaller die size, allowing more room for performance-enhancing features such as cache **memory**, memory management functions, floating-point **hardware**, etc.
- Reduced development time, because the simpler RISC-based processor requires less design and applications **programming** effort, and offers lower design costs.
- Higher performance (higher clock rate) because of design simplicity. Processors burdened with many complex instructions pay a price in slower clock rates, even when high-level functions are more efficient.
- Instruction decode logic is hardwired into the processor, unlike **CISC** processors that require large microcode ROMs to accomplish the same thing.
- Instruction execution in a single cycle, unlike CISC processors that require multiple clock cycles for completing a single instruction.

The concept of RISC-based processors originated with **John Cocke** of **IBM** Research in Yorktown, New York, in 1974. Cocke proved the Pareto Rule, which states that about 20 percent of the instructions in a computer perform 80 percent of the work. The first computer to benefit from this discovery was IBM's PC/XT in 1980. Later, IBM's RISC System/6000, made use of the idea, and is today the best-known RISC-based product.

The first commercial RISC designs in the early 1980s resulted in the *Advanced RISC Machine*, or ARM processors. Today, however, ARM has come to mean any 32-bit microprocessor based on RISC design principles. The RISC concept was also used in Sun Microsystems' SPARC microprocessors and led to the founding of what is now MIPS Technologies, part of Silicon **Graphics**. The *StrongARM®* processors from ARM, Ltd. and Intel's *XScale™* integrated microprocessors represent the latest evolution of the ARM architecture.

Early RISC technology facilitated two important properties: (1) **pipelining**, and (2) a high clock rate with single-cycle execution. Pipelining is an implementation technique in which multiple instructions are overlapped in parallel execution (sometimes referred to as *concurrency*. CISC machines have four stages: fetch, decode, execute, and write. These same stages exist in a RISC machine, but the stages are executed in parallel. Today, pipelining is key to accelerating processor speeds.

The simpler RISC design technology allowed processors to operate at clock speeds that could use all available memory bandwidth, whereas CISC devices could not (because of changes in microprocessor fabrication technologies to accommodate the necessary logic density for a single-chip processor).

Low-cost, performance-improving RISC technology is not without its drawbacks, which include the following:

- RISC processor performance depends greatly on the **code** that it is executing. If the programmer (or **compiler**) does a poor job of instruction scheduling, the processor can become stalled, waiting for the result of one instruction before it can proceed with a subsequent instruction. Scheduling rules can be complicated, so most programmers use a high level language (such as **C** or **C++**) and let the compiler take care of instruction scheduling. This makes the performance of a RISC application depend heavily on the quality of the code generated by the compiler. Therefore, compiler selection is critical to the quality of the generated code.

- Instruction scheduling can also complicate the **debugging** process. If scheduling (and other optimizations) are turned off during debug, machine-language instructions exhibit a clear connection with their corresponding lines of source code. However, once instruction scheduling is turned on, **machine language** instructions for one line of source may show up somewhere else, such as in the middle of the instructions for another line of source code. Not only does such an intermingling of machine language instructions and source code make the code difficult to read, it can also defeat the purpose of using a source-level compiler, because single lines of code can no longer be executed by themselves.

- Fixed-length **instruction set** means poor code density. With poor code density, fetching instructions consumes main memory bandwidth, which leads to higher main memory power consumption. RISC-based ARM processors address the code density issue by using what is called *Thumb* architecture. Developed by ARM Limited, Thumb architecture is a 16-bit compressed form of the original 32-bit ARM instruction set and uses dynamic compression hardware in the instruction pipeline to yield code densities higher than most CISC processors.

# RITCHIE, DENNIS (1941-   )

*American computer scientist*

Dennis Ritchie is a computer scientist most well-known for his work with **Kenneth Thompson** in creating **UNIX**, a computer operating system. Ritchie also went on to develop the high-level and enormously popular computer **programming** language C. For their work on the UNIX operating system, Ritchie and Thompson were awarded the prestigious Turing Award by the Association for Computer Machinery (ACM) in 1983.

Dennis MacAlistair Ritchie was born in Bronxville, New York, on September 9, 1941, and grew up in New Jersey, where his father, Alistair Ritchie, worked as a switching systems engineer for Bell Laboratories. His mother, Jean McGee Ritchie, was a homemaker. Ritchie went to Harvard University, where he received his B.S. in Physics in 1963. However, a lecture he attended on the **operation** of Harvard's computer system, a Univac I, led him to develop an interest in computing in the early 1960s. Thereafter, Ritchie spent a considerable amount of time at the nearby Massachusetts Institute of Technology (MIT), where many scientists were developing computer systems and software. In 1967 Ritchie began working for Bell Laboratories. Ritchie's job increased his association with the programming world, and in the late 1960s he began working with the Computer Science Research Department at Bell. It was here that he met Kenneth Thompson. Ritchie's lifestyle at Bell was that of a typical computer guru: he was devoted to his work. He showed up to his cluttered office in Murray Hill, New Jersey, around noon every day, worked until seven in the evening, and then went home to work some more. His computer system at home was connected on a dedicated private line to a system at Bell Labs, and he often worked at home until three in the morning. Even in the early 1990s, after he became a manager at Bell Labs, his work habits did not change substantially. "It still tends to be sort of late, but not quite that late," Ritchie told Patrick Moore in an interview. "It depends on what meetings and so forth I have."

When Ritchie and Thompson began working for Bell Labs, the company was involved in a major initiative with General Electric and MIT to develop a multi-user, time-sharing operating system called Multics. This system would replace the old one, which was based on batch programming. In a system based on batch programming, the programmers had no opportunity to interact with the computer system directly. Instead, they would write the program on a deck or batch of cards, which were then input into a **mainframe** computer by an **operator**. In other words, since the system was centered around a mainframe, and cards were manually fed into machines to relate instructions or generate responses, the programmers had no contact with the program once it had been activated. Multics, or the multiplexed information and computing service, would enable several programmers to work on a system simultaneously while the computer itself would be capable of processing multiple sets of information. Although programmers from three institutions were working on Multics, Bell Labs decided that the development costs were too high and the possibility of launching a usable system in the near future too low. Therefore, the company pulled out of the project. Ritchie and Thompson, who had been working on the Multics project, were suddenly thrown back into the batch programming environment. In light of the advanced techniques and expertise they had acquired while working on the

Multics project, this was a major setback for them and they found it extremely difficult to adapt.

Thus it was in 1969 that Thompson began working on what would become the UNIX operating system. Ritchie soon joined the project and together they set out to find a useful alternate to Multics. However, working with a more advanced system was not the only motivation in developing UNIX. A major factor in their efforts to develop a multi-user, multi-tasking system was the communication and information-sharing it facilitated between programmers. As Ritchie said in his article titled "The Evolution of the UNIX Time-sharing System," "What we wanted to preserve was not just a good environment in which to do programming, but a system around which a fellowship could form. We knew from experience that the essence of communal computing, as supplied by remote-access, time-shared machines, is not just to type programs into a **terminal** instead of a keypunch, but to encourage close communication."

In 1969 Thompson found a little-used PDP–7, an old computer manufactured by the **Digital Equipment Corporation** (**DEC**). To make the PDP–7 efficiently run the computer programs that they created, Ritchie, Thompson, and others began to develop an operating system. Among other things, an operating system enables a user to copy, delete, edit, and print **data** files; to move data from a disk to the screen or to a **printer**; to manage the movement of data from **disk storage** to **memory** storage; and so on. Without operating systems, computers are very difficult and time-consuming for experts to run.

It was clear, however, that the PDP–7 was too primitive for what Ritchie and Thompson wanted to do, so they persuaded Bell Labs to purchase a PDP–11, a far more advanced computer at the time. To justify their acquisition of the PDP–11 to the management of Bell Labs, Ritchie and Thompson said that they would use the PDP–11 to develop a word-processing system for the secretaries in the patent department. With the new PDP–11, Ritchie and Thompson could refine their operating system even more. Soon, other departments in Bell Labs began to find UNIX useful. The system was used and refined within the company for some time before it was announced to the outside world in 1973 during a symposium on Operating Systems Principles hosted by **International Business Machines** (**IBM**).

One of the most important characteristics of UNIX was its portability. Making UNIX portable meant that it could be run with relatively few modifications on different computer systems. Most operating systems are developed around specific **hardware** configurations, that is, specific **microprocessor** chips, memory sizes, and **input and output** devices (e.g., printers, keyboards, screens, etc.). To transfer an operating system from one hardware environment to another—for example, from a microcomputer to a mainframe computer—required so many internal changes to the programming that, in effect, the whole operating system had to be rewritten. Ritchie circumvented this problem by rewriting UNIX in such a way that it was largely machine independent. The resulting portability made UNIX easier to use in a variety of computer and organizational environments, saving time, money, and energy for its users.

To help make UNIX portable, Ritchie created a new programming language, called *C*, in 1972. **C** used features of low-level languages or machine languages (i.e., languages that allow programmers to move bits of data between the components inside microprocessor chips) and features of high-level languages (i.e., languages that have more complex data manipulating functions such as looping, branching, and subroutines). High-level languages are easier to learn than low-level languages because they are closer to everyday English. However, because C combined functions of both high- and low-level languages and was very flexible, it was not for beginners. C was very portable because, while it used a relatively small **syntax** and **instruction set**, it was also highly structured and modular. Therefore, it was easy to adapt it to different computers, and programmers could copy preexisting blocks of C functions into their programs. These blocks, which were stored on disks in various libraries and could be accessed by using C programs, allowed programmers to create their own programs without having to reinvent the wheel. Because C had features of low-level programming languages, it ran very quickly and efficiently compared to other high-level languages, and it took up relatively little computer time.

Interestingly, because of federal antitrust regulations, Bell Labs, which is owned by American Telephone & Telegraph (AT&T), could not copyright C or UNIX after AT&T was broken up into smaller corporations. Thus, C was used at many college and university computing centers, and each year thousands of new college graduates arrived in the marketplace with a lot of experience with C. In the mid and late 1980s, C became one of the most popular programming languages in the world. The speed at which C worked made it a valuable tool for companies that developed software commercially. C was also popular because it was written for UNIX, which, by the early 1990s, was shipped out on over $20 billion of new computer systems a year, making it one of the most commonly used operating systems in the world.

At the end of 1990, Ritchie became the head of the Computing Techniques Research Department at Bell Labs, contributing **applications** and managing the development of distributed operating systems. He has received several awards for his contributions to computer programming, including the ACM Turing award in 1983, which he shared with Thompson.

# RIVEST, RONALD LINN (1947- )
## *American computer scientist*

Ronald Rivest is best known for his work in **cryptography** (the RSA public key encryption system) and his co-founding of the RSA **Data Security** Group.

Ronald Linn Rivest was born in Schenectady, New York, in 1947. After growing up in the area Rivest started his university career at Yale. Rivest received a B.A. in mathematics in 1969, and in 1974 he received his Ph.D. from Stanford University, the latter in computer science. In 1974 Rivest was taken on at the Massachusetts Institute of Technology (MIT) as an assistant professor in the electronic engineering and computer science department. In 1976, while working with **Adi Shamir**, the pair came up with a system of encrypting **data**. To test the system they brought in **Leonard Adleman**. On Adleman's 43rd attempt to crack the **code** they realized they had found a system with the desired level of security. The algorithm was patented and the system, which relied on prime numbers and one-way functions (mathematical formulae that are easy to compute but almost impossible to reverse), was released. The three pioneers founded RSA Data Security Incorporated to market their product. This company was subsequently bought by Security Dynamics and the new company was called RSA Security. Eventually the patent was transferred to MIT to administer. In 1977, Rivest was promoted at MIT, becoming an associate professor—a position he was to retain until 1983. In 1981, Rivest was given the extra responsibility of being the associate director of the MIT Laboratory for Computer Science. In 1983, Rivest was made the Viterbi Professor of Electrical Engineering and Computer Science at MIT. Rivest was also the head of the Theory of Computation Group and the Cryptography and Information Security Group. As well as his interest in cryptography, Rivest is also interested in all aspects of computer and **network security** as well as **algorithms** and machine learning and inductive inference. Rivest has spent time as the director of the International Association for Cryptologic Research (the organizing body for the Eurocrypt and Crypto conferences) and as a director of the Financial Cryptography Association.

Rivest has been granted a number of awards (including several for best paper) and he is a fellow of the Association for Computing Machinery (ACM) and of the American Academy of Arts and Sciences. In 2000, with the other members of the RSA Group, Rivest was awarded the IEEE Koji Kobayashi Computers and Communications Award and the Secure Computing Lifetime Achievement Award. Rivest has written or edited three books and over 100 scientific papers, and he holds three patents, all of which are concerned with cryptography.

*See also* Cryptography

# ROBERTS, EDWARD H. (1941- )

*American medical doctor*

Edward H. Roberts is best known for his 1974 development and marketing of the MITS **Altair** 8800, widely regarded as the world's first **personal computer**.

Edward H. Roberts was born in Miami, Florida, in 1941. He was the eldest of two children. His father worked as an appliance repairman and his mother remained at home to raise the children. From an early age he had two main interests— electronics and medicine; the latter was seen when as a teenager he got a job as a scrub technician for heart surgeons in the Miami-based Jackson Memorial Hospital. Roberts went to the University of Miami to study electronic engineering. Unfortunately his academic career was cut short when, in his junior year, Roberts' first wife, Joan, became pregnant. Roberts had to leave his studies to support his new family. Roberts

chose to join the Air Force, which saw the academic potential in him. He was sent to Oklahoma State University to undertake a degree in electrical engineering—this time on full Air Force salary. Upon completing his studies Roberts was posted to the weapons laboratory in Albuquerque, where he was an officer. After several years Roberts had the desire to move his life in another direction and decided to pursue his other love, medicine. Unfortunately by this time Roberts was 27 (1968) and considered by most medical schools to be too old. Roberts remained in the Air Force and took to tinkering with electronic projects in his spare time. He proved to be very adept at this tinkering and soon produced one of the first American hand-held (pocket) calculators. Realizing the potential for such a device Roberts set up his own company—Micro Instrumentation and Telemetry Systems (MITS). MITS and its product rapidly grew beyond all of Roberts' expectations and soon he was employing 150 people. Roberts dreamed of bigger and better things— he wanted to create a personal computer.

The computer he produced (with help from Jim Bybee) in 1974 was named the Altair 8800 (after a planet in the television series *Star Trek*). This would not be recognizable as a modern PC. For example, there was no keyboard for input; instead there was a panel of switches. The Altair 8800 was based on the **Intel** 8080 chip, and it had a very small internal **memory** (256 bytes) and no external memory. Two young men were impressed by the computer and quickly wrote a version of Basic for its use. The elder of these, **Paul Allen**, was hired by Roberts. Allen's friend, **Bill Gates**, worked with MITS during his summer vacation from Harvard. Initially Roberts sold the computer either as a kit ($395) or as a fully assembled computer ($498). His first aim was to sell 400 units, which would have allowed him to break even. Due to a very favorable article in the December 1974 *Popular Electronics* 400 machines were ordered in the first afternoon. By the end of the first three months there was a backlog of over 4,000 orders. Eventually 50,000 units were sold. (It should be remembered that at the time this machine was much cheaper than any of its rivals.) The Altair 8800 pictured on the cover of the magazine was in fact a fake—the working, finished product had been lost in transit to the magazine. In 1977, Roberts sold MITS to the Pertec Computer Corporation. Roberts remained with Pertec and put forward his latest idea—a smaller version of the personal computer that could be carried around—a laptop. Pertec was not interested in this idea, believing it to be both unworkable and not wanted by computer users. Roberts resigned from the company.

By this time Roberts was a millionaire from the sale of his company. A few years later, in 1982, when Mercer University in Macon, Georgia, opened a medical school, Roberts was able to put himself through a medical degree. In 1988, aged 47, Roberts graduated as a medical doctor and set up a medical practice in Cochran. In the same year Roberts divorced from Joan, with whom he had six children. In 1991, Roberts remarried. His new wife, Donna, was a nurse from the local hospital. The fact that Roberts was now pursuing a career in medicine did not stop his interest in computers. He soon saw the advantages that would be inherent in automating some procedures in the laboratory. Since 1995, the Medical Lab

Suite of programs written and developed by Roberts has been in constant use. In 2001, Roberts was still a medical doctor working at the Bleckley Memorial Hospital, Cochran, Georgia, specializing in adult internal medicine.

*See also* Altair; Basic

# ROBERTS, LAWRENCE GILMAN (1937- )

*American computer scientist*

Lawrence Gilman Roberts is widely regarded as one of the fathers of the **Internet** via his work on ARPANet, and he is also seen as one of the creators of **e-mail**.

Lawrence Roberts was born in 1937 in Connecticut, where he went to school. His higher education was undertaken at the Massachusetts Institute of Technology (MIT), from where he received a B.S., an M.S., and a Ph.D., all in mathematics and computing. Once he had finished his education at MIT Roberts joined the Lincoln Laboratory at MIT where he was engaged in research on computer networks, initially under the directorship of J.C.R. Licklider. By 1965 Roberts, working under **Ivan Sutherland**, produced a system by which the Lincoln Laboratory TX-2 computer was able to interchange information with an AN/FSQ32 computer located at the Systems Development Corporation at Santa Monica, California, utilizing a dedicated 1200 bps telephone line. This work was funded by the **Information Processing** Techniques Office (IPTO). This organization was initially interested in military applications of computer technology and, in particular, the construction of a country-wide network for radar defense systems and a survivable electronic network to carry communications between various Department of Defense sites. This was one of the first successful demonstrations of a digital communications network. These results were announced at a conference the following year in a joint paper with Thomas Marill. In December 1966 Roberts joined ARPA (Advanced Research Projects Agency) to oversee computer communications research, and specifically to work on a wide area digital communications network (WAN). It was while employed in this position that Roberts (as program manager) and his team developed ARPANet, the first major packet-switching network—it had been widely believed that **packet switching** would not be able to work, but Roberts had previously shown it be an ideal technology for the job. In 1967 at a conference at Ann Arbor, Michigan, Roberts presented a paper (*Multiple Computer Networks and Intercomputer Communication*) summarizing the whole outline of ARPANet. In 1968 Roberts produced outlines of how everything would work and how the program would be cost effective. Cost effectiveness could be achieved by the ability of different departments to remotely use other computers and programs without having to buy their own expensive equipment. Roberts also produced a document describing communications standards for different computers that were to be connected to the ARPANet (at this time there were still many largely incompatible computer operating systems in use). The

project was approved and in 1969 Roberts became director of IPTO (a part of ARPA). ARPANet subsequently developed into the Internet.

In 1971, Roberts was already extensively using e-mail, having had the privilege of sending one of the first ever e-mail messages. In 1972, he produced software to manage e-mail—this first-ever e-mail management program was an expansion upon work carried out by Ray Tomlinson that added the ability to list, selectively read, file, forward, and respond to messages. When Roberts left ARPA he founded the first packet-switching communications carrier—Telenet—and he was CEO of this company between 1973 and 1980. In 1979, Telenet was sold to GTE and it subsequently became the **data** division of Sprint. In 1982, Roberts was president and CEO of DHL Corporation; from 1983 to 1993, he was chairman and CEO of NetExpress, a company that specialized in packetized fax and Asynchronous Transfer Mode (ATM) equipment. From 1993 to 1998, Roberts became president of ATM Systems, where he designed ATM and Ethernet switches. While there, he spearheaded several successful drives for standardization of **protocols** throughout the industry, including cells in **frames** for ATM over the Ethernet and Explicit Rate. Since 1998, Roberts has been the chairman and CTO of Caspian Networks, a company specializing in advanced IP router/switches.

Lawrence Roberts has received a number of industry awards for his work, including the IEEE Computer Pioneer Award, the IEEE Computer Society W. Wallace McDowell Award, the Association for Computing Machinery (ACM) SIGCOMM Communications Award, and the Harry Goode Memorial Award. Though he did not invent the Internet in isolation, he is recognized as one of the four founding fathers, along with Leonard Kleinrock, Vincent Gray Cerf, and Robert Kahn; all four have received a number of joint awards for their pioneering work. Outside of computing, Roberts is interested in life extension and supplements to extend age and improve performance; so far, he has identified 15 different processes in the human body that are programmed to facilitate death after the child-bearing capacity has ended.

*See also* ARPANet; E-mail; Internet; Packet switching; Wide-area network

# ROBOTICS

Robotics is the technology associated with robots. Although there is no single definition of the term, robots are generally considered to be moving programmable machines that perform tasks automatically without direct manipulation by humans. Therefore, robotics is a broad field that combines elements of mechanics, electronics, and computer engineering and **programming**. Robots and robotics began as figments of science fiction.

In 1921, Czech writer Karel Capek (1890-1938) introduced the word "robot" in a play called *R.U.R (Rossum's Universal Robots)*. The word is derived from the Czech word "robota," which means drudgery or servitude (forced labor). Robot has become a common term for an automated machine that does the work of a human. The word "robotics" was introduced in a 1942 story about robots by writer Isaac Asimov (1920-1992). The moving and thinking robots of science fiction were well beyond the technologies of the times. The real age of robotics began in the 1950s and 1960s with the invention of transistors, integrated circuits, and numerical control.

The first industrial robots were programmable manipulators developed in the late 1950s in the United States by inventor George Devol and businessman Joe Engelberger. Called Unimates, these robots were essentially mechanical arms with gripping hands that could pick up and move objects. They were controlled by a large central computer. Advances in electronics and the invention of the microchip during the next decades led to self-contained robots with computer brains. They maneuvered and navigated using pattern recognition and advanced **algorithms** built into their software.

Modern robots are sophisticated electromechanical devices. They move via gears, pulleys, or hydraulic systems and are driven by motors, power drivers, drive systems, or actuators. These systems can be complex and use a great deal of power. Robot intelligence is provided by computer controllers, such as computer chips, microprocessors, and **data memory**. State-of-the-art robots require knowledge-based or **expert systems** for their programming. They may include programs for **voice recognition** and speech synthesis, so they can "listen" and "talk" to humans.

Even the smartest robots have a difficult time doing things that are simple to humans, such as moving across a room without bumping into the furniture. Robots utilize sensors to gather information from their surroundings. Cameras and microphones serve as their eyes and ears. They also rely on sensors using radio, infrared, and sonar signals to determine the proximity and distance of nearby objects and help them navigate. The latest robots can even recognize and track objects around them. Although robots have become smarter and more mobile over time, it is still very expensive and difficult to build a robot that can, like a human, adapt to changing environments and perform multiple tasks.

The vast majority of robots in use today are robotic arms that work in factories, performing highly repetitive tasks. They move materials, parts, and tools and manufacture, assemble, and package products. Many can hold tools and utensils in their grippers, so that they can weld or paint. Robots are widely used in the automobile industry on assembly lines. Utility robots have recently been developed that can clean floors, scrub toilets, and perform other janitorial jobs.

Robots are increasingly used to perform tasks that are too dangerous for humans. They find and disarm bombs, clean up chemical spills, fight fires, go on dangerous military missions, and explore the oceans, Antarctica, and outer space. Many of these units are not considered real robots, because they are not autonomous. They have to be manipulated by humans using remote control or telepresence. Telepresence is a technology whereby a robotic device mimics the movement of a human. NASA's Robonaut is a space-going robot controlled by telepresence. A human astronaut wears a special suit containing many sensors. As the **operator** moves, the robot mimics each movement. NASA hopes to use telepresence robots to perform outside maintenance on the International Space Station.

The scientific principles of robotics are also applied in the medical field. Robotic arms are programmed to perform delicate microsurgery, particularly on the brain and eyes, where extreme accuracy and **precision** are required. The robotic assistant AESOP helps during laparoscopic surgery, in which a tube with a tiny camera at the end is inserted into a patient's body. AESOP is a robotic arm that moves the tube smoothly and steadily at the doctor's verbal orders without tiring or trembling, as a human assistant might do. Scientists are also working to incorporate robotic mechanisms into prosthetic limbs. They hope to develop prosthetics that can be controlled directly by the human brain.

A growing market share is held by robotic toys and consumer devices. There are robot dogs and cats, dolls, lawn mowers, and vacuum cleaners on the market now. These battery powered robots can do some amazing trick. Robot dogs with sophisticated sensors and computer brains can come when called, beg for treats, bark, shake hands, and chase things.

Although the idea of robots has been around for a long time, modern science has not yet been able to match the robots of science fiction. Scientists have only recently developed robots with humanlike bodies and dexterity. Humanoid robots can walk (slowly) on two legs, climb stairs, and cross a crowded room. A lifelike robot face has been developed that can mimic human expressions such as smiling and frowning. Today's robots still fall far short of the capabilities of the human brain. However, continuing research into **artificial intelligence**, **neural networks**, and biomechanics should bring about a new generation of robots that can more closely mimic human abilities to comprehend **commands** and perform tasks.

# ROUNDOFF ERROR

Roundoff error is a form of noise that pervades all calculations performed on computers (other than those dealing strictly with integers). Roundoff error occurs because computers can only use finite strings of digits to represent any given number, while many numbers are often not representable by finite strings. Numbers as commonplace as $\pi$ or 1/3, for example, cannot be perfectly represented as finite strings: 1/3 =.3333333... (the 3's repeat forever). If one represents 1/3 using, say, five digits of **precision** ($1/3 = 3.3333 \times 10^{-1}$), a *roundoff error* has been introduced of $1/3 - (3.3333 \times 10^{-1}) = 3.333... \times 10^{-6}$. Such errors may seem small, but they can and do accumulate in long chains of calculations. In some studies, including simulations of chaotic phenomena (physical processes extremely sensitive to small changes in their initial conditions), roundoff error may even lead to completely erroneous outcomes. What is more, since roundoff error may accumulate differently on different computers, completely different erroneous outcomes might be obtained on different machines.

An example of error accumulation is as follows. Consider the calculation $1/3 + 1/3 = 1/6$. If $1/3$ is represented first as $3.3333 \times 10^{-1}$, then $1/3 + 1/3$ is given by $3.3333 \times 10^{-1} + 3.3333 \times 10^{-1} = 6.6666 \times 10^{-1}$.

Not only does this result have a roundoff error of $6.6666... \times 10^{-6}$, which is double the error for either of the two operands, but if one were to calculate $1/6$ by dividing $6.0000$ directly into $1.0000$ one would obtain an answer ($6.6667 \times 10^{-1}$) with a *different* roundoff error: $1/6 - (6.6667 \times 10^{-1}) = -3.3333... \times 10^{-6}$. The most powerful computer thus calculates "$1/3 + 1/3 = 1/6$" less precisely than a sixth-grader armed with a pencil (assuming the sixth-grader knows how to add fractions).

There are two remedies for roundoff error, and they must be employed in parallel. One is brute numerical force: if enough bits are used, the roundoff error can usually be made small enough to not matter. It is for this reason that an optional double-precision form of **floating-point arithmetic** (a form using about twice as many bits) is mandated by such standards as the IEEE (Institute of Electrical and Electronic Engineers) Standard for Binary Floating-Point Arithmetic (Standard 754-1985). Variables of this type are thus available to programmers of all machines that do floating-point arithmetic. The other remedy is to choose a good technique for rounding. In the example above, rounding $1/6$ to $6.6667 \times 10^{-1}$ involved application of the rounding method always taught in schools, the "round to nearest" rule: If the digit after the rightmost digit to be retained is 5 or larger, increment the rightmost digit to be retained; if it is less than 5, do not increment. Thus 1.345 rounds up to 1.35, 1.346 also rounds up to 1.35, and 1.344 rounds down to 1.34. Alternatively, one could simply drop all extra digits, regardless of what they are (the "always round down" rule). By this method (also called *chopping* or *truncation*), even 1.346 rounds down to 1.34. Though it sounds crude some computers actually do chop, as it involves no **logical operations** and is therefore fast.

The problem with the usual round-to-nearest rule is that it is unfair. In computer calculations, results can and sometimes do land exactly halfway between two representable numbers, and by the round-to-nearest rule these halfway results will always be rounded up. Rounding up therefore occurs more often than rounding down, introducing a slight *bias* or slant. This bias can be overcome in at least two ways: (1) Round halfway numbers up or down, whichever gives the nearest even number. This will result in rounding up and down about equally often. This "round-to-even" rule is employed in many computers. (2) Decide which way to round on the basis of a random (or pseudorandom) number. This latter method has the advantage that the effects of roundoff error can be varied from one program run to the next, allowing the changing effects of roundoff error (if any) to be observed. Unlike other rounding techniques random rounding is strictly a research tool, and is not built into processor **hardware**.

***See also*** Double-precision variable; Floating-point arithmetic; Infinite-precision arithmetic

# RUNTIME

Runtime refers to events that occur while a program is executing (running). Runtime **programming** enables the logical occurrence of such events during the execution of an application, without having to go through time-consuming and error-prone cycles of the compilation of **code** and the execution of the compiled code.

When a program is executed, space is made available and the main function of the program is copied into **memory** as a sequence of executable statements. The space is called the runtime **stack**. At first the runtime stack is empty. But, as a particular function is called during program loading, the called function is also copied into the stack. The stack fills up with copies of required functions. Runtime creates virtual processors—virtual mini-processing units. These schedule the order of execution of the copied functions. As each function is executed, the copy of that function that was made is removed from the runtime stack. At the conclusion of loading of the program the runtime stack is empty.

Runtime error and runtime **library** are several runtime-associated events. A second runtime event is called the runtime library. This is a library of routines that are committed to a program during its execution.

Runtime events are operative in all operating systems, and in many programs running in these systems. So, too, are runtime errors. A runtime error is generally an error that occurs during the execution of a program. Something needed to run the program is not working properly. As a result, the program fails to execute. Common causes of a runtime error are running out of memory, of a **bug** in the program software or something that blocks the executing program, such as another program.

There are dozens of possible runtime errors. General system errors can also occur, as well as more specific errors:

- I/O system errors
- file system errors
- disk, serial ports, clock specific errors
- storage allocator errors
- resource manager errors
- scrap manager errors.

The underlying causes of the errors are numerous. The following are only a few examples:

- unimplemented core routine
- read error
- write error
- driver not found
- directory full
- disk full
- file not found
- file system error during rename
- drive not installed
- unable to correctly adjust disk speed
- resource file not found.

A malicious cause of runtime errors in the **Windows** operating system is infection with a virus known as a Trojan Horse program, specifically with species called "SubSeven" or "Backdoor." These **viruses**, typically transmitted as an attached file to an **e-mail message**, are especially insidious as they act as a conduit for the unauthorized entry of another user to the host computer. Typical viral **signature** files are "msrexe.exe," "run.exe," windos.exe," and "mueexe.exe."

Another runtime feature in object-oriented languages such as **Java** is the runtime interface. The interface serves a number of functions, including servicing **applications** that use the runtime to facilitate their functioning. An example of these applications is a mini-program called an applet that runs within another program. **Debugging** programs also utilize the runtime interface. In essence the runtime interface is a **buffer** between an application and the operating platform—the application thus need not to tied to the platform in terms of development or revision. This allows native code to continue to operate even when classes are revised.

A runtime library is a convenient collection of functions that can be invoked during the running of a program. After the program is completed, the functions are available to be used with another program. Like the other runtime aspects, the runtime library is ubiquitous in operating systems and many programs. The choice of functions in a library is vast. For example, the Free C Runtime Library, which is used in Windows operating systems, has over 100 **commands**, specifying file manipulation functions, **data** conversion functions, memory manipulation functions, mathematical functions, and more. The following few examples give a flavor for the options available:

- fgetc — reads a character from a stream
- fputchar — writes a character to stdout
- getc — gets a character from a stream
- putchar — writes a character to stdout
- remove — deletes a file
- **access**— determines file access permission
- close — closes a file
- labs — absolute **value** of log
- free — free memory block
- malloc — allocate memory block
- strcmp — compare two strings
- strstr — find the first occurrence of a **string** in another string.

***See also*** Computer language; Dataflow languages; Executable statement

# S

## SCHICKARD'S CALCULATING CLOCK

Wilhelm Schickard was born in Herrenberg, Germany, in 1592, and became a renowned astronomer, mathematician, linguist, and Lutheran minister. He is credited with building in 1623 the world's first true mechanical **calculator**, his "calculating clock" (a somewhat misleading moniker, as the device did not tell time). Schickard's hand-powered calculator was quite sophisticated, especially considering that it was the first of its kind. It was about the size of a typewriter and could add, subtract, multiply, and divide. It operated on six-digit numbers and rang a bell to announce **overflow** (i.e., a calculation result too large to represent on its readout).

Calculating aids akin to the **slide rule** had been built before (e.g., Napier's bones), so what justifies calling Schickard's clock the first "true" calculator? In using Napier's bones and similar devices, the **operator** rotates marked cylinders or slides marked sticks past each other and interprets the resulting relationship of one set of marks to another. Such devices are inherently passive; all their motions depend on the judgment of the human operator. This is also true of the **abacus**, the most ancient calculating aid. In Shickard's clock, however, numbers are represented by the states of physical devices (gears), and these devices interact with each other mechanically. In this machine the rules of arithmetic are modeled by the cause-and-effect behaviors of physical devices for the first time; the numbers stored in the calculator *actively modify one another*. This innovation is the conceptual basis of all modern computing.

Leonardo da Vinci had sketched a workable mechanical calculator a century before Schickard, but there is no evidence that his device was ever actually built. Schickard's clock was built and actually functioned.

Shickard's invention was lost when he and his entire family were killed by plague in the mid-1630s. It might not have been if the copy he was having built for the great astronomer Kepler had survived, but an unlucky fire destroyed the workshop while the copy was being made. Schickard's own copy of the machine has been lost. Only in the twentieth century was knowledge of the Schickard calculating clock recovered. In the 1950s a sketch by Schickard of his mechanism was discovered among Kepler's papers at the Pulkovo Observatory near Leningrad, Russia. Professor Bruno Baron von Freytag Loringhoff, of the university of Tübingen, Germany, used the sketch to build a working copy of Schickard's machine. This device now resides in the Computer Museum of America.

*See also* Leibniz's mechanical multiplier; Pascaline

## SCROLL BAR

A scroll bar is a bar that appears somewhere on a window, typically on the right side or along the bottom of the window. The scroll bar functions to control which portion of the document is displayed in the window's frame.

The scroll bar makes it easy to move to any desired location in a file. The speed at which this occurs is dependent on the speed at which the scroll bar is moved. When the desired area of the file is on-screen, the desired precise location can be chosen via the **mouse** manipulation of the cursor. This is accomplished much more quickly than is possible by scrolling through the document line by line.

Typically, a scroll bar has arrows at either end, a middle region, and a scroll box (also known as a thumb or elevator) that can move from one arrow to the other. This movement relates to the position in the document. Clicking on the arrows causes the document to move, or scroll, in the indicated direction. Quicker movement is possible by dragging the scroll box to the corresponding part of the scroll bar.

*See also* Windows

# SEARCHING

The **Internet** has provided an immense boost to the ability of computers to search **databases** for information on a myriad of topics. On-line searching enables the perusal of a variety of information sources. The explosive popularity of on-line searching is enhanced by the development of a number of search engines—programs that use a variety of mechanisms to search Internet sites for a requested topic, and then deliver the site to the user's computer.

Databases are often specific to one discipline, such as chemistry, physics, microbiology, or can be more general, including multiple disciplines to address themes such as energy or the environment. If a site has a number of databases and the appropriate tools, simultaneous searches across several databases is possible.

Bibliographic databases provide references to periodical articles and sometimes to other types of literature. Some of these databases provide abstracts, brief summaries, of the articles. Scientific and medical databases, such as MEDLINE, often carry article abstracts. Abstracts can be advantageous, allowing a rapid perusal of many articles, in order to focus a search to the truly germane articles. Full text databases provide the whole text of publications. A current trend is the user-pay domain site, where, for a membership or one-time fee, the user can download the text and **graphics** of an article. Databases that contain **data** are termed databanks. An example is the collection of Material Safety Data Sheets, a databank listing the properties of chemical compounds.

Aside from the search engines mentioned above, a number of search mechanisms exist. A popular search method is known as the keyword, or free-text search. This technique allows the search for the occurrence of words in any or some of the fields in a **record**. A popular key word search method is the Boolean search. A Boolean search operates based upon key words or phrases supplied by the user.

Variations on keyword searches aid the user in broadening or narrowing searches. Nesting is a variation where similar terms are placed in parentheses to specify the order in which the keywords occur. Another variation, called proximity, requires the keywords to appear within a certain number of words from each other. In effect, the words are tied together to direct the search. A related search is called adjacency. As its name implies, the keywords must appear adjacent to each other in the identified databases.

Searching can also be conducted using search trees. A search **tree** consists of so-called nodes. One is the root **node**, and the other nodes are partitioned into subtrees that are linked to the root node. If the search tree is either empty, or if each node has no more than two subtrees, than it is called a binary tree. A binary search algorithm is operative only if the data are sorted; the algorithm can then be useful to speed up a search. An instructive analogy is locating a name in a telephone book. Finding a name by sequentially searching from the beginning of the phone book is efficient only if the data entry is near the beginning. A more efficient strategy is to begin the search somewhere near where the user expects the entry to be. If the entry is not there, then the search will proceed in one direction or another. If the data is always split in half and the middle item checked, then the remaining items to be checked are halved every time. In contrast, a linear search can eliminate only one item at a time.

In a binary search, the above analogy is accomplished by the tree structure—a **parent** field, leftchild field and rightchild field. Fields at various positions allows a search of the database.

In contrast to a binary search, a sequential, or linear, search examines data items sequentially and one at a time until the target data item is identified. For example, a database could consist of a list of students and their corresponding grades. A search could be done using as the criterion the last name of a particular student. If the student exists, and their last name is in the list, the data point will be found and its corresponding grade will be retrieved. Searches can be limited to certain portions of a database, which is helpful when the databases are large.

Another way searches such as sequential searches can be made more efficient is by the use of a sentinel **value**. A sentinel value is a special value that a user assigns when the entry of a list of data is completed. Search **algorithms** incorporate the sentinel value—when the sentinel value is encountered the search is stopped. This allows a large database to be divided into smaller, more easily searched sections.

Hashing, another search technique, produces hash values. A hash value, or hash, is a number generated from a **string** of text by a formula. The number is unique; it is very unlikely that another text would produce the same hash value. Hashing enables a quick location of a data record after all the records have been treated with the formula to generate hash values for each data record. Hashes also play a role in security systems, ensuring that transmitted messages have not been tampered with. Comparison of hash values in the original **message** and the received message is accomplished. If both sets of hash values are the same, there is a high probability that the message was not altered during transmission.

***See also*** Algorithms; Boolean data type; Information retrieval; Node

# SEARCHING ALGORITHMS

The problem of **searching** involves the problem of examining a collection of N **record**s of **data**, each of which is identified by a key, and finding a data record that matches a pre-specified key. For example, if the collection of elements is a phone book, each data record consists of a name and a phone number, with the name being the key. Looking up the phone number of Jane Doe then constitutes an instance of a search problem.

A variety of data structures and search techniques are used to solve the search problem, each suited to a particular scenario. When the data records are stored in a linear fashion, one may use either an **array** or a **linked list** as the **data structure** used to hold the records. The advantage of an array is its random access property, namely that any element of the array can be accessed at will. However, arrays are not advantageous when the need arises to insert and delete data; all array elements below a given insertion point need to be moved down in order make room for the new element to be inserted. Such movement is a costly operation. In a linked list on the other hand it is easy to insert and delete elements, but the random access advantage of arrays is lost. The two desirable yet conflicting properties of ease-of-access and ease-of-insertion-and-deletion play an important role in the choice of data structure for a particular search problem.

If the data to be searched is in an array in no particular order, then one has to resort to a simple linear search, which involves looking at each element in order and comparing the keys to the key being searched for. Such an operation is O(N) in time. A slight variant of this procedure is to move popular records closer to the beginning of the list, so that records that are asked for more often will be encountered sooner in the search. Such a search is called a self-organizing search. If the records are in an array then the only really feasible option to accomplish this self-organization is by exchanging a found record with the one before it; each time a record is found it bubbles up one spot to the front. Records often searched for will thus be closer to the front, but their motion is slow. If one uses a linked list then one could simply move the searched record to the front of the list. Thus popular records move quickly to the front, but after a few searches, when the order has stabilized, these quick moves may ruin a perfectly good order—for example when an unpopular record happens to be retrieved. The conflict between speed and stability of self-organization can usually be solved by moving records up to the front in the early searches and then switching to the exchange method in later searches, after the order has stabilized.

If one has spent the computational effort to sort the data prior to searching by arranging the keys in some ascending lexicographic order, then one has vastly superior search **algorithms** available. The best known is the recursive procedure of binary search. Simply start in the middle of an array, compare the key element to the one being searched for. If it is the same, we are done. If the middle element is larger than the one we are looking for, apply binary search recursively to the top half of the array. Otherwise apply it recursively to the bottom half. By using this **divide and conquer** approach, cutting the problem size down to half in each step, binary search performs in O(lg n) time where the base of the logarithm is two.

The success of binary search hints at the use of another data structure used in the solution of search problems: the binary **tree**. The binary tree is an improvement over arrays and linked lists in that it provides for both quick access as well as ease of insertion and deletion. A binary tree is a linked data structure consisting of a set of **node**s. Each node contains a data record and a left and right pointer that each point either to another node (called the **child node** of the **parent** node to which it belongs) or to NIL, signifying that the parent node has no child in that direction. Nodes that have neither a left child nor a right child are called leaves of the tree. The top of the tree, or the node that is not a child of any other node, is called the root.

Trees that are useful in binary searches are those that satisfy a binary search tree property: namely that for any node the key of the data stored in the left child is always less-than-or-equal-to the key of the data in the parent; and likewise, the key of data in the right child is always greater-than-or-equal-to the data in the parent. If one has data arranged in this format, in order to look for a given key one simply compares that key to the root. If it is the same, we are done. If it is less than the parent's key, then move on to the left child, otherwise move on to the right child. The worst-case operation for this search is O(H) where H is the height of the tree. If the binary search tree is height-balanced—that is, for any node of the tree the left and right subtrees emanating from that node differ in height by at most one—then H = O(lg N) where N is the number of elements stored in the tree, making the whole search procedure O(lg N) like a binary search.

From the above considerations, given a set of data, it is advantageous to build a balanced binary tree. One can be constructed simply by using a variant of the binary search algorithm, but the real challenge lies in inserting and deleting data from the binary search tree in such a way as to keep it balanced, in order to accommodate modifications in the database corresponding to the binary search tree. One approach to solving this problem is that of red-black trees. These trees are binary search trees containing one extra bit of storage for each node that specifies the color of the node, red or black. This extra data, along with a set of constraints on the way the nodes can be colored along each path from root to leaf, allow for a slightly complicated method of inserting and deleting items from the tree so that the tree remains approximately balanced. Moreover, insertion and deletion are quite fast, running in O(n) time.

Finally, an alternative to searching as a way of retrieving data from large databases is called hashing. In the hashing method, a hash function H maps the set of all possible keys into the set of integers ranging from 0 to N-1. For a key K, the integer H(K) is interpreted as a location in an array, or **hash table** T, where the data associated to the key K is to be stored. In future when one wishes to lookup the key K, one simply looks up T[H(K)]. One immediate problem with this approach is that H may map two distinct keys to the same integer. In that case one says a collision has occurred and the hashing algorithm must specify a collision resolution scheme to send the second key to another location in the hash table. Much research has been done on optimal choices of hashing and collision resolution schemes, making the hashing technique an attractive method of maintaining and searching through large databases.

# SELECTOR

In **programming**, a selector is an **operation** that returns the state of an object—defining characteristics pertaining to the object—without altering that state. Typical selector operations begin with the command "get." Methods or procedures that can modify the **object** state, which are called modifiers, typically begin with the command "set."

Selectors are widely used in a number of programming languages. In a context-sensitive language like **HTML**, selectors match the desired pattern to the element that produces the pattern. Here, selectors are tags that specify what is to be achieved with a target **block of text**. A variety of selectors exist to fulfill these requirements. Contextual selectors are used when styles should be applied to an element under specific circumstances, such as specifying when a portion of text is to be blocked and manipulated in some manner, as in bolding or underlining. Other text styles, such as the size and colors of a portion of text, is specified by an alpha-numeric ID selector. Various styles can be grouped into classes. A **class** can be specified using a type of selector termed a class selector.

In the **Java** programming language, other selectors that are termed **data** selectors function in providing various options for the display of retrieved source data. Four selectors can be invoked at a time, which aids a user in extracting the maximum amount of information from data.

*See also* Attribute; Context sensitive grammar

# SEMAPHORE

Traditionally, a semaphore was an apparatus featuring colored lights and mechanical arms, which allowed for simple visual signals to be conveyed from a distance. Such a device was used, for example, to signal the **driver** of a train that the track ahead was clear for his train to proceed (or that it wasn't). Thus, a semaphore was a physical device that was used to effect **mutual exclusion** in certain real situations, most importantly involving railroads. The word is commonly used in such a sense even now outside the computing community.

In the 1960s, the problem of mutual exclusion in computing environments, where processors had to be restricted in their **access** to shared resources, arose. **Edsger Dijkstra** invented the now-classic method of using semaphores as a new approach to solving the problem. Dijkstra's semaphore is not a physical device with arms and lights; it rather is a protected **variable** or an abstract **data** type, which can only be accessed using certain well-defined operations. Access to a semaphore can be made necessary by the operating system semantics in order to use some protected or shared resource, hence the use of semaphores makes it possible to have mutual exclusion in online systems.

Dijkstra defined two operations, now abbreviated 'P' and 'V', which may be undertaken on semaphores. The 'P' stands for the Dutch 'Proberen' (to test or probe), and the 'V' for 'Verhogen' (to increment). The P and V operations on a semaphore must be 'atomic' or indivisible—if a process is performing one of these operations on a semaphore, no other process may also access that semaphore concurrently. The **value** of a semaphore is the number of units of the restricted resource that are available. A P **operation** on the semaphore grants access to a process, and decrements the value of the semaphore by 1; the V operation on a semaphore is used by a process to reset the semaphore (increment its value by 1) after it is done using the restricted resource.

In the simplest case, there is only one unit of the restricted resource available, and the semaphore can take only the values 0 and 1. Such a semaphore is called a "binary semaphore" (and is equivalent to a "spin lock" used on very short critical sections on shared-memory multiprocessors).

Semaphores have the disadvantage that they involve "busy waiting"—a process requesting a P operation is stalled until the semaphore becomes available to it. This may mean, for instance, that a process that wishes to use the semaphore is even stopped from being able to move on to other things while waiting for the restricted resource. To avoid such busy waiting, it is possible for a semaphore to have an associated FIFO **queue** of processes—if a process tries a P on a semaphore whose value is presently zero, then the process is added to the semaphore's queue. When the semaphore's value becomes non-zero because of V operations by other processes that have relinquished control of the restricted resource(s), the first process in the queue is dequeued and allowed to perform the P operation.

Semaphores can also be used to solve other standard problems in parallel **programming**, such as with shared queues. If a queue is to be shared among more than one process, then several complications arise. One obvious difficulty is the task of ensuring that no two processes try to enqueue their items of data into the same slot. (The results of attempting to do so could be garbage or worse.) The other, less obvious difficulty is to keep track of the data items and free space in such a way that every process has access to this information constantly. This particular case can be solved using two pairs of semaphores, and given some basic assumptions, the **code** is not too complicated.

Semaphores have largely grown out of favor in recent years as tools for solving complicated problems in parallel programming. This is in part because concern has shifted to achieving fault-tolerance and wait freedom. If there is any significant risk in a system that a process will crash after performing a P operation, then a semaphore is not a good choice. Semaphores are also considered to be ill-advised in user-level programs even in uniprocessors because of this, and because they tend to slow things down due to busy waiting. Many semaphore implementations also have "thundering herd" problems and lose atomicity if there is a significant amount of contention between processes; the implementation can get overwhelmed with P requests and behave in incorrect ways, thus destroying the functionality expected of the semaphore **design**.

*See also* Fault-tolerant computing; Mutual exclusion; Operating systems

# SEMICONDUCTOR

Electrical conductivity is the ability to conduct electrical current under the application of a voltage, and it is defined as the ratio of the electric current density to the electric field in a material. A semiconductor is a material whose electrical conductivity lies between that of a typical conductor, like copper, and that of a typical insulator, like rubber. Semiconducting properties are usually strongly temperature-dependent. Although most common semiconductors are of a solid, crystalline material, some semiconductors are also found in liquid and amorphous states (an amorphous state lacks a distinct crystalline structure). Semiconductors commonly produced include the chemical elements silicon, germanium, diamond (carbon), tellurium, boron, and selenium, and the chemical compounds gallium arsenide, zinc selenide, and lead telluride.

The sign of the majority of its charged carriers—i.e., its electrons—normally indicates the classification of a semiconductor. Therefore, a semiconductor with an excess number of negatively charged carriers is termed $n$-type, while a semiconductor with an excess number of positively charged carriers is called $p$-type. Many of the important semiconductor devices depend upon fabricating a sharp discontinuity between the $n$- and $p$-type materials, the discontinuity being called a $p$-$n$ junction.

In a pure semiconductor such as silicon or germanium, the outer electrons (commonly called valence electrons) of an atom are shared with adjacent atoms, producing the covalent bonds that hold the crystal together. As a result, these outer electrons poorly conduct a current (and so in this state are called "non-conduction" electrons). With the introduction of higher temperatures or radiation (such as visible light), or with the addition of impurities, semiconductors increase their electrical conductivity by several orders of magnitude; this is unlike other low-conductivity materials such as metals, which decrease their electrical conductivity in such circumstances. The increase in conductivity with temperature, radiation, or impurities is brought about by an increase in the number of conduction electrons that are the carriers of the electrical current.

In order to produce conduction electrons, temperature or radiation (but not impurities) may be used as a catalyst to excite the outer electrons out of their covalent bonds (from their occupied levels to unoccupied levels), allowing them to freely conduct electrical current. These excited electrons, along with the empty states that are left (often called "holes"), may move under the influence of an electric field, providing a means for conduction of electricity. (These holes act like electrons with positive charges.) These electron-hole pairs are the physical origin of the increase in the electrical conductivity of semiconductors with the use of temperature and light.

Another method to produce conduction electrons (the free carriers of electricity) is to add impurities to the semiconductor. The difference in the number of outer electrons between the added impurity (called the doping material, or dopant), and the host (the pure semiconducting material) provides the impetus for the negative ($n$-type) or positive ($p$-type) carriers of electricity. (As mentioned earlier, the $n$- and $p$-type carriers characterize the semiconducting material.) Adding impurities is the way that semiconductors are normally manufactured. Impurities, such as antimony, arsenic, bismuth, and phosphorous, are introduced to the semiconducting material by a chemical process called "doping" that increases the conductivity of the semiconductor. The type and level of doping

determines whether the semiconductor is $n$-type (the electrical current is conducted by an excess number of free electrons, called "donors" for extra negative charge carriers) or $p$-type (the electrical current is conducted by a vacant number of free electrons, called "acceptors" for extra positive charge carriers). Each method produces a material that, when joined to the opposite type, produces a device that conducts electricity better in one direction than the other. Specifically, when $n$-type and $p$-type semiconductor regions are placed next to each other, the combination forms a semiconductor diode, and the contact region is called a $p$-$n$ junction. Said another way, a diode is an electronic two-terminal device that highly restricts electrical current in one direction, but allows a minimal amount of electrical flow in the other direction. The conducting ability of each $p$-$n$ junction is determined by the particular direction of the voltage. As a result, this determination can be exploited in order to regulate the characteristics of electrical devices. A series of these $p$-$n$ junctions are used to make transistors and other semiconductor devices. In fact, a transistor's three-layer structure contains an $n$-type semiconductor layer sandwiched between two $p$-type layers (a $p$-$n$-$p$ configuration), or contains a $p$-type layer sandwiched between two $n$-type layers (an $n$-$p$-$n$ configuration).

In 1926 Dr. Julius Edgar Lilienfield from New York filed the first patent on what is now recognized as an $n$-$p$-$n$ junction **transistor**. The first true transistor, a point-contact germanium device, was invented in December 1947 by **John Bardeen** (1908–1991), William Bradford Shockley (1910–1989), and Walter H. Brattain (1902–1987), scientists from Bell Telephone Laboratories and co-recipients of the 1956 Nobel Prize for this invention. Beginning in the 1950s transistors began to replace vacuum tubes. Eventually they helped to start the modern computer industry, being the critical ingredient for all digital circuits within computers.

Because their conductivities can be readily and reliably manipulated in a variety of ways, semiconductors can be effectively used in the fabrication of popular electronic devices, such as the crystal diode, transistor, **integrated circuit**, **microprocessor**, photo-detector, light switch, and others. The most common method of semiconductor manufacture is chemical vapor deposition. This method is usually used in the fabrication of semiconductors because of its ability to provide for various types and concentrations of introduced impurities (or dopants, as described previously). Because of increasing consumer demands for computer and general electronic equipment, a tremendous amount of attention has been devoted to the research, development, and manufacture of high-quality, high-purity semiconductors. There is ongoing research on other materials (such as gallium arsenide) that might yield semiconductors with useful properties for computing devices, such as faster switching speeds.

## SEPARATION OF MEMORY

In modern computers there are several **memory** systems and **hardware** components that are used for the internal use and storage of **data**. These memory components are separated by different types of physical and **programming** partitions.

The principle types of system memory include, but are not limited to, random-access memory (RAM memory), **read-only memory** (**ROM** memory), programmable read-only memory (PROM), specialized types of PROM memory, and **virtual memory**. System memory is further separated into several component areas, each with their own unique block of addresses. The types of separation are, in many cases, remnants of earlier computer hardware and software designs (i.e., they are traditional designations) made necessary by the small memory capacity of early computer systems.

Conventional memory designates the first 640 KB of system memory, and it is this memory that is utilized by **DOS**-based programs. Upper memory is the next 384 KB located next to, but above, conventional memory addresses. In modern systems, upper memory is utilized by system drivers and devices. A High memory area designates approximately the first 64 KB of the second megabyte of system memory. Extended memory (in some operational schemes, also including the High memory area) consists of the remainder of system memory.

Although the traditional functional distinctions between these separations of memory are often ignored by modern programs (e.g., modern systems can use extended memory areas for running drivers and programs), almost all programs require that some part of the **code** reside in conventional memory while the code is running.

Memory located on chips (e.g. RAM memory) is linked with memory on **disk storage** mechanisms (e.g., hard disk drives used for ROM memory) via virtual memory. This separation of memory allows an overall greater storage capacity for computers. A virtual memory bridge between RAM and disk systems allows a rapid interchange of data. Virtual memory is—in accord with its name—not a hardware component or physical form of memory (e.g., a chip, disk, etc.), but rather, a system process. As a process, virtual memory links the separated forms of physical memory contained in RAM and ROM memory systems. The smooth and rapid exchange of data across the virtual memory bridge is essential because, before operations or programming instructions can be execute by a system, data blocks carrying those instructions must be loaded into the operational RAM memory. The exchange of program code and data between the RAM and ROM systems is termed swapping.

The separation of memory allows for the cost efficient storage of data. The separation allows for vastly differing sizes of memory. Large amounts of data may be maintained in larger, less expensive ROM variant systems because virtual memory systems ensure that needed blocks of programming code or data can be constantly called and put into the smaller and more expensive RAM memory as needed. Accordingly, the separation of memory allows efficient and high speed computers to be designed with much smaller allocations of relatively expensive RAM memory.

Prior to the development of modern virtual memory mediated exchanges between separated memory systems, program execution speeds and reliability were often hampered by the need for physical file swapping and the extensive fragmentation of programs.

In addition to the functional differences between the physical separation of RAM and ROM systems (RAM memory systems differs in that it is a readable and writeable form of memory), the separated forms of memory require specialized forms of maintenance, especially with regard to power supply. Ram memory chips provide a volatile memory component that requires a constant supply of electrical current to maintain the integrity of the system. RAM systems experience a steady decay in charge state and, without a steady current input, readily degrade, or corrupt. Accordingly, an interruption in current or high variation in the power supply will result in a loss of the data or programming code maintained in RAM memory.

Apart from the functional differences in ROM memory, the hard disks housing ROM provide a long term stable (non-volatile) form of memory able to maintain it's integrity even after an interruption or loss of power. Although by strict definition, ROM systems are "read-only" forms of memory, there are variations of ROM that reside on programmable read-only memory (PROM) chips that may be erased and reused.

The separation of memory has been an important feature of computing systems since first utilized in the **Atanasoff-Berry Computer**, constructed by **John V. Atanasoff** and graduate student **Clifford Berry** in the late 1930s and early 1940s.

Some modern computer security systems rely on the separation of memory to fragment code. In such systems, the **algorithms** themselves never exist as a single file, but rather exist in fragmented states that reside in separate memory components.

*See also* Multitasking; Software management; Thrashing

# SEQUENTIAL CONTROL

Sequential control refers to the execution of statements in the order in which they were written by the programmer. Typically, sequential execution occurs in subroutines that, when combined, form the complete program **code**. The sequential execution is important as the execution of one statement can depend on the execution of a preceding statement.

In most programs, the sequential control is the default function. Unless otherwise commanded by the programmer, a computer will execute statements in stepwise order and will continue until a termination command is read. If a nonsequential order of statement execution is desired, this order must be written into the code by the programmer.

The use of a sequential control is especially beneficial in longer programs. In short programs, where only a few lines of code may be present, the execution of statements by the computer and the comprehension of the code by the programmer are easy. However, as the length of **programming** codes reaches thousands of lines, understanding the code becomes difficult. Breaking a program code into a series of blocks, which are called subroutines, helps alleviate confusion on the part of the programmer. The subroutines can be invoked, or called, as needed during the execution of the program. Within a **subroutine**, the execution of statements occurs sequentially. The final statement of a subroutine directs the computer to the next line of code. This step need not be sequential; the computer may not necessarily proceed sequentially, but can "jump" backwards or forwards to the next line of code. Put another way, sequential control permits an orderly and symmetrical function to be set up in a very non-symmetrical way. Sequential control flow of computation orders the computation process to save programming effort and time.

The use of sequential control within a subroutine can save programming time and the writing of code that is redundant. One of the advantages to the sequential control is that it allows an **operation** to be executed in a **loop**. If a subroutine can be invoked for various functions in a program, then the computer requires only to be guided to that subroutine. The same set of statements need not be re-written at various points in the code. The computer can be looped back to a subroutine and, because of sequential control within the subroutine, a common set of actions can be invoked. For functions that are required repeatedly in different **applications**, iterations followed by a programmed sequence of executable statements can save programming time and decrease programming error.

Sequential control has been used extensively in so-called concurrent programming languages, such as SR (Synchronizing Resources), Tempo, and **Java**. However, despite its benefits and applications, sequential controls have limitations. They are not well suited to the description of **hardware**, for example.

*See also* Programming

# SERVLETS

Servlets are a special kind of "server-side" **Java** application. While Java **applets** are special Java programs that are downloaded from a webserver and run by the web client, a servlet is a piece of Java software that is run by the server itself on behalf of the client. A servlet is a generic server extension—a Java class that can be loaded dynamically to expand the functionality of a server. Servlets most are commonly used with web servers, where they can take the place of **CGI** scripts.

Servlets are most commonly known as replacements for the older (but still current) technique of CGI scripts, and have advantages over CGIs, the most obvious being that since Java is a fully functional programming language while a CGI is created using a basic scripting language like **Perl**, a Java servlet has the full power of an **application** program, and can be used for creating artistic skins, or otherwise improving the presentation of content over the web in manners not possible using CGI. At this time servlets are mostly used on webservers, but they can be used to extend the functionality of any server that runs Java. Most servlets developed at the present time are designed for use with the **HTTP** protocol used on the web, but other uses are very likely as newer **protocols** for other client-server applications are realized.

Since servlets run on the server itself, there is no question about their interpretation by the client—which is an issue, it may be noted, with applets and CGIs alike. Applets are run on the Java Virtual Machine provided by the client **browser**, and since the JVM implementations of various browsers may not be alike, the applets may not run just the same way on all of them. Likewise, CGI scripts may not produce exactly the same functionality on different browsers and systems. However, a servlet running on a certain server will always produce the same behavior, regardless of variations in the client's software. This uniformity is a big help to web designers.

As servlets are built using Java, they can be ported to any server that runs Java, with a minimum of fuss involving compiling and configuration. Servlets work on all the major web server types in current use. To make it easy to develop servlets, Sun Microsystems has made a set of servlet classes publicly available—these provide basic servlet support. All common web server software vendors support these classes, and some even provide additional functionality.

*See also* Applets; CGI; Client-server interaction; Computers and art; Java; World Wide Web

# SGML (STANDARD GENERALIZED MARKUP LANGUAGE)

SGML is an acronym for Standard Generalized Markup Language. This language was developed and organized by the International Organization for Standards in 1986 as a means for organizing and identifying elements of a document that are destined to be formatted. The identification process is termed marking up. To markup a document is to indicate with symbols or **code** how a particular piece of text should be formatted; that is, what its appearance will be in the final version. For example, in a **word processing** document text can be formatted with respect to font, alignment and size, among others considerations.

SGML can also be described as a metalanguage—a means of formally describing a language. As a markup language, SGML specifies what markup is allowed, what markup is required, and how the markup will be distinguished from text. The meaning of the SGML markups is standard, having been developed by the **ISO**.

SGML is popular for the management of large documents that undergo many revisions and hard copy production in various formats. Many such **applications** are confined to large computer systems. The complexity of the SGML system has restricted its use on personal computers. However, the explosive use of the **World Wide Web** has rekindled interest in the use of SGML by personal users, as the World Wide Web uses a language called HyperText Markup Language (**HTML**). HTML is a means of identifying and interpreting the SGML format tags in a document.

There are three characteristics of SGML that are different from other markup languages: the use of descriptive rather than procedural markup, the document type concept, and its **data** independence.

The first of these features, descriptive markup, refers to the use of codes to categorize parts of a document. For example, <para> identifies the following portion of a document as a paragraph and </para> indicates that the current paragraph has ended. In contrast, a procedural markup system defines in greater depth what is to be done at certain points in a document. An example of a procedural markup is "move the left margin 2 quads left, skip down one line, and go to the new left margin." SGML is not as detailed because those sort of detailed formatting instructions are resident in separate programs, which can be applied to the document in question. Different processing programs can key on different markup codes within a document. Thus, depending on its intended use, a document can be formatted in various ways.

The second feature, document type, refers to a system whereby documents can be defined according to their component sections and the order of these sections. For example, a report may be defined as consisting of a title, author(s), an abstract and descriptive text and/or **graphics**. If one or more of these features are not present the document is not recognized as a report and formatted accordingly. The advantage of document type is that documents can be prepared without concern to their format, as formatting will be done automatically afterwards. Technically, this is done using what is known as an SGML parser.

The third feature of SGML, data independence, means that documents can be transferred between different **hardware** and software environments without loss of information or presentation appearance. This is accomplished by a mechanism called **string** substitution—a machine-independent way of designating that a particular sting of characters will be replaced by another sting of characters upon document processing.

SGML is most commonly used in electronic publishing in the public, private and academic sectors.

*See also* Computers and literature; HTML (HyperText Markup Language); Parser and parsing

# SHAMIR, ADI (1952- )
*Israeli mathematician and computer scientist*

Adi Shamir is best known for his work in **cryptography**, specifically the construction of the RSA public-key encryption system and the subsequent co founding of the RSA Group. Subsequent to this work Shamir has also produced a number of cryptographically important advances.

Adi Shamir was born in Tel Aviv, Israel, in 1952. After schooling in the local area he went to university at the Weizmann Institute of Science, Rehovoth, Israel, where he studied mathematics. He was awarded his Ph.D. in 1977. Upon completion of his studies Shamir moved to the United States and the Massachusetts Institute of Technology (MIT), where he worked in the Laboratory of Computer Science as an instructor. Here Shamir met Ronald L. Rivest and found one of his new tasks was to teach an advanced algorithm course—an area of which he only had a basic knowledge. Shamir obtained all of the library books on **algorithms** and quickly brought himself up to speed on the subject. Shamir's new-found knowledge fit in well with the work of Rivest and together they developed an algorithm for public-key cryptography (the ability of two people who had never met to communicate via computers in a secure manner), based on the work of **Whitfield Diffie** and **Martin Hellman**. The pair brought in a third researcher, **Leonard Adleman**, to test the system they had devised. Some of the initial systems they developed proved very easy to solve but on their 43rd attempt they found they had a level of encryption that was felt to be sufficient by all members of the group. The system, based on prime numbers and one-way functions (mathematical formulae that are simple to compute but almost impossible to reverse), was patented and the California-based RSA **Data Security** Incorporated was formed to look after the system. Eventually the patent was transferred to MIT (where all three were working at the time of development) and the company was taken over by Security Dynamics and the new company was called RSA Security.

In 1980 Shamir moved back to Israel to work at the Weizmann Institute of Science and in 1981 he was made the Paul and Marlene Borman Professor of Applied Mathematics and Computer Science. During his time at the Weizmann Institute Shamir has been responsible for the Fiat Shamir identification scheme and many other cryptographic systems, including a visual cryptosystem, zero-knowledge proofs (a system where proof is given that the key is held without the key being given over), secret dispersion, and differential cryptanalysis. At the end of the twentieth century Shamir announced TWINKLE (The Weizmann Institute Key Locating Engine). TWINKLE is an electro-optical device that will execute sieve-based factoring algorithms several times faster than a **personal computer** can achieve. The practical use of this system is that it could be utilized to break computer generated codes that have previously been regarded as secure, such as those used by financial and government systems. As of 2001 this idea has not been made reality.

In 2000, with the other members of the RSA Group, Shamir was awarded the IEEE Koji Kobayashi Computers and Communications Award and the Secure Computing Lifetime Achievement Award. Shamir also won the Kennedy prize in 1975 (the Weizmann University award for best Ph.D.) and the IEEE W. R. G. Baker prize in 1986—this was a solo award for Shamir for a paper entitled *A Polynomial-Time Algorithm for Breaking the Basic Merkle-Hellman Cryptosystem*. Adi Shamir has nearly 100 publications to his name.

During the development of the RSA key one or two unexpected problems were encountered—in 1977 *Scientific American* published a **message** encoded using the key and offered a $100 reward to anyone who could crack the **code**. As part of the competition readers were invited to write to the original authors for a copy of the scientific paper; all three then sent out thousands of copies of the paper. Unfortunately when the National Security Agency (NSA) heard about this the leadership saw serious implications for national security in the unlimited and partially overseas distribution of such a powerful method of encryption (the NSA's consternation was compounded by the fact that Shamir was not an American citizen). The NSA attempted to ban the exporting of encryption technology, but the distribution of this information was eventually allowed—due to the fact it had already been published and distributed so any further action would merely serve to publicize it's existence, and those who wanted to use it for nefarious purposes would have already seen it. Problems with official concerns over national security have shadowed much of Shamir's work.

*See also* Cryptography

# SHANNON, CLAUDE ELWOOD (1916-2001)
*American information and computer scientist*

Claude Elwood Shannon is commonly referred to as the father of **information** sciences.

Claude Shannon was born in Petoskey, Michigan, in 1916. His father was a businessman and his mother a language teacher at the local high school. Shannon went to Gaylord High School (where his mother eventually became principal) until he was 16. From there he went to the University of Michigan where he was awarded a degree in mathematics and electrical engineering in 1936. This interest in mathematics and electronics had developed during his early school years. Shannon had constructed many radio-controlled toys and even made a telegraph system that connected to a friend's house some half a mile distant (his system utilized a barbed-wire fence that ran between the two properties). To fund these projects Shannon took to repairing radios in Gaylord. Having obtained his degree from the University of Michigan Shannon took a position as a research assistant at the Massachusetts Institute of Technology (MIT) Department of Electrical Engineering. Shannon worked part-time for the department while undertaking graduate studies, and in 1937 he was awarded an M.S. in electrical engineering. He then received a Ph.D. in mathematics in 1940 after transferring to the mathematics department in 1938. The awarding of Shannon's doctoral degree was at times in doubt due to his inability to meet the language requirements of MIT. Eventually, with the aid of a personal tutor, Shannon was able to pass muster in both French and German. Shannon's master's thesis was in **Boolean algebra** (looking at the analysis and synthesis of switching and computer circuits), while his doctoral thesis (*An Algebra for Theoretical Genetics*) was in statistical genetics. While at MIT Shannon worked with **Vannevar Bush** on the differential analyzer (at the time one of the most advanced calculating machines known). In 1941 Shannon published a paper on the mathematical theory of this machine. A brief period of work at Princeton followed, and it was there that Shannon started to devote his research interests to information theory and communications systems. At the end of 1941 Shannon joined AT&T Bell Telephones as a research mathe-

matician (he had also spent the summers of 1937 and 1938 working there). With the publication of *A Mathematical Theory of Communication* in the Bell System Technical Journal in 1948, Shannon founded the subject of information theory. In the paper Shannon proposed a linear schematic model of a communications system—he thought that information could be sent as a series of off and on signals rather than as an electromagnetically controlled wave, a digital system of transmitting **data**. This paper also introduced the idea of a "**bit**" in computing and is widely regarded as Shannon's most important contribution to computing science. The publication in 1949 of *Communication Theory of Secrecy Systems* set **cryptography** on a more rational basis than had previously been the case. In 1950 Shannon wrote one of the very first papers showing how a computer could be programmed to play the game of chess, and many chess programs still operate on the basic principles outlined in this paper. Also in 1950 Shannon developed Theseus—a maze-solving **mouse** that was actually one of the earliest attempts at **artificial intelligence**: it had the ability to learn from trial and error. In 1956 Shannon was made a visiting professor of communication science and mathematics at MIT. In 1957 he was appointed to the faculty, although he remained on as a consultant for AT&T. In 1958 Shannon was made Donner Professor of Science at MIT. Throughout all of these changes Shannon continued his work in communication theory. Specifically he studied systems with feedback mechanisms to try to increase their reliability. Through his work Shannon defined many of the limits on communication rates in telephone channels and optical and wireless communications. In 1972 Shannon left his position at AT&T. After this period he became an emeritus professor at MIT and continued his own pursuits, building many more machine toys and attending a number of conferences as the honored guest and speaker.

Shannon married Mary Elizabeth Moore (who also worked at Bell) in 1949 and together they had three sons and one daughter. While working Shannon was largely considered a loner, but he was also willing to help other people with their problems if they approached him. One of his great loves in life was unicycling and he frequently rode to work on his unicycle (often juggling three balls at the same time). Shannon's other hobbies tended towards the science and computing sphere. He developed a pocket **calculator** that carries out all computations in roman numerals, an automatic juggling machine, and an army of "turtles"—small independent machines that roam around the floor. Throughout his life he received many awards including the Alfred Nobel American Institute of Engineers Award (1940) for his master's thesis, the Morris Liebmann Memorial Award of the Institute of Radio Engineers (1949), the National Medal of Science (1966), the IEEE Medal of Honor (1966), the Audio Engineering Gold Medal (1985), as well as honorary degrees from 11 Universities. Claude Shannon died at age 84 after a long battle with Alzheimer's disease.

*See also* Boolean algebra; Information and information theory

## SHAREWARE AND FREEWARE

Shareware is a trial version of a program, posted by a vendor on the **Internet**. The version may not possess all the capabilities of the final version. Users who approve of the trial version may be induced to send payment once the final version is available. Freeware is software that is available for free on the Internet. In recent times, the most well-known example of freeware has been the **Linux** operating system.

In the 1970s, when the computer user community was small, user-written programs were routinely circulated among users. Following the introduction of the International Business Machine **personal computer** in 1981, the number of users skyrocketed, making such communal sharing of programs not feasible. The following year, two programmers, Andrew Fluegleman and Jim Knopf wrote a communications program and a database program, respectively, for use on the **IBM** PC. They decided to distribute these programs over existing computer distribution networks. Although they intended to be remunerated for their programs, Fluegleman coined the term (and trademarked the name) "Freeware" to designate the programs. Because the source **code** (which specifies the **operation** of a program) was also distributed, however, the control over the freeware programs by the two programmers was lost.

Other **programming** entrepreneurs followed in Fluegleman's and Knopf's footsteps, and within a few years, freeware had developed a reputation for quality. In 1984, a computer magazine sponsored a contest to find a name for this burgeoning class of freely available programs. The most popular choice for a name was "shareware." Eventually, the term freeware became public property, and both terms worked their way into the computer lexicon.

The terms shareware and freeware are somewhat misleading, because such programs are not truly public property. Because a copyright automatically accrues to any software that is distributed, even over networks, for a program to be in the public domain, the programmer has to specifically label it as such. So, while freeware does indeed include some public domain software (Linux, for example), most freeware is software that can be freely used without payment to the programmer, but for which the programmer retains the copyright.

As the popularity of shareware and freeware grew, organizations formed to review the software and provide catalogues of emerging programs. This tact proved popular. For example, one group, the Houston Area League of PC Users, which began in 1982 with a handful of members, currently has over 10,000 members world-wide.

Presently, there are thousands of shareware programs for every conceivable application. The advent of the Internet, and particularly the increasing popularity of inexpensive high speed modems, which enable the rapid transmission of large amounts of **data**, has fueled an explosion in shareware and freeware popularity.

*See also* IBM; Modem

## SHAW, MARY (1943- )
*American computer scientist*

Professor of computer science and dean of professional programs at Carnegie-Mellon University in Pittsburgh, Pennsylvania, Mary Shaw has made major contributions to the analysis of computer **algorithms**, as well as to **abstraction** techniques for advanced **programming** methodologies, programming-language architecture, evaluation methods for software performance and reliability, and software engineering. She has also been involved in the development of computer-science education. She was elected to the Institute of Electrical and Electronic Engineers in 1990 and the American Association for the Advancement of Science in 1992; she received the Warnier Prize in 1993.

Mary M. Shaw was born in Washington, D.C., on September 30, 1943, to Eldon and Mary Holman Shaw. Her father was a civil engineer and an economist for the Department of Agriculture, and Shaw attended high school in Bethesda, Maryland, at the height of the Sputnik—the first artificial satellite—era, when the country was making a concerted effort to bolster science and mathematics education. Her father encouraged her interest in science with books and simple electronic kits when she was in the seventh and eighth grades, and her high-school years provided opportunities to delve more deeply into both computers and mathematics.

An **International Business Machines (IBM)** employee named George Heller from the Washington area participated in an after-school program which taught students about computers; he arranged for the students to visit an IBM facility and run a program on an IBM 709 computer. This was Shaw's introduction to computers. For two summers during high school, as well as during the summer after she graduated, she worked at the Research Analysis Corporation at the Johns Hopkins University **Operation** Research Office. This was part of a program begun by a woman named Jean Taylor to give advanced students a chance to explore fields outside the normal high school curriculum. "They would give us a system analysis problem and ask us to investigate," Shaw told contributor Rowan Dordick. Among the problems she worked on was a study of the feasibility of using irradiated foods to supply army units.

Shaw entered Rice University with the idea of becoming a topologist, having become enamored with Moebius strips and Klein bottles while in high school. She quickly changed her mind, however, after looking through a textbook on topology. Though there were no courses at that time in computer science, there was something called the Rice Computer Project, a group which had built a computer—the Rice I—under the leadership of an electrical engineering professor named Martin Graham. Shaw wandered into the project area one day and asked a question about the computer. By way of an answer, she was given a machine reference manual and was told to read it first and then come back. She surprised the project members by doing just that. It was a small group, consisting mostly of faculty and graduate students, and Shaw ended up working with the project part-time during her last three years, under the mentorship of Jane Jodeit, the head programmer. Shaw gained valuable experience on the Rice I; she worked on a programming language, wrote subroutines, and helped figure out ways to make the operating system run faster.

After her junior year, Shaw attended summer school at the University of Michigan, where she met **Alan Perlis**, a professor at Carnegie Mellon University. After receiving her B.A. *cum laude* in mathematics from Rice in 1965, she entered Carnegie Mellon, where Perlis became one of her advisors. She received her Ph.D. in 1971 in computer science, with a thesis on compilers—programs that translate language a human can easily understand into language that the computer understands. Shaw was invited to join the faculty after receiving her degree. One of her first notable accomplishments, in collaboration with Joseph Traub, was the development of what is known as the Shaw-Traub algorithm, an improved method for evaluating a polynomial which allows computers to compute faster. This effort was part of a general interest Shaw had in finding ways to formalize computations in order to make them more efficient.

Shaw's focus on improved software **design** led her to pursue an approach to the organization of computer programs called **abstract data types**. This approach is one of the foundations of **object-oriented programming**. Large programs are difficult to read or modify unless there is some intrinsic structure, and this is the problem abstract-data-type programming was designed to address. Abstract data **types** is a method of organizing the **data** and computations used by a program so that related information is grouped together. For example, information about electronic details of a telephone-switching network would be grouped in one part of the program, whereas information about people and their telephone numbers would be grouped in another part.

Shaw's work in this area came to fruition in two ways. The first was in the creation of a programming language called Alphard that implemented abstract data types; she developed this language with William A. Wulf and Ralph L. London between 1974 and 1978. The second, more theoretical result, was the clarification of abstractions in programming. Shaw made it easier to design programs that are more abstract—the word "abstract" in this context means that elements of the program are further removed from the details of how the computer works and closer to the language of the problem that a user is trying to solve. This work can be viewed as a continuation of the trend in programming languages, begun with **FORTRAN**, to write programs in a higher-order language that reflects the nature of the problem, as opposed to programming in the binary machine language—ones and zeros—that the computer understands.

Shaw's concerns with abstraction proved a natural bridge to a more general issue, which she posed to herself as a question: What other ways are there of organizing programs? The answer emerged as Shaw came to realize that what she was really looking for was the organization of software engineering. In "Prospects for an Engineering Discipline of Software," she wrote: "The term 'software engineering' was coined in 1968 as a statement of aspiration—a sort of rallying cry." The problem, as she and others realized, was that the

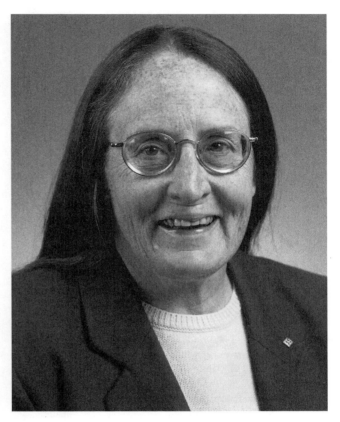

**Mary Shaw**

term was not so much the name of a discipline as a reminder that one did not yet exist.

Through historical study of the evolution of civil and chemical engineering, Shaw has developed a three-stage model for the maturation of a field into a complete engineering discipline. She has shown that an engineering discipline begins with a craft stage, characterized by the use of intuition and casually learned techniques by talented amateurs; it then proceeds through a commercial stage, in which large-scale manufacturing relies on skilled craftsmen using established techniques that are refined over time. Finally, as a scientific basis for the discipline emerges, the third stage evolves, in which educated professionals using analysis and theory create new **applications** and specialties and embody the knowledge of the discipline in treatises and handbooks. Shaw has concluded that contemporary software engineering lies somewhere between the craft and commercial stages, and this conclusion has led to an effort on her part first to promote an understanding of where software engineering should be headed and second to develop the scientific understanding needed to move the discipline into the third stage.

The transformation of a discipline proceeds through its practitioners, so it is natural that Shaw has devoted much of her career to improving computer-science education. She was a coauthor of the first undergraduate text to incorporate the concept of abstract **data structures**, and she led a group that redesigned the undergraduate computer-science curriculum. She was also involved in the execution of an innovative Ph.D. program that has been widely adopted.

Shaw's accomplishments are not limited to computer science. She was the National Women's Canoe Poling Champion from 1975 to 1978, and she placed in the Whitewater Open Canoe National Championships in 1991. Her marriage to Roy R. Weil—a civil engineer, software engineer, and commercial balloon pilot—spurred an interest in aviation. She has become an instrument-rated pilot, a single-engine commercial glider pilot, and a Federal Aviation Administration (FAA) certified ground instructor.

## SHOCKLEY, WILLIAM (1910-1989)

*American physicist*

William Shockley was a physicist whose work in the development of the **transistor** led to a Nobel Prize. By the late 1950s, his company, the Shockley Transistor Corporation, was part of a rapidly growing industry created as a direct result of his contributions to the field. Shockley shared the 1956 Nobel Prize in physics with **John Bardeen** and **Walter Brattain**, both of whom collaborated with him on developing the point-contact transistor. Later Shockley became involved in a controversial topic for which he had no special training, but in which he became avidly interested: the genetic basis of intelligence. During the 1960s he argued, in a series of articles and speeches, that people of African descent have a genetically inferior mental capacity when compared to those with Caucasian ancestry. This hypothesis—which was not new and had long been discredited—became anew the subject of intense and acrimonious debate.

William Bradford Shockley was born in London, England, on February 13, 1910, to William Hillman Shockley, an American mining engineer, and May (Bradford) Shockley, a mineral surveyor. The Shockleys, living in London on a business assignment when William was born, returned to California in 1913. Shockley did not enter elementary school at the usual age, however, because, as he told *Men of Space* author Shirley Thomas, "My parents had the idea that the general educational process was not as good as would be done at home." As a result, he was not enrolled in public schools until he had reached the age of eight.

Shockley's interest in physics developed early, inspired in part by a neighbor who taught the subject at Stanford and by his own parents' coaching and encouragement. By the time he had completed his secondary education at Palo Alto Military Academy and Hollywood High School at the age of seventeen, Shockley had made his commitment to a career in physics. Shockley and his parents agreed that he should spend a year at the University of California at Los Angeles (UCLA) before attending the California Institute of Technology (Caltech), where he earned a bachelor's degree in physics in 1932. Offered a teaching fellowship at the Massachusetts Institute of Technology (MIT), Shockley taught while working on his doctoral dissertation, "Calculations of Wave Functions

for Electrons in Sodium Chloride Crystals," for which he was awarded his Ph.D. in 1936. Shockley later told Thomas that this research in solid-state physics "led into my subsequent activities in the transistor field."

Upon graduation from MIT, Shockley accepted an offer to work at the Bell Telephone Laboratories in Murray Hill, New Jersey. An important factor in that decision was the opportunity it gave him to work with Clinton Davisson, who was to win the 1937 Nobel Prize in physics for proving Louis Victor Broglie's theory that electrons assumed the characteristics of waves. Shockley's first assignment at Bell was the development of a new type of vacuum tube that would serve as an amplifier. But, almost as soon as he had arrived at Bell, he began to think of a radically new approach to the transmission of electrical signals using solid-state components rather than conventional vacuum tubes. At that time, vacuum tubes constituted the core of communication devices such as the radio because they have the ability to rectify (create a unidirectional current) and multiply electronic signals. They have a number of serious practical disadvantages, however, as they are relatively fragile and expensive, and have relatively short life-spans.

As early as the mid–1930s, Bell scientists had begun to think about alternatives to vacuum tubes in communication systems, and by 1939 Shockley was experimenting with semiconducting materials to achieve that transition. Semiconductors are materials such as silicon and germanium that conduct an electrical current much less efficiently than do conductors like silver and copper, but more effectively than do insulators like glass and most kinds of plastic. Shockley knew that one **semiconductor**, galena, had been used as a rectifier in early radio sets, and his experience in solid-state physics led him to believe that such materials might have even wider application in new kinds of communication devices.

The limited research Shockley was able to complete on this concept of alternative conductors was unsuccessful, largely because the materials available to him at the time were not pure enough. In 1940, war was imminent, and Shockley soon became involved in military research. His first job involved the development of radar equipment at a Bell field station in Whippany, New Jersey. In 1942, he became research director of the U.S. Navy's Anti-Submarine Warfare Operations Research Group at Columbia University, and served as a consultant to the Secretary of War from 1944 to 1945.

In 1945, Shockley returned to Bell Labs as director of its research program on solid-state physics. Together with John Bardeen, a theoretical physicist, and Walter Brattain, an experimental physicist, Shockley returned to his study of semiconductors as a means of amplification. After more than a year of failed trials, Bardeen suggested that the movement of electric current was being hampered by electrons trapped within a semiconductor's surface layer. That suggestion caused Shockley's team to suspend temporarily its efforts to build an amplification device and to concentrate instead on improving their understanding of the nature of semiconductors.

By 1947, Bardeen and Brattain had learned enough about semiconductors to make another attempt at building Shockley's device. This time they were successful. Their device consisted of a piece of germanium with two gold contacts on one side and a tungsten contact on the opposite side. When an electrical current was fed into one of the gold contacts, it appeared in a greatly amplified form on the other side. The device was given the name transistor (for *trans* fer re*sistor*). More specifically, it was referred to as a point contact transistor because of the three metal contacts used in it.

The first announcement of the transistor appeared in a short article in the July 1, 1948 edition of the *New York Times*. Few readers had the vaguest notion of the impact the fingernail-sized device would have on the world. A few months later, Shockley proposed a modification of the point contact transistor. He suggested using a thin layer of P-type semiconductor (in which the charge is carried by holes) sandwiched between two layers of N-type semiconductor (where the charge is carried by electrons). When Brattain built this device, now called the junction transistor, he found that it worked much better than did its point contact predecessor. In 1956, the Nobel Prize for physics was awarded jointly to Shockley, Bardeen, and Brattain for their development of the transistor.

Shockley left Bell Labs in 1954 (some sources say 1955). In the decade that followed, he served as director of research for the Weapons Systems Evaluation Group of the Department of Defense, and as visiting professor at Caltech in 1954–55. He then founded the Shockley Transistor Corporation to turn his work on the development of the transistor to commercial advantage. Shockley Transistor was later incorporated into Beckman Instruments, Inc., and then into Clevite Transistor in 1960. The company went out of business in 1968.

In 1963, Shockley embarked on a new career, accepting an appointment at Stanford University as its first Alexander M. Poniatoff Professor of Engineering and Applied Science. Here he became interested in genetics and the origins of human intelligence, in particular, the relationship between race and the Intelligence Quotient (IQ). Although he had no background in psychology, genetics, or any related field, Shockley began to read on these topics and formulate his own hypotheses. Using **data** taken primarily from U.S. Army pre-induction IQ tests, Shockley came to the conclusion that the genetic component of a person's intelligence was based on racial heritage. He proposed that people of African ancestry were inherently less intelligent than those of Caucasian lineage. He also surmised that the more "white genes" a person of African descent carried, the more closely her or his intelligence corresponded to that of the general white population. He ignited further controversy with his suggestion that inferior individuals (those whose IQ numbered below 100) be paid to undergo voluntary sterilization.

The social implications of Shockley's theories were, and still are profound. Many scholars regarded Shockley's whole analysis as flawed, and they rejected his conclusions. Others were outraged that such views were even expressed publicly. Educators pointed out the significance of these theories for their field, a point pursued by Shockley himself when he argued that compensatory programs for blacks were doomed because of their inherent genetic inferiority. For a

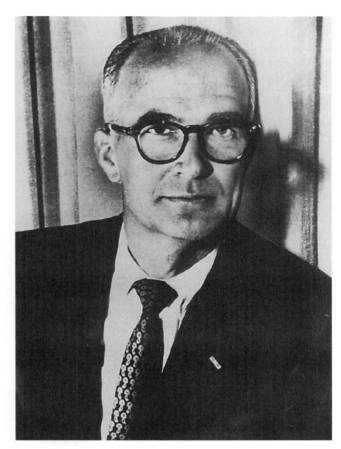

**William Shockley**

number of years, Shockley could count on the fact that his speeches would be interrupted by boos and catcalls, provided that they were allowed to go forward at all.

During his life, Shockley was awarded many honors, including the U.S. Medal of Merit in 1946, the Morris E. Liebmann Award of the Institute of Radio Engineers in 1951, the Comstock Prize of the National Academy of Sciences in 1954, and the Institute of Electrical and Electronics Gold Medal in 1972 and its Medal of Honor in 1980. He was named to the National Inventor's Hall of Fame in 1974. Shockley remained at Stanford until retirement in 1975, when he was appointed Emeritus Professor of Electrical Engineering. In 1933, Shockley had married Jean Alberta Bailey, with whom he had three children, Alison, William, and Richard. After their 1955 divorce, Shockley married Emily I. Lanning. He died in San Francisco on August 11, 1989, of prostate cancer.

## SHORTEST SUPERSTRING PROBLEM

The shortest superstring problem, often abbreviated SSP, is a computational problem whose answer is the shortest **string** which contains each string from a given set of strings. In other words it is a problem involved with finding a superstring, a string containing each member of a set of strings in order, of minimum length. The shortest superstring problem has applications in **data compression**, sparse matrix compression, and computational biology, namely DNA-sequencing. It is a pure classical optimization problem.

An example of the shortest superstring problem is as follows: Given a collection of strings $S=\{s_1, s_2..., s_n\}$ over a finite alphabet find the shortest superstring $\Sigma$ that contains each $s_i$ as a substring.

$s_1$ = babab

$s_3$ = abcba

$s_2$ = ababc

$s_4$ = babca

In this case $\Sigma$ = abcbababca and is ten characters long.

Undoubtedly two of the most common applications of the shortest superstring problem are in **data** compression and DNA-sequencing. The motivation for using this approach in data compression is that one is able to use textual substitution and then **macro** encoding to solve such a problem. Using this one can select macros from a string and replace them by pointers. For the best performance it is best to try to overlap the macros as well as possible. DNA is a double-stranded, oriented sequence of four types of nucleotides and can be viewed as a string over the alphabet of four characters, each representing a different nucleotide. Reading a long string of DNA is the sequencing problem in molecular biology. There exist laboratory procedures for reading short DNA strands and so this is employed, along with the shortest superstring problem, in deciphering the long strings of DNA. In order to implement this many copies of the longer strands are made and cut into many, overlapping short pieces. These pieces are read and yield a set of strings. Then the shortest common superstring is found and the longer strand of DNA can be reassembled from this information. The short, common superstrings preserve the important biological structure and are good models of the original DNA sequence.

There are several methods of approach to solving shortest superstring problems. Some of these include families of three-stage **algorithms**, **learning algorithms** or **automatic programming** systems, and the GREEDY procedure. The GREEDY procedure is widely utilized and appears to do well with the shortest superstring problem. The GREEDY procedure consists of first picking two strings that overlap the most number of characters and then merge them. Then GREEDY finds a string of length at most twice optimal. This means that it achieves at lest half of the optimal compression. Although this method is widely accepted some have suggested the use of heuristic methods.

## SIGNATURE

The term signature refers to a signature file, or "sig" file, and is the on-line equivalent of a business card. A signature file is a short file typically containing information including the sender's contact addresses and number and, if desired, a salutation, which can be attached to outgoing **e-mail** messages.

Additionally, the term signature is also increasingly being used to designate the addition of a digitized hand-written signature to documents.

The purpose of a signature file is to identify the user. The sender's name, company name if appropriate, the sender's position in the company, phone and fax numbers, mailing address, and a Web site **URL** (Uniform Resource Locator) are typically part of a signature. A business or personal salutation can be included as well. Another common inclusion is known as **ASCII** art—a drawing made using the symbols on a standard keyboard. ASCII characters are the medium of choice for simplicity and because, in general, e-mail messages contain only these characters.

Typically, a signature file is built in Note Pad or other text editor by typing the file as it will appear. The file is saved as a text file (.txt). Depending on the e-mail program, that program can be configured to automatically input the new sig file into any outgoing mail.

Signatures are often used judiciously, and are brief. A generally accepted rule is that signatures should be no longer than six lines. Presentation is important, given the wide potential distribution for e-mail via the **Internet**. A well-designed signature can become a powerful marketing tool for a business.

Linked e-mail addresses and URL are often automatically recognized as a link. Recipients are thus provided a convenient means of linking to the sender's e-mail address or Web site, simply by clicking on the highlighted links.

The other meaning of the term signature concerns a digital signature—a digital **code** that can be attached to an electronically transmitted **message**, be it an e-mail or a **word processing** document. As with a written signature, the purpose of a **digital signature** is to guarantee that the person sending the message is who he or she claims to be. Digital signatures are especially important in electronic business transactions. To be effective, digital signatures must not be easily copied, or vulnerable to forgery. The legality of digital signatures on documents on the open Internet network is currently under consideration. For example, the American Bar Association Section of Science and Technology Law has produced a legal overview of cryptology and electronic signatures.

*See also* Computers and intellectual property; Cryptography; E-mail

## SIMON, HERBERT A. (1916-2001)

*American computer scientist*

Generally considered one of the fathers of **artificial intelligence**—computer programs capable of complex problem-solving—Herbert A. Simon made distinguished contributions in a number of fields, including computer science, the psychology of learning, business administration, political science, economics, and philosophy. Recipient of the 1978 Nobel Prize in economics for his work on human decision-making, he also, in 1986, became the first person to receive the National Medal of Science for work in the behavioral sciences. In addition to his varied professional interests, he also painted, played the piano, and enjoyed mountain-climbing, traveling, and learning foreign languages. He died February 9, 2001 from complications following surgery to remove a cancerous tumor from his abdomen.

Simon was born in Milwaukee, Wisconsin, on June 15, 1916. His father, Arthur Simon, was a German-born electrical engineer and his mother, Edna (Merkel) Simon, was an accomplished pianist. After being skipped ahead three semesters in the Milwaukee public school system, Simon was just seventeen when he enrolled in the University of Chicago, where he would earn his B.A. in political science in 1936. As an undergraduate, Simon conducted a study of the administration of the Milwaukee Recreation Department. This study sparked Simon's interest in how administrators make decisions—a topic that would be a focal point of his career. In 1937, Simon married Dorothea Isobel Pye, also a graduate student in political science at the University of Chicago; they would have three children, Katherine, Peter, and Barbara.

After graduating, Simon was hired by the International City Managers' Association (ICMA) in Chicago as an assistant to Clarence Ridley, who had been his instructor in a course on evaluating municipal governments. Ridley and Simon became widely recognized experts on mathematical means of measuring the effectiveness of public services. While at the ICMA, Simon had his first experience with computers. As an assistant editor of the *Municipal Yearbook,* Simon started using **IBM** keypunch, **sorting**, and tabulating machines to prepare statistical tables. His consequent fascination with these machines would play a major part in his research and his career.

In 1939 Simon moved to the University of California at Berkeley to head a three-year study of local government funded by a grant from the Rockefeller Foundation. While at Berkeley, Simon completed the requirements for his Ph.D. from the University of Chicago. His dissertation, on decision-making in organizations, later evolved into his first book, *Administrative Behavior.* In 1942, Simon joined the faculty of the political science department at the Illinois Institute of Technology, where he remained for seven years, becoming department chair in 1946. Then, in 1949, he was tapped by the Carnegie Institute of Technology (later known as Carnegie-Mellon University) in Pittsburgh, Pennsylvania, to teach in its new graduate school in business administration. Simon would play a major role in shaping the curriculum, which was designed to provide students with the basic tools necessary for independent learning and problem-solving.

In his autobiography, *Models of My Life,* Simon describes 1955 and 1956 as the most important years of his scientific career. It was at this time that Simon, along with **Allen Newell** and Clifford Shaw of the RAND Corporation, began using computers to study problem-solving behavior. To do this, they observed individuals as they worked through well-structured problems of logic. Subjects verbalized their reasoning as they worked through the problems. Simon and his colleagues were then able to **code** this reasoning in the form of a computer program. The program was not subject-matter specific; rather, it focused on the problem-solving process. Together, Simon, Allen, and Shaw developed Logic

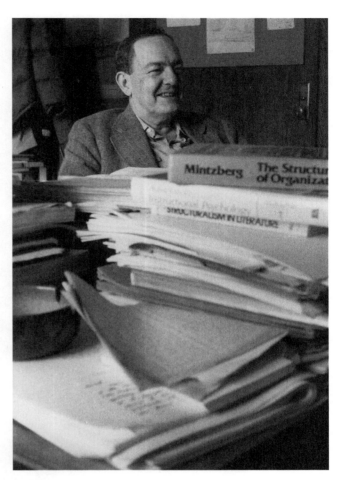

**Herbert A. Simon**

Theorist and General Problem Solver, the first computer programs to simulate human reasoning in solving problems. This work was at the forefront of the newly developing field of artificial intelligence. Simon and J. R. Hayes later developed the "Understand" program, which was designed to allow computers to solve even poorly structured problems. The program first worked to define the problem, and then focused on the problem's solution. Simon's work in artificial intelligence would lead to his being named Richard King Mellon University Professor of Computer Science and Psychology at Carnegie-Mellon University in 1966.

In 1957 Simon released a second edition of *Administrative Behavior.* In the new edition, Simon built on his original contention that because of the complexity of the economy, business decision-makers are unable to obtain all of the information they need in order to maximize profits. As a result, he had argued, most companies try to set goals that are acceptable but less than ideal—a behavior he termed "satisficing." In the second edition, Simon pointed out that his findings undermined a basic assumption of classical economic theory that the decision maker in an organization has access to all of the information needed to make decisions and will always make rational decisions that maximize profits. Simon's conclusions met with resistance from many economists, although those specializing in business operations were more accepting.

Simon's distinguished career received significant recognition in the 1960s and 1970s. He was elected to the National Academy of Sciences and became chairman of the Division of Behavioral Sciences for the National Research Council in 1967; the following year, he was appointed to the President's Science Advisory Committee. In 1969, Simon received the American Psychological Association's Distinguished Scientific Contributions Award, and in 1975, he shared the Association for Computing Machinery's A. M. Turing Award with his long-time collaborator Allen Newell. This string of awards and honors culminated in 1978 when he was awarded the Nobel Prize in economic science for his research into the decision-making process within organizations.

In the 1980s, Simon continued to be an active researcher, with his work including a study of short-term **memory** with colleagues from China. He continued his activity with the National Academy of Sciences and published a second volume of *Models of Thought* in 1989. In 1991, he published his autobiography, *Models of My Life*. In the introduction to this book, Simon commented on the varied academic paths he has chosen: "I have been a scientist, but in many sciences. I have explored mazes, but they do not connect into a single maze. My aspirations do not extend to achieving a single consistency in my life. It will be enough if I can play each of my roles creditably, borrowing sometimes from one for another, but striving to represent fairly each character when he has his turn on stage."

# SIMPLE DATA TYPES

**Data** are simply pieces of information, and an individual piece of information is a datum. Common usage, however, allows "data" as both the singular and plural form of the word. In the **hardware** of computers, data exists as **bits** and **bytes** stored as electronic **memory**. The function of a program or application (software) is to manipulate data. Each program formats data in a specific way that classifies a particular type of information. Humans learn to do this automatically and can easily distinguish between a number or a letter or what a percentage (%) character means. Computers, however, must be told what these data **types** mean within each **programming** language; therefore, the programmer has to declare the data type for every data **object**. Typical data types are numeric, alphanumeric (a mixture of alphabetic letters), numbers and special characters, dates, and logical (true/false) data types. If data is assigned a particular data type, it can never be treated like another type. Thus alphanumeric data, like an address, can never be calculated.

Simple data types, some of which are also referred to as atomic types, include all types of numbers, and, usually all types of any data built into the specific programming language itself. In some languages, the user is allowed to create extensions of the Simple types. Although it is limited, these extensions will work as if they were built in. Generally, any type that can be returned as a **value** from a function **operation** can be considered a simple type. In algebra, a function is like a black box that does some type of operation on the data put into it. For example, for every value of x add the value one, as in the function y = x + 1. If the value of the **variable** is assigned to be 1, then y is equal to 2, and only two. There can be only one answer to a function **operator**.

The **Java** programming language has eight simple types that can be divided into four groups:

- Integers—"byte," "short," "int," and "long."
- Floating point—also known as real numbers—used when fractional **precision** is needed. "Double" is used for transcendental functions like sine, cosine and square root.
- Characters—"char" represents symbols a character set like letters and digits (a digit is a single number such as 1, 2, 3...). A character can represent a digit. An integer is a numeric value, such as 1,2,3,4,5,6, and can contain one or more digits.
- Boolean—Boolean logic is a form of algebra where all values are reduced to either TRUE or FALSE. This type of logic is especially important to understanding computers because it fits comfortably with the binary numbering system, where each bit has a value of 0 or 1.

*See also* Atomic data types; Character sets

# SIMULA

Simula (as in "SIMUlation LAnguage") is based on the **Algol60** programming language. It is highly standardized, allowing it to be portable between different computing platforms. Many important object-oriented concepts like classes, objects, **abstract data types**, and **inheritance** were introduced in Simula. Although Simula has never been widely used, the Smalltalk, **C++**, and **Java** programming languages have been influenced by Simula.

### History

Simula was designed and built by Ole-Johan Dahl and Kristen Nygaard at the Norwegian Computing Centre in Oslo between 1962 and 1967. The first **iteration** of Simula is now referred to as Simula I. The first prototype of Simula I was implemented in 1964 for discrete event **simulation**, which, in essence, tells how to generate new values for variables and the times the new values should take effect. Simula I was geared toward problems in operations research, which is the study of quantitative (that is, statistical) methods like linear programming and simulation in the analysis and solving of organizational problems. Use of Simula I spread through Sweden, Germany, and the Soviet Union in the next few years.

During the 1960s, special-purpose programming languages were on the decline. Programming languages that could be used for multiple applications were becoming more popular. Simula was expanded and re-implemented as a general-purpose programming language in 1967. This version is referred to as Simula 67. The latest Simula language definition was adopted in 1986 and is maintained by the Simula Standards Group (SSG).

### Programming in Simula

Simula is a procedural, block-structured language. Features of Simula include strong typing, procedures, conditional statements, repetitions, **list processing**, and file input/output functions. Simula's **syntax** and **data types** are similar to Algol. The basic data types include integer, real, Boolean, and character.

Programs consist of sequences of instructions called blocks. The simplest program may have only one block. Each block starts with the word *begin* and finishes with the word *end*. The block structure results in modularized programs. Within each block, programming instructions include **declarations** and statements. Declarations reserve and name **memory** locations for data types, and statements tell Simula what the program is to do. There are two basic types of statements: assignments and procedures. Assignments tell Simula to place a data **value** in a location specified by the declaration. Procedures are a sequence of steps or actions to be performed. Certain procedures are predefined by the system, and others can be defined within the program by the programmer.

Programmers create the source **code** in a text editor, compile the code through a Simula **compiler**, and link the resulting **object** code to any required run-time libraries. Most errors are detected during the compile process, but additional checking occurs when the program runs. Simula is not case-sensitive, meaning that programs can consist of any combination of upper-case and lower-case letters.

*See also* Algol60; C++; Java; Object-oriented programming; Programming languages, types

# SIMULATION

One of the most fancy and cutting-edge **applications** of computer technology is in the building of simulations that emulate the behavior of real-life or theoretical systems or situations. Such simulations can serve a variety of purposes such as training and education, research, and entertainment. To take an easy example, certain experiments in psychology or behavioral sciences are either unethical or impossible to conduct—for instance, the assessment of how a particular person would react given certain accident situations often cannot be known well using standard means because accident situations cannot be created at will. The military may wish to train its soldiers in war, but does not wish to needlessly expose them to the actual bloody horrors of battle. A pilot may need to be trained to fly a new type of aircraft, but there is little sense in risking the plane and her own life during the training process itself.

For all these and many other such applications, it is desirable to create a simulation of the actual scenario and to then train or test the human subject or user on the simulation.

This method is commonly used for training crews for the space shuttle, advanced jet fighter aircraft, and the like, and the creation of simulation equipment that realistically emulates the real situation is a complex and involved task.

There are a great many challenges to the creation and use of simulations, but the major ones continue to concern traditional computer science issues. For a long time, the **design** of realistic simulations was limited for the reason that **hardware** required to operate the simulation in real time was either unavailable or prohibitively expensive. However, with the rapid growth in processor speeds in recent years, that is not a serious problem any more, and processor support for realistic simulations is inexpensively available. However, many other technical concerns remain that prevent simulations themselves from yet being commonplace and inexpensive.

If a simulation is to convey a sense of reality and emulate the real world, it must operate in real time from the perspective of the user. The CCITT G.114 Delay Recommendations (CCITT is the acronym for the old French name for the International Telecommunication Union, ITU—see http://www.itu.int; the acronym still survives in the literature and the standards prescribed under the former name) for systems that interact with human users are as follows:

- 0 to 150 milliseconds—"acceptable for most user applications"
- 150 to 400 ms—"may impact some applications"
- above 400 ms—"unacceptable"

In addition, users in a simulation must be able to perceive the effects of their own actions within 100 ms, else dissatisfaction and disorientation result.

The available bandwidth can be a critical factor in deciding the speed of the response obtained, and thus in deciding the richness of a simulation, hence having a large bandwidth available would appear to be desirable. This is especially true since a simulation typically would be expected to carry some sort of image **data**, which in turn typically require enormous amounts of bandwidth.

However, larger bandwidth can come with its own assorted set of problems, especially so over larger networks. On LANs, bandwidth has not been a major issue because standard Ethernet (10 Mega bits per second) appears to work relatively well and is inexpensive; however, the demand for LAN (**Local-Area Network-** ) simulations is rather limited. The far greater demand is for **Wide-Area-Network** and **Internet**-based simulations, where the bandwidth currently is generally limited to T1 speeds (1.5 Mbps) and where increasing the bandwidth creates new problems.

Current **protocols** such as the Ethernet do not scale well to high bandwidth requirements, at least given current hardware capabilities. The Ethernet protocol requires each **node** to look out for a collision between its transmission and that of any other node on the network, and re-transmit if a collision occurs. In order to detect a collision, however, the network must have a minimum packet size, which is proportional to the desired bandwidth and the distance of transmission. For example, for a 10 megabit Ethernet running over 300 miles, the minimum packet size should be about 6400 bytes. Current architecture however cannot support such a large packet size. If one uses standard packets (40 to 60 bytes in size) and pads them with overhead bytes to reach the minimum size required for collision detection, one ends up wasting a large majority of the available network bandwidth, and no advantage is achieved for the simulation. Achieving high bandwidths is thus a critical bottleneck in building successful simulations, and continues to be one of the chief reasons why simulations are generally too expensive for widespread use.

For these reasons, simulations continue to remain restricted for the most part to military and highly specialized applications, and much research interest at present focuses on making them widely and inexpensively available to the general public.

*See also* Central processing unit (CPU); Computer architecture; Graphics; Real-time computing

# SLIDE RULE

A slide rule is a hand-held, manually operated calculating tool that allows the user to perform multiplication, division, exponentiation, extraction of roots, and various other algebraic operations. The slide rule makes use of a set of logarithmical scales that slide alongside each other in order to perform its function. The computational accuracy of the slide rule depends on its size and on the **precision** of the printed scales. For instance, a typical 10-inch slide rule allows accuracies of about 0.1%, which is acceptable for many engineering calculations. The slide rule remained an important instrument in the mathematics of science, engineering, and business until the easier-to-use and more accurate electronic **calculator** replaced it in the 1980s.

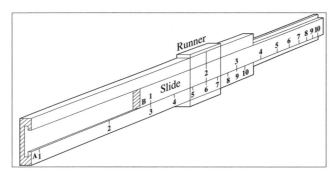

**Figure 1. Slide rule.**

The basic slide rule, as shown in Figure 1, consists of two adjacent logarithmical scales (*A* and *B*) mounted to slide along each other, and so arranged that a reading on one scale can be added to a reading on the other scale. This represents the addition of logarithms when multiplying numbers. The slide rule looks very much like a heavily calibrated ruler (scale *A*) with a movable midsection (scale *B*). The midsection, called the "slide," is engraved with precise lines to allow

the user to quickly and efficiently align different logarithmic scales. A glass or clear plastic "runner" with a finely marked vertical line is provided for easier alignment of the scales.

In 1614, research by **John Napier** concerning the simplification of mathematical calculations resulted in his creation of logarithms. Napier discovered that the logarithm made it possible to perform multiplications and divisions with the use of addition and subtraction. This is shown from the fundamental properties of logarithms (1) $log\ ab = log\ a + log\ b$, (2) $log\ a/b = log\ a - log\ b$, and (3) $a^n$ = n log a. The logarithm L of any other number N is defined as $L = log_B N$, where $N = B^L$ and the number B is the base of the system of logarithms. For example the log (base 10) of 1,000 is 3 and the log of 0.001 is -3. Napier's logarithms and the computation and publication of tables of logarithms eventually made possible the invention of the slide rule. As can be seen from the equation $N = B^L$, a logarithm L is an exponent. A base of 10 (i.e., B = 10) is probably the one most often employed in science and business.

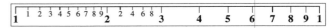

**Figure 2.**

Englishman Edmund Gunter created a logarithmic scale in 1620, as shown in Figure 2. Previously, mathematicians looked up two logs, added them together, and then looked for the number whose log was the sum. Gunter's rule, as it was called, consisted of a straight number line in which the positions of numbers were spaced at intervals proportional to their common logarithms (logs). The scale started at one because the log of one is zero ($log\ 1 = 0$). Two numbers could be multiplied by measuring the distance from the beginning of the scale to one factor with a pair of dividers, then moving the dividers to start at the other factor and reading the number at the combined distance.

Based on Napier's logarithms and Gunter's rule, Englishman William Oughtred developed in 1650 what is considered the first slide rule. It is also often called the first analog computer of modern times since multiplication and subtraction were determined by physical distance. Soon afterwards Oughtred simplified measurements further by taking two Gunter scales and sliding them relative to each other thus eliminating the dividers, as shown in Figure 3. In this example, since the upper scale's origin of 1 is set above the lower scale's 3, the multiplication of 3 x 2 is shown to be 6; that is, the 2 on the upper scale is directly above the 6 on the lower scale.

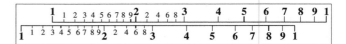

**Figure 3.**

The first known slide rule where the slide worked between parts of a fixed stock was made in 1654 by Robert Bissaker. Later, French military officer Amédée Mannheim invented in 1859 what is often considered the first modern slide rule, the one that was used and modified up to present times. This very simple slide rule, produced for more than a century, had scales on one face only, and contained three pieces: the stock, the slide, and the cursor (indicator). Then, in 1890, William Cox introduced a revolutionary construction providing for scales on both the front and back of the slide rule. An indicator with glass on both sides made it possible to refer to all the scales on both sides of the rule simultaneously.

As explained earlier, the principle of the slide rule is the translation of all computations to equivalent additions or subtractions that can be carried out on a set of scales sliding over each other. Thus, two uniformly graduated marked scales can be used for addition or subtraction, for example 2 + 3 = 5, as shown in Figure 4. If 2 and 3 are to be multiplied, it follows from the definition of logarithm that $log\ 2 + log\ 3 = log\ 6$. Accordingly, a scale that is laid out logarithmically, as shown in Figure 5, can be used to add (or subtract) logarithms and therefore to multiply (or divide). Figure 5 illustrates the principle of multiplication by the slide rule, with the example of 2 x 3. Two logarithmic scales, A and B, are arranged on a slide rule so that they may be mechanically added; that is, the end of the B scale is aligned over the 3 on the A scale. Thus, under the 2 on the A scale, one reads the product of 2 x 3 = 6 on the A scale.

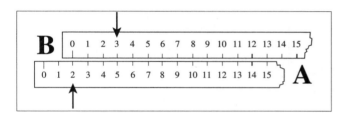

**Figure 4.**

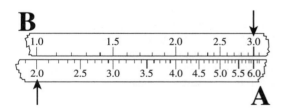

**Figure 5.**

Later developments of the slide rule added improvements, such as the "runner" mentioned earlier, to the original scales so they operated more effectively together, and increased the number of scales so more calculations could be made. These improvements also bettered the relationships among the scales, enabling them to more effectively work together. These improvements gave added speed and flexibility to the solving of simple and complex problems, since it produced solutions by continuous **operation**, without the need of intermediate readings.

# SLIP/PPP (SERIAL LINE INTERNET PROTOCOL / POINT-TO-POINT PROTOCOL)

SLIP is short for serial line **internet** protocol, which is a method for connecting to the Internet. PPP is short for Point-to-Point Protocol, another method of Internet connection. They both permit **data** communication via a transient dial-up connection of via a dedicated point-to-point connection. PPP is the more stable of the two **protocols** and provides more error checking features. SLIP is an older and simpler protocol. Practically, however, there is little difference between SLIP and PPP in connecting to the Internet.

With SLIP, the establishment and breaking of links is done manually. PPP accomplishes linkage automatically. PPP was proposed as a standard to replace SLIP in 1990, in recognition of its improved features.

SLIP preceded PPP as a means of relaying Internet Protocol (IP) packets of information over dial-up lines (where the connection between the computer and the Internet is via a telephone line). SLIP is limited in features, as compared to PPP. It typically only contains a mechanism permitting the **operation** of a process called **encapsulation**, where elements are combined to create something new. PPP has more features, and so has largely supplanted SLIP.

PPP is a so-called layered protocol, meaning that it accommodates several protocols for the establishment of a link between a computer and the Internet and for the transport of information over the link. The initial establishment of an Internet link is via a Link Control Protocol. Once this protocol is initialized, or ready to assume its function, one or many of several Network Control Protocols can be used for the information transport. The type of network protocol varies, depending on the nature of the transportation route, network, computer and information. Network Control Protocols exist for Appletalk, OSI, DECnet Phase IV, Vines, XNS and Ethernet connection.

PPP provides features, such as error checking, that is not part of SLIP. Address notification permits a server to inform a client linked via a dial-up connection of its IP address for the particular link. This is also called dynamic address assignment. Other IP addresses can be provided as well. These features are provided automatically; with SLIP, similar information is obtainable, but is a manual process. Another PPP feature is called **authentication**. Through either the **Password** Authentication Protocol or the Challenge-Handshake Protocol the authenticity of the connection and the client can be checked and verified. A third PPP feature allows multiple protocols, and so multiple functions, to operate simultaneously on the same Internet link (multilink). A fourth feature called Link Monitoring permits a periodic check of the quality and efficacy of the link. Other PPP features are the automatic retrieval of links, the dropping of links that have not been used for a set time, and the ability to function in network protocols that are based on something other than IP.

While both protocols are still utilized, PPP willmost likely continue to grow in popularity as the standard of choice for Internet connection.

*See also* Dataflow; Internet protocol (IP) address

# SOCKET INTERFACE

A socket interface, one of the most fundamental technologies of computer networking, facilitates communication between **applications** using standard mechanisms built into network **hardware** and operating systems. Socket interface technology has been employed for about two decades but is mainly used today in conjunction with the **Internet protocols**. A socket interface is a single connection between exactly two pieces of software. For more than two pieces of software to communicate effectively multiple socket interfaces are required. Although most socket-based software usually runs on two separate computers on the same network they can also be employed for local communication between programs on a single computer. Since either side of the socket interface is capable of both sending and receiving **data** they are called bi-directional. Sometimes the terms client and server are employed depending on which applications initiates communication but this type of terminology can be confusing in a non-client/server atmosphere and so should be avoided. There are three categories of socket interfaces: **stream** sockets, datagram sockets, and raw sockets. These are discussed below. Usually programmers **access** socket interfaces using **code** libraries packaged with the operating system. There are many such libraries that implement standard application **programming** interfaces such as the Berkeley Socket Library, developed in 1982 and widely in use with **UNIX** systems, and the **Windows** Sockets Library, developed in 1993 and used with **Microsoft** operating systems.

The stream socket interface, the most commonly used type, uses connection- oriented semantics. That is, the two communicating applications first establish a connection. After the connection is established any data passed from one application to the other is guaranteed to arrive in the same order in which it was sent. This type of socket interface uses not only Internet Protocol addresses to identify specific computers but also **port** numbers on those computers to distinguish multiple applications from each other. The code libraries that use this type of socket interface use Transmission Control Protocol.

The datagram socket interface uses semantics that are not connection oriented. That is the connections are implicit rather than explicit as with stream socket interfaces and so an application simply sends a datagram as needed and waits for the other application to respond. Messages can be lost in transmission or received out of order but it is the application's responsibility, not the socket interface, to deal with those problems. This type of socket interface can boost the performance of some applications as well as giving added flexibility as opposed to stream socket interfaces. This type of socket interface also uses port numbers as well as IP addresses to identify not only the specific computers involved in the communica-

tion but also the specific applications. The code libraries using this type of socket interface use User Datagram Protocol.

The third type of socket interface, the raw socket interface, effectuates communication between applications in a way that bypasses the code libraries packaged with the operating system. This means that the built-in support for standard communication protocols, such as TCP and UDP, are not used and that these sockets require much more sophisticated programming. These socket interfaces are usually used for custom, low-level protocol development because of the complexity involved.

Although traditionally socket interfaces have been of interest to mainly computer programmers new, emerging networking applications have led to a whole section of network savvy Web surfers that are learning and understanding how these interfaces operate. The socket application programming interfaces are relatively simple and small and as such many of the functions are similar to those used in file input/output routines. As computer networking becomes more ubiquitous socket interfaces will, no doubt, become more mainstream in their understanding.

# SOFTWARE—HISTORICAL OVERVIEW

The basic idea of computing—that is, the use of machines to perform tasks that require "intelligence"—is not new. Adding machines and the like have existed for generations now. In the early nineteenth century, a chess-playing machine was the rage, and was demonstrated to the French ruler Napoleon Bonaparte. That the machine was later shown to be fraudulent (as it repeated the moves of a hidden human operator) did not lessen the desire of humans to build and use intelligent devices. Later in the nineteenth century, the Englishman **Charles Babbage** designed a computer he called the **Analytical Engine**.

However, if one thinks about it, there are a great many tasks requiring some modicum of skill that one could ask a machine to perform. To have a separate machine for each such task is clearly too expensive. Even if one could afford the expense, the use of many machines would be rather cumbersome, and other inefficiencies and difficulties would be involved in the transfer of **data** from one machine to another. The notion of a universal computing device that captures the notion of **computability**, and which can thus carry out any computation whatsoever, was proposed by **Alan Turing** in 1936. The concept had an influence on the great 20th-century mathematician **John von Neumann**, who extended it in a seminal 1945 paper, and called it the stored program concept. It basically says that a machine should not, of itself, have a proclivity for just one type of task, but instead should carry out whatever instructions it is given, i.e., it should execute a stored program. The program, which defines a carefully defined procedure to accomplish a certain task, would direct the machine to carry out the task the user wanted to perform in that instance. In present day terminology, we would say that the device or machine that has capabilities but no particular fixed objective, is the **hardware**, while the **stored program**, which guides the hardware to perform its task, is software.

Therefore, we may say that the advances of Turing and von Neumann created the very concept of software, and made the widespread economical use of computers possible. It is important to understand that but for software that makes it possible to carry out different tasks on the same device, computing as we now know it would simply not exist.

Since von Neumann's time, software of course has greatly increased in its complexity and variety, and a great many of the activities of everyday life are constantly dependent upon it. We of course know about software that we commonly use for tasks like reading e-mail, **word processing**, or the like, but personal software isn't all there is. Software is used in banking and financial transactions to hold and transfer trillions of dollars, in electric power supply where a single error could bring a large city and all its critical services to a halt, and so on. To achieve a great degree of reliability in software is a constant and major research effort, and has been for decades.

The creation of software is also an exceedingly complex task, much more so than we may commonly suppose. Many people think creation of software is just the same as computer **programming**, but there's really a lot more to it. A major software program to control an electric power grid, or to help stabilize the space shuttle during launch, or even to make modern word processing possible, is never the work of one person. Based on long experience we know that a good programmer may write, on average, a few dozen lines of program code per working day, yet such a major software program typically has millions of line of program **code** that must all be thoroughly tested and debugged. Clearly, this is a task that requires a large team of dedicated software professionals to work in cooperation. Issues of human relations, personal compatibility and attitudes, and the like, therefore play a critical role, and software development is a task that requires as much people skills as technical know-how.

In addition, modern software development relies on sophisticated tools to manage programs, i.e., programs that manipulate other programs to monitor change, keep track of alternate versions, integrate modifications from different team members, etc. The use of these tools led to the celebrated quip by a Stanford student: "I'd rather write programs that help me write programs than write programs."

The discipline of software engineering has therefore evolved over the years to help make possible the efficient and speedy creation of reliable and useful software. Software vendors, and others such as large companies or the government, who need to create large software programs or packages for their own use or to sell in the marketplace, need to apply the best techniques of management and planning, with the specific experiences gained from many software development efforts past, and this is what software engineering is all about. Software, once created, does not exist unchanged for ever either. It is constantly necessary to upgrade it (come up with newer versions, with more features or with bugs removed), or else to replace it with entirely new software. Planning and managing all these things in a dynamic setting with unex-

pected changes, new technologies, unforeseen needs and shortcomings, and so on is not easy, and is also something that software engineering helps achieve.

***See also*** Applications; Hardware; Object-oriented programming; Program design; Programming; Verification

# SOFTWARE ARCHITECTURE

Software is very important to computing, and software architecture, as an aspect of software engineering and the **design** and construction of working computer systems, is a central concern to computer science and information technology. However, there unfortunately is not a single universally accepted definition for what software architecture itself is! Authors have used the term in various related but distinct ways. An important definition among these is that by Booch, Rumbaugh, and Jacobson, the "Three Amigos" of software engineering: "An architecture is the set of significant decisions about the organization of a software system, the selection of the structural elements and their interfaces by which the system is composed, together with their behavior as specified in the collaborations among those elements, the **composition** of these structural and behavioral elements into progressively larger subsystems, and the architectural style that guides this organization—these elements and their interfaces, their collaborations, and their composition." (*The UML Modeling Language User Guide*, Addison-Wesley, 1999)

Just as building architectures are best envisioned in terms of a number of styles or building models, so also with software architectures, which are split along a few major styles. Structural perspectives help document and communicate the details of the architecture in terms of the structure of the system—the specific components and their functional inter-relationships. This type of perspective is most useful in assessing structural qualities such as extensibility. Behavioral perspectives are useful in considering component interactions, the effect of component malfunctions, and so on. Execution perspectives help in communicating distribution options, and in documenting the system.

The importance of software architecture is summarized in a well-known quote from Barry Boehm, one of the renowned gurus of software engineering: "If a project has not achieved a system architecture, including its rationale, the project should not proceed to full-scale system development. Specifying the architecture as a deliverable enables its use throughout the development and maintenance process."

In defining a system's architecture, it is necessary for the designers to define the rationale of the proposed system—what it will be and what it will achieve—and to determine who the stakeholders of the system are going to be. The stakeholders of a system are, simply put, any parties who have a stake in the construction and running of the system—these include entities such as the corporate customer, the maintenance subcontractor, the human users (possibly the customer's employees), the programmers who may have to write patches, upgrades, or special local features for the system, the social group or community served by the customer, any political pressure groups or individuals associated with or interested in the proposed system in some way, and so on. Each stakeholder in the system has a specific perspective of the system, and to a certain extent does not care a great deal about other perspectives. The architecture should, at the outset, allow the system to be successful in the eyes of all its stakeholders, or at least to achieve a reasonable degree of compromise that allows for the system to be at least passable from as many perspectives as possible. The software architect may have to give greater weightage to perspectives felt to be more important—for example, a political stakeholder may be regarded more highly than others.

The concept of **modularity** is widely applied in software architecture—the grand task is broken up into components or modules, each of which is designed separately. The breakup of the total system into components must be done in accordance with accepted principles of modularity such as **information hiding**. The modular structure of the system prescribes the structure of the system being developed. That structure also determines the allocation of the system development work and hence the organization structure of the project development effort.

Software architecture is a highly iterative process, requiring prototyping, testing, measurement, and analysis. The architecture should be specified in a manner that is unambiguous and clearly specifies the working of the proposed system. The architecture must also be clear to all the stakeholders of the system, to prevent future trouble due to misunderstandings. The software development team must clearly understand the work that is required, and must be able to share tasks specifically among individuals and groups. The management of the software development team must have a clear grasp of the scheduling implications and the like.

The **UML** (**unified modeling language**) proposed by the Three Amigos (Booch, Jacobsen, and Rumbaugh) is widely applied as a tool of software architecture.

*See also* Modularity; UML

# SOFTWARE DESIGN, ENGINEERING, AND TESTING

The term "software engineering" was first used as the title of a convention held in Garmisch, Germany, in 1968 that was convened to address an emerging "software crisis." NATO called the conference because of its concern with the state of **the software industry**, which had begun to have great difficulty providing the large, complex software systems that governments and businesses required, on time and within budget. Some advocated an "engineering" approach to the software crisis, bringing the discipline of time-proven engineering methods to the relatively new field of software in order to put the new field on a more secure footing.

In the early 1970s software engineering came to be recognized as a field of study and practice that was distinct from

hardware engineering. However, early software development models were based on hardware development models. In 1976 Barry Boehm published a paper titled "Software Engineering" in which he defined the term as "The practical application of scientific knowledge in the **design** and construction of computer programs and the associated documentation required to develop, operate, and maintain them." A later author, Bruce Blum, built on Boehm's definition to define software engineering as "the application of tools, methods, and disciplines to produce and maintain an automated solution to a real-world problem."

In his 1976 paper Boehm described a software life-cycle model that came to be known as the waterfall development model. The **waterfall model** is made up of a series of stages that are completed one after another, in order. Similar to the stages of hardware development, the stages of the waterfall model are:

- Requirements analysis and definition—Developers and users of the proposed system determine its purpose and functions
- System and software design—Developers determine how the system and software will actually perform the required functions and meet its purpose.
- Implementation and unit testing—Developers build and test the units of the system.
- Integration and system testing—Developers integrate the system's units and test the entire system.
- **Operation** and maintenance—Developers and/or users put the system into operation and maintain it.

Boehm's paper is a landmark in the history of software engineering, but the waterfall model of software development has fallen under criticism for its failure to take into account the differences between software and hardware and the way those differences impact the software development process.

New methods of software development have been proposed and successfully used. Some of the new methods are:

- Incremental design—With this model a basic working system is built as soon as possible, and then further developed and refined until it works as required.
- Prototyping—The prototyping method also produces an early system that is then used to establish system requirements. Once the requirements are agreed on, a new, functional system is built to meet the requirements.
- Spiral model—Boehm proposed the spiral model as a refinement of the waterfall model in 1988. In the spiral model, the steps of thee waterfall method are accompanied by a series of risk analyses and prototypes that enable developers to produce a set of low-risk system requirements.
- Formalism—The formalism or "formal transformation" method seeks to develop a set of formal requirements and then flesh those out in increasing level of detail until the system is completely built.

The design phase of software development is the process of determining and documenting the architecture, interface, components, **algorithms**, and **data** structures, etc. necessary to satisfy the requirements specification. (The requirements specification may be modified as part of the design process.)

There are two basic types of software designs: function-oriented and object-oriented. Until the mid-1980s most software designs were based on the functions the software was to provide. Recently many designers have designed software as sets of objects rather than as sets of functions. Whereas function-oriented design centralizes system state, object-oriented design allows each **object** to have its own state and operations that act on the basis of its state. In **object-oriented** design, objects interact by sending messages or by calling other objects' procedures. When working on large software systems, designers may take both function- and object-oriented approaches at different points in their work.

Just as current approaches to software engineering and design have evolved over time, so have approaches to software testing. In the early days of software development, testing software involved programmers modifying the **code** to remove known bugs from the software product. In the late 1950s testing came to be viewed as a process that included detecting new bugs—a process that was entirely separate from **programming**; testing was performed only after initial programming was completed.

In the late 1960s along with the awareness of a "software crisis" and the development of software engineering as a discipline, there was a growing emphasis on the importance of testing throughout the software development process. In the 1970s early testing methods were proposed. Quality standards for software were established by different groups in the 1980s, providing a basis for testing. In the 1990s automated testing tools became commercially available. Although many organizations now use accepted standards, methods, and tools, testing is still frequently short-changed in the software development process.

Definitions of testing have changed as the field has evolved, and there is still a range of perspectives on the purpose of testing. In general, though, testing involves ensuring that software:

- Is error free
- Meets the requirements specification
- Meets quality standards
- Is reliable
- Is acceptable to the user(s)

Testing is often referred to as "verification and validation" or "V&V." V&V addresses the entire software development process to validate that the software meets requirements and to verify that it functions accurately and reliably.

# THE SOFTWARE INDUSTRY

The software industry has grown to become one of the cornerstones of the world economy, with nearly 10,000 independent publishers ringing up sales approaching $10 billion annually. It is an industry that is becoming most identified as a supplier of consumer goods, but it has equally served, and

was in fact founded for, applications in the military, scientific research, and engineering realms.

With software engineers responsible for creating and maintaining systems that have become indispensable for communications, manufacturing, and finance, as well as for land, sea, and air travel and a broad array of safety systems, it is difficult to imagine a world without the software industry. But since this is an industry whose ascendance has been linked, self-evidently, to that of the practical applications of electronic computing, it is always instructive to remind ourselves that the software industry is still more or less in its adolescence.

If we define software as media in the form of input **data** designed to carry instruction sets, then the history of the software industry can probably be traced to the development of the **Jacquard loom** in the 1820s. Of course this programmable textile tool had no computing applications, but it is certainly the earliest known example of an attempt to program repetitive functions for the sake of commercial automation.

Practically speaking, software development began with work carried out during and after World War II. First-generation computing consisted of the most practical applications of logic and arithmetic operations, but the advantage of finding a way to streamline the input and processing of routine functions was clear to engineers early on. Efforts were hindered, however, by the limitations of the first generation of machine languages, which were extremely error prone.

By the 1950s **programming** languages had become much simpler, but mass-marketed software products had still not yet been conceived. Standardization among the few computer manufacturers was unheard of, so cross-platform programming, with all its commercial implications, remained impossible.

This problem was overcome with the advent of *high-level* and *very high-level* **assembly languages**, which enabled programmers to adapt their work to different computer systems. These languages were also among the first to incorporate functions for identifying **syntax** errors and for defining the reusable objects of **code**, thus significantly reducing the number of lines of code required for standard operations. We can see then that software development evolved toward the era of commercialization not so much through the zeal of entrepreneurship—at least not yet. These early important advances were instead inspired by strictly utilitarian work designed to streamline extremely specialized applications.

What made the meteoric rise of the software industry inevitable was the public's fascination, dating from the earliest days of computing, with the fantastic "thinking machines." Even as the first commercially deliverable models of computers were still a decade and a half away, a few visionary programmers foresaw the day when they would be writing code for consumers instead of the government, and they began to prepare. Their most important efforts in paving the way for the multinational, multi-billion dollar industry that would follow was developing the scores of languages that would serve it.

Of the more than 200 **computer languages** that have been developed over the years, **BASIC** (Beginners' All-Purpose Symbolic Instruction Code) can probably be credited most with helping to create a commercially viable industry.

BASIC was quickly recognized as an ideal language for both operating systems and broadly marketable utilities. As programmers became more and more engaged in creating suites of nonproprietary (and thus mass-marketable) business software, utilization of BASIC spread across platforms and across the burgeoning industry. It also gained the notice of the as-yet-small but growing ranks of computer hobbyists.

The real breakthrough for independent software developers came in 1970 when **IBM** ceased bundling software with their **hardware** sales. Up until this time little distinction was made between hardware and software by casual users. Now armed with both a market and market awareness, the software industry was ready to make true consumer inroads.

Also in the early 1970s the industry was struggling to find some sort of standardization among the myriad of operating systems in use and being developed. This goal was never completely accomplished, but the field of contenders was reduced enough to allow both specialized and cross-platform software development to begin in earnest.

By the 1980s IBM was emerging as the industry leader for PC sales, and their **DOS** operating system was supporting a growing software industry. The software industry's consumer offerings now largely consisted of an array of utility programs designed to enhance the performance of DOS; however the industry was also selling applications such as **databases**, spreadsheets, **word processing** and, increasingly, entertainment.

The 1990s saw a major industry shift in operating systems, with the various **Windows** versions and **Apple**'s Mac overtaking DOS's position of primacy. The independent software developers, by now quite adept at publishing releases for whatever platforms promised the greatest returns, took the change in stride. They were much more challenged by the all but unforeseen rise of the **Internet**. Although networks of varying sizes had been served by the software industry for at least two decades, few programmers had prepared themselves for a **World Wide Web** flooded with computing novices. As the market stabilized somewhat for the traditional utilities and applications, a new market emerged for the lucky few able to mass market user-friendly browsers, **e-mail** apps, search engines, and content filters.

The Internet continues to transform the software industry. Concepts like **shareware and freeware**, which would seem to go against the grain of a consumer-driven industry, have actually been shown to boost sales. With on-line shopping, software consumers no longer need to trek to the store to shop for software; and, with the wide availability of high-speed, broadband connections, the same shoppers can receive their purchases in just minutes. Technical evolutions of the Internet, along with emerging media such as DVD and compact flash, represent the next likely challenges to the software industry.

# SOFTWARE LIBRARIES

Nearly all software systems today are designed and built to be modular; that is, they consist of separate components or modules that are connected together to form the larger system. The beauty of modular architecture is that it is possible replace or add any one component (module) without affecting the rest of the system. The opposite of a modular architecture is an integrated architecture, in which no clear divisions exist between components. The integrated architecture is not preferred for larger projects requiring more than a very small number of developers, because it requires every developer to have a comprehensive view of the total system, which is impossible for large systems and many developers.

Although the basic principles of modular **design** can apply to both **hardware** and software, modular software design in particular is based on a design strategy in which software is composed of relatively small and autonomous routines that fit together. The software modules are used must all fit a functional specification which is often made in terms of its behavior and other things such as the applicable user interface.

As large artifacts such as cars or houses are built from smaller components that can often be obtained off-the-shelf or sub-contracted, it is likewise possible for software to be generated in part using modules that already exist, using only a small amount of system-specific "glue" **code** to hold them together. The advantages of doing this are that modules can be re-used from old versions of the software (not every module need be replaced with every upgrade of the system). It is also possible for modules to be built by different teams of developers, with the possibility then being of sub-contracting specific modules to other companies or programmers.

There are sizeable libraries of software artifacts that can be applied in development efforts, based on the concept of modularity. The advantages indicated above for modular software development of course obtain, but additionally, such libraries help make individual programmers' lives easier by helping them as well. For often-used programming languages like **C**, vast libraries of routines, header files, and programs to solve well-known problems exist, that can be used by individual programmers. This means, for example, that a researcher working on a straight-forward implementation of a certain kind of graphic **simulation** using B-splines does not have to worry about the involved task of coding and **debugging** a routine that will create the B-splines—such a routine is there already, and all she has to do is to make sure the rest of her code works with it.

Most software that is made available is shareware—software that is available over the **Internet** and usable for any purpose, but which comes with no guarantees. This kind of software has in turn led to the "open-source" model of software development, wherein applications are released along with their source code, so that other programmers can modify the source code to make improvements, or to create compatible **applications**, drivers, etc. Software libraries are a critical resource in the open-source model of software development, as they facilitate exchange of source code and modules among developers. A concept called "copyleft" (a pun on "copyright") has been evolved for the open source model of development. Source code or software that has a 'copyleft' on it is copyrighted by its author and made freely available, but with the caveat that any further development using it must remain free also. Thus, there is a restriction against any further restrictions being added when it is improved or modified. This ensures that no proprietary or non-open-source applications are developed using the work of an author who had meant his work to be available to all without charge. The most common form of legalese that goes with the "copyleft" restriction is the "GNU Public License" created by the Free Software Foundation and now used widely.

Other kinds of license may apply in respect of software artifacts obtained from libraries. The most common of them are:

- non-exclusive license, meaning that the library artifact is given with the understanding that it may also be made available to others (useful to know in case the buyer has to compete with other developers for a product that will use the artifact from the library).

- non-commercial license, meaning that the artifact obtained from the library may not be used for development of a commercial product, but may only be used for in-house software.

- limited-use license, meaning that the provider of the artifact places some restrictions on the use of any software that uses it.

Software libraries exist which support both high-level abstractions (routines for implementing **algorithms** or solving specific kinds of problem) and low-level device control, user interfaces, and such. Higher-level libraries may contain dynamically loaded routines that are invoked by software at run time, or may contain shared object implementations. **Object** implementations usually cover software interaction with peripheral devices, because such device specifications are standard, and libraries can easily be designed to work with them; the creators of applications can then use these libraries without having to work on the interactions.

*See also* Object-oriented programming; Program design; Programming

## SOFTWARE METRICS

Software metrics are measures of the quality of software. They typically include measures of the complexity, understandability, testability, description and intricacy of **code**. The main function of software metrics is to improve the quality of computer software. In the past software metrics has focused on reliability and quality of the final software product but now the emphasis is moving more towards management of the software creation process as well as evaluation of intermediate software products. This is probably because software is becoming more and more complex and the human hours needed to write such complex software is ever increasing. In order to make the most effective use of time and resources many developers are seeking successful metrics that can be employed to facilitate such activities and make the most of the resources available to them.

One of the first software metrics was the number of lines of source code or the very similar delivered source instructions. It is not surprising that this was one of the first metrics since there are automated tools to measure the number of lines of code and the **value** of the result is inherently obvious to experienced programmers who are usually able to give reasonably accurate estimates of the number of lines of code necessary for a specified task before the code is written.

Measures in general are categorized by measurement theory into direct and indirect measures. Direct measures are those whose outcome is independent of the measurement outcome of any other **attribute** whereas an indirect measure is one whose outcome is inherently linked to the measurement of one or more other attributes. The number of lines of code is a direct measure. One of the main criticisms of the metrics extracted by measuring the number of lines of source code was that these became available only at a late stage of the project's development hence are of limited value when planning the crucial early phases of a project.

In an attempt to gain a better evaluation handle on software creation another approach utilizing software metrics divided into product and process metrics has been developed. They are metrics that are involved in the measurements of products created in the process and those resources used to create the products. Product metrics are often called **design** metrics as well and focus on the complexity, size and robustness of the software design being used for a specific application. They measure characteristics related to the source code, final executable program as well as analysis or design documentation. Process metrics, or project metrics as they are often called, are those metrics designed to quantify issues relating to management such as application size, staffing size and human effort expended over the process, scheduling of deliverables, number of defects, and the costs associated with fixing those defects. From these metrics it is clear that the measure of software quality is complex in that it is multidimensional, hierarchical and sometimes abstract. Because of this it is likely that no single metric is ever likely to be completely and accurately descriptive as a single expression of software quality.

## SOLID-STATE MEMORY STORAGE TECHNOLOGY

Solid-state **memory** storage technology refers to the development of computer **hardware** that is capable of storing large amounts of information, and retain that information in the absence of power. The demands for nonvolatile memory—memory that retains its contents without power—are increasing, with the expanding need to transfer information between computers, hand-held personal digital assistants, digital cameras, and multi-media devices. The term solid-state refers to the hardware aspect of this technology. Solid-state disks are plug-in storage devices that have no moving parts.

**Data** is stored in solid-state memory devices in Dynamic **Random Access Memory** (DRAM), the same **semiconductor** devices used to make the main memory for the computer's

**Central Processing Unit** (**CPU**). They appear to the host computer the same as a magnetic rotating disk, such as is used for conventional memory storage, even though they do not contain a rotating magnetic platter. Solid-state disks were originally designed in the 1980's for use in real-time industrial and military systems. They were popular because the increased performance of the computers in which they resided, and provided increased reliability because of their robust, shock-resistant construction. Their solid-state construction protected them from shock, vibration, dust and harsh temperatures, which would destroy conventional disk drives with their rotating magnetic information storage platforms.

Today, solid-state disks are popular principally because their **access** time—the time needed for the storage of information—is typically 200 times faster than the faster hard drives. Solid-state disks can double the response time of a computer. They have been most effective when used for sever **applications** and server systems, where response time is critical. The data stored on solid state devices is typically anything that could slow down the performance of a system, such as **databases**, files that are used for several different applications, library files, index files, and information concerning authorization and login.

Conventional hard drives and solid-state devices are identical in the way they connect with the computer and in their operating software. This makes solid-state devices literally plug and play—they simply plug into a computer's I/O controller, and no special operating features or programs are required to use them.

Solid-state storage devices are marketed under names such as CompactFlash, DataFlash, SmartMedia, and Memory Stick. These are powerful information storage devices. For example, Sony's Memory Stick is about the size of a stick of chewing gum and can hold 20 times as much data as a 3.5-inch floppy disk. All these solid-state storage devices are based on the same fundamental idea, **ROM**. ROM stands for **read-only memory**, which refers to one of its features, that the data stored on it cannot be altered. This is in contrast to another form of memory storage, RAM, or random access memory. The other important feature that distinguishes ROM from RAM is that ROM does not require power to maintain the data. The switches used to store data in ROM are fixed in position and cannot be changed. The switches in RAM require a current to maintain their state as on or off. ROM is nonvolatile memory; its contents remain intact when the power is turned off.

Originally, ROM data was an integral part of a chip, permanently forged onto the chip during fabrication. More flexibility in **data storage** was created with the development of the programmable ROM, PROM for short. In this chip, the data was burned into different memory locations on the chip. The data could not be changed, but chips could, allowing the replacement of one chip with another carrying different information. Next came an erasable form of the PROM chip (EPROM). Writing information to the memory could be done. But, if changes were necessary, the entire contents of the chip had to be erased and everything begun again. A large advance came next—the creation of an electrically erasable, program-

mable read-only memory (EEPROM) chip. This chip operated like the EPROM chip, except for one added advantage; it could be erased by running a higher than normal voltage through the chip. The ROM could be changed as operations proceeded.

In the present day, the standard is flash memory, which is also called flash ROM or flash RAM. Flash memory is very similar to EEPROM, but it does not require higher voltage. This allows it to be used in the three to five volts normally available in computers, personal digital assistants, and digital cameras. While flash memory is not capable of infinite write and erase cycles, a million cycles or more are feasible, making this form of memory storage robust and convenient. Flash memory is standard for bios chips, which are vital for the operations of computers and modems. This is because they can be updated easily. Downloaded information can be written onto the chip after a utility has erased the old information from the chip. New information can be added selectively, so that erasure need not be total. The solid state construction of flash memory cards has been a boon to users of personal digital assistants, portable devices that necessarily experience rough handling.

***See also*** Data storage; Dynamic programming; Memory; Random-access memory (RAM); Read-only memory (ROM)

# SORTING

In many cases it is necessary to take a sequence of values and sort them in some specified order. For example, a list of class examination scores may be sorted by decreasing order of scores, or by the identification number of the students in the class. In most cases, there is a **record** with several fields, such as student's name, number, score, and grade. A field such as the score which is sorted against is called a key, while other fields are considered ancillary to it and are referred to as satellite **data**. When a sorting algorithm rearranges the order of the key fields, it rearranges the satellite fields as well. However, these details are often irrelevant in considering the question of the methods to be used for sorting, as details of implementation are usually left to the programmer. For purposes of understanding the **algorithms**, we pretend that the key fields are the only ones that exist.

The simplest sorting algorithm is called bubble sort. Here, the list is scanned in order, and when a key **value** is found to be in the wrong position relative to its immediate neighbor, the two are switched. The sorting is not accomplished in one pass over the entire sequence, however, and as many passes are needed as there are values to be sorted. The algorithm is given its name because a value that needs to move into a different position in the sequence "bubbles through" the sequence one step at a time.

Another simple sorting algorithm is called insertion sort, which proceeds the way people sort a hand of cards while playing a game like gin rummy. The algorithm simply starts with an empty sequence, and inserts each element into its right place respective to the others. This algorithm has the disadvantage of requiring greater storage space, and is not as efficient as possible.

Merge sort is another algorithm that uses the divide-and-conquer approach by breaking up the sequence to be sorted into smaller subsequences, and then sorting them using simple methods. In fact, when the size of each individual subsequence is 1, there is no real work to be done, as each such subsequence is trivially sorted. Using the divide-and-conquer approach, it is then possible to combine the smaller sorted sequences to obtain the total solution.

Two of the other commonly used **sorting algorithms** are **heap** sort and quick sort.

Heap sort relies on a special **data structure** called a heap, which is a complete binary **tree** with values stored at the nodes, such that each **node** in the tree has a value no larger than its parent. Because the root of the heap holds the largest value, one can obtain the largest value in the heap immediately simply by reading the root. After the root is read, its value is destroyed, and a value from another node is moved up to take its place. This disturbs the heap so that the "heap property" that no node can be smaller than its child no longer holds, so it is necessary to heapify the data structure again by switching any **parent** and child wherever the parent is smaller than the child. In this way, the heap is restored again. By repeatedly reading the root and restoring the heap, it is possible to obtain the elements in decreasing order. Alternatively, we could define the heap to have the property that no parent is larger than its child, and obtain them in increasing order as well.

Quicksort is very similar to merge sort in its use of the divide-and-conquer method and recursive solution.

- Divide—the **array** to be sorted is partitioned into two parts such that every element in the first part is less than or equal to every element in the second part.
- Conquer—the two parts are sorted by recursive calls to quicksort.
- Combine—since the parts are in the correct positions relative to each other, no further work is required, and the final array is readily obtained.

The previous sorting algorithms all involve comparisons between the sequence of values that are to be sorted. In some cases, it is not necessary to carry out comparisons in sorting, and there is a well-known result that says that if one does use comparisons in sorting, then the performance achieved is not going to be proportional to the size of the input array but will be larger, while if comparisons are not used, then such proportional results could be achieved. If one has an input array of size 10000, for instance, the difference could be of a factor of between 4 and 10000 in the time taken. For this reason, in some cases, it is preferable to use methods like counting sort and radix sort, which do not involve comparisons. For example, if it is known that all student identification numbers in a school run from 1 to 2300, then it is not necessary to compare values while sorting student records by identification number; one may place each value appropriately simply as determined by its correct value.

*See also* Abstract data type; Divide and conquer algorithm; Program design; Programming; Recursion

# SORTING ALGORITHMS

*Sorting* is the process of taking an initially unordered **array** of records and arranging them in some specific *target order*. The target order is specified by a *comparison function* which, given two records, decides which **record** should come first. For example, if the records are two integers, the comparison **function** may be the rule: "put the smaller number earlier in the list." There are many sorting **algorithms**, and some can be quite computationally complex. The main justification for going through the process of **sorting** is that once it is done it is relatively easy to find records in the sorted list using fast algorithms such as binary search.

An important criterion used to rate sorting algorithms is their *running time*. Running time is measured by the number of computational steps it takes the sorting algorithm to terminate when sorting n records. We say that an algorithm is $O(n^2)$ (read, "of order *n*-squared") if the number of computational steps needed to terminate as *n* tends to infinity increases in proportion to $n^2$

An important theoretical constraint on the speed of sorting algorithms can be obtained from the following reformulation of the sorting problem. For *n* records there are *n*! possible linear arrangements, only one of which is the correct, sorted set of records. ($n! = 1 \times 2 \times 3 \times ... [n -2] \times [n - 1] \times n.$) One may imagine these *n*! arrangements as the leaves of a binary **decision tree**. The process of sorting then involves starting at the root of the **tree** (the unordered initial list) and traveling down the nodes, choosing either the left or right **node** based on results of comparisons. (In this terminology, the "root" of a tree is at the *top*, and all the branches expand downward.) The maximum number of steps needed would correspond to the height of the tree, which is log *n*!. Using Stirling's approximation of log *n*! for large *n*, this process would be $O(n \log n)$. This is the fastest we could hope for in a sorting algorithm based on comparisons.

Examples of some comparison-based sorting algorithms are *bubble sort, selection sort*, and *insertion sort*, all of which run quite slowly since they are $O(n^2)$. *Selection sort* is arguably the simplest. This algorithm simply scans the list for the smallest record (assuming, for this example, that record magnitude is the relevant sorting criterion) and switches that record's position with the record in the first position. Then it scans through the remaining *n* - 1 records, finds the smallest, and switches it with the record in second position, and so on until all the records have been arranged in ascending order.

*Bubble sort*, instead of going directly for the smallest record, works on the premise that whenever two adjacent records are out of order, they should be switched. On the first pass bubble sort goes down the array of records and compares each pair of records. If record *i* + 1 is smaller than record *i* than it switches them. On a single pass the list will not be sorted, but the largest record will definitely be at the end. After *n* such passes the list is ordered. The name "bubble sort" is derived from the image of smaller items bubbling up to the top of the list. Although both bubble sort and selection sort are $O(n^2)$, bubble sort is usually slower, since more exchanges are involved on average, and exchanging large records can be an expensive **operation** in terms of computation time.

*Insertion sort* is the algorithm most people use automatically when ordering a deck of cards. At any given point in the algorithm, insertion sort maintains in the first $j$ occupied positions of the record array a sorted list of records. The remaining $n - j$ records are unsorted and need to be inserted into the sorted list one by one. The first record in the unsorted list, in position $j + 1$, is inserted into the appropriate place in the sorted list, moving any records down if needed to make room. As the algorithm continues in this manner, the sorted list gets larger and the unsorted list gets smaller until the whole list is sorted.

All these algorithms are $O(n^2)$, far short of the theoretical limit for comparison searches, which is $O(n \log n)$. *Heap sort* is an algorithm that approaches this limit. The key to its success is the underlying **data structure** of a **heap**, which is a complete binary tree, that is, a binary tree where each node has 0 or 2 children, except possibly nodes at the next to highest level. The nodes themselves contain the **data** to be sorted and satisfy the *heap property*, which states that for every node other than the root, the **value** of that node is larger than or equal to that of its parents. Note that this forces the root to contain the largest record. One can put the nodes of the heap into one-to-one correspondence with positions in an array simply by numbering the nodes in order level by level from top to bottom and from left to right within each level. Under this scheme the root (at the very top) is the first element in the array, and the rightmost leaf at the lowest level is the last element of the array. Thus the heap and the array of data to be sorted can be implemented in exactly the same locations in **memory** and no extra memory is needed. In fact one should think of the heap and the array as one and the same **object**; the heap is just another way of looking at the array.

We will now see how to use this heap data structure to order the array. We first assume that we can somehow impose a heap structure on the array by rearranging the array elements so that the heap condition is satisfied. Then the largest record will be at the root of the heap or, equivalently, in the first position in the array. If we switch the first record with the last record, the largest record will be in the last position. Now if we ignore the last position, which is equivalent to ignoring the rightmost leaf of the lowest level of the heap, we are left with a smaller heap except for one problem: the root node does not satisfy the heap property since it cannot be larger than its children. A procedure called *heapification* fixes this problem. Heapification merely amounts to letting the root node contents bubble down the tree by successively exchanging them with the contents of its immediate children until the heap property is satisfied. Then we are left with the original situation where the root note contains the largest element. We again exchange it with the record in position $n - 1$, ignore the last two positions, and heapify to get a smaller heap. After repeating this $n$ times we get a fully sorted array. The process of heapification is $O(\log n)$ since $\log n$ is the height of the binary tree, or the longest distance the root contents can bubble down in order to satisfy the heap property. Thus the whole algorithm is $O(n \log n)$, provided we can build the initial heap quickly. It turns out that the initial heap can be built in $O(n)$ time by iteratively

using the heapify algorithm from the bottom up. Heap sort thus achieves the theoretical limit.

Whereas heap sort achieves its $O(n \log n)$ efficiency by making use of a binary tree structure, another algorithm, *quicksort*, achieves the same efficiency on average by using a recursive divide-and-conquer strategy. The idea behind quicksort is that the given array is first partitioned into two nonempty subarrays such that each element of the first subarray is less than or equal to each element of the second. The two subarrays are then themselves sorted by recursive calls to quicksort. It is clear that this recursive process will completely sort the array. The partitioning itself is done simply by choosing the first element of the array to be partitioned as an element around which to pivot. Any element less than or equal to this first element is inserted directly below it. This achieves the partitioning. Although in the worst case scenario, this strategy can yield an $O(n^2)$ algorithm depending on how unbalanced or unequal in size the resulting partitions are, on average the partitions are usually quite balanced and the average behavior is $O(n \log n)$.

# SPREADSHEET PROGRAMS

A computer spreadsheet is an automated ledger book. The spreadsheet—a large piece of paper with columns and rows that shows details about transactions—predates computers by hundreds of years. Computerized technology has provided the electronic replacement of the accountant's columnar pad, pencil, and **calculator**. Spreadsheet programs use columns and rows to display both numbers and text, and allow calculations to be performed on the numerical **data**. In addition to number-crunching, spreadsheet programs allow editing of data, graphical representation of data and financial modeling.

The development of the electronic spreadsheet began in 1961 with Richard Mattessich. Practically, the electronic spreadsheet originated with VisiCalc, the first such program, which was developed in 1978 by **Daniel Bricklin**, and refined with the assistance of Robert Frankston. Frankston's accomplishment was to package the program such that it occupied relatively little machine **memory**. This allowed VisiCalc to run on a **personal computer**, which proved very popular. In the jargon of the computer user VisiCalc is now recognized as the first "killer application" for personal computers. The program was discontinued in 1985.

In 1980, the dif format was introduced. This allowed spreadsheet data to be shared or imported into other programs, including text-based **word processing** programs. Three years later, Lotus 1–2–3, which was based on Visicalc, was developed by Lotus co-founder Mitch Kapor. Lotus 1–2–3 introduced naming cells, cell ranges and spreadsheet macros. It became the premier spreadsheet program for many years following its release. Towards the end of the 1980s, **Microsoft** and Corel released the spreadsheet programs Excel and Quattro pro, respectively. These emphasized the **graphical user interface** technology, with pull down menus and a point and click capability using a mouse-pointing device. Currently, Excel **commands** the biggest market share, although many other vendors have spreadsheet programs as well.

The columns and rows of a spreadsheet make up a grid pattern on each page (a page can also be called a worksheet). A number identifies each row, and a letter identifies each column. The intersection of a particular row and column is called a cell. Each cell is identified by its column and row number. The number of cells can be huge. Lotus 1–2–3 contains 8192 rows and 256 columns, which translates to over two million cells, and the latest version of Excel has 255 pages containing more than four million cells. Once the cells have been defined and the formulas for linking them together have been written, data can be entered in the cells. Each cell can contain a label, which is a text entry, or a value, which can be a number, formula or a formula's result. The active cell is indicated by the cursor. A new active cell can be selected, or the cursor can be used to drag the data from one cell to another cell.

Cells are linked mathematically by formulas. For example, D1 = B1 + F4 would display the sum of B1 and F4 in D1. The sum of data in designated cells in rows or columns can be programmed. Mathematical short cuts are also possible, with statistical designations such as SUM, AVERAGE, MEAN, MIN, and MAX being invoked for the assigned cells. These and other tools (copying, calculating a numerical difference between two cells) allow the spreadsheet data to be rapidly manipulated and analyzed. Selected values can be modified to explore how other values will change, and are called what-if scenarios.

Most spreadsheets are described as being multidimensional; one spreadsheet can be linked to another. A three-dimensional spreadsheet can be thought of as a **stack** of spreadsheets, connected mathematically to one another via formulas. A change made in one spreadsheet will automatically affect the other spreadsheets. Tax preparation software is one such example.

Another useful tool is the ability to represent numerical data in graphical form. For the Excel **programming**, this tool is called the Chart Wizard. Bar **graphs**, line graphs, column graphs, pie charts, area plots, and scatter plots can be constructed in two or three dimensions. This aids in perceiving trends or patterns that would otherwise be difficult to discern from a chart of numerical data, and the graphical representation of data is always appreciated by an audience in a presentation.

The educational value of electronic spreadsheets has been enormous. They have been most valuable for completing repeating tasks and for exploring the effects of different arrangements of data.

*See also* Computer science and corporations; Data base; Data storage

# STACK

A stack is a dynamic **data structure** that can store records of **data** and that supports two primary functions usually called PUSH and **POP**. The **operation** PUSH is used to add elements to the stack, while the operation POP removes a prespecified element off the stack. A key property of a stack is that it implements a last in, first out (LIFO) policy; namely the last ele-

ment pushed onto the stack must be the first element popped off the stack. One should compare this policy to that of another data structure, the **queue**, which implements a first in, first out (FIFO) policy.

An important way to visualize the operation of a stack is to think of it literally as a stack of cafeteria trays, with each tray corresponding to a **record** of data. The PUSH operation corresponds to pushing a tray, or new piece of data onto the top of the stack, while the POP operation corresponds to removing, or popping, the top tray off the stack. In this visual analogy, it is clear that the last tray pushed onto the stack is the first tray popped off and hence the LIFO policy is obeyed.

In actuality, in a computer a stack of at most n elements can be implemented simply by an n element **array** called STACK[0..n-1]. The top of the stack corresponds to the last nonempty spot in the array, whose index could be remembered by an auxiliary **variable** called TOP. Pushing an element on the stack simply involves placing that element in the array location STACK[TOP+1], and then incrementing TOP by 1, first checking of course that TOP does not exceed n-1. Popping an element off the stack similarly involves returning the data in STACK[TOP] and decrementing TOP. If TOP equals 0 then the stack is empty and the POP **function** should return some sort of error. If one does not know the maximum number of elements to be held by the stack in advance one could alternatively implement the stack using a **linked list** with PUSH and POP corresponding to appending and deleting the last element in the list.

In terms of their applications, stacks as data structures are ubiquitous in all modern computing tools. For example consider some of the early calculators which use postfix notation. In such a notation one would type in the number 4, then the number 5, and then some operation, say +, and the **calculator** would read out 9. In the **hardware** what is happening is that each time the user enters a number, it is pushed onto the top of the stack. Whenever a binary operation, such as +, -, *, or / is entered, the first two elements at the top of the stack are popped off and taken as input to the binary function, whose output is printed on the screen. This elegant implementation of a calculator obviates the need for using parentheses to specify the associativity structure of a calculation. Instead, the act of pushing and popping takes care of everything, albeit forcing the user to think in postfix.

As another elegant example of the use of a stack, consider the implementation of a parenthesis checker, a program that takes as input a mathematical statement and checks whether all the parentheses match up. Such a **subroutine** would be useful in a **compiler** for example. The checker could be implemented simply using a stack. First it starts off with an empty stack. Every time it encounters an open parenthesis "(" it pushes some symbol onto the stack. Also every time it encounters a closed parenthesis is pops the same symbol off the stack. If at any point the checker has to POP a symbol off an empty stack, the parentheses cannot be well matched. Assuming such an error does not occur, if the stack is empty after the the last symbol is read, it is guaranteed that the parentheses match up correctly. From these simple examples once can see the utility of stacks, which explains their presence in almost all hardware implementations of modern computing tools.

# STALLMAN, RICHARD MATTHEW
## (1953-   )
### American computer scientist

His stringy brown hair and mesmerizing green eyes once inspired the computer trade publication *LinuxWorld* to describe him as "Rasputin-like." At times during his controversial career, Richard Stallman lived in his ninth-floor office at the Massachusetts Institute of Technology (MIT), surrounded by books, printouts, and a blinking computer terminal. But *Wired* magazine has declared him "one of the greatest programmers alive."

Stallman, recipient of a $240,000 MacArthur Foundation "genius" grant in 1990, authored principal parts of the GNU/Linux operating system, estimated at the turn of the millennium to have more than 10 million users worldwide. He also founded the GNU Project and is founding president of the non-profit Free Software Foundation.

Stallman was born in New York City, two years after **UNIVAC** I (the machine that started the modern era of general-purpose commercial computers) was completed for the U.S. Bureau of the Census. His passion for the computer first developed during his high school days. It began at a summer camp, where Stallman devoured computer manuals borrowed from counselors. He returned to Manhattan and pursued his newfound interest at a computing center there. By the time Stallman finished high school, he was considered an expert in computer operating systems, assembly languages, and text editors.

In 1971, as an undergraduate at Harvard University, Stallman walked into MIT's **Artificial Intelligence** Lab in Cambridge, Massachusetts, where he so impressed administrator Russ Noftsker that he was offered work as a systems programmer. He developed improvements to a computer operating system called ITS (Incompatible Time-Sharing).

Because he worked mainly at night, Stallman's coworkers at the lab were unaware that he was also a student by day. "When the people in the lab discovered after the fact that he was simultaneously earning a magna cum laude degree in physics at Harvard, even those master hackers were astonished," Steven Levy wrote in a chapter devoted to Stallman in his 1984 book, *Hackers: Heroes of the Computer Revolution.*

Speaking to students at Stockholm's Royal Institute of Technology in 1986, Stallman recalled a refreshing openness at the MIT lab: "The terminals were thought of [as] belonging to everyone, and professors locked them up in their offices on pain of finding their doors broken down....Many times I would climb over ceilings or underneath floors to unlock rooms that had machines in them that people needed to use, and I would usually leave behind a note explaining to the people that they shouldn't be so selfish as to lock the door." Unlocked doors were just one manifestation of an entire philosophy at the AI laboratory, which also deliberately avoided protecting its computer files.

In the 1970s, however, MIT began requiring passwords to access many of its computers. Stallman worked to undermine this development. "In the old days on ITS, it was con-

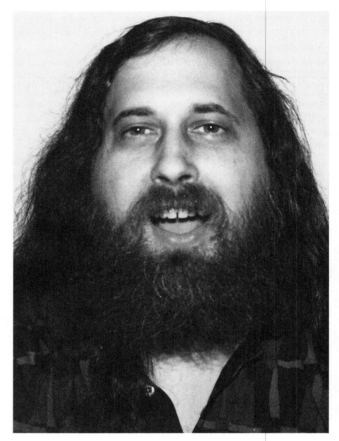

**Richard Stallman**

sidered desirable that everyone could look at any file, change any file, because we had reasons to," he recalled during his Stockholm speech. He infiltrated MIT's **password** system, and sent messages to users, encouraging them to switch their passwords to a simple carriage return. "It's much easier to type, and also it stands up to the principle that there should be no passwords," he told the system users. "Eventually I got to a point where a fifth of all the users on the machine had the Empty **String** password," he later told Levy.

Since those days at the AI lab, Stallman has clung to his controversial belief that computer software should not be owned or copyrighted. This conviction was to be deeply tested. Stallman's boss, Russ Noftsker, left MIT in 1973 with the intention of starting a company that would develop artificial intelligence machines. The result, formed in 1977, was Symbolics, a company that offended Stallman by hiring away many of MIT's brightest hackers, then persuading MIT to buy its machines. Determined to get revenge, Stallman helped a rival company, LMI, by producing enhancements to LMI's operating system that matched those introduced by Symbolics.

Then, in 1984, he left MIT to start the Free Software Foundation (FSF). Stallman's idea was to create an operating system compatible with the popular **UNIX** system, but one that users would be free to copy, redistribute, or change. To allow modifications, the system's source **code** would also be freely available. He called this proposed operating system GNU (a recursive acronym: GNU's Not Unix). The foundation was established to promote the development of GNU, and to work to eliminate restrictions on the copying, redistribution, understanding, and modification of computer programs.

Stallman was the principal or initial author of some critical components of GNU, including GNU Emacs (a widely used text editor), GNU C **Compiler** (which supports seven **programming** languages and more than 30 computer architectures), as well as a GNU **debugging** program. The many pieces of the GNU system were finally brought together by a "kernel" written by **Linus Torvalds**. The name of this kernel, **Linux**, is now widely used to describe the full GNU/Linux operating system.

In a 1999 interview with *LinuxToday,* Stallman said that a free operating system had been achieved, but more free application software was needed. "I know that many of the companies that make proprietary **applications** are now starting to release versions of them that run on GNU/Linux. It's a step forward.... But it's only the first step. It's not the same as fully having freedom. To fully have freedom you've got to be using a free application instead of a proprietary one. So, we need to develop large numbers of free applications."

Now considered a legendary computer hacker, Stallman derives much of his income from speaking engagements. "Fortunately, I live cheaply," he told Joe Barr from *LinuxWorld.* "I've resisted acquiring the expensive habits that some other people pick up as soon as they get enough money to. You know, like houses and cars and children and boats and planes."

However, Stallman has picked up some other, less-expensive interests. His **Internet** home page lists these as: "affection, international folk dance, flying, cooking, physics, recorder, puns, [and] science fiction fandom."

## STATE TRANSITION DIAGRAM

A state **transition** diagram is a graphical representation of the states of an **object** as well as the transitions the object may pass through during its lifetime. State transition diagrams are used in object-oriented modeling and **design** to represent a finite-state machine.

In a state transition diagram circles represent states and directed line segments represent transitions between the states. A state is an observable mode of behavior of an object. At any time a particular object can only be in one state. Transitions can be internal events or events external to the system that have an effect on object states. Transitions may have conditions attached to them, meaning that a transition only occurs if a condition is true.

State transition diagrams were originally introduced by G. H. Mealy and E. F. Moore in the 1950s. Today's state transition diagrams are descendants of these models. The most popular implementation of state transition diagrams is the Harel statechart, developed by David Harel in 1983. On top of the basic state transition diagram concept, the Harel statechart

includes the notions of hierarchy of state transitions as well as the ability to abstract common states into super-states. The Harel statechart has been adopted in the **UML** (**Unified Modeling Language**).

Creating a state transition diagram involves identifying all the possible states of the object, identifying all transitions between states, identifying the state the object is in when it is created, and identifying the state the object is in before it is destroyed.

State transition diagrams are best at describing the behavior of a single object. Since systems generally contain multiple objects, system analysis and design would consist of multiple state transition diagrams. Interaction diagrams (also called activity diagrams) are also used for describing behavior involving several objects.

*See also* Finite-state machine; State; UML (Unified Modeling Language)

## STATIC

The term static is defined within computer processing as the condition of being fixed or stationary. The opposite condition to being static is the condition called *dynamic;* that is, occurring immediately or constantly changing. Both terms can be applied to a number of different types of computer-related items, such as **hardware**, Web pages, **programming** languages (or its components), and application programs. For example, a **memory buffer** (a temporary holding place for **data**) that is static remains invariant ("fixed") in size throughout program execution. On the other hand, computer operations are often performed dynamically ("on-the-fly") and are based on decisions made while the program is running rather than beforehand. For example dynamic memory buffers are dynamically created; that is, the storage space is created when actually needed, and not reserved ahead of time.

Static can also be defined as a *piece of hardware* that does not need to be refreshed. Such a device retains its contents without having to be refreshed by the **central processing unit** (**CPU**). Main memory, which is usually high-speed **random access memory** (RAM), is memory in which specific contents can be accessed directly in a very short period of time regardless of the sequence (and hence location) in which they were recorded. Two types of main memory are possible. Static random access memory (SRAM) retains the data within its structure as long as there is enough power in order to run the device. On the other hand, dynamic RAM (DRAM) stores information within integrated circuits that contain capacitors. Because capacitors lose their charge over time, dynamic RAM must include logic to refresh ("recharge") itself continuously.

The term static can also refer to *Web pages* that are requested by a computer user when clicking on a hyperlink or entering a **URL** (**Uniform Resource Locator**). In some cases, when the server returns the **HTML** (HyperText Markup Language) document page from where it was stored and the Web **browser** displays it on the monitor screen, the user is able to interact with the page through whatever links or **applets** (small programs) that are available. But, the user has no capacity to return information that is not pre-formatted. In this case the Web page is static in nature. However, on a dynamic Web page, the user can make data requests (often through a blank form) contained in a server's database that will be assembled "on-the-fly." For example, the user might request information on a sporting event played at a certain date and location. When the user requests such information, the request is relayed to the server and an Active Server Page (ASP) script becomes embedded in the HTML page. In this instance, the Web page is designated as dynamic.

There are also static (and dynamic) *programming languages*. In a static programming language, such as **C** or **Pascal**, a developer must declare the type of each **variable** before the **code** is compiled, making the coding less flexible, but also prone to less errors. In a dynamic language, such as **Perl** (acronym for Practical Extraction and Reporting Language) or **LISP** (acronym for **LISt Processing**), a developer can create variables without specifying their type. This creates more flexible programs and can simplify prototyping and some **object-oriented** coding.

*See also* Dynamic data structure

# STIBITZ, GEORGE R. (1904-1995)
*American mathematician and computer scientist*

George R. Stibitz joined the Bell Telephone Laboratories as a mathematical engineer in 1930. His work at Bell Labs convinced him of the need to develop techniques for handling a large number of complex mathematical operations much more quickly than was currently possible with traditional manual systems. His research eventually led to the development of one of the first binary computers ever built. Stibitz was also the first to transmit computer **data** long-distance. Later in his life the mathematician became especially interested in the application of mathematics and the computer sciences to biomedical problems.

George Robert Stibitz was born on April 20, 1904, in York, Pennsylvania. His mother was the former Mildred Amelia Murphy, a math teacher before her marriage, and his father was George Stibitz, a professor of theology. Stibitz's childhood was spent in Dayton, Ohio, where his father taught at a local college. Because of the interest in and aptitude for science and engineering that he had exhibited, Stibitz was enrolled at an experimental high school in Dayton established by Charles Kettering, inventor of the first automobile ignition system.

For his undergraduate studies, Stibitz enrolled at Denison University in Granville, Ohio. After earning his bachelor of philosophy degree there in 1926, he went on to Union College in Schenectady, New York, where he was awarded his M.S. degree in 1927. After graduating from Union, he worked as a technician at General Electric in Schenectady for one year before returning to Cornell University to begin his doctoral program. Stibitz received his Ph.D. in mathematical physics from Cornell in 1930.

Stibitz's first job after graduation was as a research mathematician at the Bell Telephone Laboratories in New York City. His job there was to work on one of the fundamental problems with which modern telecommunication companies have to deal: How to carry out the endless number of mathematical calculations required to **design** and operate an increasingly complex system of telephones. At the time, virtually the only tool available to perform these calculations was the desktop mechanical **calculator**. It was obvious that this device would not long be adequate for the growing demands of the nation's expanding telephone network.

In the fall of 1937 Stibitz made the discovery for which he is now best known, the use of relays for automated computing. A relay is a metallic device that can assume one of two positions—open or closed—when an electrical current passes through it. The relay acts as a kind of gate, therefore, that will control the flow of electrical current, and was a common device used to regulate telephone circuits.

In November 1937 Stibitz decided to see if relays could be used to perform simple mathematical functions. He borrowed a few of the metal devices from the Bell stockroom, took them home, and assembled a simple computing system on his kitchen table. The system consisted of the relays, a dry cell, flashlight bulbs, and metal strips cut from a tobacco can. He soon had a device in which a lighted bulb represented the binary digit "1" and an unlighted bulb, the binary digit "0." The device was also able to use binary mathematics to add and subtract decimal numbers. Stibitz's colleagues later gave the name "K-Model" to this primitive computer because it was built on his kitchen table.

When Stibitz first demonstrated his K-model computer for company executives, they were not very impressed. "There were no fireworks, no champagne," he was quoted as saying in *The Computer Pioneers*. Less than a year later, however, Bell executives had changed their minds about the Stibitz invention. An important factor in that decision was the increasing pressure on Bell to find a way of solving its increasingly complex mathematical problems. The company agreed to finance construction of a large experimental model of Stibitz's invention. Construction on that machine began in April 1939, and the final product was first put into operation on January 8, 1940. Called the Complex Number Calculator (CNC), the machine had the capacity to add, subtract, multiply, and divide complex numbers—just the kinds of problems that were particularly troublesome for engineers at Bell.

Nine months later, Stibitz recorded another milestone in the **history of computer science**. At a meeting of the American Mathematical Society at Dartmouth College, he hooked up the new Complex Number Calculator in New York City with a telegraph system. He then sent problems from Dartmouth to the CNC in New York, which solved the problems and sent the answers back to Dartmouth by means of the telegraph. This type of data transmission has now become commonplace in a modern day society of modems and fax machines.

During World War II, Bell Labs permitted Stibitz to join the National Defense Research Council. There the demands of modern military artillery convinced Stibitz even more of the need for improved computer **hardware**, and he spent most of the war working on improved versions of the CNC, also known as the Model 1. The Model 2 computer, for instance, used punched tapes to store programs that would give the computer instructions; in this manner the computer could perform the same complex calculations many times on different sets of numbers. This proved useful in calculating weapons trajectories.

At the end of World War II, Stibitz decided not to return to Bell Labs. Instead he moved with his family to Vermont where he became a consultant in applied mathematics. After two decades in this line of work Stibitz was offered a job at Dartmouth's Medical School, where he was asked to show how computers can be used to deal with biomedical problems. He accepted that offer and was appointed professor of physiology at Dartmouth; in that capacity he investigated the motion of oxygen in the lungs and the rate at which drugs and nutrients are spread throughout the body. In 1972 he retired from his position and was made professor emeritus; nevertheless, he continued to contribute his knowledge to the department.

Stibitz was married on September 1, 1930, to Dorothea Lamson, with whom he had two daughters, Mary and Martha. Among the awards he has received are the Harry Goode Award of the American Federation for Information Processing (1965), the Piore Award of the Institute of Electrical and Electronic Engineers (1977), and the Babbage Society Medal (1982). He was also the recipient of honorary degrees from Keene State College and Dartmouth College. The holder of 35 patents, Stibitz was named to the Inventors Hall of Fame in 1983. He died in his Hanover, New Hampshire, home on January 31, 1995. He was 90.

# STORED-PROGRAM PRINCIPLE

The stored-program principle, also known as the stored program concept, refers to the storage of both **data** and **programming** (i.e., instructions) within in a single, uniform **memory** structure known as main (or primary) memory. Main memory is the general-purpose storage area that is directly accessible by the computer's **central processing unit (CPU)**; main memory is synonymous with "RAM," which stands for "random access memory."

Nowadays it is taken for granted that a programmer writes a computer program, which is then read into main memory for execution. However, such was not the case for the first electronic computers, which were created starting in the late 1930s until the close of the 1940s. During that period there were two competing technologies for performing advanced digital computing: *relay* computers and *electronic* computers. The terms "relay" and "electronic" referred to the kinds of devices that the computer used to perform its computations. Relay-type computers used a switching device, borrowed from the telephone industry, which controlled the flow of electricity by the opening and closing of metal contacts. The **Bell Laboratories relay computers**, produced from 1939 to

1949, constitute an excellent example of these "electro-mechanical" digital computers. Like modern computers, most Bell computers held their data (which consisted of numbers) in internal memory inside the computer. However, unlike modern computers the instructions that directed the computer's computations were represented as punched holes in a paper tape, and those instructions were not stored in memory, but rather executed as they were processed by an input device. A result of this architecture was that computations could be performed no faster than the instructions could be fed in via paper tape from the input mechanism. This limitation to the computer's processing speed made sense for relay computers since they were inherently slow (as compared to electronic computers).

In contrast to relay computers, electronic computers used vacuum tubes that controlled current flow without the need for moving parts. Electronic computers using vacuum tubes could generally perform computations much faster than computers that used relays. For instance, the Bell Laboratories Model V relay computer, made around 1945, could perform about one multiplication per second, while the electronic computer **ENIAC** (**Electronic Numerical Integrator and Computer**), also completed in 1945, could perform some 357 multiplications per second. By the late 1940s, electronic computers had eclipsed relay computers with their far greater processing speeds.

Upon becoming operational in 1945, ENIAC became the world's first general-purpose, electronic computer. Though probably the most powerful computer (in terms of computations per second) at the time of its debut, its creators realized it had several limitations. One of the biggest drawbacks to the efficient use of ENIAC concerned its programming. For each new program ENIAC was to execute, it had to be physically reconfigured by human operators who turned dials, connected and disconnected electric plugs, and so on. In other words, a program for ENIAC was input through **hardware** settings, and not (as is the case today) by storing the program as instructions in the computer's electronic memory. Since the hardware settings that represented ENIAC's programming could take hours or even days to complete, ENIAC's creators decided that a better method of program input was needed.

Even before ENIAC's completion, its successor was being planned. **EDVAC (Electronic Discrete Variable Automatic Computer)** was designed with a much more efficient and cost effective memory system than its predecessor ENIAC. This meant that, as compared to ENIAC, the newer EDVAC would have much more main memory available. Several of the people designing EDVAC, including Hungarian-American mathematician **John von Neumann**, proposed that the additional memory available to EDVAC be used to implement the stored-program principle (i.e., the storage of both data and instructions in the same area of the computer's main memory). The storage of data and instructions in main memory meant that EDVAC could perform computations at electronic speeds without the need for the "hard-wiring" (i.e., the setting of switches, dials, etc.) used by ENIAC. Von Neumann first laid out his vision for the structure of EDVAC, including the stored-program principle, in a 1945 paper entitled "The First Draft of a Report on the EDVAC." This report was widely circulated and had an almost immediate, worldwide impact on **computer architecture** (i.e., structure). The vast majority of computers in use today incorporate the stored-program principle.

Computers laid out along the lines of von Neumann's 1945 report are said to possess **von Neumann architecture** and are called *von Neumann machines*. The stored-program principle is a cornerstone of von Neumann computers. A von Neumann computer uses a *control unit* to distinguish between data and instructions in main memory (i.e., RAM). The **control** unit directs the retrieval of instructions from RAM at the appropriate times and in the proper sequence for processing by the arithmetic logic unit (**ALU**). In modern electronic computers the control unit and ALU have been combined into the **microprocessor**, or CPU.

***See also*** Bell Laboratories relay computers; EDVAC (Electronic Discrete Variable Automatic Computer); ENIAC (Electronic Numerical Integrator and Computer); Memory; Random-access memory (RAM); von Neumann architecture

## STRACHEY, CHRISTOPHER (1916-1975)

*American computer scientist*

Christopher Strachey co-founded the field of denotational semantics that provided a strong mathematical foundation for computer **programming** languages. *Denotational semantics* is a technique for giving precise meaning to a programming language. While the *syntax* (grammar) of a programming language is formally specified in various texts and user guides, the more important part of defining its *semantics* (the relationship between words or symbols and their intended meanings) is normally left to natural language, making it open to interpretation when used in programming languages. To create a better understanding, the programming language is defined by a *valuation function* that maps programs into mathematical objects considered as their *denotation* (i.e., meaning).

Strachey was the first professor of computation at Oxford University in Oxford, England. During his tenure, Christopher Strachey invented the term "currying," meaning to turn an "uncurried" **function** into a "curried" function. (A curried function is defined as a function that returns a function as a result, thus an uncurried function does not return a function as a result.) Strachey used the term in his lecture notes on programming languages in the 1960s. During this time, Strachey also became the first director of the Programming Research Group (PRG) (founded in 1965), under the direction of the Oxford's Computing Laboratory (set up in 1957).

While in charge of the PRG, Strachey was very vocal when he stated:

> It has long been my personal view that the separation of practical and theoretical work is artificial and injurious. Much of the practical work done in computing, both in software and in **hardware design**, is unsound and clumsy because the people who do it have not any clear understanding of the fundamental design principles of their work. Most of the abstract mathematical

and theoretical work is sterile because it has no point of contact with real computing. One of the central aims of the Programming Research Group as a teaching and research group has been to set up an atmosphere in which this separation cannot happen.

This quotation accurately sums up Strachey's basic philosophy, and the continuing philosophy of the Computing Laboratory.

The PRG obtained its early reputation under Strachey's direction for its (1) pioneering research on programming languages by concentrating on their logical foundations (including Scott-Strachey denotational semantics, where computer scientist Dana Scott was the other co-founder of denotational semantics), (2) development of the Communicating Sequential Processes (CSP) approach to concurrent processes, and (3) Z specification language and algebraic theories of programming. Paralleling Strachey's philosophy of intellectual strictness, the PRG research projects relied on a strong interaction of mathematical theories with their experimental processes, and crossed many other disciplines such as the social sciences. Still today the PRG is focused toward the free interchange among its members and with many other disciplines working on different theories or on different applications. The intermingling of practical application and comprehensive theory of problems and concepts continue to justify the earlier wisdom of Christopher Strachey.

Some of Strachey's important publications are *A Theory of Programming Language Semantics* (with R.E. Milne, in 1976), *Toward a Mathematical Semantics for Computer Languages* (with Dana Scott, in 1971), *Fundamental Concepts for Programming Languages* (in 1967), *Towards a Formal Semantics* (in 1966), and *Time Sharing in Large, Fast Computers* (in 1959). The Strachey Memorial Lecture at Oxford University is named after Christopher Strachey.

***See also*** Programming; Syntax definition

## STREAM

The term stream has two meanings in the context of computing and computer science, both of which refer to the flow of **data**.

First, in **programming**, stream refers to an order flow of programming entry and execution. It is an ordered set of records or elements in which information is added to the end of sequence of data and execution of data occurs at the beginning. Streams can be used to produce an ordered **access** to data.

In the programming language known as **C**, data can be read to a stream without knowledge concerning the destination of the information. A **library** routine that is part of the program acts to receive the information and then to route the information onward.

The second meaning of stream relates to electronic communication. Here, stream refers to any flow of data from a source, such as the sender, through an established electronic connection to a single destination. As its name implies, a stream of data is usually sent in a continuous and connected way. This contrasts to the transfer of data via so-called packets, where portions of the data can be addressed and routed to their destination separate from other portions.

*See also* Dataflow; Library; Packet switching

# STRETCH

STRETCH was the **code** name for the **International Business Machines** (**IBM**) Corporation's first line of **supercomputers**, the IBM Stretch 7030; where the first unit was completed in 1961. A *supercomputer* is a large, very fast, and expensive computer used for quite complex calculations. Unlike conventional computers, supercomputers usually contain several **central processing unit**s (**CPU**s).

The story of the STRETCH supercomputer started in 1954 when IBM began a project called "Datatron" with the intention of growing into a leader of high-performance computers. Remington-Rand, which at the time was a dominant computer manufacturer and IBM's main competitor, won a contract (over IBM) to build the Livermore Automatic Research Computer (**LARC**) by promising a fast delivery time. IBM's bid was based on a renegotiation clause for its proposed machine that would be four to five times faster than requested and cost $3.5 million rather than the requested $2.5 million. When IBM lost the bid on its high-performance decimal (base-10) computer system the company decided to begin a redesign of the project, and the STRETCH project was begun in 1955. In the following year, IBM aggressively bid a binary (base-2) computer at the Los Alamos Scientific Laboratories (LASL) in New Mexico that was described to possess a "speed at least 100 times greater than that of existing machines." In 1956 IBM won the contract (with delivery beginning in 1960) for what would become the IBM Stretch 7030.

Heading the STRETCH project was Stephen Dunwell, who oversaw the assembly of the first machine at IBM's Poughkeepsie Laboratory, and its delivery in April 1961 to LASL. In use for the next ten years, the eight IBM Stretch 7030 supercomputers were IBM's initial attempt at building computers with transistors designed to "stretch" the speed of its current vacuum tube technology. The machine was very sophisticated for its time, providing simultaneous execution of business instructions with **floating-point arithmetic**. IBM lost an estimated 40 million dollars in developing the STRETCH, but acquired extensive knowledge from its development that led to large profits with its subsequent computers.

The IBM Stretch 7030 possessed an advanced machine **design** for its time that included many forward-looking computer technologies (even by today's standards) such as: core **memory**, **transistor** circuit design, and circuit packaging. The supercomputer also introduced many innovative computer architectural features such as: predecoding, memory operand prefetch, out-of-order execution, speculative execution (based upon **branch prediction**), branch misprediction recovery, memory interleaving, multiprogramming, **pipelining**, and (precise) **interrupts**. The organization structure used by the STRETCH for preprocessing the instruction **stream** to handle

branches and memory loads was a precursor of later high-end IBM **mainframe** computers.

The IBM Stretch 7030 contained 169,100 transistors and 96,000 64-bit words of core (main) memory. Instructions that flowed through the supercomputer were routed through two processing elements: (1) an "indexing and instruction" unit that fetched, predecoded, and partially executed the instruction stream and (2) an "arithmetic" unit that executed all mathematical instructions and those not executed by the indexing and instruction unit. The processing units (without its memory banks) filled a volume of about 9,000 cubic feet, about the size of a small three-bedroom house.

The first manufactured IBM Stretch 7030 turned out to be functionally slower than what was designed, and it was delivered a year later than planned. However, the first STRETCH (along with the other seven computers) provided IBM with great technological advances in transistor design and computer organization principles (such as multiprogramming, memory protection, generalized interrupts, and the 8-bit **byte**). Even though it did not achieve its full commercial potential the IBM Stretch 7030 was still the fastest computer in the world from 1961 to 1964.

*See also* Floating-point arithmetic; IBM (International Business Machines); Supercomputer

# STRING

A string is a unique sequence of **byte**s representing specific characters. Strings are often referred to as text strings or character strings.

Depending upon the particular program or **operation** in which the string is utilized, the relationship (mapping) between bytes and characters (e.g., eight-**bit** characters) is predetermined by the character set (e.g., **ASCII**) in use. Accordingly, strings are interpreted in with regard to the environment in which they are used.

The most common text strings encountered in modern computer usage result from the use of the ASCII character set or some other character set (e.g., **Unicode**). In contrast to numerical **data** upon which mathematical operations may be performed, text strings that result from character mapping are simply series of linked characters that can be manipulated as a group. Much as words are formed from combinations of letters, strings are unique combinations of characters that can be interpreted or manipulated as a group. (akin to words or sentences).

Just as the length of a word or sentence is determined by the number of letters or words in it, the length of a string is determined by the number of characters in it. Moreover, these linked characters are different from numerical data and are treated differently by most **programming** languages.

The following text enclosed in quotes, "System" contains six characters. Some programs may add an additional blank space as a leader or end (string terminus) to the string and thus increase the string length in the example used to seven characters. The string "operational" contains 11 regular characters.

To concatenate strings is to join two or more text strings into one string. A concatenation of the examples used above, the strings "system" and "operational" would result in a new string, "system operational" that contains 18-19 characters depending on leading or trailing spaces included.

One-way hash functions are **algorithms** that may be used to turn string messages into numerical data upon which algebraic operations may be performed. Such transformations—from string to numerical data— are often utilized by security or encryption programs. In addition, whenever data intended to be used numerically, is entered as a string (e.g. "4" representing the number four) such a displayed character must be transformed into numerical data before it can be used in mathematical operations.

Programs often work on the principal of string matching. Although it may not be possible to perform the operation IF A>"dog" THEN... it is certainly possible to look for strings that match (e.g., the command IF A="dog" THEN...). In such a search operation, a character set matching the character set defined with the quote marks (not including the quote marks) is sufficient to match and to initiate the THEN command.

*See also* Character input and output; Character sets; Data structure; Reserved words; String-matching; String variable

# STRING-MATCHING

One of the important basic tasks in computing is the finding of all occurrences of a particular alphanumeric **string** in a document, or the finding of all documents that have one or more occurrences of a given alphanumeric string. One common example where such a task needs to be carried out is on the **World Wide Web**, where search engine software needs to find all occurrences of a given query term or keyword, and return the results based on some rules of priority and relevance. It is also common for there to be find-and-replace macros or features in text-editing programs, allowing for all occurrences of a certain string to be replaced with another string. For example, in writing many form letters having the same nature, it is possible to just change the salutation: Dear Ms. Smith, Dear Mr. Jones, Dear Mrs. Fowler, Dear Dr. Koopman, etc., while keeping the rest of the letter the same. String-matching **algorithms** are also applied in genetic engineering to find matching patterns in DNA sequences.

The applications of string-matching are thus diverse, but they all have a common point—the efficiency of algorithms used is extremely important. This is especially true in cases like web searches—search engines receive thousands of search requests each minute, and even with the software running on very high-end computing equipment, it does not pay to delay the results. The algorithm must return results very quickly to free up the **hardware** to service other queries. It is also possible that users of search engines will be disappointed and turn away, if their queries are not answered very quickly. Thus, there is in such cases a very great need for speed, so the algorithms used must be designed with this in mind.

The naive string-matching algorithm simply uses a brute-force comparison by sliding the test string along the string to be compared with, and making a comparison at each and every possible point. This is a meaningful but very inefficient way of determining a match. A more efficient method was created by **Richard Karp** and Michael O. Rabin; their algorithm is almost as bad as the naive algorithm in the worst case, but has much better best-case and average performance. Other algorithms have also been proposed; the best deterministic one known and accepted widely at this time is the Boyer-Moore algorithm of Robert S. Boyer and J. Strother Moore.

In many cases, it is necessary to have fast on-line approximate string matching. This is the problem of **searching** a pattern in a text allowing errors in the pattern or in the text. Algorithms to do this are commonly based on a very fast string-matching kernel which is able to search short patterns using a nondeterministic finite automaton. A number of techniques and **heuristics** are possible to extend this kernel for longer patterns. However, the techniques can be integrated in many ways and there is no single optimal solution.

In many applications, it is necessary to determine the similarity—or lack thereof—of two strings. Similarity is in a broad sense vague and intuitive, but a practical definition of the abstraction that is widely used is the so-called edit distance—the minimum number of insertions, deletions, and substitutions required to transform one string into the other. A number of stochastic models have been proposed to determine the string edit distance.

A more important general case of the problem of string matching is that of **pattern matching**. This is a combinatorial problem that addresses issues of searching and matching strings and more complicated patterns such as trees, regular expressions, **graphs**, point sets, and arrays. The goal is to derive non-trivial combinatorial properties for such structures and then to exploit these properties in order to achieve improved performance for the corresponding computational problem of matching patterns.

The area of pattern matching has attracted a great deal of intensive research; the subject itself has thus changed from a sparse set of isolated results into a full-fledged area of algorithmics with some important practical applications. The subject is expected to grow even further due to the increasing demand for speed and efficiency that come from molecular biology and genetic engineering, but also from areas such as **information retrieval**, pattern recognition, biometric **authentication** (such as speech and speaker recognition, feature recognition, and the like), program compilation, **data compression**, program analysis, and system security.

*See also* Algorithms; World Wide Web

# STRING VARIABLE

A string variable is a set of alphabetical or alphanumeric characters used to represent a **value**. Examples of **string** variable are firstname, first_name, 1_name, 1stname, 1st_name. The string **variable** is invaluable to computer **programming**. For example, let's say that Joe Smith had to write a program that printed his students' last name, first name and social security number for his math class. Depending on the computer program he was using, his string variables might be first_name, last_name and ss_number. After writing his program, he would enter all of the students' names and social security number. The program would read the **data** that he entered and then print out the students' names and social security numbers in the ordered specified.

> Jones, Matt, 123-456-7895
>
> Anderson, Marian, 456-123-7895
>
> Simon, Paul, 896-456-4568
>
> Hines, Duncan, 897-546-1235
>
> Simpson, Bart, 456-357-9861

Here is Joe's program.

> Open Mathclass
>
> ...
>
> Read last_name, first_name, ss_number
>
> Print last_name, first_name, ss_number
>
> ...
>
> End

Without string variables, Joe's program would look like this.

> Read Jones, Matt, 123-456-7895
>
> Print Jones, Matt, 123-456-7895
>
> Read Anderson, Marian, 456-123-7895
>
> Print Anderson, Marian, 456-123-7895
>
> Read Simon, Paul, 896-456-4568
>
> Print Simon, Paul, 896-456-4568
>
> Read Hines, Duncan, 897-546-1235
>
> Print Hines, Duncan, 897-546-1235
>
> Read Simpson, Bart, 456-357-9861
>
> Print Simpson, Bart, 456-357-9861
>
> ...
>
> End

Also, Joe would have to create the same program for each of his 7 classes. With the string variable, he only has to create one program, and he only has to create one data file for each class as opposed to 7 programs.

## STRUCT DATA TYPE

The "struct" **data** type is specific to the **C** and **C++ programming** languages. The original data **type** came from C and then was subsumed into C++. While the C++ version retains the original semantics and **syntax** of the original, it has been extended to make C++ structs bona-fide objects in their own right.

Structures contain a set of contiguously allocated member variables that can be of any type, including other structures. In C++ structures may have member functions, too. C++ structures are identical to C++ classes except that the **access** rights to a structure's functions and data members are public rather than private unless the programmer says otherwise. The reason for this is that the conceptual difference is that a structure is a collection of related data elements whereas a **class** is a tightly bound cohesive unit or **object**.

The struct keyword is short for "structure" and is followed by one or more **variable declarations** within a set of braces (the "{" and "}" characters respectively). A typical C structure declaration is shown in the **code** fragment below:

```
struct roadVehicle {
  int engineSize;
  int wheelCount;
  int seatCount;
};
```

This fragment declares a structure that might represent a road vehicle. Once it has been declared, it can then be used as a type blueprint from which the programmer can create roadVehicle objects. For example the code below declares two unique and separate variables:

```
struct roadVehicle car;
struct roadVehicle truck;
```

The syntax is a little cumbersome, so C has the "typedef" keyword that associates a simple **identifier** with a complex declaration. So if the structure had been declared as

```
typedef struct {
  int engineSize;
  int wheelCount;
  int seatCount;
} roadVehicle;
```

it would be possible to write

```
roadVehicle car;
roadVehicle truck;
```

In C++ the typedef keyword is not needed here although it is supported for backwards compatibility with C; in other words it would have been possible to have the struct declared like this

```
struct roadVehicle {
  int engineSize;
  int wheelCount;
  int seatCount;
};
```

and then to write

```
roadVehicle car;
roadVehicle truck;
```

The method used to access a structure's members in both C and C++ depends on whether the structure is being accessed by **value** (as an object), or via a pointer. In C++ it is also possible to access a structure's members by reference, in which cases the syntax is the same as for access by value.

For example:

```
roadVehicle car;
roadVehicle truck;
roadVehicle van;
roadVehicle* carPtr = &car;
```

roadVehicle& vanRef = van; // C++ only

To assign a value to the number of wheels of each vehicle the code could look like this:

vanRef.wheelCount = 3; // must have hit a drain

carPtr→engineSize = 400;

truck.seatCount = 2;

The only type of variable a structure cannot contain is its own type, so the following declaration is illegal:

```
struct roadVehicle {
roadVehicle vehicle;
int engineSize;
int wheelCount;
int seatCount;
};
```

However, it can contain a "pointer" to its own type like this:

```
struct roadVehicle {
roadVehicle* next;
int engineSize;
int wheelCount;
int seatCount;
};
```

Why this is useful is not perhaps immediately apparent, but on closer examination it can be seen that "next" can point to another roadVehicle, which can point to another roadVehicle,... and so on. Thus the structure is the basic element of linked lists in C.

A special kind of structure is a "union." A union is a set of overlaid structures that all begin at the same address. A union is really only of any use as "containers" of structures that can have more than one "view" of them. For example, a programmer may wish to store a set of integers or characters in a structure of a single type:

```
typedef struct {
int a;
int b;
} integers;

typedef struct {
char a;
char b;
} characters;

typedef union {
integers i;
characters c;
} values;
```

What this union does is give two "views" of integer values. If the programmer accesses an object of type "values" via an "integer" structure, he will get integer values out; if he access it via a "character" structure, he will get char values out.

Structures provide an extremely powerful way of building very complex data types in C and it is almost impossible to create a program of any real utility without them. Their use in C++ has been somewhat attenuated by the **class declaration**, but they still have their place where a full class would be considered overkill.

## STRUCTURED PROGRAMMING

Computers always execute programs in a fixed, sequential order only, with no intelligent choice or discretion. Most **algorithms**, however, require the application of certain procedures or execution of certain blocks of **code** repeatedly—for instance, the **sorting** of an **array** usually involves recursive application of the sort procedure a number of times. When an algorithm which asks for such repetition is translated into a program that is executed in sequential order, the tendency of computers to execute in strict sequential order must be altered on purpose—this is done by specifying "branches" or other instructions.

Branches are of two kinds, conditional or unconditional. A conditional branch has the form, "Check for this condition to be true; if it is, then do the following." A conditional branch thus causes execution to jump to a specific block of code if a certain condition is fulfilled. In commonly used **programming** languages, such branches are specified by the use of *if* and *while* statements in the program. The program evaluates a controlling **expression**, and carries out a certain execution *if* it is true, or *while* it is true, as the case may be. After the branch has been completed, the control of the program execution is returned either to the point where it started, or else to another predetermined point in the program.

Unconditional branches transfer execution to another point in the code, without providing a means by which it can be returned to the starting point. Most programming languages have a "goto" statement that fulfills this purpose. The **syntax** of this statement usually is of the form:

goto *Label*

The *Label* is one that is given to a labeled statement, and the effect of the above is to unilaterally transfer control to that statement. Since no conditions are evaluated before such transfer, this is an unconditional branch. Control does not return to the point of origin unless some special provision is made; execution simply continues with the statements following the labeled statement to which control has been transferred.

Older programming languages such as **FORTRAN** and **COBOL** were used in the 1950s and later to produce code that used unconditional branching liberally. Such programs were found to be very difficult to read, debug, and maintain, and such use of unconditional branching earned a very bad name, and is now referred to as "spaghetti code." Beginning computer programming classes no longer teach use of goto statements as an essential feature, and programming language theory classes actively discourage its use, though the statement often survives in some form even in modern languages such as **Java**.

Along with the problems of spaghetti code, programming languages borrowed too many of each others' features and became increasingly involved and hard to produce workable code in. In order to solve these problems, **Edsger W. Dijkstra**, **Tony Hoare**, and other leading computer scientists of the late 1960s embarked on an effort to bring discipline to programming, by means of a technique they called structured programming. This technique rested on three important principles that they showed to be true:

- Only three control structures—sequence, selection, and repetition, are necessary for writing of programs.
- Unconditional branching is not necessary for any program.
- Programs written using just the three essential structures are easier to read, write, debug, and maintain compared to those that also use unconditional branching.

Structured programming therefore is the practice of creating programs using only the three essential structures, while eschewing the use of unconditional branches completely. A computer program that has been produced in accordance with the principles of structured programming is a structured program—such a program has a simpler **design**, is less complex, is more readable, and is easier to maintain. The structured programming paradigm also enforces a discipline on programming in general, and thus makes it easier for programmers to cooperate and to understand one another's code.

*See also* Programming; Sorting

## STUB

A stub is a skeleton program or routine used early in the software development process to substitute for a fully functional program that has not been developed yet. Stub programs are temporary sections of **programming code** that assist in testing interfaces to and from the complete program.

Minimal programming code is written in a stub. A stub must contain enough code to be compiled and linked with the other related programs as well as test **data** values being passed to and from other programs. To do this the stub must include at least the **declarations** of variables and functions. In addition programmers sometimes include simple functionality or text **debugging** messages that allow them to view the sequence of logic being executed by the stub.

As the development process proceeds, stub functions are replaced one at a time with the real functions. This allows the programmer to isolate errors, improving the quality of development.

## SUBROUTINE

A subroutine, which can also be commonly called a routine, is a section of a computer program that performs a particular task. Subroutines are sets of computer instructions that exist and run within a program.

Computer programs can be written as a single document. However, this format can be cumbersome when checking for **programming** defects. Accordingly, many programs are now written in more easily managed sections. Each of these sections, which can also be termed a module (or modulus), is made up of one or more subroutines/routines. The concerted performance of the various tasks specified by the subroutines enables the program to function.

Subroutines can be used repeatedly during the execution of a program. This makes a program shorter and easier to write, as redundant sections are eliminated. A subroutine can be invoked during the running of a program and, when finished, that subroutine can branch back to the next instruction following the one that branched to it.

Subroutines are often parts of computational programs. Following a prompted format, the user inputs **data** (for example, a number specifying a temperature in degrees Celsius) the program then immediately accesses a conversion subroutine to add 273.15 to the number to convert the number to the Kelvin scale) the use of the input and conversion subroutine saves many programming lines that would otherwise be dedicated to performing this repetitious task for separate data entry items. Branching to subroutines also permits programs to directly **access** needed programming steps without having to run through unneeded **code**.

A subroutine may also be useful in more than one program and a subroutine code may be capable of being shared by multiple programs. Subroutines may also be packaged together with an interface to allow their use for a specific function such as those exemplified by Library routines.

*See also* Library; Programming

## SUPERCOMPUTERS

Supercomputing is a concept that has evolved rapidly. Computers developed under that description have existed only since the early 1970s. For most of the time since, supercomputers have been widely imagined to be expensive, arcane devices, employed in only the most esoteric functions of theoretical science and government research.

Since the mid-'90s, however, supercomputers have become more efficient, less expensive, and available for applications in all walks of life. Supercomputers are currently relied upon for computer-generated animation, for advanced **design** of automobiles and other complicated machinery, and in the more complex areas of medicine such as microbiology. These are in addition to the established roles of supercomputing in creating weather models, making population-growth projections and in digitally simulating nuclear detonations.

So what is a supercomputer? No universally accepted definition exists, other than that of a vague class of exceptionally fast computers. *Parallel processing*, that is, the practice of directing multiple processors toward the completion of a common task, is usually identified closely with supercomputing. It is true that most supercomputers make use of **parallel processing**, or its cousin, *vector processing*. But since supercomputing predates parallel processing, and since it is likely that coming generations of supercomputers might evolve beyond it, a working definition of supercomputing must embrace a wider scope. Supercomputers, then, are simply whichever computers are the most powerful of a given generation.

Although a widening field of manufacturers are engaged in supercomputer production—among these are **IBM**, Fujitsu Ltd., NEC Corporation, **Intel**, Hitachi Ltd., and Thinking Machines Corporation—a single name is most often identified with both the birth of supercomputing and with the state of the art. **Seymour Cray** (1925-96), backed by the handful of companies he founded, has consistently developed and delivered some of the most advanced supercomputing concepts and practices in the world. From the installation of the first Cray-1 at Los Alamos National Laboratory in 1976, to the creation of the Cray-4 (the first supercomputer which was smaller than a human brain), Cray endeavored always to advance the science of supercomputing with only the most cursory attention paid to commercial success.

The key to Cray's designs have always been efficiency. Cray has been adept at tapping the most advanced technology of the era in the name of better and faster computers. One of his earliest systems, the CDC1604 created for **Control Data Corporation** in the late 1950s, was the first transistorized scientific computer—developed at a time when all IBM computers were still utilizing punch-card systems. Later, in 1972, Cray Research was the first to utilize the **integrated circuit** in computer design. Cray systems tend to be designed with physical efficiency in mind as well. The "horseshoe" shape of several of the Cray systems was intended to bring all components closer together, and allowed for all elements of wiring to be no longer than four feet in length. Cray has been innovative in peripheral systems as well, such as cooling. Early Cray designs incorporated their own Freon reservoirs, which might have been only partially successful when one considers that employees of Cray Research in Minnesota were known to run a supercomputer or two simply to heat the office. Later designs, such as the Cray-4, utilized as a coolant the same chemical used in medical applications as artificial blood. Finally, Cray has even innovated the technology of chip manufacturing. Since the early '90s, Cray has eschewed the use of silicon in favor of gallium arsenide (GaAs). While gallium arsenide has proven to be a more efficient platform for circuitry, its utility is so complicated that Cray Research was forced to build their own gallium arsenide foundry.

Historically, the world's most powerful computers were gauged by their ability to complete instruction sets—measured in MIPS (millions of instructions per second). As software became more and more distinct from the **hardware**, however, it became clear that the MIPS measurement could too easily be skewed by vagaries in the software **code**. A new benchmark, based upon pure computing power, had to be formed.

The current standard is the FLOP, or floating-point **operation**. Today's supercomputers are classified by their capabilities in floating-point operations per second in the millions (megaflop), billions (gigaflop) and most recently, trillions (teraflop). The teraflop barrier was first broken in the mid-'90s, although there is some contention as to which super-

computer was the first to sustain operations in the teraflop range. It's interesting to note that a truly unconventional design may hold pride of place as the world's largest supercomputer, operating in the seven-teraflop range. SETI (Search for Extraterrestrial Intelligence), upon having their funding cut by the U.S. Congress in the early '90s, issued a worldwide appeal for computer users to donate their systems' downtime for the analysis of billions of intercepted stellar radio waves. More than one million processors in 223 countries make up the components of this global "supercomputer."

Like all computer manufacturers, the world's supercomputer providers are engaged in an undeclared yet ongoing competition for faster and better machines. Most have 100 teraflop systems on their drawing boards that could be ready for distribution in a decade or less. And before he died in an automobile accident in 1996, Seymour Cray reported a government initiative to conquer the petaflop ($10^{15}$ FLOPS) realm. As unimaginable as that number might be, the history of supercomputing—with all its innovations and its penchant for defying the odds—instructs us to discount no such possibilities.

## SUPERCONDUCTOR TECHNOLOGY

A superconductor is a material that loses all resistance (called "zero resistance") to the flow of direct electrical current and nearly all resistance to the flow of alternating current when three conditions are met: (1) the material is cooled below a characteristic temperature, known as its critical temperature; (2) a current passing through a given cross-section of the material must be at, or below, its (characteristic) critical current density; and (3) the magnetic field to which the material is exposed must be below its (characteristic) critical magnetic field. Superconductivity of a material is activated only when those three critical conditions are met, which vary with the material used. Some examples of materials that are capable of exhibiting superconductivity are mercury, zinc, magnesium, lead, aluminum, iridium, tin, vanadium, and many alloys.

The research and development of superconductors (sometimes called cryogenic conductors) is called superconductor technology. Superconducting materials include both high temperature superconductor (HTS) materials, which exhibit superconductivity at critical temperatures above 23 Kelvin (denoted 23K), and low-temperature (or classical) superconductor (LTS) materials, which exhibit superconductivity at critical temperatures equal to or below 23K materials. Both classes of materials need to be cooled to cryogenic (very low) temperatures in order to exhibit the property of superconductivity.

The discovery of superconductivity was made in 1911 by Dutch physicist Heike Kamerlingh Onnes, called "the gentleman of absolute zero," who found that the resistance of mercury suddenly dropped to zero at a temperature of 4.2K (-268.8°C/-451.8°F). The first successful theory pertaining to superconductivity was not realized until 1957, when American physicists **John Bardeen**, Leon Cooper, and John Schrieffer announced the BCS theory of classical superconductors. The three were awarded the 1972 Nobel Prize in physics for their theory that describes superconductivity as a quantum-mechanical phenomenon in which at very low temperatures electrons in an electric current move in pairs. This pairing allows them to move through a crystal lattice without their motion being interrupted by lattice collisions, resulting in zero electrical resistance. After the BCS theory there were a series of announcements about other LTS materials that became superconducting near absolute zero (0K, equaling -273°C/-459°F).

In 1962 British physicist Brian Josephson investigated the quantum nature of superconductivity, proposing the existence of oscillations in the electrical current flowing through two superconductors separated by a thin insulating layer in a magnetic or electric field. This *Josephson effect* was developed into a fast switching technology that uses superconductors where circuits are immersed in liquid helium to obtain near absolute zero temperatures. This "ultra-fast" switching takes place in a few picoseconds (one picosecond equals one-trillionth of a second). Although Josephson junctions have not materialized for computer circuits, they have been used for selected medical instruments.

Up until 1986, the critical temperatures for all known superconductors did not exceed 23K (-250°C/-418°F). These LTS materials only worked with refrigeration to a few degrees above absolute zero. These temperatures were achieved with liquid helium, an expensive, inefficient coolant that is costly to maintain. As a result, very low temperature operations place a severe constraint on the efficiency of a superconducting device. Thus, before the discovery and development of HTS materials, the use of superconductivity had not been practical for widespread commercial applications.

A breakthrough occurred in 1986 when scientists K. A. Müller and J. G. Bednorz, at **International Business Machines** Corporation's (IBM's) Zurich research laboratory, announced the discovery of a ceramic oxide compound that was shown to be superconductive at 30K (-243°C/-406°F). This created a new class of superconductors called high temperature superconducting (HTS) materials that contain copper and oxygen atoms, which form planes or chains of atoms in the crystal. Their superconducting properties are anisotropic; that is, dependent on the direction of current flow and of magnetic field with respect to the planes and chains of atoms. The work of Müller and Bednorz, which earned them the 1987 Nobel Prize in Physics, started the discoveries of related materials such as copper oxides, barium, lanthanum, and yttrium that have higher critical temperatures up to 125K (-148°C/-234°F). In 1987 American physicist Paul Chu, at the University of Houston, raised the critical temperature for a superconductor to 94K (-179°C/-290°F). This achievement, for the first time, showed that new superconductors could lead to lucrative new superconductor technologies, including a dramatic impact on the future of computing. Further discoveries at other universities and research laboratories began to radically alter the impracticability of using superconducting materials for commercial uses. Ceramic metal-oxide compounds containing rare earth elements were found to be superconductive at temperatures high enough to permit using liquid nitrogen as a coolant.

Because liquid nitrogen, at 77 K (-196°C/-321°F), cools 20 times more effectively than liquid helium and is 10 times less expensive, a host of potential applications began to hold the promise of economic profitability.

The properties of these new HTS materials are sensitive, however, to the amount of oxygen in them. Problems of brittleness, instabilities in some chemical environments, and a tendency for impurities to segregate at surfaces of the crystals have yet to be overcome. Theoretically, superconducting wires provide significant advantages over conventional copper wires because they conduct electricity with little or no resistance and associated energy loss and can transmit much larger amounts of electricity than conventional wires of the same size. Thin films of normal metals and superconductors that are brought into contact can form superconductive electronic devices, which can replace transistors in some applications.

The discovery of better superconducting compounds is a significant step toward a far wider range of applications, including faster computers with larger storage capacities, magnetic energy-storage systems, computer parts, and very sensitive devices for measuring magnetic fields, voltages, or currents. The main advantages of devices made from superconductors are low power dissipation, high-speed **operation**, and high sensitivity.

# SUTHERLAND, IVAN (1938-   )
*American computer scientist*

Ivan Sutherland is a pioneer in the field of computer **graphics**. His 1960 "Sketchpad" system contributed to the development of computer graphics, computer **simulation**, and video games as we know them today.

Ivan Edward Sutherland was born in Hastings, Nebraska, on May 16, 1938. His first experience with computing was in high school, where as a young student he build various relay-driven machines. In the early 1950s, computers were exciting and exotic devices, and many bright students set their sights on that field.

Sutherland received his B.S. from Carnegie-Mellon University in 1959, his M.S. from the California Institute of Technology in 1960, and his Ph.D. in electrical engineering from the Massachusetts Institute of Technology (M.I.T.) in 1963. Throughout college Sutherland was always interested in logic and computing; he held a summer job with **International Business Machines (IBM)** after he got his bachelor's degree, and he switched from Cal Tech to M.I.T. for his doctoral studies because of the latter's superior computer department. His doctoral thesis committee comprised some of the biggest names in computing at the time, including **Claude Shannon**, **Marvin Minsky**, and Steven Coons. At M.I.T., Sutherland worked at the Lincoln Laboratory. There he had the use of a large, modern computer called the TX–2, which played a significant role in the research for his doctoral dissertation, entitled "Sketchpad."

"Sketchpad" was arguably Sutherland's greatest work and the basis for much of what he subsequently accomplished.

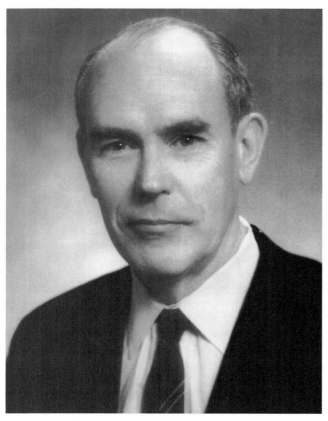

**Ivan Sutherland**

The principle behind "Sketchpad" is that of a pencil moving on paper, but instead it uses a light-sensitive pen moving on the surface of a computer screen. By measuring the vertical and horizontal movements of the pen by means of a grid system, the computer could recreate the lines on the computer screen. Once on the screen, lines could be manipulated (lengthened, shortened, moved to any angle) and connected to represent solid objects, which could then be rotated to display them at any angle, exactly as if they were true three-dimensional artifacts. (Previously existing graphics systems were strictly two-dimensional.) Sutherland documented his dissertation research with a film called *Sketchpad: A Man-Machine Graphical Communication System*, and the film became very well known in the computer research community of the time. The concept of "Sketchpad" was revolutionary, and its direct repercussions extend down to this day.

From M.I.T., Sutherland went into the army, due to a Reserve Officers Training Corps commitment left over from Carnegie-Mellon. After brief assignments with the National Security Agency and a radar and infrared tracking project called Project Michigan, he was made director of the **Information Processing** Techniques Office (IPTO) of the Defense Advanced Research Projects Agency (DARPA), where he stayed for two years. This was a heady assignment for the 26-year-old lieutenant, and it had a profound influence

on his later career; virtually every business partner he subsequently had was someone he had met at DARPA.

From DARPA he went to Harvard as an associate professor of engineering and applied physics. He remained at Harvard for almost three years, during which time he developed computer graphics tools that became invaluable to his later work on computer simulation. In 1967, he was recruited by David Evans, a contractor he had worked with at DARPA, to join the computer science program at the University of Utah. Evans, who had recently moved to Utah from Berkeley, also had in mind developing a company that would exploit some of the exciting developments in computer graphics.

At the University of Utah, Sutherland worked with a group of brilliant graduate students, and the computer department became an experimental center for computer graphics. Sutherland and his students refined the animation of their simulated figures; they developed "smooth curves" and lighting and highlight effects that began to replace the original "wireframe" models. One of Sutherland's students, Nolan Bushnell, eventually went on to develop the original video arcade and home video game Pong.

In 1968, Evans and Sutherland formed the firm Evans & Sutherland in Salt Lake City. Computers at that time were being used for well-understood routine tasks, such as billing, filing, and information processing. Evans and Sutherland, however, recognized that computers had exciting possibilities as **design** and training tools, a potential that was not being exploited anywhere. As Evans noted in an Evans & Sutherland newsletter, computers are essentially simulators that can "replace real objects on occasions when a simulation can be built more cheaply than the physical model can be."

Evans & Sutherland's first products were **computer-aided design** tools, which they sold in small quantities. The company did not begin making a profit until its fifth year of **operation**, but by the mid–1970s it was beginning to develop a broad range of products for several market niches, principally in flight training and computer-aided design. Evans & Sutherland remains in business today. Although Sutherland left the company's day-to-day operation in 1974, he remains on the board of directors.

From 1976 to 1980, Sutherland headed the department of computer science at the California Institute of Technology. In 1980, he joined forces with Robert Sproull, the son of one of Sutherland's superiors at DARPA, to form Sutherland, Sproull & Associates in Pittsburgh, Pennsylvania, later moving to Palo Alto, California. Sutherland's last written work in computer graphics was a joint paper with Sproull titled, "A Characterization of Ten Hidden Surface Algorithms." Sutherland would say in a 1989 interview that this "seemed to tidy up a loose end," and he counts it as the time at which he stopped being involved with computer graphics for good.

Sutherland remains associated with Sutherland, Sproull & Associates, doing research in **computer architecture** and logic circuits. Married, with two children, he is a plain-spoken man who avoids publicity and rarely grants interviews. He has, however, been frequently honored by his peers in the computer industry. He has received many honorary degrees and has won many prestigious honors and awards, including the first Zworykin Award from the National Academy of Engineering and the first Steven Anson Coons Award.

## SWAP FILE, SWAP SPACE, PAGE SWAPPING

A swap file is a file used by an operating system, or a specific program, as part of the **virtual memory** exchange of information between the RAM chip drives and the **ROM** disk drives. Swap files occupy swap space that is located in a specialized region of the **hard drive** reserved for use by the virtual **memory** system.

The movement of swap files is often coordinated by a scheduler or virtual memory system that mediates the transfer of files from the hard drive to RAM memory. The portion of the hard drive reserved for swap files is isolated from the remainder of the hard drive and is usually not fragmented. Because swap files are maintained in one localized region of the hard drive, their close physical proximity reduces the time required to find and **access** swap files. **Hardware** and software manufacturers recommend varying minimum and maximum values for the optimal size of the swap space allocated to swap files depending on the particular operating system in use. Usually the maximum size is determined as a function of the available RAM (e.g., a typical maximum size allocation recommendation might specify that swap files should be located in swap space no more than two or three times the size of the available RAM memory).

Although swap files differ from page files used by demand **paging** systems to transfer only a portion of a program file, the use of swap files also allows for use of programs larger than RAM memory space. Before a process can be executed, it must first load or move into RAM memory from the swap space on the hard drive via the virtual memory system. For example, **programming code** can only be executed after it is loaded into RAM memory. Virtual memory systems use swap files and swap space to rapidly interchange programming code between RAM and ROM memory. Using this system of file transfers, the entire programming code is not required to be in RAM memory in order to execute the program. The seamless exchange of swap files means that only the portion (block) of code actually needed by the system must be in RAM memory. Accordingly, the use of swap files and swap space allows the use of larger programs than could be held in RAM memory. In addition, the use of swap files and swap space enables those programs to run more quickly and efficiently.

The use of swap files essentially means that the maximum program size is dictated not by the smaller available RAM memory space, but rather by the size of the larger physical memory locate on the hard drive.

The virtual-memory systems in modern operating systems have replaced the need for earlier forms of physical file swapping and fragmentation of programs.

A page is a fixed number of bytes recognized as a related group by the operating system. In paging systems (typ-ically virtual memory systems), the area of the hard drive dedicated to storing blocks of **data** to be swapped via virtual memory interface is also termed the page file. The exchange of these types of files is termed page swapping. As with swap files, in most operating systems, there is a preset size for the page file area of the hard disk. Page files, however, are able to exist on multiple drives (separate physical disks or other types of ROM memory storage). As with the page file size, although the actual size of the pages is preset, modern operating systems usually allow the user to vary the size of the pages swapped, but typical page sizes range from a thousand bites to many megabytes.

Page swapping allows an entire block of data or programming (e.g., an application process) to reside in virtual memory, while only the part of the code being executed is in RAM physical memory. Accordingly, the use of virtual memory allows operating systems to run many programs and thus, increase the degree of multiprogramming within an operating system.

Virtual memory exchanges between ROM and RAM memory are accomplished through either a process termed demand-segmentation or through another process termed demand-paging. Demand-paging processes, more common because it is simpler in **design**, do not swap pages from disk to RAM until the program calls for the page. With page swapping, paging processes track memory usage and constantly **call** data back and forth between RAM and the hard disk. Page states (the state of availability to the **CPU**) are monitored by the virtual page table. When **applications** attempt to access invalid pages, a virtual-memory manager that initiates page swapping intercepts the page fault **message** and initiates a swap into RAM memory. If the page needed is not available, the application is usually aborted through one of several **interrupt** sequences.

***See also*** Multitasking; Physical and virtual memory; Software management; Thrashing

## SYNTAX

Syntax is simply the rules that define the structure of a **programming** language. These rules specify how the words, symbols, and punctuations are used to form a statement. Each program, thus, has its own set of syntactical rules. The format used by a program governs which words are meaningful to the computer, how they are spelled, in what combination they are to be written, and what punctuation is necessary. In human languages these rules are rather relaxed, but in computer programming languages these rules are inflexible. If the rules of syntax are not followed exactly, the computer will not understand it, and the user will get a syntax error **message**.

A syntax error is basically any error that breaks one of the strict rules of grammar imposed by any language. All errors must be "caught" and corrected before the program will run. An example of a syntax error would an error in logic. This would be something like defining a set of operations that are not permitted. To illustrate, adding together the two Boolean

　　　　　　　　　　　　　　　　　　•　　　　　　　　　　　　　

**types**. In Boolean logic, all operations produce one of two possible alternative values—either something is true or it is false. Obviously, something cannot be true and false at the same time.

Finding every syntax error in a document can be a tedious process. There are programs available, however, that are able to check for syntax problems during compilation. The **compiler** is that portion of the program that reorganizes the source **code** and turns it into the **object** code, which is what the computer understands. This would be the equivalent of translating the human language into the **machine language**. The process for tracking down syntax errors is called parsing, or syntax analysis. Once an error is found these programs are able to locate where the error is within the code and also indicates what rule has been broken—punctuation, incomplete statement, etc. Logic errors, however, are more difficult to discover and often require a skilled human programmer to detect them.

*See also* Computer language; Parser and parsing

# SYSTEM RELIABILITY

Distributed computer systems and networks have brought about big changes in the way modern society functions in its commercial, educational and research activities. Critical infrastructures such as banking and commerce, telecommunication, transportation, power distribution and medicine, are all increasingly dependent on networked systems. It is estimated that technology glitches in the U.S. cost at least $100 billion a year in lost productivity. This has led to a surge of interest in techniques for making network and software systems highly secure and reliable.

Increasing complexity in modern systems necessitates much greater reliability even to maintain the same apparent performance. For example, contemporary versions of Microsoft's **Windows** operating system have a mean time between failures (MTBF) of around 1 day. It is expected that by Moore's law, **personal computer** chip speeds will increase within ten years to over 10 GHz, in comparison with about 500 MHz at present. This means that a computer running the same software but running at the higher speed would crash about once every hour instead. However, since software also may be expected to increase in complexity over the duration, and assuming that the rate of bugs in software stays the same, it may be estimated that the operating system will crash almost every five minutes, rendering it effectively useless.

Interest in system reliability or dependability has been there for the longest time, of course, but the formulation now commonly accepted was introduced in 1985 by Jean-Laude Laprie at an IEEE Computer Society Symposium on **Fault-Tolerant Computing**. In this formulation, a reliable system is one in respect of which it is possible to make formal guarantees of performance on certain aspects of the quality of service that it delivers. The quality of service encompasses both its **correctness** (conformity with requirements, specifications, and expectations) as well as continuity of delivery.

A departure from the quality of service that is expected of a system constitutes a failure—therefore, a reliable system may be thought of as being one that does not fail. However, not all failures are to be treated equally. A benign failure is one where the consequences are insignificantly dissimilar to the benefits of normal system **operation**, while a catastrophic failure is one whose consequences are far worse than the benefit of normal system operation. Catastrophic failures are further subdivided into various kinds such as crash failures (where the system stops functioning), Byzantine failures (where the system behavior can be arbitrarily malevolent and erratic), etc.

Failures in systems are attributable to underlying causes called faults—a failure is a property of the external system behavior when it stops delivering the desired quality of service, while a fault is a property of the system state itself at the time of failure. Faults are broadly classified into two types, physical and logical. Physical faults may be further subclassified as being either due to operation or manufacture. Examples of operational faults include wearing out of machine components, and anomalies in the system environment. A well-known operational fault of recent times was the improper sealing of the O-rings around the main boosters of the Challenger space shuttle due to extreme adversity of weather, which resulted in a spectacular and tragic disaster. Instances of manufacturing faults include flawed components shipped from a factory being installed on a system instead of being rejected. Logical faults are further subclassified as either **design** faults or operational faults. Design faults incude bugs in chip design or software, and errors in tolerances or margins for physical components. The best-known design fault in recent times was the FDIV **bug** in the original Pentium chip, which caused incorrect results on division by some operands because of incorrect values in a lookup table; the chip's maker **Intel** took a $450 million writeoff to deal with the problem. Operational faults include intrusions by unauthorized users, use of the system for purposes other than the one it was designed for, and **operator** error.

It is possible for a fault to remain in a system without causing an overt failure. Such a fault is called a latent error, and much interest in system reliability is in detecting and correcting latent errors before they cause catastrophic failures. Even if a single fault is not itself significant, it is possible that it will leave a system much more vulnerable to failure should further faults occur.

Once an error is detected, error recovery is attempted—this consists of replacing the erroneous state with a valid state. The valid state may be generated by repairing the erroneous state, or by copying over some previously archived state that is known to be acceptable. The first method is called forward error recovery, while the second is called backward error recovery.

Fault-tolerant systems attempt to maintain system performance even in spite of the occurrence of faults. The classical means of doing this is by modular **redundancy**, with multiple independent components performing the same task, and the result being taken on the basis of majority voting, thus allowing a minority to fail safely. Although most complexity in modern system arises from software, traditional fault tolerance focuses for the most part on hardware fault tolerance, which severely limits the application of the concept.

The current trend in system design for reliability and fault tolerance is to use commercial, off-the-shelf components to reduce cost. Repair activities are sought to be minimized, and modules are meant to be used and thrown away. It may be possible to use certain application-specific techniques to aid in fault-tolerance; these include **data** integrity checking, control flow checking, and executable assertions.

*See also* Verification

# SYSTOLIC ARRAY

A systolic **array** is a type of parallel **computer architecture** that uses a large number of processors simultaneously to achieve a high flow of **data** through the system, and provide a fast **stream** of outputted results. Systolic arrays are best suited for repetitive tasks with a high degree of regularity, but can cope with large numbers of computations. While such arrays have generally been limited to **supercomputers**, as computer technology progresses they are likely to have much broader usage.

Systolic arrays are a development of the **pipelining** approach to processor **design** and architecture. Pipelining works in much the same way as an actual pipeline, or an assembly production line. Data is fed into a linked chain of processors, and moves through each processor in the pipe, until it is outputted at the other end. A single step in the computation is carried out at each processor, which immediately passes the result on to the next processor in the pipe. Just like a water pipe, if the pipe is empty it will take a long time for anything to come out at the other end. However, once the pipe is full then the output flows out just as fast as the input comes in. The speed of the flow is limited only by the speed of the slowest task in the array. An analogy is a car assembly line, where each uncompleted car must go through a number of stations, having some small process done at each one. Each car has to stay behind the next in the **queue**, and so the overall pace of the line is determined by the slowest stage in the assembly line. While it may take a long time for a single chassis to pass through the factory, at the end of the assembly line the new cars come out at a constant and fast pace. A specific piece of data may take a long time to pass through a pipeline array, yet the flow of results at the output can be very high.

Systolic arrays can be thought of as interconnected pipelines, where data can flow in different directions. Each processor can take data from one or more neighbors (for example top and left), process it, and then pass the results on in the direction of the flow (bottom and right). As with pipelin-

ing, once the system has been filled the results flow out quickly.

Other parallel computing architectures are usually based on data partitioning, where each output is computed on one processor only. In a systolic architecture, each cell (processor) usually handles only a small amount of data (such as one data word from any direction) and the **input and output** of each processor is directly connected to its neighbouring processors. In a classic **message-passing** architecture, the input and output go through the **memory** before being passed to the processor, and a larger **message** (a number of words) is typically used.

The name derives from the systolic pumping action of the heart. A systolic array operates in a pulsing action. Simultaneously all the processors (or cells) alternately compute and then pass the data to the next cells. Just as blood is pumped through the body in pulses, data is regularly pumped from one cell to the next.

H. T. Kung and Charles Leiserson published the first paper on systolic arrays in 1978. They have been confined to supercomputers, and often the array is designed for a specific task. Systolic arrays are best suited for repetitive computations that are highly regular, such as mathematical applications. Examples include matrix multiplication, least squares calculations, polynomial arithmetic, and eigen-value computations, where the individual computations at each cell are simple and regular, but the overall computation may be complex and large. Systolic arrays have also been used in signal and image processing, such as digital filters, encoding and decoding for compression, and error detection. **Searching, pattern matching**, regular language recognition, **relational databases**, and complex graph and geometric calculations are tasks that can also benefit from systolic array computation.

The advantages of systolic arrays include the ability to perform many operations simultaneously. The simplicity and regularity of each step requires only simple and uniform processors (cells), and systolic arrays can be built in modular, and therefore expendable, units. However, the need to control the many simultaneously acting processors makes the construction and **operation** of such arrays a sophisticated and highly technical process.

As software and **hardware** technology improves, the use of systolic arrays may become more widespread, just as the use of pipelining architecture has become more common. While systolic arrays are not suitable for all computing tasks, they provide a simple and efficient parallel structure that has the ability to provide a high-speed output for many computationally demanding problems.

*See also* Computer architecture; Parallel processing; Pipelining

# T

## TANENBAUM, ANDREW STUART (1941-  )
*American computer scientist*

Andrew Tanenbaum is best known for his work on **computer architecture**, operating systems, and networks.

Andrew Stuart Tanenbaum was born in New York in 1941 and grew up in White Plains, New York, where he attended the local high school. His undergraduate degree was obtained at the Massachusetts Institute of Technology (MIT) in 1965 and his Ph.D. came from the University of California at Berkeley in 1971. Both degrees were in computer science. During his undergraduate period Tanenbaum spent a summer working at **IBM**, and this experience put him off working in industry for the rest of his life. For his postdoctoral studies Tanenbaum went to Amsterdam, where he has remained ever since. His postdoctoral studies were carried out jointly at Mathematisch Centrum and Vrije Universiteit between 1971 and 1973. In 1973 he took a permanent position at Vrije Universiteit where he rose to the position of professor of computer science in the Division of Mathematics and Computer Science. In 1981 he wrote the textbook *Computer Networks*, which outlines the **International Organization for Standardization (ISO)** open systems interconnection network model. At Vrije Universiteit he is director of the Computer Systems Group as well as being the Scientific Director and dean of the Advanced School for Computing and Imaging, the graduate school at the university. Tanenbaum's research projects include Amoeba, Paramecium, Globe, and the Orca project. Amoeba is a micro kernel–based distributed operating system; Paramecium is an extendable operating system; and the Globe and Orca projects are parallel **programming** systems based on shared objects. Tanenbaum is also responsible for the MINIX software system. MINIX is an operating system similar to **UNIX**, but due to its small size it is easily runnable on even modest specification PC systems.

Tanenbaum is a member of the Royal Dutch Academy of Science and Arts (1994), a fellow of both the IEEE (1997) and the Association of Computing Machinery (ACM) (1995), and he is also the recipient of the 1994 ACM Karl V. Karlstrom Outstanding Educator Award and the 1997 ACM Outstanding Contributions to Computer Science Education Award. For relaxation Tanenbaum lists as his hobbies playing with a computer, genealogy, travel, and photography. Tanenbaum is interested in distributed and parallel systems, computer networks, and portable compilers. Although Tanenbaum has spent most of his working life in Amsterdam, he has had various work and study periods in other countries and research organizations including Bell Laboratories, New Jersey (1979, 1980, and 1983), and a period of time during 1979 as a visiting scholar at the University of Guelph in Ontario, Canada.

*See also* International Organization for Standardization (ISO); Operating systems; UNIX

## TAPE STORAGE

In addition to the storage of **data** on a computer's **hard drive** or on a server, the storage of a copy of the data on a removable media is prudent strategy. In the event of the computer's failure or destruction, the data is safe for subsequent retrieval and use.

Prior to the development of solid **data storage**, such as CD- and DVD-ROM, the use of tape as a storage medium was widespread. Tape has always been the least expensive storage medium at less than a penny per megabyte, versus five cents for optical or magnetic storage. Tape storage, however, acquired the reputation of being very slow. Now, faster and more efficient tape technologies are available from a number of companies. If the time required for backup is not a factor, tape storage can still be the best option for a user.

The most popular tape devices for smaller commercial users are those based on the digital audio tape (DAT) format. DAT devices are grouped under another specification called digital data storage (DDS). Some DDS devices can hold up to

24 GB of compressed data. Other tape products offer more storage capacity. The Advanced Intelligent Tape (AIT) is a magnetic tape that uses 8–mm cassettes with built-in **memory** chips to speed the process of data retrieval. Another magnetic tape technology, digital linear tape (DLT), can hold up to 70 GB of data. Finally, 8–mm tape, named for its width, was first introduced in 1987. Improvements in the ensuing years have boosted its storage capacity to 40 GB.

With DLT, the data recording process involves the routing of the tape out of the cassette, around the rotating read/write drum assembly, and finally back into the cassette.

Data can be written onto DLT and other tapes in several ways. In linear recording, the data track goes the entire length of the tape (about 1,800 feet). When the end of the tape is reached, the heads are repositioned and the tape runs back the other way, recording the entire length. This pattern continues until the tape is full. In a newer modification, the head assembly can be rotated three ways during the back-and-forth motion to create a highly condensed herringbone pattern of data. By contrast, the helical scan method, used in the AIT for example, writes data to the tape in diagonal stripes running across the tape. The angled position allows the storage of more information per area of tape.

Among the new tape storage products, which debuted in the past several years, the most prominent is called Linear Tape Open (LTO). The first generation LTO drives can store 200 GB of compressed data per tape. By the fourth generation, it is anticipated that the storage capacity could reach 1.6 TB of compressed data. Researchers are also exploring the use of a brand of ordinary commercial adhesive tape as a storage medium. The structure of the tape may be suited to the **holographic storage** of data.

*See also* Data; Holographic storage technology

# TASK BAR

A task bar is a graphic tool bar used in most **Windows** applications (such as Windows 2000) to select, through the **mouse**, one of a number of active or open applications and programs. (The *tool bar* within a **graphical user interface (GUI)** is a row, column, or block of on-screen buttons or icons. When these buttons or icons are clicked on with the mouse, certain functions of the application are activated. The task bar is just one type of tool bar.) The task bar usually consists of a row of buttons or graphical controls on a computer screen, and is normally a bar that is located at the bottom of the Windows's desktop. However, the task bar can be moved to any of the four corners of the screen and adjusted in size. The task bar can also be set to disappear or reappear when so desired. The components of the task bar can also be rearranged to accommodate the needs of the user. The task bar has two primary functions: it is a *program launcher* and a *task switcher*. By going into "Start," then "Programs," a user can "launch" programs that are already installed inside the computer. When programs are already active, the user can "switch" between tasks by using the icons normally located near the center of the task bar.

The *Start* button is a major feature of the task bar. It is located in the far left end on the task bar (or on the top when the bar is located vertically on the side of the screen). It is responsible for launching applications, opening documents, and making settings. Clicking on the Start button opens the Start menu. The Start menu is used to access programs and other features in Windows that are frequently used. Within the Start menu are such features as Programs, Favorites, Documents, Settings, Find, Help, Run, and Shut Down. Pointing and clicking on one of the Start features opens a nested menu. For instance, the Programs feature contains a nested Programs menu that lists the programs and groups of programs installed on the computer.

Some buttons located on the task bar represent currently running Windows application programs or open folders. They are used for task switching, meaning the user can switch among these currently running programs by clicking on appropriate buttons. Clicking on a particular button makes that window active, and displays it on the display screen.

The task bar also contains several secondary status functions such as a clock (usually in the far-right corner), and small icons to indicate such things as waiting electronic-mail (**e-mail**), that the computer is online with the **Internet**, the printing of a document, volume settings for sound, the battery condition (for laptop computers), the Web **browser**, the email application, and other applications that are activated during startup of the computer. Clicking on one of the icons typically brings up a related settings box.

*See also* Graphical user interface (GUI); Macro; Tool bar; Windows

# TAYLOR, ROBERT WILLIAM (1932-    )
*American Computer scientist*

Robert William Taylor is best known for initially conceiving, and then directing, the development of **ARPAnet** in the 1960s. Taylor was also involved in fostering many new technologies that eventually became widely accepted essentials of computer and communication systems.

ARPAnet, the acronym for Advanced Research Projects Agency network, was the "supernetwork" of defense research networks that eventually evolved into the **Internet**. While working as the director of the Information Processing Techniques Office at the Department of Defense's Advanced Research Projects Agency (ARPA), Taylor saw enthusiastic users crowd around each group of interactive terminals that were connected to three separate computer systems. Taylor felt that the projects he was overseeing could be more efficient if these three isolated systems would merge. He therefore proposed the creation of ARPAnet.

ARPAnet covered a fairly large geographical area that eventually consisted of about 60,000 computer systems. The original ARPAnet—the first computer network—was established in 1969 for the free interchange of information between universities and research organizations, and for communications amongst the United States military. Although ARPAnet began as a slow, academically oriented computer network, over a fifteen-year period of time it turned into today's powerful Internet.

During his tenure at ARPA, Taylor organized the funding of new and ongoing research on fundamental computing technologies, such as time-sharing, networking, computer **graphics**, pointing devices (i.e., **mouse**), teleconferencing, and **artificial intelligence**. With **J.C.R. Licklider**, Taylor co-authored the original 1968 paper *The Computer as a Communications Device*, which was one of the first published articles to communicate the **value** of networks.

In 1970, after leaving ARPA, Taylor founded the Computer Science Laboratory (CSL) at Xerox's Palo Alto Research Center (**Xerox PARC**). CSL was the birthplace for the Ethernet (the first **local-area network**, or **LAN**) and for PARC Universal Packet protocol (PUP, the first "internetwork" technology that was needed to convert the limited ARPAnet into the more comprehensive Internet). **Graphical-user interfaces** (**GUI**s) developed under Taylor's leadership led to operating systems such as the Macintosh and **Windows** operating systems. Other inventions that were overseen by Taylor were laser printing and WYSIWYG (acronym for What You See Is What You Get) **word processing**.

In 1984 Taylor moved to **Digital Equipment Corporation** and founded the now-famous Systems Research Center (SRC), which he managed until his retirement in 1996. Under Taylor's guidance, SRC's numerous accomplishments were the first multiprocessor workstation, the first fault-tolerant switched local-area network (LAN), and the first electronic notebook.

Taylor assembled innovative teams of talented researchers and motivated them to accomplish ambitious technological projects. Early in his career, Taylor saw the potential of the computer when, as a research manager at the National Aeronautics and Space Administration, he arranged financing to **Douglas C. Engelbart**, a young researcher at the Stanford Research Institute (SRI), for his work inventing the computer mouse. From the research laboratories that Taylor created and staffed numerous people went on to become founders and leaders of computer companies. Some of these people included Bob Metcalfe of 3Com; John Warnock and Chuck Geschke of Adobe Systems; and Charles Simonyi of the Applications Division of **Microsoft**. In addition, the companies of **Apple** Computers, Silicon Graphics, Inc., Cisco Systems, Novell, and Sun Microsystems built successful businesses on the published and demonstrated work that originated from Taylor's research laboratories.

Butler Lampson, an architect at Microsoft Corporation and an adjunct professor of **computer science and electrical engineering** at Massachusetts Institute of Technology, said about Taylor, "When you write something on your WYSIWYG word processor, print it on your laser **printer**, store it on a file server, or **e-mail** it to a colleague, you're enjoying the fruits of Bob Taylor's research labs. Much of the growth of Silicon Valley has been tied to the Internet, workstations, and local area networks. All these technologies started in labs that were founded or sponsored by Taylor."

Robert William Taylor was one of four individuals awarded the 1999 National Medal of Technology™, the United States's highest technology award. At that time, Taylor was cited for "visionary leadership in the development of modern computing technology."

*See also* ARPAnet; Internet; Local-area network (LAN)

# TCP/IP

TCP/IP, which stands for Transmission Control Protocol/Internet Protocol, is a suite of **protocols** built into the **Unix** operating system and is the standard used to connect computers over the **Internet**. The term TCP/IP actually refers to a whole family of protocols, of which TCP and IP are just two. TCP and IP were first developed in the 1970s in connection with a United States Department of Defense (DoD) research project to connect numerous separate networks designed by different companies into a network of networks, the **ARPAnet**, named for the DoD's Advanced Research Projects Agency (ARPA).

Tracing the history of TCP/IP therefore leads back to the inception of the Internet. TCP as a suite of communications protocols providing end-to-end network communication was first proposed and implemented in 1974 throughout the ARPAnet, which formed the core of the modern Internet. The emergence of packet-switching technology at the time ensured that ARPAnet was designed (in 1968) to be a **packet switching** network with a proposed line speed of 50 Kbps. Packet switching, still the fundamental technology driving the Internet, comprises a **data** network in which all components (i.e., hosts and switches) operate independently. Data is transmitted in a series of discrete packets (containing both data and header information) across complex networks and can be switched dynamically across nodes. This results in fast, economical networks.

ARPAnet started with four University nodes in 1969, spanned the continental U.S. by 1971, and had connections to Europe by 1973. In 1974, following a trail of other protocols, TCP, offering a new and robust suite of end-to-end protocols, was introduced for use throughout the ARPAnet. However, since an end-to-end protocol was widely seen as unnecessary for the gateways (known as routers today) at intermediary points in the network, a new **design** came into use in 1978, splitting responsibilities between a pair of protocols: the new Internet Protocol (IP) was intended for intermediate data routing and host-to-gateway or gateway-to-gateway communication; and TCP was intended for reliable end-to-end host communication. Since TCP and IP were originally intended to function as a single protocol, the protocol suite, which actually refers to a large collection of protocols and **applications**, is referred to simply as TCP/IP. Original versions of TCP and IP in common use today were written in September 1981, although both have undergone several modifications. In addition, the IP version 6, or IPv6, specification was released in December 1995.

TCP/IP's usage profile has undergone a few transformations. In 1983, the DoD mandated the use of the TCP/IP protocol suite for all long-distance communications. TCP/IP became the protocol suite of choice for the evolving Internet, and it developed during the late 1980s as the Internet grew. Meanwhile the OSI (Open Systems Interconnect) protocols also came into prominence, and in 1988 the DoD and most of the U.S. Government chose to adopt OSI protocols, since OSI products were believed to be only a couple of years away. TCP/IP then ran only on limited platforms. The DoD mandated that all computer communications products would use OSI protocols by August 1990 and use of TCP/IP would be phased out. Subsequently the U.S. Government OSI Profile (GOSIP) excluded TCP/IP when defining the set of protocols to be supported in products sold to the federal government.

Despite this mandate, TCP/IP development continued in an open environment at ARPA/NSF (National Science Foundation) sites. OSI products were still a couple of years away, and TCP/IP became the de facto open systems interconnection protocol suite. In 1990 the DoD created an environment to allow OSI applications to operate over TCP/IP. Meanwhile the Internet and OSI communities worked together to combine TCP/IP and OSI; many TCP and IP features started to migrate into OSI protocols. The National Institute for Standards and Technology (NIST) suggested in 1994 that GOSIP incorporate TCP/IP and drop the "OSI-only" requirement. Interestingly it is often noted that OSI represents the ultimate sliding window since OSI protocols have been "two years away" since about 1986.

The IP portion of TCP/IP is the most fundamental protocol on the Internet, responsible for both the transmitting of data packets from one system to another, and for the system of numeric IP addresses, which determines destination points for data on a network. IP operates on **gateway** machines that move data internally from departments to enterprise networks and then externally to regional networks and finally across the world on the global Internet. The associating of natural language host names with IP addresses established the **domain name system** (**DNS**), a distributed database of IP addresses and their host names.

TCP is the protocol that ensures correct delivery of data from client to server. Since data can be lost or delayed across networks, TCP provides support to detect errors or lost data and to initiate retransmission until the data is correctly and completely received. This design allows the construction of large decentralized networks. The TCP protocol provides both a virtual connection between two systems (over the base network of physical connections), as well as connection guarantees like retransmission of dropped packets, sequential receipt of packets (though each packet may take a different route to reach its address), and integrity of data content. Designed initially by the Department of Defense to withstand battlefield damage to communications networks, TCP/IP is built to be robust and to recover automatically from phone line or **node** failure.

A protocol often substituted for TCP by applications requiring speedy transmission and high performance (as opposed to reliability and integrity) is UDP, or User Datagram Protocol. UDP sends data one chunk at a time in a "datagram" and does not provide a virtual connection or make the guarantees TCP does. Datagrams can be lost, arrive out of sequence, or be dropped if corrupted. Despite these drawbacks, UDP, being lighter and faster, is useful for some bulky applications like audio/video streaming, and Internet phone applications. TCP, though more reliable, is slower because of all the extra information required by its guarantees.

## TELEDESIC

Teledesic is a company that is building a broadband **internet** network that will provide global communication links via a constellation of 288 LEO, low-earth-orbit, spacecrafts. The service, backed by **Bill Gates** and Craig McCaw, will act like a network **operator** linking customers worldwide by supporting communications from high quality voice channels to broadband channels supporting videoconferencing, interactive multimedia and real-time two-way digital **data** flow. Service is planned to commence in 2005.

Teledesic was founded in Bellevue, WA, a suburb of Seattle, in June. Most of the funding has come from Bill Gates and Craig McCaw. By 1994 Teledesic had the initial system **design** completed and a Federal Communications Commission (FCC) application to get a large chunk of the Ka-band, the communication band they planned to use, filed. Because Teledesic felt that the digital revolution is just as fundamental as the industrial revolution their initial goal was to create a system that would provide affordable **access** to advanced network connections to all of those parts of the world that will never get such advanced services through current capabilities. They believe that such a system will change all aspects of our societies. By March of 1997 Teledesic had obtained an FCC license for the communication spectrum they wanted to use as well as having the World Radio Conference designate the corresponding necessary international spectrum for their service. In 1998 Motorola, whose Celestri project was seen as one of the major competitors to the Teledesic system, joined forces with Teledesic. The solution to another aspect, seen as a major hindering problem to the Teledesic system, was solved in 1999 when Teledesic signed a major launch contract with Lockheed Martin.

Teledesic's global service is planned to begin in 2005. They plan to offer worldwide access to high-level communication links that will support downlink speeds of 64 Mbps and uplink speeds of 2Mbps. Some higher-speed terminals will be able to offer 64 Mbps or greater speeds in a two-way capacity. 64Mbps represents access speeds in excess of 2,000 times faster than a typical 28.8kbps analog **modem**. This service is planned to operate through a constellation of 288 LEO satellites where each satellite acts as a **node** in a large-scale packet-switching network. The entire project is estimated to cost about $9 billion.

# TELNET

Telnet is a simple **Internet** program for connecting users to remote hosts (computer systems accessible at distant locations) and servers (network devices that manage network resources). The Telnet program contains a set of procedures (commonly called a "protocol") that enables an Internet user to log on to and enter **commands** on a distant (remote) computer in order to simulate a user who is directly attached to the computer. Telnet, sometimes abbreviated TN, is one of the oldest activities on the Internet, being used primarily to **access** online **databases** and to read articles stored on university servers.

Telnet uses *terminal emulation*, a program that allows personal computers (PCs) to respond like a **mainframe terminal** that is connected, and able to access, a mainframe computer or **bulletin board** service. (A *mainframe terminal* is a device consisting of a combination of keyboard and display screen that allows a user to communicate with a mainframe computer. When a user uses a **personal computer** in terminal **emulation** mode the mainframe interacts with the PC as it would with any mainframe terminal.) Transmission Control Protocol/Internet Protocol (**TCP/IP**), a suite of communications **protocols** used to connect hosts on the Internet, supports Telnet. TCP/IP is built into the **UNIX** operating system that is used by the Internet as a standard format for transmitting **data** over networks. Users enter text-based commands through the Telnet program and the commands are executed as if they were directly being entered through the server console. This enables the Telnet user to remotely manipulate the server and communicate with other servers on the network. Generally the user must possess a valid user identification (ID) and **password** for the remote computer. Features generally included with Telnet are electronic mail (**e-mail**), program downloads, and "chatrooms" with other Telnet users. Many computer systems, like those associated with libraries, allow Telnet users to access their large databases in order to perform searches and other needed activities.

It is also possible to activate Telnet within a Web **browser** by changing the *http://* to *telnet://* and entering the site's address. Normally a login prompt will appear to allow the user to enter that site; that is, if the correct login identification is provided. A better way to enter a Telnet site is to download a Telnet program onto a computer, open an Options menu on the computer's Web browser, and add it as a "helper" application or as an external "viewer." Most commercial online services do not allow users to use Telnet, but there are a few workarounds. For example, the Spry **Mosaic** browser that is included with the CompuServe Internet package works just like Netscape, so a Telnet helper program can be added.

Telnet originated before the Internet. However, it has been generally overshadowed by the more comprehensive and easier to use Internet so that it is now merely a component of the Internet. Today users are able to connect to web sites and other peoples' computers with other programs besides Telnet. Telnet's main advantage is that it allows users to log on to a remote system and run programs on that system just as if it were an actual connected mainframe terminal. But the main disadvantage of Telnet is that the actions available are very limited. For instance, files cannot be saved.

*See also* Emulation; Host system; HTTP (Hypertext Markup Language); TCP/IP protocol / Transmission Control Protocol / Internet Protocol; Terminal; UNIX

# TEMPLATE

The term template has several meanings in computer science. All relate to a means of summarizing information in a standard form, to eliminate the repetitive addition of information.

A template can be a plastic or paper diagram designed to fit over a computer keyboard. Displayed on the template are the meanings of specific keys—such as the F series at the top of a standard keyboard—for a particular program. This display of information can speed up the keying in and processing of **data**.

A related type of template is used for a digitizing tablet, a combination of an electronic tablet and an electronic pen (or stylus), which is used to enter drawing and sketches into a computer. Here, the template is typically a plastic sheet that has menus and command boxes drawn on it. Menus and **commands** can be selected by positioning the stylus over the appropriate box and pressing the underlying key.

A third form of a template is blank form or style sheet, on which fields into which information can be put are defined in terms of, for example, location, length, format, style, and linkage to other fields. Put another way, a style sheet defines the layout of a document. **Word processing** templates eliminate the need to fill out the same information (addresses or salutations, for example) for repetitively similar documents. The same style sheet can be used for many documents. For example, a style sheet could be defined for personal letters, another for official letters, and a third for reports. In spreadsheet and database **applications**, the template is typically a spreadsheet in which all of the cells have been defined but no data has yet been entered.

A fourth form of a template relates to computer operating systems and Web pages. In **operating systems**, the template is a temporary storage area where commands reside. In operating systems other than **DOS**, such as **UNIX**, the template is referred to as the command **buffer**. Templates for Web pages and for various communication forums (such as word processing, facsimiles, and computer presentation software) exist, and are obtainable commercially. The basic **design** and layout of the page is supplied, often including buttons where links to other sites can be programmed. The user adds the unique information in the appropriate fields.

Finally, the term template also applies to images that can be cut and pasted into document; so-called clip art. As for the word processing and spreadsheet functions, the clip art templates provide a ready made graphic that is available for use.

The increasing use of computers for presentations is creating a demand for innovative and head-turning images. Entrepreneurs have responded to the demand, with a variety of **Internet** sites now marketing templates that can be downloaded by customers.

*See also* Class

# TEMPORAL LOGIC

The phrase "temporal logic" has been used in a broad sense to denote all approaches to the representation of temporal information within a logical framework, and also in a restricted sense to refer specifically to the modal-logic type of approach introduced around 1960 by Arthur Prior, who used the name Tense Logic.

Temporal logic literally means the logic of time, i.e., a logic that describes the flow of real events in time, which common **propositional logic**, etc., do not. For example, A & B is the same as B & A in standard sentential logic, but if A is the statement "X got married," and B is the statement "X had three children," then one conveys "X got married and had three children," while the other, "X had three children and got married," not quite the same thing necessarily. Temporal logic may thus be regarded as an enrichment of propositional logic by the addition of operators that denote time. In addition to the usual operators known from propositional logic (AND, OR, NOT, XOR, etc.), temporal logic introduces others that relate solely to time.

Temporal logic has a great many applications, including as a formalism for clarifying philosophical issues about time, as a framework within which to define the semantics of temporal expressions in natural language, as a language for encoding temporal knowledge in **artificial intelligence**, and as a tool for handling the temporal aspects of the execution of computer programs and **hardware**.

With Temporal logic one can specify and verify how components, **protocols**, objects, modules, procedures and functions behave as time progresses. The specification is done with temporal logic statements that make **assertions** about properties and relationships in the past, present, and the future.

As already noted, tense logic was introduced by Arthur Prior around 1960 following in the footsteps of the Megarian philosopher Diodorus Cronus (340-280 B.C.), who spoke of a relationship between tense and modality. The logical language of Tense Logic contains, in addition to the usual truth-functional operators, four "modal operators" with intended meanings as follows:

- P—"It has at some time been the case that..."
- F—"It will at some time be the case that..."
- H—"It has always been the case that..."
- G—"It will always be the case that..."

P and F are known as the weak tense operators, while H and G are known as the strong tense operators. The two pairs are generally regarded as interdefinable. Although this is an early formulation and has since been greatly extended, it gives a flavor for the sorts of temporal operators that are generally added. The logic to which temporal operators are added would be propositional logic at the most basic, level, but more recent efforts start with **First-Order logic** or similar.

Temporal logic is useful in describing and proving properties of systems such as "safety" and "liveness," especially in the context of concurrent or **distributed systems**. "Safety" describes the lack of occurrence of a certain type of unwanted even in a system, i.e., that "something bad will not happen."

"Liveness" is the continual occurrence in a system of a certain desirable event, i.e., that "something good always happens." In systems where dependability or security is an issue, safety is paramount, as undesired events may include dangerous faults or failures, intrusions into the system by unauthorized parties, and the like. Safety can sometimes be trivially achieved simply by shutting down the system and not allowing any progress, so to avoid this trivial and unacceptable solution, the liveness condition is to be maintained also.

Another area where temporal logic has been applied is in the context of the "frame problem" in Artificial Intelligence. That problem has to do with knowing not only what things change upon the carrying actions, but also with knowing what things do not. This is taken almost for granted in our everyday life, but can be very difficult in the context of automated systems. For instance, a human does not have to be told that when one presses the brake pedal while driving a car, only the velocity of a car changes but not its color, but a computer does not realize this obvious fact. Thus, the "frame" of the problem has to be defined in a way that allows the computer to understand exactly what aspects of the problem domain remain unchanged, and in this temporal logic is found to be useful.

Recent flavors of temporal logic that have gained wide attention include Leslie Lamport's Temporal Logic of Actions (TLA), the UNITY formalism of K.M. Chandy and J. Misra, and other formulations such as Interval Temporal Logic.

***See also*** Artificial intelligence; Deadlock; Verification

# TERMINAL

The term terminal has two meanings in computer science, relating to an individual computer and to a computer network.

In the context of an individual computer, a terminal is a device that enables the user to communicate with the computer. Generally, the device is a combination of a keyboard and a display screen. There are three classes of terminals with respect to their processing speed and **data** handling capability: intelligent terminal, smart terminal, and dumb terminal.

An intelligent terminal is a device that can process information. It has **memory** and a processor. In contrast, a dumb terminal has no processing capabilities. A dumb terminal can only accept data from the **central processing unit** of the computer to which it is linked. It is also the slowest operating of the three terminal classes. Nevertheless, a dumb terminal is adequate for most applications for which terminals are required. The third class of terminal, the smart terminal, has features that position in between the intelligent and dumb terminals. A smart terminal does have its own processor and built-in logic, which enables it to perform functions like bold and blinking characters.

In the context of networking, a terminal refers to a **personal computer** or a workstation that is connected to a **mainframe** computer. Typically, each personal computer runs what is termed terminal **emulation** software that makes the mainframe think each terminal is another mainframe terminal. This enables a personal computer to be part of the mainframe network. An example of such a setup is the SETI (Search for Extraterrestrial Intelligence) project. In SETI, individual's personal computers can emulate a mainframe terminal, so that many more individuals than those residing in the SETI facility can do the analysis of incoming signals from outer space. The speed of analysis is increased by such a configuration.

Another well-known example of network terminals is the **Telnet**. Telnet, the Network Terminal Protocol, is a two-way communication network. It was implemented so that users could communicate with computers, users could communicate with other users, and computers could communicate directly with other computers, all using the same protocol and rules. A useful feature of Telnet is the ability of a user at a terminal to gain **access** to an application that is not on the Telnet server. For example, if a user does not have an **e-mail** program, as would be the case using a dumb terminal, Telnet can be used to send e-mail messages. The user can establish a Telnet connection to the recipient. Then, using text **commands** from the computer to which the terminal is connected, the user can identify themselves as a sender, enter a text **message** and have the message delivered.

*See also* Telnet

# TEXAS INSTRUMENTS

Texas Instruments Incorporated (TI) is an electronics developer and manufacturer with a **design**, manufacturing, or sales presence in 28 countries and more than 30,000 commercial and industrial customers worldwide. Headquartered in Dallas, Texas, TI is one of the world's largest **semiconductor** manufacturers and is the market leader in designing and supplying digital signal processors (DSPs) and analog **integrated circuit** technologies. TI's DSPs are inside over 50% of wireless telephones and are also found inside such devices as modems and videocassette records. TI's semiconductor products include standard logic devices, application-specific integrated circuits, reduced instruction-set computing microprocessors, microcontrollers, and digital imaging devices. They are used in cellular telephones, personal computers, digital cameras and audio-players, and automobiles. TI produces millions of integrated circuits daily in numerous fabrication centers worldwide. In addition to semiconductors, TI also sells electrical and electronic controls, sensors, radio-frequency identification systems, and graphing and educational calculators. TI engineers have produced major advances in the electronics field, including the commercial silicon **transistor**, the integrated circuit, and the hand-held **calculator**.

Texas Instruments started operations in 1930 as Geophysical Service (GS), a Texas oil exploration company founded by John Karcher and Eugene McDermott. GS pioneered the use of sound-wave technology (reflection seismology) to locate oil deposits. GS soon incorporated as Geophysical Service, Inc. (GSI), and began working with the world's largest oil companies. The company quickly expanded, with a history of efficiency, honesty, and reliability. As a result of its success, management separated its oil pro-

duction and oil exploration businesses in 1938. The parent company was renamed Coronado Corporation and GSI became a subsidiary. Just before World War II, cofounder Eugene McDermott, C. H. Green, J. E. Jonsson, and H. B. Peacock bought GSI. During the war, GSI expanded into research on electronic military equipment and production of submarine detection devices.

In order to emphasize the diversity of its electronic products the company's name was changed to General Instruments, Inc., but when a name conflict arose it was renamed Texas Instruments Inc. in 1951, with GSI as a subsidiary. McDermott became TI's first chairman and Jonsson its first president. At this time the company set three goals: (1) to continue developing and producing geophysical equipment and providing seismic services, (2) to become a major military systems provider, and (3) to enter emerging electronics technologies. TI's fateful moment came when Pat Haggerty suggested to Jonsson that they manufacture germanium transistors, a new Bell Laboratories invention. A license was purchased for $25,000, and in 1952 TI began to develop the transistor. By 1954 TI announced the production of the first commercial, portable, transistor radio, the Regency Radio. Its semiconductor devices occupied less than 1/10th of a cubic inch apiece, heralding the miniaturization of consumer electronics.

In 1954, while manufacturing the germanium transistor, TI developed the first commercial silicon transistor. It was smaller, less expensive, and operated more reliably than germanium transistors. This same year TI supplied transistors to the first United States satellite, Explorer 1. TI's electrical engineer **Jack Kilby** came to work for TI in 1958 in order to develop technology for circuit miniaturization. This research resulted in the integrated circuit, which more than any other single invention has made possible the microelectronics revolution of the last few decades.

In the 1960s Texas Instruments expanded globally, establishing facilities in South America, Europe, Asia, and Japan. In 1961, TI delivered its first integrated circuit (IC) computer to the Air Force, a machine 150 times smaller and weighing 48 times less than previously available computers of equivalent computing power. The computer showed that semiconductor networks were suitable for military equipment because of their reduced size, weight, and cost and increased reliability. In 1964, TI introduced the first IC consumer product, a hearing aid. The IC hearing aid out-performed the amplification of conventional devices and was more reliable. After two years of development TI released in 1967 the first electronic hand-held calculator. The battery-powered device could accept a number of up to six digits, performed the four basic arithmetic functions, and printed its results on a thermal **printer**. Also in the late 1960s TI provided **precision** switches, thermostats, transistors, and other semiconductor products for the Apollo missions to the Moon.

In 1971 TI built the first microcomputer structured around a single-chip logic circuit. In 1972 TI offered its TI-2500 portable calculator (along with the TI-3000 and TI-3500 desk models). In 1973, TI received a patent for the single-chip **microprocessor**, and the next year introduced the TMS-1000 single-chip microcomputer. TI also introduced the first single-chip speech synthesizer, the Speak & Spell, marking the first time the human voice was electronically duplicated on a silicon chip. In 1975 Texas Instruments produced the world's first inexpensive digital watch. In 1978, TI was awarded a patent for the microcomputer, the first integrated circuit with all computer elements on a single silicon chip.

During the 1980s TI introduced (1) a high-speed (5 million instructions per second), single-chip digital signal processor, (2) a specialized chip for intense mathematical computing, (3) the first single-chip 32-bit microprocessor specifically for **artificial intelligence** applications, and (4) the first quantum-effect transistor, 100 times smaller and 1,000 times faster than conventional transistors.

Despite TI's many landmark inventions, it began to have difficulty with less expensive Asian competition. However, in 1989 a Japanese court upheld the patent for Kilby's integrated circuit and, as a result, a number of major electronics corporations were ordered to pay TI royalties. In the late 1980s and early 1990s the company entered into strategic partnerships to produce custom-designed electronic components.

Innovations by TI during the 1990s included (1) 125 million transistors placed on a chip; (2) digital signal processing application design-and-development tools on the **Internet**; (3) a silicon-based monolithic spatial light modulator, the "digital micromirror device"; and (5) the first optoelectronic integrated circuit.

TI is presently focusing on digital signal processors. and analog devices. Digital signal processors and analog semiconductors are at the heart of a wide range of communication achievements, from wireless cellular phones to high-speed broadband information access to the home, Internet-downloadable music devices, and digital cameras.

*See also* Integrated circuit; Microprocessor; Semiconductor; Transistor

# THOMPSON, KENNETH LANE (1943- )

*American computer scientist*

Kenneth Lane Thompson studied **programming languages**, **operating systems**, and **computer games**. He was one of the inventors of the **UNIX** operating system, perhaps the most widely used computer system in the world. He also invented the **C** programming language and co-developed several chess-playing machines.

UNIX is well known for its simplicity, generality, and portability. Thompson conceived of the system in the late 1960s, and together with **Dennis Ritchie**, a colleague working with him at Bell Laboratories, developed UNIX as an alternative to the old batch programming systems that dominated the industry at the time. Although Thompson created UNIX while working at Bell Labs, the system was developed independently by the two programmers. It was very unusual because it was not commercially marketed like other systems. Instead UNIX gained in popularity through a network of researchers

long before it was released commercially, and it has had one of the longest gestation periods of any computer program. UNIX is now believed to be one of the most widely used systems in the world, supporting over twenty million dollars of equipment.

Kenneth Thompson was born on February 4, 1943 in New Orleans, Louisiana, the son of Lewis Elwood Thompson, a fighter pilot in the U.S. Navy, and Anna Hazel Lane Thompson. He majored in electrical engineering at the University of California, Berkeley, also working at the computer center as well as participating in a work-study program at the General Dynamics Corporation. Thompson received his B.S. in electrical engineering in 1965 and his M.S. in electrical engineering in 1966, both from Berkeley.

Though Thompson's formal education was in electronic **hardware** and he built a lot of computers, he was very accomplished in developing computer software, and this is what he pursued professionally. After receiving his master's degree, Thompson went to work for the Computing Science Research Center at Bell Laboratories in New Jersey. He married his wife Bonnie on July 2, 1967, and they had one son, Corey. Bell Labs was famous for its research productivity, and for the unconventional looks, dress, and work habits of some of its scientists. Thompson fitted in well—bearded, bespectacled, and long-haired, he wore a tee-shirt in one published picture. His work habits were also unusual, and he would sometimes put in thirty hours in a row without sleep while working on a project.

One of Thompson's greatest achievements at Bell Labs was inventing and then developing the UNIX with Ritchie. A computer operating system manages the housekeeping functions within a computer. By enabling the user to create, open, edit, and close **data** files, as well as move data from a disk to the screen or **printer**, and to store data on disks in addition to activating and using other programs, an operating system makes computers easy to run and fast. While at Bell Labs in the late 1960s, Thompson had been assigned to work on developing such a multi-tasking and multi-user system. Together with engineers from General Electric and the Massachusetts Institute of Technology (MIT), Thompson and other Bell Lab programmers began working on what was called Multics.

This multi-tasking and multi-user system would contrast in important ways with existing batch-operation computers. Batch computers required a user to create a stack of pre-punched data cards which were then run through the computer at one time. During this process, the computer could only apply its programming abilities to the one user's stack of cards, requiring all other users to wait for their jobs to get done. After waiting an hour or longer a user would get a printout of results on paper. If users wanted to make any changes after seeing the results on the print-outs, they would have to punch out another stack of cards and wait to resubmit them to the computer for processing. Getting the results from simple changes in a data request could take a long time.

On the other hand, multi-tasking, multi-user computer systems would be structured in such a way that the flow of data inside the computer would allow it to process many jobs at once for numerous users. The benefits were obvious: users could get their results back quickly and get much more work done. Also, if a computer screen **terminal** was used as an **input and output** device, users could key their requests into the terminal, and the computer could display its response to the requests on the screen. Changes and revisions could be made immediately, while the computer could still run other programs. Multi-tasking, multi-user computer systems like UNIX have replaced batch processing almost completely, and when Thompson invented the program at Bell Labs in 1969, he started the ball rolling to create that change. In late 1988, American Telephone & Telegraph (AT&T) licensed its millionth UNIX system.

In 1978 Thompson stopped working on UNIX and began other projects. Some of his later projects included another operating system called Plan 9, and computer chess. Chess had been one Thompson's boyhood hobbies, and he carried it into his adult years by making computers and computer programs that could play chess. One of these programs was so good that it became three-time American champion. Thompson also built a chess-playing computer, which he named "Belle." Besides programming, Thompson was also involved in teaching computing. During a 1975 sabbatical he taught upper division and graduate courses in computer science, including a seminar on the UNIX operating system, at the University of California at Berkeley. On another break in 1988, he taught computer science at the University of Sydney in Australia.

In 1993, after working for years on computer chess and another operating systems, Thompson began to work on digital audio encoding. He has received a number of awards for his contributions to computer programming, including the famous Turing award in 1983 from the Association for Computing Machinery, which he shared with Ritchie. The citation for the Turing award read as follows: "The success of the UNIX system stems from its tasteful selection of a few key ideas and their elegant implementation. The model of the UNIX system has led a generation of software designers to new ways of thinking about programming. The genius of the UNIX system is its framework, which enables programmers to stand on the work of others." Lane was elected to the National Academy of Sciences in 1985.

Lane is now a distinguished staff member at Lucent Technologies, the parent company of Bell Labs. Bell Labs is considered the most famous research and development and organization in the world.

## THRASHING

Thrashing occurs when a computer spends too much time loading **data** into **random access memory** (RAM) and not enough time computing. In extreme cases, a computer's time may be virtually monopolized by thrashing.

What causes thrashing? Suppose one wishes to run a program too large to fit into available RAM. In principle, it is easy to do so: one simply loads and runs fragments of the program in sequence, as needed (perhaps repeatedly), until the whole program has been run. Suppose further that the program in question tends to alternate between two subroutines (chunks of **code**) for long stretches of computing time. If both subroutines can fit into RAM at once, all is well; otherwise, every time the computer finishes one routine it must load the other. In the latter case, since loading code from a **hard drive** or other archival **memory** device is time-consuming by computer standards, the computer may start to spend most of its time loading code into RAM (thrashing). Since memory is generally divided into "pages," thrashing is also called "page thrashing."

There is no sure way to prevent thrashing except to install enough RAM to hold the largest program that a machine might will ever be required to run. There would also have to be enough RAM to hold the all the data to be manipulated by any given program. This much RAM is not generally feasible, so computer designers have developed the concept of the "working set." The working set of a program changes from moment to moment during run-time. It is that set of pages (code, data, or both) which a program references, typically, during the time required to fetch a single new page from disk memory (call it T seconds). In other words, if a working set is present in RAM the computer can run for about T seconds without having to **access** disk memory. At the end of that time, it usually finds that it needs a fresh page of code or data from disk; the page is fetched, which takes T seconds. Having updated its working set the computer can now run for another T seconds (on average) without fetching a page. This cycle repeats until the program terminates. In other words, a computer that always has enough RAM for a working set wastes no more than half its time fetching pages. (Even half is a lot, but at least the program is running.) To avoid thrashing, therefore, a computer's available RAM must be at least as large as the typical working set of any program it is expected to run.

*See also* Random access memory (RAM); Virtual memory

## THREAD

A thread is a portion of a program that runs separately during execution. As a program runs it spawns off separate functions as threads. Threads cannot run independently; they remain under the control of the program. Threads are sometimes referred to as "lightweight processes." Both threads and processes are each a sequential flow of control, but a thread is lightweight because it is running within the context of a complete program. It must share system resources belonging to the program of which it is a part.

A thread contains the information needed to serve a particular service request. If multiple users are using the program or concurrent service requests occur, a thread is created and maintained for each of them. Thread information is stored in a special **data** area, the address of which is recorded in the **register**.

Most operating systems support both **multitasking** and multithreading. Multithreading is the ability to run multiple threads simultaneously, with each thread performing a different task. This allows for faster execution of an application, especially when the application is run on a computer with multiple processors.

An application must be written in a certain way to take advantage of a multithreaded operating system. Some **programming** languages have built-in support for threading, and others require the use of **application programming interfaces** (APIs). An example of a multithreaded application is a web **browser** that allows a user to scroll up or down on a web page while downloading additional images.

Multithreaded **applications** are complex to manage. Because threads share system resources, it is easy for one thread to tie up the **CPU** and prevent other threads in the program from executing. Different operating systems have different mechanisms for thread management.

*See also* API (Application Programming Interface); Multithreaded operation; Register

# THROUGHPUT

Throughput refers either to (1) the number of operations which a computer or component of a computer can perform in a given period of time or (2) the speed with which **data** can be passed through a communications **channel**. There is no single, precise definition of throughput, but a range of definitions adjusted to different uses.

First consider computer throughput. To give a precise meaning to "the number of operations which a computer or component of a computer can perform in a given period of time" one must first specify what is meant by an "operation." At the **hardware** level, this may be a single floating-point **operation** (i.e., the multiplication of two floating-point numbers); at the system level, it may be the completion of an entire program. Regardless of the sort of "operation" under consideration, computer throughput has units of operations per second. For a processor, millions of floating-point operations performed per second (MFlops) or millions of instructions executed per second (MIPS) are common measures of throughput. Throughput for entire systems is often measured by running benchmark programs (standard computing tasks). The complement of throughput is latency, the time that elapses from commencement of an operation (however defined) to the availability of its result. Shorter average latency means faster net throughput. In computer science, throughput is also referred to as bandwidth.

The throughput of a digital communications channel is the number of bits, characters, or words passing through that channel per second. Common units are millions of bits per second (megabits per second or Mbps) and billions of bits per second (gigabits per second or Gbps). Channel throughput has also been defined as the number of *meaningful* bits or other data units passing through a channel per second; in this usage, non-informative bits such as those used solely for framing purposes would not be counted.

It should be noted that in communications, in contrast to computer science, throughput and bandwidth are not equivalent. In communications, bandwidth is a frequency interval having units of cycles per second (Hertz)—a measure of the range of frequencies which a channel uses to communicate—whereas throughput is an performance measure having units of, say, bits per second. Bandwidth may be "wide" or "narrow"; throughput may be "low" or "high." A wide-bandwidth channel will often have high throughput, but not always. In spread-spectrum radio, for instance, a very-wide-bandwidth channel might have fairly low throughput (see entry for **Long-Distance Communication**).

# TIME-SHARING COMPUTER SYSTEMS

Time sharing enables large computers to interact with and perform tasks for many users at such a fast rate that users are practically unaware the computer's time is divided. Before the development of time-sharing systems in the 1960s, computers were generally large and expensive and ran only one program at a time. Users took turns on the computer. Running a single program could take hours because it involved manually setting up the whole computer system: computer, tape drives, card punchers and readers, and printers. An iterative computer task, such as **debugging** a program, could take many lengthy sessions with the computer. During setup, the computer itself sat idle—a waste of an expensive, valuable resource.

**Operating systems** (OS) and batch processing were early developments that made computers more efficient. Operating systems were developed in the mid-1950s as sets of special computer programs that controlled peripheral devices. While the OS handled the **peripherals** for one program, the processor moved on to address the next program. Eventually, methods were developed for running sets of several programs in quick succession. This was called "batch processing," and it greatly increased computer efficiency. Batch-processing computers were often managed by special departments within organizations. Computer users submitted their "jobs" to the batch-processing department and returned later to pick up the results. So, while batch processing improved the efficiency of computers, it also put a distance between computers and users. This distance was particularly irksome to programmers for whom direct interaction with computers was the better, faster way to develop, test, and debug programs.

Another advance in computer efficiency was realized in the development of "multiprogramming" in the late 1950s. Multiprogramming makes use of an executive program to run several programs at once and to generally organize the computer's processing functions for maximum efficiency.

In the early 1960s, a group of computer experts centered at the Massachusetts Institute of Technology (MIT) who had worked on early, interactive computers began to seek ways to allow multiple users to interact with computers simultaneously. They built upon advances made in the development of multiprogramming to create the first time-sharing systems.

The first time-sharing system was proposed by **John McCarthy** of MIT and developed by McCarthy and Herbert Teager, also of MIT. The purpose of this first system was to allow programmers to debug their programs while other users were running production programs or debugging other programs. The system was operational at the MIT Computation Center in early 1960. It was an exciting success, and MIT decided to meet all its computing needs with a large, time-sharing computer system that would be remotely accessible from several locations on the campus.

While planning for a campus-wide time-sharing system was still underway, another group at the MIT Computation Center, led by Fernando Corbato, began developing a new time-sharing system in late 1960. This system, called the Compatible Time-Sharing System (CTSS), was operational in 1961. CTSS marked a step forward in time sharing in that it supported up to 21 simultaneous users by 1963. CTSS stored programs in its main **memory**. Users requested jobs to run via remote terminals. CTSS ran the programs and sent the results to users at the terminals. As soon as one job was complete, the CTSS processor began work on another, so that users were not aware the system was running other jobs. The final version of CTSS included powerful utilities for editing, testing, and debugging programs.

At Bolt Beranek and Newman (BBN), a Cambridge, Massachusetts, company with strong ties to MIT, Edward Fredkin developed a time-sharing system on a smaller computer than those used at MIT. The BBN system included the innovation of dividing the computer's memory into short-term and long-term and of achieving time-sharing by swapping users in and out of short-term and long-term memory. **J. C. R. Licklider**, another employee at BBN, worked on this system and became a time-sharing enthusiast. Licklider later became the first director of the Information Processing Techniques Office (IPTO) of the Department of Defense's Defense Advanced Research Projects Agency (DARPA). Licklider made research and development in time sharing the primary focus of IPTO when it opened in 1961. With the funding it provided companies and universities to research and develop more advanced time-sharing systems, IPTO became the most important proponent of time sharing.

One of Licklider's first actions as director of IPTO was to alter the only current project—a command and control project with Systems Development Corporation (SDC) of Santa Monica, California—to a time-sharing project. Later, Licklider approved IPTO funding for other time-sharing projects on the west coast, at the University of California at Los Angeles, University of California at Berkeley, the Stanford Research Institute, and Stanford University. Researchers for these projects were able to connect to the SDC time-sharing system when it was completed in 1963.

Licklider also sought to increase existing interest in time sharing on the east coast, specifically at MIT and BBN. With encouragement from Licklider, Robert Fano of MIT received IPTO funding for an MIT time-sharing project. He and Licklider called it Project MAC, for "Multiple Access Computer" and "Machine Aided Cognition." The Project MAC system was operational in 1963. It was based on the CTSS system but quickly outpaced that system.

In 1964 leaders of Project MAC began to plan significant improvements to the system. They contracted with General Electric (GE) and Bell Laboratories to build a new system using a GE computer and Bell software. This new project was called MULTICS, for "Multiplexed Information and Computing Service." MULTICS was to be a cutting-edge system that advanced time-sharing research and development to the next level, while providing MIT with the very best computing services available. However, achieving the next level of time sharing proved to be much harder than anyone had anticipated. MULTICS was expected to be complete in 1965; it was operational—but not complete—by 1969. Interest in and work on MULTICS gradually faded, and the project was never completed.

At the time the MULTICS project began, the major computer manufacturers, including **IBM** and **DEC**, offered time-sharing computers and large, mature time-sharing systems were in use in commercial as well as research settings. The promised benefits of time sharing, however, were increasingly viewed with skepticism. Some argued that batch-processing systems were more reliable and more economical than time-sharing systems, and, when designed with enough computing power, could provide turnaround times that were acceptable to programmers as well as general users. It was not batch-processing systems, however, that overtook time-sharing systems. It was the increasingly available small, cheap, yet powerful computer that ended the dominance of time-sharing systems in computing research, development, commercialization, and use.

Although time-sharing systems did not become the dominant method of computer use, they are still used in some settings and they have influenced the nature of current computer use. Time-sharing systems are still used in situations where there is a large computer or peripheral device that needs to be shared by multiple users. And the interactive, shared elements of time-sharing systems have become important, substantial elements in contemporary computer systems.

# TIME SLICE

Time slice is a short interval of time during which a particular task (or process) is allowed to run uninterrupted within a **microprocessor** in a pre-emptive **multitasking** operating system. Multitasking is a type of microprocessor that is able to process multiple tasks apparently at the same time by piecing out the microprocessor's time among different tasks. Pre-emptive multitasking is a type of multitasking where a scheduler within the operating system uses the computer's **central processing unit** (**CPU**, commonly also called the microprocessor) to **interrupt** and suspend (or "swap out") the currently running task in order to start or continue running ("swap in") another task. The length of time for which a process runs is known as its "time slice" and may depend on the priority of the task or its use of resources such as **memory** and I/O (input/output). Time slices are typically in the order of fractions of seconds, with several milliseconds being a common time slice. The scheduler is run once every time slice in order to choose the next process to run. If the time slice is too short then the scheduler itself will consume too much processing time, but if it is too long then processes may not be able to respond to external events quickly enough.

In order to efficiently schedule tasks, each task in time slicing is given the attention of the microprocessor for a fraction of a second. To maintain order, tasks are either assigned priority levels or processed in sequential order. Because the user senses time much slower than the processing speed of the computer, time slice multitasking operations seem to be simultaneous. An example of an operating system that uses time-slice multitasking is Microsoft's **Windows** 2000.

*See also* Operating systems, types; Multitasking; Microprocessor

# TOOLBAR

A toolbar operates in a **graphical user interface** environment, where it functions as a repository of selectable buttons for desktop or application functions. The toolbar is positioned as a horizontal or vertical row. By selecting and clicking on a button within the toolbar, the particular task is activated.

There are a myriad tasks that can be activated using toolbars, such as saving or printing a document or moving pages forwards or backwards within a Web **browser**. Customization of toolbars is easy to accomplish, allowing the user to construct a toolbar that suits their specific needs. The toolbar is a standard feature of **word processing**, spreadsheets, and many other types of application programs. In addition, a burgeoning software development industry exists to supply supplementary toolbars to address very specific functions. For example, toolbars as portals to news, weather and sports groups, search engines, and completion of forms such as income tax, are available for purchase from numerous vendors.

*See also* Graphical user interface (GUI); Menu bar; Windows

# TOP-DOWN DESIGN

Top-down **design** is a phrase from the field of software engineering, and refers to a strategy used in designing a product, such as a software program.

Top-down design in software **programming** is similar to the concept of outlines in the design of documents, in that the structure of the document, or the software, is the central emphasis. Software top-down design, however, is unique from a document that is written once and is not changed. Software undergoes multiple revisions and improvements following its initial design. Top-down design makes the maintenance process easier.

A design project is divided into a series of hierarchies, or levels, ranging from the entire project to the smallest aspect of the project. These project components are arranged in a logical progressive order and relationships are established—what must be done at one level before the next level can be accomplished,

for example. In principle, top-down design involves starting at the uppermost level and working down, level by level

The design begins at the conceptual level, with a model of the project; software or database. The next stage is the design of operations—how exactly to go about achieving the goal. By organizing a project into inter-related hierarchies, a flow diagram, also called a structure diagram, is generated. This can be a pictorial representation, and a mathematical one, in the form of an algorithm and programming instructions. A working form of the model is then generated, followed by refinements.

There are two broad categories of top-down design: the complex **object** approach and the grammar-based approach. The complex object approach uses an algebraic approach to link aspects of the project together. While useful with complex objects, the approach can be too complex for many users, and the conversion of text information to algebraic information can introduce loss of information. The grammar-based approach is, as the name implies, a grammatical way of linking objects. This approach is generally more user-friendly.

**HTML** documents often benefit from top-down design. The design process provides a roadmap of the directories and files that will be needed. As cross-referencing becomes necessary, the user can easily identify the file that contains the relevant reference, even if the file has yet to be written. Thus, referencing can be done as the document is being written, rather than returning later and add references in the appropriate spots.

If conducted properly, top-down design instills accountability in the development process. This, in turn, results in a logical process and produces an end program that is user-friendly. In practice, top-down design is difficult to achieve. Projects tend to proceed on multiple fronts, rather than sequentially from one project level to the next. Also, various aspects of a software development project may not be undertaken by one programming team.

*See also* Architecture (software); Benchmarks; Bottom-up design; Design

# TORRES Y QUEVEDO, LEONARDO (1852-1936)

*Spanish scientist*

Spanish scientist Leonardo Torres y Quevedo constructed during the late nineteenth century and early twentieth century several relay-activated, electromechanical calculating machines that "played" chess. The mechanical machine, or "automaton," that Quevedo built in 1890, which he named "El Ajedristica," is often called the first true chess computer. It performed algorithmic calculations by mechanical means, similar to an adding machine. The machine automatically played a king and a rook endgame against an opposing king (played by a human opponent) and was able to achieve checkmate from any initial position in a few moves. The machine consisted of a metal base that made contact with the squares of the board to enable the automaton to identify the king's square by electric currents. (Quevedo's name is appropriate for his invention since "*torres*" is Spanish for "rooks.") **Programming** was relatively simple because a limited set of rules could be input for making satisfactory moves in such an endgame. However, this elementary end game was seen as quite advanced for that period of time.

Quevedo's machines were later publicly acclaimed when one machine competed against and defeated a cyberneticist (a person involved with the theoretical study of control processes in electronic systems) by the name of **Norbert Wiener**. Although its function was limited to particular chess endgames, Quevedo proved that further advancement in computer technology was possible at a time when information about "artificial intelligence" was very limited. At the time of his invention Torres was the president of the Academy of Sciences in Madrid, Spain. His 1890 machine can still be viewed, in working order, at the Polytechnic Museum in Madrid.

Quevedo was directly influenced by the work of English mathematician **Charles Babbage** (1791–1871) and his **analytical engine**. That knowledge helped Quevedo to play a significant role in the history of the development of program-controlled computers. A civil engineer, logician, and automation expert, Quevedo was also the author of numerous inventions and international patents in such things as suspension bridges, analog computers, ferries, and airships. In addition, in 1906 Quevedo designed a complex number multiplier device, and in 1907 developed a language for defining mechanical drawings. However, Quevedo saw little future in his chess-playing machines because, like Charles Babbage, he felt restricted by the existing mechanical constraints.

Quevedo is especially remembered as the 1915 author of the fundamental work *The First Modern Treatise on the Automatism* that described the basic functions of automatic sensors. Within the article Quevedo also analyzed one of Charles Babbage's machines. Today the publication is considered to have contributed an important role in numerous computer achievements during the twentieth century. The experiments and inventions of Leonardo Torres y Quevedo provided the evidence that eventually led to the understanding that technology could advance and someday take over basic duties of humans in the form of **artificial intelligence**.

*See also* Artificial intelligence; Cybernetics

# TORVALDS, LINUS (1970-  )
*Finnish software engineer*

Software engineer Linus Torvalds is the creator of the **Linux** (pronounced LIH-nucks) operating system, a program that by the late 1990s was getting attention as a potential competitor to the powerful **Microsoft Windows**, which runs about 85 percent of the world's computers. This would be intriguing enough if Torvalds was a software guru out to topple Microsoft as a leader in this market, but astonishingly, after cobbling together the project on his own time for his own use as a computer science student at the University of Helsinki,

the Finnish programmer posted the system and all its **code** (the set of instructions used to create it) on the **Internet**, free to anyone who wanted it. His motivating factor, then, was not to earn money from a superior product, but just simply to build a better quality, more reliable operating system. "People have grown used to thinking of computers as unreliable, and it doesn't have to be that way," Torvalds told Amy Harmon in the *New York Times Magazine*. "I don't mind Microsoft making money. I mind them having a bad operating system."

Though Linux has made Torvalds a hero among the technically savvy, he is quick to point out that he only supplied a "kernel" of the program. By opening the source code, users around the globe continue to work on it on a volunteer basis, fixing any bugs that hamper its performance and making enhancements as they wish, as long as they post their code back to the community of users for perusal. Thus, its users claim, Linux runs faster and is more stable than other operating systems, specifically Microsoft Windows for networks (the program is far more popular on computer servers than on individual machines). Despite the fact that the system lacks a user-friendly graphical interface and the code remains free, some companies are finding ways to make a profit off of it. Red Hat Software, for example, charges about $50 for their version of Linux and it offers technical support for users. Those who download Linux on their own, on the other hand, have no central source to contact if they need assistance.

Although Linux was sprung from hacker origins and it shows in its lack of slick graphic **design**, its more reliable nature and its growing accessibility are helping it gain a wider range of fans, including many businesses and governmental bodies. Many still think it has a while before it becomes a serious contender, especially since it cannot run many of the more popular desktop software programs yet that will be necessary to make it appealing to home users. However, more and more big-name firms are supporting its growth by offering Linux on systems and investing in companies that are selling their versions of Linux, and Torvalds holds the hope that someday it will be a viable option to Windows.

Torvalds was born in about 1970 and named after physicist Linus Pauling as well as the intellectual Peanuts comic character. He grew up in Helsinki, in a family of journalists, but his grandfather, Leo Toerngvist, had the biggest influence on him. He was a mathematician and statistics professor at the University of Helsinki who bought one of the first personal computers in order to use it as a programmable **calculator**. Enlisting his grandson to help out with the Commodore VIC-20, Toerngvist taught Torvalds the basics of writing programs. Before he had reached his teen years, Torvalds was devoting most of his time to writing code for **computer games**. "I liked the challenge of making a computer do what you wanted it to," he mentioned to Leslie Helm in the *Los Angeles Times*. He also admitted, "I was a geek."

As a computer science student at Finland's University of Helsinki, in 1991 Torvalds felt he needed a better operating system to perform his work. Microsoft's MS-DOS was simply not technologically up to snuff, but as a poor undergraduate, Torvalds could not afford to spend the $6000 to $9000 for the more advanced **Unix** system, which runs large mainframes in

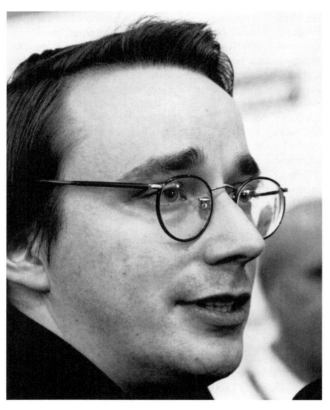

**Linus Torvalds**

the corporate and academic arenas. So he figured he would write his own version. As Torvalds put it to Elizabeth Simnacher in the *Dallas Morning News*, "Reliability was an issue, but the systems were very messy. There was essentially no philosophy. They didn't fit my notion of what an operating system should be." He explained further, "When you don't have some kind of a plan, the end result is such that nobody can understand how it works and there aren't any clear rules about how to use it."

Torvalds was dedicated to his pursuit. "Forget about dating! Forget about hobbies! Forget about life!" he exclaimed to Janice Maloney in *Time*. "We are talking about a guy who sat, ate and slept in front of the computer." When he mentioned his project to an Internet discussion group, one person offered him some space on a university computer to post the program. One of the members dubbed the program "Linux," after its original creator and the program he based it on, Unix. The decision to unleash the Linux program for free over the Internet was astounding enough, but Torvalds went a step further when he also posted the source code so that other programmers could play with the version on their own, making modifications at will. This is what is known in the industry as open source software (OSS), a movement that is gaining steam even in the commercial sector because of the fact that more minds being applied to the product will yield superior programs. Sure enough, a few people soon downloaded and puttered around with the code and e-mailed modifications to

Torvalds. "When I released Linux, I thought maybe one other person would be interested in it," Torvalds related to Harmon.

Before long, the handful of Linux enthusiasts grew to somewhere between 100 and 200, and by 1994, Torvalds felt it could be considered a complete operating system. At this point, about 100,000 people had downloaded it and were running it on personal computers. To keep the it free, Torvalds had right away used the GNU General Public License, a licensing system developed by **Richard Stallman**, a pioneer in the free software movement, which required anyone who modified the program to offer their code at no charge to anyone else who wanted it. Stallman dubbed this a "copyleft," instead of a copyright, license, in homage to its liberal philosophy.

By 1998, seven to eight million users were running Linux. A few million converts to this renegade system was still along way from the roughly 250 million using Windows, but Linux won over more than just a loose-knit collection of disgruntled techno-geeks. Linux became the operating system preferred by people running Internet servers, the computers that route traffic on the **World Wide Web** and provide web sites to users. Smaller servers on local area networks began using it, too, and it started to seep into businesses as computer network administrators got word of it and its reliable nature. Soon, some big players had begun installing Linux, helping transform it from an underground, cultish product for the techno-elite to one with a promising future for the masses.

In April of 1998 Linux was installed on 68 personal computers combined together into a "supercomputer" at Los Alamos National Laboratory in order to run a program to simulate atomic shock waves. In addition, Linux was installed on machines at NASA, the United States Postal Service, and in administrative offices for the U.S. Navy and the Boeing Company, and is also the operating system that runs computers at Digital Domain, a special effects firm hired for the film *Titanic*. The telecommunications giant Southwestern Bell also installed Linux and found that it helped decrease their costs because of its stability—when a network goes down, productivity is stalled, and thus profits are chipped away. Whereas most Windows users find they need to reboot their systems at least weekly or more, Linux users are finding that their computers can run for months without a reboot.

Linux still has a ways to go before it will be competitive with Microsoft or Unix. Some naysayers counter that Linux is difficult to install and use, and that the only means of technical support is by time-consuming communications with other users via the Internet. A solution to the support dilemma came along when companies like Red Hat and others offered their own version of Linux and accompanying technical support for $50, thus providing a more efficient way to obtain answers. This made the system more commercially viable. In 1996 a version of Linux released by Red Hat Software won the award for best desktop computer operating system from *InfoWorld*, a trade magazine. Red Hat also began working on a graphic interface it dubbed GNOME to make it more user-friendly.

The future for Linux seemed sealed when technology behemoths Netscape and **Intel** each purchased a stake in the tiny, North Carolina–based Red Hat in late 1998. Intel vice president Sean Maloney said at the time, "The investment in

Linux is clearly a reflection of (its) growing importance and influence in the business community," according to an article by Karlin Lillington in the *St. Louis Post-Dispatch*. In April of 1999, Dell computers purchased an interest in Red Hat as well, and announced it would start selling a line of computers running Linux. Meanwhile, Microsoft Corporation president Steve Ballmer indicated that his firm considered Linux a threat, and hinted that Microsoft may even consider eventually making available some of its code for Windows.

Torvalds is married; his wife's name is Tove, and she was the reigning karate champion of Finland for six years. They have two daughters, Patricia and Daniela, and live in a tract house in Santa Clara, California, which is filled with stuffed penguins—the mascot of Linux, because Torvalds finds them friendly and sympathetic. Though he is one of the most popular icons among the computer-savvy, Torvalds has not made a cent from his creation. However, his reputation earned him a job at Transmeta, a secretive start-up firm in Santa Clara in 1997. The company is partially financed by Microsoft cofounder **Paul Allen**, and is reportedly involved in chip design or operating systems. He and his family left Finland so he could accept the six-figure salary in Silicon Valley. Torvalds's hobbies include reading and playing snooker.

# TRANSISTOR

The transistor is the fundamental component of most analog and digital circuits. A transistor consists of a piece semiconducting crystal (usually silicon, but sometimes germanium or gallium arsenide) with which impurities such as antimony, bismuth, arsenic, and phosphorous have been mixed by a process called *doping*. Doping increases the semiconductor's conductivity (tendency to carry electric current) by introducing free electrons that act as negatively-charged current carriers or, conversely, by introducing positively-charged gaps in the **semiconductor** crystal's electron structure, *holes*, which act as positively-charged current carriers. The difference between the number of electrons in the outermost orbital of the added impurity (*dopant*) and that of the host semiconductor determines whether the dopant introduces extra electrons (producing regions of "*n*-type" semiconductor) or extra holes (producing regions of "*p*-type" semiconductor).

In 1926 Julius Edgar Lilienfield of New York filed a patent on what is now acknowledged as the blueprint for an *n-p-n* junction transistor. Lilienfield's title for his proposed device was *Method and Apparatus for Controlling Electric Currents*, but it was never developed into a commercial application. In the mid-1940s, in order to expand and improve its telephone business, AT&T's Bell Telephone Laboratories began to develop a solid-state semiconductor switch to replace the vacuum tube. As a result, a team of scientists led by experimental physicist **Walter Brattain** (1902–1987), theoretical physicist **John Bardeen** (1908–1991), and theoretician and project team leader **William Shockley** (1910–1989) developed the first practical transistor in December 1947, a *point-contact*

device made from gold foil and a chunk of germanium. Upon learning of this invention Shockley developed the *bipolar junction transistor*, which was sturdier and easier to manufacture than Bardeen's and Brattain's device. For these achievements the three scientists shared the 1956 Nobel Prize in physics. Today Shockley is generally noted as the initiator and director of the research program that led to the transistor's discovery, and Brattain and Bardeen are credited with the actual invention of the transistor. The word *transistor* was formed at this time from TRANSfer resISTOR. The company publicly announced the transisto" on June 30, 1948, but its announcement received little attention. Nonetheless, by the 1950s transistors began to rapidly replace vacuum tubes, especially in radios, and eventually became one a key ingredient of all computers.

There are two basic types of transistors, the *bipolar junction* transistor (BJT) and the *field effect* transistor (FET). Both BJTs and FETs exploit the properties of *p*-type and *n*-type doping to enable a *control voltage* to control a current flow, much as a faucet valve controls the flow of water through a pipe. Imagine that a strong flow of water is passing through a faucet: twisting the faucet knob rapidly back and forth will produce a corresponding series of ups and downs in the water flow, turning a fairly small physical signal into a much larger one. This is essentially how analog signal amplification using transistors works. Or, one could simply use the valve to turn the water ON and OFF; this is mode in which transistors are used to process binary signals representing 1s and 0s.

The faucet-control effect is achieved by BJTs and FETs as follows. Both *n*-type and *p*-type regions of doped silicon conduct electricity (i.e., allow charges to flow through them), but differently: An *n*-type region conducts current by passing negative charges—electrons—through its crystal structure, and a *p*-type region does so by shifting holes as if they were mobile positive charges. The central feature of a transistor is the "*p-n* junction"—a plane where a *p*-type region touches an *n*-type region, like cheese lying on bread. The holes in the *p*-type region tend to steal electrons from the parts of *n*-type region they are nearest to (since opposite charges attract), which deprives a thin layer of the *n*-type material at the *p-n* junction of electrons. But without free electrons, *n*-type material has nothing to carry current with; the electron-free layer of *n*-type material thus acts as an insulator, a barrier to current flow, *especially* to current flow which tries to make electrons move further into the *n*-type region, which widens the *depletion layer* (layer depleted of electrons). The *p-n* junction is thus a one-way barrier to electron flow. If a three-layer *n-p-n* sandwich is made, there will two such junctions, one on either side of the *p*-type layer. (One could also build a *p-n-p* sandwich, but for simplicity's sake this discussion will be restricted to the *n-p-n* case.) Clearly, no matter which way one tries to make current flow through two back-to-back *p-n* junctions, one of them will tend to block the current.

The current-valve structure of the transistor is now almost complete. Both BJTs and FETs exploit the *n-p-n* (or *p-n-p*) sandwich structure, but in different ways. (1) A BJT is arranged so that the large current to be controlled tries to flow from one *n*-type layer to the other. Because of the back-to-back *p-n* junctions in the *p-n-p* sandwich, however, it cannot. Therefore wires are attached to the edges of the *p*-type layer in the middle of the sandwich and a control voltage is used to inject electrons into it. Each electron fills in a positively-charged hole; if enough electrons are injected, the *p*-type layer is temporarily and reversibly transformed into a *n*-type layer, possessing extra electrons for conduction. As far as current flow is concerned, there is now an *n-n-n* sandwich, the *p-n* junctions have disappeared, and current can flow through freely. Varying the control voltage varies how many electrons are injected into the *p*-type layer, which in turn controls the amount of current that can flow through the transistor, just as a valve varies the water flowing through a pipe. (2) An FET arranges current to flow *sideways* through the *n-p-n* (or *p-n-p*) sandwich, through the *p*-type layer. Normally the current has no problem doing so, because it can slip easily between the depletion layers above and below the *p-type* layer. But by applying an appropriate voltage to both the *n*-type layers of the sandwich, one can cause the nonconducting depletion layers of the two *p-n* junctions to thicken inward, squeezing the conductive *p-type* path in the middle—perhaps shutting it off completely. Thus, as in the BJT, control of the *supply of charge carriers* implements a current valve.

Although FETs are somewhat slower than BJTs, they are cheaper, smaller and used less power. FETs are used as amplifiers, oscillators, and switches, being very suitable for the amplification of very small signals.

Until the invention of the transistor in 1947, digital circuits were composed of vacuum tubes, which also function as valves for current flow. (British engineering slang for vacuum tubes was "valves.") Compared to tubes, transistors are durable, small, resistant to physical shock, and inexpensive. They also use less energy. At one time, only *discrete* (physically separate) transistor devices existed; normally these were sealed in ceramic or plastic "cans," with wires poking out that could be connected to an **electric circuit**. Although discrete transistors are still used, the vast majority of transistors are built into integrated circuits as parts of microprocessors, **memory** chips, and the like. State-of-the-art microprocessors contain millions of tiny transistors (mostly FETs). Today, transistors are used in virtually every electronic device, including radios, televisions, computers, and communication satellites.

*See also* Integrated circuit; Semiconductor

# TRANSITION

The term transition refers to the property of objects in **object-oriented programming**. Specifically, transition refers to the change in an object's state (the way an **object** is, as determined by the properties of the object) due to the **action** of other objects on it. This can also be referred to as state transition.

An example of transition from the real world concerns the filling of a glass. Initially the state of the glass is empty. A jug of water is used to pour water into the glass. This action of the jug changes the state of the glass from empty to full. If someone pours the water out of the glass, then the state of the glass has been changed yet again, this time back to the original state. Thus, the state of an object (the glass) is affected by the performance of actions associated with other objects.

In object-oriented **programming**, defining all the possible states of a system can be exceedingly complex, because of the myriad of object interactions that might occur. Defining the possible interactions within object classes is commonly done using state transition diagrams.

Programming transition is described as a "goto" **function**. This can be accomplished using the following **operation**: <tab>proceed state. The "state" **attribute** contains the specified **value**. This **argument** defines the new state and so invokes a transition.

In the **Java** programming language, a method called transition specifies a transition from one generation to the next. Functions involved in this type of transition include loops, "if" statements, or the construction of arrays for storing tables.

*See also* Class; Object-oriented programming; State transition diagram

# TRANSVERSAL

Transversal is a computer science term that relates to the dissemination of information via computer networks such as the **Internet**. In a transversal information system, the transfer of information occurs between parties in more of a spider web pattern. This pattern contrasts to the radial pattern of information transfer, where information originates from a central point and radiates outward, through bureaucratic layers, for example.

Transversal dissemination of information can be a people-related process, not a machine dependent process. People communicate with other people, sharing ideas. Computers are merely the tools of information transmission. The information is also organic, capable of change and refinement as two-way communications continue.

Other forms of transversal information systems do require harmony between communicating computers, such as is found in a network. An example is the network of shared information and coordination of **data** that is required in urban traffic control. Transversal communication between traffic sensors provides real-time information about road conditions and traffic flows in order that traffic signal timing can be adjusted to permit smooth movement of vehicles. The systems for traffic control, trip planning, and emergency management require extensive data collection and transmission devices to process this data and to provide operators with timely information on which rational decisions can be made.

Another, similar example is the development of an information system for the sharing of information between municipalities. The data that resides in the myriad **databases** in community's information networks can be shared with other communities. The discussions arising out of the perusal of the data will help formulate new municipal development and regulatory programs. Currently such a system, known as the Cities Agency, is being developed in Europe.

The transversal property of two-way communication facilitating execution of an **action** has been exploited in the development of software termed middleware. Middleware functions to permit program modules or software packages that normally have dissimilar applications to be integrated into a functional package.

A final example of transversal concerns the evolving patterns of service provision by many governments. Traditionally, departments have developed their information infrastructure somewhat independently. Each of these information systems is transversal, with the pattern of information flow being shared and two-way. Now, with the realization that efficiency can be increased by having a "one stop shopping" service, the need for a common site at which the individual information networks can be tapped for information is more pressing. The central repository does not alter the organic nature of the transversal systems. Rather, it attempts to synthesize relevant information so as to convey the important essence of the individual systems to clients. As with the traffic control example, **hardware** modifications are necessary to support the **operation** of the overall system. Computer-telephone software linkage and call distribution machinery are two examples of the necessary hardware.

*See also* Dataflow; Information and information theory

# Traveling salesman problem

Imagine that a salesman must travel to $n$ cities and wants to take the shortest route possible. Assume that the salesman can start from any city on his itinerary and that the distance from city X to city Y is the same as the distance from Y to X (i.e., there exist no one-way shortcuts).

For small values of $n$, the traveling salesman problem (TSP) is simple. With three cities, for example, there is only one possible route; with four cities, three routes exist. Unfortunately, as the number of cities increases, the number of possible routes grows immensely. In general, for $n$ cities, there exist $((n - 1)!) / 2$ routes to consider. (The factorial $(n - 1)! = (n - 1) \cdot (n - 2) \cdot ... \cdot 3 \cdot 2 \cdot 1$.) For a tour of nine cities, there are 20,160 different routes; for $n = 15$, the number of possible routes surpasses one trillion.

Although the traveling salesman problem has been solved for some large values of n, the best algorithm known to date is of order $2^n$, which means that the time required to solve the TSP grows exponentially with the size of the problem. For each 30 cities added to the salesman's route, the time required to solve the problem with today's **algorithms** increases by a factor of one billion, since $2^{30}$ is approximately $10^9$.

Since an exponential algorithm requires too much time to produce a precise answer to the TSP, one might instead turn to a **heuristic** or **greedy algorithm**. A heuristic is a rule or procedure that almost always delivers the right answer. Almost always won't be good enough in some circumstances, but in many occasions a fast, almost-certain-to-be-correct answer will be better than a slow, absolutely correct one.

The TSP is equivalent to a class of mathematical problems called **N-P ("nondeterministic polynomial") complete problems**, which are often used to create security features on computers and networks. No one has proved that a fast algorithm for the TSP, or N-P complete problems in general, doesn't exist, and in the unlikely event that one is discovered, alternative security measures would have to be put into place quickly.

*See also* Algorithm; Greedy algorithm

# Tree

A tree is a type of **data** structure. Data structures are ways for programmers to store and organize data while a program is running. Different data structures are used to perform different tasks on data efficiently.

A tree is composed of nodes. Each **node** has an item of data and a connection to other nodes. There are many types of trees, such as binary, B+, **heap**, AVL, and red-black. Every tree is a collection of nodes that is identified by a special node known as the *root*. The root of a tree (usually drawn at the top) is connected to other nodes. These are known as *internal nodes*. The internal nodes are connected to more internal nodes. The structure continues to branch down until the bottom nodes are reached. These nodes, to which no more nodes are connected, are called *leaves*. When drawn with the root at the top, and the leaf nodes at the bottom, the structure resembles a family tree. For this reason, a node is called the **parent** of the nodes that branch down from it. The root has no parents, and the leaves have no children.

All nodes in a tree, including the root and leaves, are simply nodes that each contain an item of data. The root and leaves are only special in that they are at the top and bottom of the tree, respectively. Every node can be thought of as the root of a small tree. That tree contains the node itself, and all its children, grandchildren, and so forth, down to the leaves.

A tree node may have any number of children. Sometimes children are all treated as equals, and sometimes the children have a special ordering to them. In either case, there are two main ways to traverse a tree. A traversal of a tree is the process of accessing every node and doing something with the data at that node, such as displaying it on the screen.

A breadth first traversal consists of first accessing the data at the root. Then data at the children of the root is accessed. Then the data at the root's grandchildren is accessed, until finally, the data at the leaves is accessed. This causes each level of the tree to be reached in turn from top to bottom.

A depth first traversal first follows a single path from the root to one of the leaves, accessing the data at each node along the way. Then a path from the root to a different leaf is chosen. Any nodes that were already accessed along a previous path are not accessed again. Successive paths differ as little as possible. Once all the leaves (and thus all other nodes) have been accessed, the traversal is complete.

There are three variations of depth first traversal: *pre-order*, *post-order*, and *in-order*. During a pre-order traversal, the data of a parent is accessed before any of its children's data is accessed. During a post-order traversal, the data of a parent is accessed after all of its children's data has been accessed. During an in-order traversal, the data of a parent node is accessed after some of its children, and before others.

The simplest, and perhaps the most useful, tree is a *binary tree*. Every node has 2 children: a left child, and a right child. Sometimes one or both of the children are not present for a specific node, such as the leaf nodes. Binary trees are an efficient way to store data for a binary search. To accomplish this, every node's data is always "greater" than the data of its left child, and "less" than the data of its right child. "Greater" could mean larger if the data is a number, or later alphabetically if the data is words, or any other meaningful way to order the items of data stored at the nodes. A binary search on a binary tree consists of checking for the desired **value** (search key) in the root. If the search key is greater than the root's value, the search continues to the right child. Otherwise, it continues to the left child. The search key is compared to each node's value along the way until a match is found. Each time a match is not found, the search continues to the correct child. Due to the properties of a binary tree, there is no **backtracking** in this algorithm. An in-order depth first traversal of a binary tree accesses all the data in sorted order.

A general tree with an arbitrary number of children to each node is a useful **data structure** for evaluating possible moves of a game such as chess. The data at each node is a configuration of the board. The root contains the start configuration. The children of any node are the configurations after performing a possible legal move. Therefore, the children of the root each represent one possible opening move. A typical game of chess has an average of 25 possible moves per play. However, some board configurations are so bad that the children of that node are never explored. That is called *pruning* the tree. Some board configurations are better than others, and they should be explored first. When two children of the same parent are explored in a specific order for reasons such as the one mentioned above, the procedure is called *node ordering*.

Trees are efficient because in general, data can be extracted or inserted by taking a direct path from the root to one of the leaves. This path contains log n nodes, where n is the total number of nodes in the tree. This is only true when the tree is well balanced. If every node of a binary tree only has a left child, then the tree degenerates into a linear linked-list. A path from the root to the leaf contains *every* node. There are ways to keep trees balanced, such as using red-black, or AVL trees, which ensure that there are about as many left children as right children.

Implementing trees and **algorithms** for traversing or **searching** them ranges from very simple, to extremely complex. Usually trees are made only as complex as they need to be to assure that the implementation will be correct and efficient. Most of the algorithms that use trees are recursive because of the recursive nature of trees. Like **linked-lists**, and **arrays**, trees are an indispensable data structure.

# TUNNICLIFFE, WILLIAM (1922-1996)
*American engineer*

William Tunnicliffe was one of the founders of **Standard Generalized Markup Language** (**SGML**), and is often remembered as the father of generic coding. Historically, electronic manuscripts contained control codes ("macros") that caused the document to be formatted in a manner called "specific coding." In contrast, *generic coding*, which began in the late 1960s, uses descriptive tags (for example, "heading" rather than "format-17"). Generic coding eventually evolved into Generalized Markup Language.

*Generalized Markup Language* (GML), created by **International Business Machines**'s (**IBM**'s) Charles Goldfarb, Edward Mosher, and Raymond Lorie, was based on the generic coding ideas of Stanley Rice and Tunnicliffe. GML was invented to describe a document in terms of the relationship between organization structure and content parts. Instead of a simple tagging scheme, GML introduced the concept of a formally defined document type with an explicit nested element structure. Major portions of GML were implemented in specific IBM **applications** and achieved considerable industry acceptance. GML eventually evolved into Standard Generalized Markup Language.

*Standard Generalized Markup Language* is a generic "markup" language used by publishers and multimedia companies for organizing and tagging documents in order to solve problems arising from incompatibility between text editing, formatting, and database applications. A document encoded in SGML has information that directs how the text is formatted. For instance, the beginning of a chapter is marked with the text **string** <chapter>, while the chapter's end is marked with </chapter>. The computer interprets this markup in order to process the encoded information for the desired output format. The web-based Hypertext Markup Language (**HTML**) is an example of an SGML-based language. Tunnicliffe provided superb diplomatic and negotiating skills during the development of the SGML international standard while a member of the **American National Standards Institute** (**ANSI**) and **International Organization for Standardization** (**ISO**) committees.

Tunnicliffe was born and raised in Washington, D.C., but lived most of his adulthood in Winchester, Massachusetts. He graduated from Worcester Polytechnic Institute (WPI) in 1943 and Harvard in 1951, where he received degrees in applied physics and engineering sciences. Between college programs, Tunnicliffe enlisted in the United States Navy, attaining the rank of captain that he held until 1982 while in the Navy Reserves. Tunnicliffe worked with Raytheon Corporation and the Courier Citizen newspaper in Lowell, Massachusetts before leaving to start Tunnicliffe Associates, a Winchester-based engineering firm that he operated for 10 years before retiring.

Many historians credit the start of the generic coding movement to a presentation made by William Tunnicliffe while chairperson of the Graphic Communications Association (GCA) Composition Committee. During a meeting at the Canadian Government Printing Office in September 1967

Tunnicliffe presented his now-famous topic involving the separation of information content of documents from their format.

*See also* Code; SGML (Standard Generalized Markup Language)

# TURING, ALAN (1912-1954)
*English mathematician*

Mathematician Alan Turing is recognized as a pioneer in computer theory. His classic 1936 paper, "On Computable Numbers, with an Application to the Entscheidungs Problem," detailed a machine that served as a model for the first working computers. During World War II, Turing took part in the top-secret ULTRA project and helped decipher German military codes. During this same time, Turing conducted groundbreaking work that led to the first operational digital electronic computers. Another notable paper was published in 1950 and offered what became known as the "Turing Test" to determine if a machine possessed intelligence.

Alan Mathison Turing was born on June 23, 1912, in Paddington, England, to Julius Mathison Turing and Ethel Sara Stoney. Turing's father served in the British civil service in India, and his wife generally accompanied him. Thus, for the majority of their childhoods, Alan and his older brother, John, saw very little of their parents. While in elementary school, the young Turing boys were raised by a retired military couple, the Wards. At the age of 13, Turing entered Sherbourne school, a boys' boarding school in Dorset. His record at Sherbourne was not generally outstanding; he was later remembered as untidy and disinterested in scholastic learning. He did, however, distinguish himself in mathematics and science, showing a particular facility for calculus. Turing also developed an interest in competitive running while at Sherbourne.

Turing twice failed to gain entry to Trinity College in Cambridge, but was accepted on scholarship at King's College (also in Cambridge). He graduated in 1934 with a master's degree in mathematics. In 1936 Turing produced his first, and perhaps greatest, work. His paper "On Computable Numbers, with an Application to the Entscheidungs Problem," answered a logical problem staged by German mathematician David Hilbert. The question involved the completeness of logic—whether all mathematical problems could, in principle, be solved. Turing's paper, presented in 1937 to the London Mathematical Society, proved that some could not be solved. Turing's paper also contained a footnote describing a theoretical automatic machine, which came to be known as the **Turing Machine**, that could solve any mathematical problem—provided it was give the proper **algorithms**, or problem-solving equations or instructions. Although it may not have been Turing's intent at the time, his Turing Machine defined the modern computer.

After graduating from Cambridge, Turing was invited to spend a year in the United States studying at Princeton University. He returned to Princeton for a second year—on a

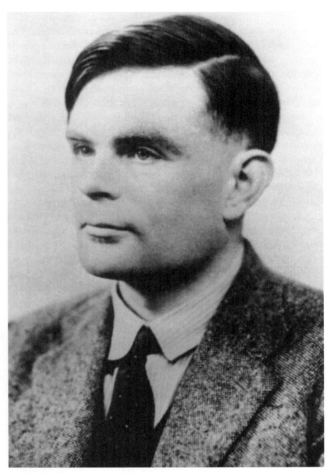

**Alan Turing**

Proctor Fellowship—to finish his doctorate. While there, he worked on the subject of **computability** with Alonso Church and other mathematicians. Turing and his associates worked with binary numbers (1 and 0) and **Boolean Algebra**, developed by **George Boole**, to develop a system of equations called logic gates. These logic gates were useful for producing problem-solving algorithms such as would be needed by an automatic computing machine. From the initial paper exercise, it was a simple matter to develop logic gates into electrical **hardware**, using relays and switches, which could—theoretically, and in huge quantities—actually perform the work of a computing machine. As a sideline, Turing put together the first three or four stages of an electric multiplier, using relays he constructed himself. After receiving his doctorate, Turing had an opportunity to remain at Princeton, but decided to accept a Cambridge fellowship instead. He returned to England in 1938.

Cryptology, the making and breaking of coded messages, was greatly advanced in England after World War I. The German high command, however, had modified a device called the **Enigma machine** that mechanically enciphered messages. The English found little success in defeating this method. The original Enigma machine was not new, or even secret; a basic Enigma machine had been in **operation** for several years, mostly used to produce commercial codes. The Germans' alterations, though, greatly increased the number of possible letter combinations in a **message**. The Allies were able to duplicate the modifications, but it was a continual cat-and-mouse game; each time Allied analysts figured out a message, the Germans' changes made all of their work useless.

In the fall of 1939, Turing found himself in a top-secret installation in Bletchley, where he played a critical role in the development of a machine that deciphered the Enigma's messages by testing key codes until it found the correct combinations. This substitution method was uncomplicated, but impractical to apply because possible combinations could range into the tens of millions. Here Turing was able to put his experience at Princeton to good use; no one else had bridged the gap between abstract logic theory and electric hardware as he had with his electric multiplier. Turing helped construct relay-driven decoders (which were called Bombes, after the ticking noise of the relays) that shortened the code-breaking time from weeks to hours. The Bombes helped uncover German movements, particularly the U-boat war in the Atlantic, for almost two years. Eventually, however, the Germans changed their codes and the new level of complexity was too high to be solved practically by electrical decoders. British scientists agreed that although a Bombe of sufficient size could be made for further deciphering work, the machine would be slow and impractical.

Yet other advances would prove advantageous for the decoding machine. Vacuum tubes used as switches (the British called them thermiotic valves) used no moving parts and were a thousand times faster than electrical relays. A decoder made with tubes could do in minutes what it took a Bombe several hours to accomplish. Thus work began on a device which was later named Collosus. Based on the same theoretical principles as earlier Bombes, Collosus was the first operational digital electronic computer. It used 1800 vacuum tubes, proving the practicality of this approach. Much information concerning Collosus remained classified by the British government in the early 1990s. Some claimed that Turing supervised the construction of the first Collosus.

Many stories were circulated about Turing during the war; mostly surrounding his eccentricity. Andrew Hodges noted in his book *Alan Turing, The Enigma,* "With holes in his sports jacket, shiny grey flannel trousers held up with an ancient tie, and hair sticking out at the back, he became the cartoonist's 'boffin'—an impression accentuated by his manner of practical work, in which he would grunt and swear as solder failed to stick, scratch his head and make a strange squelching noise as he thought to himself." Unconvinced of England's chances to win the war, Turing converted all of his funds to two silver bars, buried them, and was later unable to locate them. He was horrified at the sight of blood, was an outspoken atheist, and was a homosexual. Still, for his unquestionably vital role in the British war effort, he was later awarded the Order of the British Empire, a high honor for someone not in the combat military.

In the waning months of the war, Turing turned his thoughts back to computing machines. He conceived of a device, built with vacuum tubes, that would be able to perform any function described in mathematical terms and would carry instructions in electronic symbols in its **memory**. This universal machine, clearly an embodiment of the Turing machine described in his 1936 paper, would not require separate hardware for different functions, only a change of instructions. Turing was not alone in his ambition to construct a computing machine. A group at the University of Pennsylvania had built a computer called **ENIAC (Electronic Numerical Integrator and Computer)** that was similar to, but more complex, than **Colossus**. In the process, they had concluded that a better machine was possible. Turing's **design** was possibly more remarkable because he was working alone out of his home while they were a large university research group with the full backing of the American military. The American group published well before Turing did, but the British government subsequently took a greater interest in Turing's work.

In June of 1945 Turing joined the newly formed Mathematics Division of the National Physical Laboratory (NPL). Here he finalized plans for his Automatic Computing Engine (ACE). The rather archaic term "engine" was chosen by NPL management as a tribute to **Charles Babbage**'s **Analytical Engine** (and also because it made a pleasing acronym). Turing, however, was unprepared for the inertia and politics of a bureaucratic government foundation. All of his previous engineering projects had been conducted during wartime, when time was of the essence and no budget constraints existed. More than a year after the ACE project was approved, though, no engineering work had been completed and there was little cooperation between participants. A scaled-down version of the ACE was finally completed in 1950. But Turing had already left NPL in 1948, frustrated at the slow pace of the computer's development.

In 1950 Turing produced a widely read paper titled "Computing Machinery and Intelligence." This classic paper expanded on one of Turing's interests—if computers could possess intelligence. He proposed a test called the "Imitation Game," still used today under the name "Turing Test." In the test, an interrogator was connected by teletype (later, by computer keyboard) to either a human or a computer at a remote location. The interrogator is allowed to pose any questions and, based on the replies, the interrogator must decide whether a human or a computer is at the other end of the line. If the interrogator cannot distinguish between the two in a statistically significant number of cases, then **artificial intelligence** has been achieved. Turing predicted that within fifty years, computers could be programmed to play the game so effectively that after a five-minute question period the interrogator would have no more than a seventy-percent chance of making the proper identification.

Turing's personal life deteriorated in the early 1950s. After leaving NPL he took a position with Manchester College as deputy director of the newly formed Royal Society Computing Laboratory. But he was not involved in designing or building the computer on which they were working. By this time, Turing was no longer a world-class mathematician, having for too long been sidetracked by electronic engineering, nor was he an engineer: The scientific world seemed to be passing him by.

While at Manchester, Turing had an affair with a young street person named Arnold Murray, which led to a burglary at his house by one of Murray's associates. The investigating police learned of the relationship between Turing and Murray; in fact Turing did nothing to hide it. Homosexuality was a felony in England at the time, and Turing was tried and convicted of "gross indecency" in 1952. Because of his social class and relative prominence, he was sentenced to a year's probation and given treatments of the female hormone estrogen in lieu of serving a year in jail.

Turing committed suicide by eating a cyanide-laced apple on June 7, 1954. His death puzzled his associates; he had been free of the hormone treatments for a year, and, although a stigma remained, he had weathered the incident with his career intact. He left no note, nor had he given any hint that he had contemplated this act. His mother tried for years to have his death declared accidental, but the official cause of death was never seriously questioned.

# TURING MACHINE

In 1936 English mathematician and computer theorist **Alan Turing** (1912–1954), while studying at Cambridge University, began work in predicate logic. His studies led in 1937 to a proof that certain mathematical problems could be solved by automation. Turing postulated a universal machine—the Turing machine, which would function by passing through a series of discrete states or steps, assuming only one of a possibly infinite list of internal states at any given moment.

Turing described his machine in the paper *On Computable Numbers with an Application to the Entscheidungsproblem* ("decidability problem"). The Turing Machine consists of the following components: (1) An infinitely long *input/output tape* stretched like a scroll between rollers so it can be wound forwards and backwards. The tape is marked off into squares, each marked with a 0 or 1. (2) A *read/write head* that sits above the tape, scanning one symbol at a time, and is always in a particular internal state (which it indicates by displaying a number on its exterior). The head has the ability to read, write, or erase any single square on the input/output tape, and may change to another internal state at any moment. (3) The *rule list*, stored in the read/write head, which determines the machine's changes of state at any particular point.

The machine begins computation in some given state. It then scans a 0 or 1 from the tape, either leaving that symbol alone or replacing it with its opposite state; finally, it moves to the next square on the tape (scrolling the tape left or right, depending on the machine's internal state). The machine's behavior thus depends on three factors: (1) The machine's *state*. (2) The *number* on the scanned square. (3) The *rule list*. The rule list specifies, for each internal state and binary input, what the machine should write, which direction it should move in, and which state it should go into. For example, suppose the machine is in state 32 and the head reads a 0. The machine consults its rule list and finds rule "32-0-17-R," which means: "If you are in state 32 and read a 0, then change to state 17 and advance the tape head to the right." The output of the machine could be read off the appropriate parts of the tape once the machine had stopped.

One problem with Turing machines, it seems, is that a different machine would have to be constructed for every new computation: that is, a new rule list would have to be built into the device. But Turing realized that any algorithm, or set of procedures for accomplishing some computational task, can be written as a set of instructions. A "universal" Turing machine can thus be constructed to do, if supplied with the proper sequence of instructions (on the tape), what any other particular Turing machine can do. In other words, one machine can be programmed for all possible tasks, for the 1s and 0s on a tape can the behavior of any machine.

The concept of the Turing machine is the foundation of the modern theory of computation. Indeed, the universal Turing machine embodies the essential principle of the computer: a single machine can perform any well-defined task if supplied with the appropriate program. The Turing machine is considered the theoretical prototype of the digital computer because it incorporates the computer's key processing features: (1) *input/output device* (tape and reader), (2) *memory* (read/write head or control mechanism storage), and (3) *central processing unit* (control mechanism that interprets the rules vis-à-vis the input bits). Although an actual Turing machine would never be built, as a thought-experiment which reduces the concept of computation to its ultimate, stripped-down extreme it has proved essential to the theory of computation.

# TURING TEST

The Turing test was developed by British mathematician **Alan M. Turing** as a means of assessing the capabilities of a computer to process information like a human brain. Turing devised a subjective test to answer the question "Can machines think?"

In a 1950 paper entitled "Computing Machinery and Intelligence," Turing argued that computers would, in time, be programmed to acquire abilities that would rival human intelligence. This would be possible if the operations in the human brain were executed in a computational manner. The Turing test arose from this paper.

In the test, a human questioner is placed in an isolated environment. In the original Turing test, the human used a computer **terminal** that was, in turn, connected to two unseen terminals. One of these unseen terminals was under human control, while the other was controlled by computer software. The task of the interrogator is to pose questions and to use the answers to distinguish between a computer and a human. If a distinction cannot be made, then the computer is considered intelligent.

Over the years, the number of questions submitted for use in the Turing test has increased to over 9,000. Some of these questions are:

- Are you a computer?
- How old are you?
- What is your favorite flavor of ice cream?
- Do you believe in life after love?
- What do you like to do in your spare time?

With time, the Turing test has broadened in its application. Now a machine passes the Turing test if it can convince the interrogator that it is human; another human need not be part of the test.

*See also* Artificial intelligence; Turing machine

# TURNPIKE PROBLEM

The term turnpike problem relates to the transmission of information via electronic networks such as the **Internet**. Specifically, a turnpike problem refers to the congestion that can arise on an electronic route, typically involving **e-mail**, because of the electronic traffic that is on the route.

The derivation of the term turnpike problem is the problem with congestion of vehicular traffic on high-speed turnpikes. Traffic flow proceeds smoothly and swiftly when relatively few vehicles are moving along the turnpike and when no obstructions are present. However, traffic flow can slow or even stop when the number of vehicles present exceeds the capacity of the system or when an obstacle, such as an accident or construction, blocks a portion of the route or exit.

When messages are sent from one destination to another, they can take a circuitous route from one **Internet Service Provider (ISP)** to another. For example, the following is an actual route an e-mail **message** might take from an ISP in Rutland, Vermont to a location in Texas. When the message is sent from the sender's computer, it moves to a Postal Service Protocol (**POP**) in White River Junction, Vermont. The message continues to the ISPs main POP in Lebanon, New Hampshire. From there it moves onto a super high speed Internet backbone, a broadband connection, and a sort of electronic superhighway on which much electronic information is moving. This and other high speed connections route the message to Manchester, New Hampshire, then Boston, Massachusetts, then New York City, then to several other locations until it arrives at the ISP used by the message recipient. At this point the message is handled by that ISP that, in turn, routes the message to their mail server and, finally, into the recipient's computer mailbox.

Similar circuitous routes can be taken when information is requested from a web site.

This entire process can take only seconds. However, slowdowns can occur in times of heavy electronic traffic, such as during business hours and in the evenings. There are many places where the packets of information can slow down or halt, due to obstructions. This is the turnpike problem.

One cause of the turnpike problem relates to the communication between the different ISP **hardware** along the route. The transfer of information packets involves the "passing off" of the information from one server to another. The speed at which one computer connects with another and releases the information packet can be prolonged. Since the speed of delivery is governed by the speed of the slowest component, the transmission will slow.

This bottleneck is exacerbated when many packets are passing through the same point. The nature of the electronic highway is a one-dimensional, source to point set-up, where the packets lie on a line. If information could enter and exit the highway randomly and in three dimensions, then problems associated with 'points on a line' would disappear. For the present, however, the identification of bottlenecks caused by slow servers and remediation efforts are the most cost effective methods to insure maximum transmission speed.

*See also* Client-server interaction; Data flow

# TWO'S COMPLEMENT ARITHMETIC

The on-and-off voltages manipulated inside a digital computer are, by convention, usually interpreted as "ones" and "zeroes." Strings of ones and zeroes are, by a further act of interpretation, usually held to represent larger numbers. However, no one system of interpretation is mandatory. For example, "0000" is always, in practice, read as decimal 0, and "0001" as decimal 1, but it could have been the other way around. Any mapping of voltages to numbers is, ultimately, arbitrary.

There are practical consequences to this freedom of interpretation. Consider the question of representing positive and negative integers using N bits. N bits allow for $2^N$ different orderings of ones and zeroes. How should one interpret each of these $2^N$ strings? There are three basic answers: (1) the sign-and-magnitude (S&M) system, (2) the radix complement system (of which two's complement arithmetic is a special case), and (3) the digit complement system. The first two are discussed below; a version of the third, the *one's complement* system, is also used in computers but will not be described here.

The S&M system is the most intuitive. In it, one interprets the leftmost (most significant) **bit** not as "1" or "0" but as "+" or "-." (By convention, the same physical device state is used for "0" and for "+.") One uses the remaining N-1 bits to represent positive magnitudes; for example, if N = 5 then the 4 digits to the right of the sign bit are interpreted as 0001 = 1, 0010 = 2, 0011 = 3, and so on. In this system, 00001 = +1 (leading 0 specifies plus sign), 10001 = -1 (leading 1 specifies minus sign), and so on. The S&M system has the peculiarity that there are two zeroes, a positive zero and a negative zero (00000 and 10000, respectively, for 5-bit word length)—two distinct binary numbers which are computationally equivalent.

Consider the addition of two S&M numbers, say +2 and -10:

$$
\begin{array}{rl}
0\ 0\ 0\ 1\ 0 & [2] \\
+\ \underline{1\ 1\ 0\ 1\ 0} & [\text{-}10] \\
1\ 1\ 0\ 0\ 0 & [\text{-}8]
\end{array}
$$

It is notable here that the simplest way of adding the operands (i.e., bit by bit, starting with the rightmost, or least significant, bit) would produce a wrong answer, namely 11100 (-12). On the other hand, adding +2 and *positive* 10 proceeds as follows:

$$
\begin{array}{rl}
0\ 0\ 0\ 1\ 0 & [2] \\
+\ \underline{0\ 1\ 0\ 1\ 0} & [10] \\
0\ 1\ 1\ 0\ 0 & [12]
\end{array}
$$

Here the correct result *is* achieved by ordinary bitwise addition starting with the least significant bit. It follows that when performing addition in the S&M system, one must apply *different addition rules to the individual bits of the operands depending on their signs*. This increases complexity—more **hardware** or more computation or both. Since binary multiplication and division of integers are achieved by repeated additions, the need for a more complex **adder circuit** affects the other basic numerical operations as well. Is there a number system that allows use of the same rules for any two numbers?

There are at least two such. The one in almost universal usage is the two's complement system, which may be understood in terms of *modulo arithmetic*—that is, arithmetic which uses a closed or circular number system. A familiar example of such a system is the numbering of the hours on an analog clock face.

Imagine the face of a clock with its numbers in the usual places, only with a 0 at the top instead of a 12. As an adder, such a clock has odd properties. Two o'clock plus 3 hours is five o'clock (2 + 3 = 5), but ten o'clock plus 3 hours is *one* o'clock (10 + 3 = 1?). In the latter case, adding a relatively large number actually has the effect of a *subtraction*—of adding a negative number. This property can be used to advantage as follows.

Define all the hours from 0 to 5 literally—that is, let 2:00 stand for +2, 3:00 for +3, and so on. The rest of the clock shall be used to represent negative numbers. Consider what happens if we declare that 11:00 codes for -1. To add -1 to 3 we would then *physically* add 11 to 3, which means starting at 3:00 and moving 11 hours clockwise to 2:00. This gives the correct answer (-1 + 3 = 2). (If this not clear to your mind's eye, sketch a clock.) All the hours later than 5:00 can be used to "code" for negative numbers in this fashion as follows:

-1 = 11:00
-2 = 10:00
-3 = 9:00
-4 = 8:00
-5 = 7:00
-6 = 6:00

Each number on the dial thus has a *complement* or negative version of itself on the other side. (The exceptions are 0, which needs no complement, and -6, which has none in this system.) Note that the numbers to be *physically* added are always the hours themselves, and that all additions are performed by the same physical process, namely clockwise movement around the dial, which recalls our desire to use only one kind of adding mechanism in the digital realm. Note also that in this system no additions are valid that give results greater than 5 or less than -6; for instance, "5 + 4 = 9" cannot

be calculated on this very crude processor because there is no way to represent a 9. (9:00 is reserved to **code** for -3.) In digital computing, any such attempt to produce a non-representable result is called an *overflow*.

To avoid **overflow** in practical computations, we need a bigger clock. This is exactly, in effect, what the two's complement number system provides. In the two's complement system, all $2^N$ binary numbers are treated (in effect) as if they were arranged around a vast clock face, starting with 0 at noon and continuing clockwise in order of magnitude. Half these $2^N$ numbers (those with a "1" for most significant bit) occupy the space from 6:00 to noon and are defined as negative. Arithmetic proceeds exactly as in the 12-hour system described above, only with many more numbers (for a 32-bit word, over 4 billion numbers). Just as the most negative number on the clock (-6) had no positive complement, the most negative number in two's complement has no positive complement. In the binary system, too, just as on the clock, the same procedures apply to adding all numbers, whether positive or negative. Note that in two's complement representation the most significant bit of every word can (as in the S&M system) be viewed as a sign bit, in the sense that every number with a leading 1 is negative. However, to change a number from positive to negative or vice versa it does *not*, in two's complement, suffice to reverse its sign bit.

The two's complement of a binary number may be produced very simply, in hardware or by hand, without resorting to visualizations of clocks or circular number systems. Given a binary number M, start with the rightmost bit and copy all bits up to and including the first 1 encountered; then complement (flip from 0 to 1 or vice versa) all the remaining bits. The two's complement of 010110, for example, is obtained as follows:

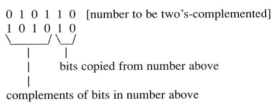

Reversing the sign of a number thus is more complex in the two's complement system than in the S&M system (where flipping the sign bit is all that is necessary). However, sign reversal can still be accomplished in a single clock cycle by a simple circuit.

Because the computational tasks involved in manipulating floating-point numbers are different from those for manipulating fixed-point numbers, such as the integers treated above, two's complement is not used to code floating-point numbers.

*See also* Floating-point arithmetic; Overflow

# TYPE CAST

A type cast is an instruction from the programmer to the **compiler** for it to treat a **variable** or **object** of one type (see entry on types) as if it were of another. The "type" of a variable or object is a classification of what kind of **data** or real-world "thing" it represents. Type-casting is a feature mostly associated with statically-typed languages, where the compiler needs to know the type of all objects in the program before it can create the executable **code**.

Typically, a type-cast is indicated to the compiler like this:

<type a> variable = (<type a>) object

where "object" is of a different type from "type a." By example, to cast from a char to an integer:

char a = 'a';

int b = (int)a;

Type-casting is potentially very dangerous because the programmer is relieving the compiler of the responsibility of ensuring that objects are being used only where and how they are supposed to be used. Because of this, the compiler still makes some checks and, depending on the language, will forbid type-casts that are outside its set of internal rules.

**C** and **C++** have a very relaxed set of rules and will happily cast between pointers to data structures and classes that are of completely unrelated type, integers, and characters without complaint. The trouble is that the compiler will believe what it is told and if the programmer has made an error and at run-time the program tries to do the wrong thing with an object, the best that can happen is catastrophic failure.

**Java** has a more robust method in that not only will it forbid certain casts at compile-time, but it will also check again at run time to make sure the object can do what it has been told it can do. If it detects the wrong type of object, it can report an error that the programmer can arrange to trap rather than having the whole program die horribly.

# TYPES

One of the fundamental issues in **programming** languages is the "types" of objects or **data** primitives they afford to programmers. Fundamentally, these **object** types fall into the following categories:

- Boolean—this is a type, sometimes abbreviated BOOL, for representing truth **value**, which can take the logical values True or False (sometimes represented as 1 and 0, but without the normal numeric connotation). A Boolean type typically cannot be converted to anything else.

- Integer—this is a type, sometimes abbreviated INT, for representing whole numbers, either positive of negative. The integer type has siblings SHORT and LONG (sometimes called SHORT INT and LONG INT), vide infra.

- Floating point—this is a type, sometimes abbreviated FLOAT, used to represent rational numbers. The float type has siblings DOUBLE and LONG DOUBLE, vide infra.

- Character—this is a type, sometimes abbreviated CHAR, used to represent alphanumeric strings.

The basic integer object type in **C**, **C++**, **Java**, and other programming languages is called INT. Generally, the specification of the programming language itself does not specify the size of an INT—that depends on the **hardware** and on the **compiler** used. Thus, the size of an INT may be said to be "implementation dependent," to mean that the creator of the compiler is free to choose this size given the constraints of the hardware and the needs of his intended market. On most contemporary PC systems, INT is a 32-bit signed number; "signed" because it always has a positive or negative sign associated with it, to show whether a positive integer or a negative integer is being referred to. On larger systems, INT may be a 64-bit signed number. Some programming languages also provide for types SHORT and LONG—these are also implementation dependent, but the specification usually requires that INT be no shorter than SHORT and no longer than LONG.

The basic rational number object type is FLOAT, the floating-point type. There is no type for real numbers such as $\pi$ (because infinite fractional expansions cannot be handled on a computer), so real numbers are approximated by using FLOAT. Analogous to the INT case, greater **precision** may be obtained by use of DOUBLE and still greater by LONG DOUBLE. The sizes of these types are generally not dictated by the programming language specification, and are compiler dependent—most commonly, FLOAT is a 32-bit IEEE 754 floating-point number, while DOUBLE is a 64-bit IEEE 754 floating-point number.

The character object type CHAR is related to the integer object type. Each character (such as letters a-z, A-Z, &, %, #, @, etc.) is encoded as an integer; there is a table or encoding scheme where an integer in a certain range represents a particular character. The encoding scheme used is called the character set. Early **IBM** mainframes used the **EBCDIC** character set with each character represented by an 8-bit integer; the **ASCII** character set, in much wider use, uses a 7-bit integer. The CHAR data type traditionally used an 8-bit integer, even with ASCII, but newer languages like Java use an 16-bit **Unicode** character set, to allow for the use of special symbols, characters from languages other than English, and so on. It is important to note that the CHAR type can hold numbers as well, as long as they are treated as mere strings rather than entities to be manipulated for computation.

A programming language is said to be "strongly typed" if it requires that all variables be defined as being of a certain type before they are first used in a program, and that no **variable** be used in a manner corresponding to a type other than the one it is declared as (such as declaring a variable to be a CHAR, but then using it as an integer). A "weakly typed" language has the opposite quality and allows variables to be used without first being defined, and also may allow variables to be used in a maner inconsistent with their **declarations**. Java is an example of a strongly typed language, and C is an example of a weakly typed language. The advantage of strong typing is considered to be a reduced risk of careless mistakes on the part of programmers—because every variable must be declared before first use, a certain accounting of procedures and ideas is forced, which may be useful in larger programs with many variables that interact in complex ways. Strong typing is also considered to improve the security features of the language. Weak typing is the more traditional approach, and is preferred by some programmers for the greater freedom it affords them.

*See also* ASCII; Compilers; Computer architecture; Programming; Unicode

# TYPESETTING

Typesetting once literally meant the setting of type, that is, the arrangement by hand or machine of narrow slugs of metal, usually lead, bearing on their ends the raised images of individual characters. A readable text was produced when the set type was inked and pressed against paper. Today, however, the term typesetting often refers to computer methods for producing a printer-ready image of a document: that is, an image of the document exactly as it is supposed to look on paper. Here the word printer refers not to a desktop **printer** but to an industrial workshop that can produce a journal, bound book, or other printed **object** of professional quality. Printers no longer rely on moveable metal type to put ink on paper, but on flexible sheets of metal on which text and **graphics** have been produced as a raised pattern by photoresist techniques. These metal sheets are fixed to cylinders and rolled against paper at high speed.

Typesetting is thus located toward the end of the document-production process, just before actual printing. **Word processing**, on the other hand, is located at the other end of the process—the compositional or creative end. Word processors are computer **applications** used to record, display, organize, spell-check, and otherwise manipulate writing. Today's word processors can also incorporate graphics and Web links into the documents they produce, and will soon routinely incorporate sound and video as well.

Because word processors allow users to control so many aspects of the final appearance of their documents, there can be no neat dividing line between typesetting and word pro-

cessing. However, the absence of a line does not always mean the absence of a difference. Typesetting and word processing remain distinct activities. One important distinction is that word processing consists, primarily, of writing, which is a personal, creative act—a specialized form of speech or conversation—and can therefore receive only marginal assistance from a machine. A word processor, for all its hundreds of features, is primarily passive, a fancy piece of paper. Typesetting, on the other hand, involves the final arrangement of all the visual elements of a document, including font, justification, spacing, margins, indents, captions, character spacing, section heads, and many more. Professional typesetters have generally devoted thousands of hours to developing expertise in their field, and produce professional results; word-processor users who attempt to typeset complex documents (or who over-embellish simple documents) usually produce obviously amateur results.

On the positive side, the fact that word processors give their users control over many of the aspects of document appearance, and to print their documents on desktop devices, makes it possible for users to quickly produce highly legible letters, reports, proposals, and more—a positive result. An outstanding *negative* result is that untold hours are wasted on amateur typesetting that could have been spent on productive work (or on breaks from work). This wastage probably contributes its share to what economists have long called the "productivity paradox"—the fact that although the amount of computing power purchased by U.S. businesses has increased by a factor of hundreds since the 1970s, white collar productivity (profit produced per worker-hour) has by many measures not increased at all—it may even have decreased. As Nobel Prize–winning economist Robert Solow said in the early 1990s, "we see computers everywhere except in the productivity statistics." The time wasted by many word-processor users on irrelevant typesetting is a typical result of the computer's tendency to make the unnecessary easy.

*See also* Word processing

# U

## UIMS (User-interface management system)

UIMS is an acronym for User-Interface Management System. This system supports the development and performance of user-interfaces.

Typical features of a UIMS include a **graphics** system, a widget **library** (tools that enable the user to construct **graphs**, **trees**, etc.), a layout editor (another construction aid), and various **programming-language** and **operating-system** extensions. These components support the development of larger-scale projects such as constraint-maintenance systems (where the relationship between two objects is established and maintained).

UIMS is associated with older systems where an interface is specified in a formal language. Thus, most UIMSs are concerned with a special textual or graphical language for programming the user-interface. Also, a UIMS is a one-way process—it involves input from the user to the computer, not the reverse.

The development of user-interfaces can be complex, with contradictory goals present. For example, on one hand it is desirable to have a portable the interface **code** so that the same code can be run on different host systems. On the other hand, commercial users demand a code that meshes closely with their particular system

The **design** of a UIMS must be done with the requirements of the system uppermost in importance. For example, the information stored in the database may be complex, capable of presentation in textual, graphical, or video formats, and may have many overlapping linkages to related information. The design and mapping of different so-called logical models to different types of **applications** and interfaces is the main task for UIMS researchers and designers.

The development of a UIMS is a multi-stage process, with different development tools employed at each step. The first stage is the design of the interface. Here, analysis tools for the various software **protocols** to be used are important. Next comes the actual construction of the interface. In this second step, various tools are used to construct the components that will be operative in the interface, such as icons and a dictionary. A particularly important tool is the interface builder. The interface builder is itself an interactive interface, having palettes of prototypes of graphical objects, which can be used to construct the graphical elements of the UIMS. Various vendors market interface builders. The third step is called the **run-time** execution step. Essentially, the runtime execution is a testing and performance step. The tools employed at this stage of development help the developer to ascertain the performance of the system and to correct any deficiencies. Finally, comes the evaluation of the user-interface, where performance is evaluated under real operating conditions. Appropriate analysis tools are used during the final step.

Interface builders are, in general, designed to be used for **static** data—data that is unaltered once entered into a database. Some **data** can change, however, depending upon factors such as time or, in the case of scientific experiments, physical factors pertaining to the environment in which the experimental subject resides. In such cases, the UIMS program code must allow for the insertion or **deletion** of objects during the application, and to map the data to the drawing attributes. One method of achieving this operational flexibility is to make the graphical objects sensitive to **mouse**-driven **commands** such as "CUT" and "PASTE."

A well-designed UIMS also contains associations between the objects within a window. For example, when the size of a window is changed by the user, the size and spatial relationships of the objects or icons within the window should automatically change, so as to maintain the same spatial perspective. In the case of text, this may necessitate an automatic change in font size.

Maintenance of the relationships between the data demands a number of features of the UIMS. Control over the various data may require control at different times—asynchronous control. Also, because the applications built with an object-oriented database must be able to present inter-related and overlapping information, the management of multiple views in the user interface is necessary. Finally, the user should have the ability to browse and update the data.

Operationally, the inter-relationships between data and user activities is addressed in several manners. One is the use of a hierarchy of menus, known as dialog trees. Another tact utilizes what is known as a **transition** network. Here, text or a diagram can be used to link tasks.

There are now many commercially available UIMSs. The choice of a system depends on a myriad of factors, including the users principle need ("hard" scientific versus social scientific data, for example), required manipulation of the data, number of users (including simultaneous usage), price, compatibility with present and future operating platforms, and vendor support.

*See also* Data; Design; Software architecture

# ULTRA-LARGE SCALE INTEGRATION

Ultra-large scale integration, or ULSI for short, refers to the ability to position more than one million integrated circuits on a single computer chip. An **integrated circuit** is a circuit whose components are etched onto a slice of **semiconductor** material.

The ability to pack more integrated circuits onto a chip increases the computational power and speed of the computer or other machine in which the chip resides. The use of ULSI in a device permits **operation** at a lower voltage, lowers the power consumption and provides a higher speed of operation. Some of the devices that utilize ULSI technology are processors, scanners that convert printed information to coded **data**, semiconductor **memory**, semiconductors (such as the Metal Oxide Semiconductor Field Effect **Transistor**, or MOSFET), and the bipolar transistor, which amplifies analog and digital signals. The widely used **Intel** 486 and Pentium **microprocessors**—silicon chips that contain the computer's central processing unit—use USLI technology.

USLI is the largest type of integrated circuit. The other types rang in size from less than 100 circuits (small-scale integration) to between 100,000 and 1,000,000 (very-large scale integration, or **VLSI**). Operationally, the dividing line between VLSI and ULSI integrated circuits is often difficult to determine.

*See also* Central processing unit (CPU); Computer architecture; Integrated circuit

# ULTRASONIC MEMORY

Ultrasonic **memory** is a form of acoustic delay-line memory. Acoustic delay-line memories were developed as rapid-access **data storage** devices in the mid-1940s, before affordable electronic memory in the form of vacuum tube arrays or transistors existed.

The acoustic delay memory principle is a simple one. A tube one or two meters long and about an inch across is filled with warm (liquid) mercury and capped at each end with a piezoelectric quartz crystal, one for sending waves through the tube and the other for receiving them. (Piezoelectric crystals expand or contract when a voltage is applied across them, and produce a voltage when stretched or squeezed.) **Data** to be stored in the delay-line memory are transmitted along the mercury in the tube as a series of sound waves. When these waves arrive at the receiving end, the crystal there translates them into electronic pulses. (Only at this time are the data available electronically to the computer.) If the data are to be stored unchanged, the electronic pulses from the "read" end of the memory tube are looped back unaltered to the "write" end and regenerated as waves in the mercury. If the data are to be changed, a control line intervenes in this feedback **loop**, altering the series of waves to be transmitted into the tube.

Such a device is called a "delay-line" memory because it takes time for the waves representing the stored data to travel from one end of the tube to the other (.5–1 millisecond, in a typical **design**). By using the feedback principle described above to keep the data circulating in the line, information can be stored indefinitely. The term "ultrasonic" is used because the frequency of the sound waves used in such devices is beyond the range of human hearing, and all such waves are ultrasonic by definition.

The mercury-based ultrasonic memory concept was originally developed by **William Shockley** of Bell Laboratories, co-inventor of the **transistor**. Mercury-based ultrasonic memories were used in several important early computers, most notably the 1949 British computer **EDSAC (Electronic Delay Storage Automatic Calculator)**, which was named for its use of this type of memory. The EDSAC's ultrasonic memory consisted of 16 steel tubes filled with mercury; each stored 32 words of 17 bits each for a total of 8,704 bits—about twice what it takes to store this article in memory.

Mercury proved a troublesome material. Since the velocity of sound in mercury depends on temperature, the delay lines had to be kept in special warming ovens. Less temperature-sensitive alternative materials were investigated, including mixtures of alcohol and water. **Alan Turing**, one of the founders of modern computer science, is said to have suggested seriously that London Dry Gin might provide an optimal delay-line medium.

By the 1960s, compact acoustic delay lines using nickel wire rather than mercury (or gin) had been developed. These were still in use in special applications, such as video **terminal** control, as late as 1975. By the end of the 1970s integrated-circuit memory chips had taken over all high-speed electronic data storage.

*See also* EDSAC (Electronic Delay Storage Automatic Calculator)

# UML (UNIFIED MODELING LANGUAGE)

The Unified Modeling Language (UML) is a graphical language used to visualize, specify, construct, and document an object-oriented or component-based software system. It is a notation for expressing analysis and **design** that supports many **programming** languages but is independent of programming language itself.

Before the UML, a number of similar analysis and design methods with slight differences were used for object-oriented development, including the Booch method, **Object** Modeling Technique (OMT), the Rational Unified Process (RUP), and Object-Oriented Software Engineering (OOSE). Each of these methods was evolving along its own path, and no clear leader had emerged. In the 1990s Rational Software Corporation and leading methodologists Grady Booch, James Rumbaugh, and Ivar Jacobson began an effort to fuse the best practices of existing methods into a single modeling language. The UML is a successor to these earlier methods.

The foundation of the UML is that developing a model of a system is essential to the construction process. Much like a blueprint for building a house, models ensure consistency and structural soundness. Models capture the structure and behavior of the system. A system model is developed jointly by developers and customers to communicate the design and behavior of the system.

As a modeling language the UML consists of a collection of concepts with a notation (**syntax**) and rules for usage. The notation for UML includes a set of shapes that can be combined in specified ways to create system diagrams. These diagrams help communicate and integrate multiple perspectives of the system under construction. Common UML diagrams include **use-case** diagrams, **class** diagrams, and implementation diagrams. Systems projects may use some or all of the UML depending on the nature of the system, the development tools being used, and the methodology being followed.

The system development process typically involves documenting a problem, solving the problem, and documenting the solution. The UML aids in gathering system documentation throughout the development process. As an industry standard the UML is independent of programming languages, software tools, and development processes. Although the UML is process-independent, it encourages the use of a development process that is use-case driven, architecture-centric, iterative, and incremental.

A consortium of industry leaders contributed to the UML specification; it also incorporated feedback from user and scientific communities. The UML v1.1 specification was adopted by the Object Management Group (OMG) in November 1997 as a standard for developing object-oriented applications (e.g. **Java**, **C++**, IDL). The OMG has assumed responsibility for further development of the UML.

*See also* Use case

# UNDECIDABILITY

Certain problems that occur in the theory of computation and elsewhere do not have solutions. In those cases it is not that a solution cannot be found easily, nor even that a solution, if found, would be too hard, or perhaps take too long, to implement on a real existing computer. It is simply that there is no well-defined procedure guaranteed to answer the question "yes" or "no" in all cases. In logical terms, neither a well-formed statement nor its negation may be logically implied by a logical system, so it is possible that the **algorithm** may not halt on either a "yes" or a "no." Problems for which a solution exists, but where the solution cannot be efficiently implemented on existing computers, are called *intractable* problems. Those for which no general solution exists at all, are called *undecidable* problems. The study of undecidable problems—or, more generally, the question of which problems are undecidable—is called undecidability.

The earliest and best-known result in undecidability is the famous **Halting Problem** for Turing machines. **Alan Turing**, a British mathematician, defined an abstract mathematical model of a computer, which has become known as a **Turing machine** in his honor. In layman's terms, the Halting Problem simply says that a Turing machine cannot predict or model its own behavior. It is thus always meaningful to ask, "Will this computer program halt if given such-and-such input?"; it is intuitively obvious, however, that there is no computer program that would always be able to answer that question, because it would have to be able to answer the question about itself as well. Turing's genius was in perceiving this now obvious result and proving it in rigorous mathematical terms in the 1930s, even before there were any computers or computer programs. One obvious consequence of the undecidability of the Halting Problem, as evident here, is that human programmers are always necessary, that computer **programming** cannot be left entirely to computers themselves.

One of the most significant aspects of undecidability is that it extends well beyond questions of mere logic or computation. Many interesting questions in number theory, algebra, combinatorics, graph theory, linguistics, physics, and so on have been shown to be undecidable. Undecidability proofs usually take the form of showing that a certain problem is reducible to the Halting Problem, i.e., that if one were able to solve that certain problem, then one could use that fact to find a solution for the Halting Problem as well. And since we know that there is in fact no solution for the Halting Problem, there must be none for the other problem under consideration as well. Similarly, one is able to build up a group of undecidable problems, and whenever a question arises about a new candidate problem, one can find a proof of undecidability simply by showing that the candidate is reducible to one of the known undecidable problems.

At first it may appear that undecidability is a very negative and depressing thing to know, since it forever places the answers to certain important and useful questions beyond the pale of our understanding. However, mathematicians and computer scientists may welcome proof that a certain question is undecidable because it frees them from the task of finding a solution for it. Indeed, it is better also to be aware early that a task one is attempting is not feasible, than to discover the fact after one has expended a great deal of wasted effort. For this reason, undecidability has been at the forefront of topics of research since the time of Turing. An important result in undecidability, probably the best-known to computer scientists other than the Halting Problem itself, is called Rice's Theorem, after the mathematician who first proved it. Essentially this theorem states that no non-trivial question one could ask about an infinite set is decidable.

It is important to note, however, that proving that a problem is undecidable does not mean that we give up all hope whenever it arises. In most cases this only means that a general solution cannot be found for all cases of the problem. However, it is quite likely that specific cases of the problem will have solutions. For example, there is no computer program that will tell us if *any* computer program has errors; but there certainly can be a program that will answer the question for a certain large class of useful programs. Having such a program, known in the programming community as a debugger, is of such great benefit that very few working programmers devote any thought to the question of undecidability.

# UNICODE

Unicode is a standard for the representation of characters as integers. Another means of character representation, **ASCII**, is a more commonly used form of character representation. Although ASCII uses only eight bits for each character, Unicode uses 16 bits to represent each character. This means that Unicode is capable of representing more than 65,000 unique characters. By comparison, ASCII's capacity is only 128 characters. For the English language and Western-European languages, the full character capability of Unicode is not utilized. However, languages such as Greek, Chinese and Japanese cannot be fully represented without the power of Unicode.

The Unicode standard was created in 1991 by a team of computer professionals, linguists and scholars. Since the first version (1.0) several versions have been released (1.1, 2.0, 2.1, and 3.0). Version 4.0 of Unicode is expected within the next several years.

In its inception, provision was made in Unicode for every character, punctuation mark, and symbol for every spoken language. In fact, currently there are over 29,000 unused codes. This will allow for expansion of Unicode to include new characters such as hieroglyphics.

Fundamentally, computers deal with numbers. They store letters and other characters by assigning a number for each one. Before Unicode was invented, there were hundreds of different encoding systems for assigning these numbers. This was because no single encoding, such as ASCII, could contain enough characters. Even for English, no single encoding was adequate for all the letters, punctuation, and technical symbols in common use. A number of coding systems can also cause problems, as encoding systems can **conflict** with one another.

Unicode is able to provide a unique number for every character in a way that is independent of the operating system or **programming** language being used. The **design** of Unicode is currently controlled by two co-operating organizations. The first organization is the Unicode Consortium, a nonprofit special interest group founded in 1991 to promote Unicode. The Consortium is comprised mainly of American software manufacturers with an interest in Unicode. The second organization is a sub-committee of the **International Organization for Standardization** and the International Electrochemical Commission.

Unicode is growing in popularity. The Unicode Standard, which specifies the design and modifications to Unicode, has been adopted by prominent companies such as **Apple**, **Hewlett-Packard**, **International Business Machines**, JustSystem, **Microsoft**, Oracle, SAP, Sun, and Sybase. Furthermore, Unicode is required by modern programming standards including **XML**, **Java**, CORBA, and WML. The emergence of the Unicode Standard, and the creation of programming tools to support it, such as software for Arabic, Russian, Hebrew, Japanese Kana and Korean languages, is one of the most significant global software trends of recent times.

As **the software industry** continues to orient more globally, the need for Unicode will continue to grow. Some analysts have predicted that Unicode will someday supplant ASCII as the standard character-coding format.

*See also* Class

# UNIVAC (UNIVERSAL AUTOMATIC COMPUTER)

UNIVAC (Universal Automatic Computer) was the first mass-produced commercial computer. UNIVAC was the result of a collaborative effort between computer pioneers **John Mauchly** (1907–1980) and **J. Presper Eckert** (1919–1995). Their partnership in building advanced computers began in the early 1940s at the University of Pennsylvania's Moore School of Engineering. At the Moore School, Mauchly and Eckert took lead roles in building **ENIAC (Electronic Numerical Integrator And Computer)**, the world's first general-purpose electronic computer, and its successor **EDVAC (Electronic Discrete Variable Automatic Computer)**, one of the first computers to implement the **stored-program principle**. The two men drew heavily on their experiences with ENIAC and EDVAC in the creation of UNIVAC.

In 1946 Mauchly and Eckert jointly applied for a patent for "the automatic, digital computer" (i.e., ENIAC). When the Moore School disputed their patent rights, they left to form the Electronic Control Company, which was the first company in the United States dedicated solely to the manufacture of electronic computers. From the beginning of their commercial partnership, Mauchly and Eckert held a clear idea of what their company's mission would be: to build a **data** processing computer for business and government that would be standardized and mass produced. These notions were quite inno-

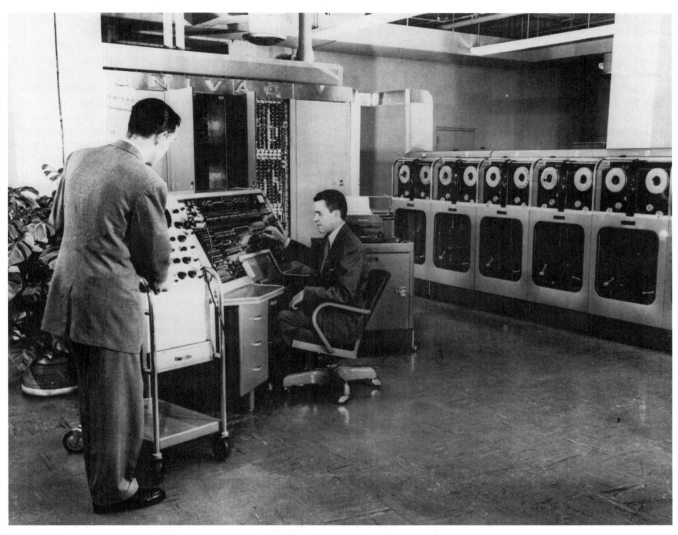

**UNIVAC**

vative in the mid-to-late 1940s, since advanced computers of the era were custom-built and designed to solve scientific and engineering problems. In 1946 the United States Census Bureau agreed to purchase Mauchly's and Eckert's as-yet-unnamed, and unproven, computer for the tabulation of the upcoming 1950 census data. In 1947 the company was incorporated as the Eckert-Mauchly Computer Corporation (EMCC), and the corporation's main product was christened "UNIVAC." Though not one UNIVAC had been built, EMCC received additional orders throughout the late 1940s. In spite of the many firm orders for UNIVACs, cost overruns meant that by late 1949 EMCC was in serious financial difficulty.

To fend off bankruptcy, Eckert and Mauchly looked for a buyer for their corporation, and eventually approached **International Business Machines (IBM)** Corporation; but IBM was prevented from purchasing EMCC by anti-trust laws. The Remington-Rand Corporation, however, did not have such restrictions and in 1950 EMCC became the UNIVAC Division

of Remington Rand. Eckert and Mauchly were retained to lead the new division, and the first UNIVAC was delivered in mid-1951 to the United States Census Bureau.

UNIVAC had much in common with the two advanced computers that Eckert and Mauchly had been so instrumental in creating, namely ENIAC and EDVAC. Like those two computers, UNIVAC performed its electronic computations using vacuum tubes (it was not until the late 1950s that all-transistor computers were commercially available). Like ENIAC, UNIVAC performed computations using a decimal (i.e., base-10) architecture, versus the binary (i.e., base-2) system that would eventually dominate modern computing. UNIVAC's primary (or main) **memory** was provided by "mercury delay line" technology, which had been developed by Eckert for use in EDVAC. Though considerably smaller than ENIAC, UNIVAC was nonetheless a large machine—it weighed approximately 8 tons, used over 5,000 vacuum tubes, and consumed around 120,000 watts of electrical power. But UNIVAC went beyond using tried-and-true technology from previous computers; it incorporated new technologies and techniques, such as magnetic tapes for secondary memory.

For the American public of the early-to-mid 1950s, UNIVAC was the prototypical computer. This was in no small part due to its appearance on the CBS television network on election night in November 1952. Early that evening, with only a small percentage of the total vote actually counted, an election-prediction program co-written by Mauchly and run on a UNIVAC correctly predicted a landslide for presidential candidate Dwight Eisenhower. This prediction was at first discounted because conventional opinion polls had predicted a close race. Eventually, UNIVAC's successful prediction was released to the public and the potential of computers became clear, even to the layman. Up until 1955, Remington Rand enjoyed a near-total dominance in the large, general-purpose computer market. But in spite of this tremendous lead, IBM became the dominant computer manufacturer by the late 1950s. IBM's answer to the UNIVAC, the IBM 702, possessed several advantages over UNIVAC. For example, UNIVAC was a rather monolithic computer, whereas the 702 was of modular construction, and hence easier both to assemble at the customer's site, and to customize to suit the customer's needs. IBM also provided better customer support through its well-trained technical and sales staffs. Nevertheless, UNIVAC was a successful product for Remington Rand (which in 1955 merged with Sperry Gyroscope to become Sperry Rand Corporation). Though UNIVAC introduced new technologies (e.g., magnetic tape used for secondary **data storage**), its biggest impact on the future of computing was to demonstrate that large **mainframe** computers had an important role in data processing fields, like accounting and inventory control, and not just in the engineering and scientific arenas. Subsequent computers were built under the UNIVAC name; for instance, the UNIVAC 1108, which debuted in the mid-1960s, was a successful mainframe computer incorporating IC (**Integrated Circuit**) technology. In order to avoid confusion the original UNIVAC model is sometimes called UNIVAC I. An original UNIVAC I is housed at the Smithsonian Institution in Washington D.C.

*See also* EDVAC (Electronic Discrete Variable Automatic Computer); ENIAC (Electronic Numerical Integrator and Computer); IBM (International Business Machines); Primary and secondary memory

# UNIX

Unix is an operating system that was developed by **Kenneth Thompson** and colleagues at AT&T Bell Laboratories in the late 1960's. The program was originally intended for scientists and engineers, although its use has expanded since the inception of Unix. There are now several modifications to the AT&T standard, mostly because Bell Labs distributed the operating system in its source language form. This allowed anyone to modify the system for his or her own purposes.

Now, Unix is the operating system on which many network **protocols**, such as **TELNET** and FTP, are based.

There are two main types of Unix. System V is produced by AT&T and BSD4.1– 4.3 are produced by The University of California at Berkeley.

Operating systems, including Unix, determine how a computer is to operate, and provide the link between the user and the computer resources. An operating system schedules tasks and allocates computer resources, including **hardware** such as the **central processing unit**, system **memory**, disk and **tape storage** systems, printers, terminals, modems, and any other internal or external peripheral.

The core of Unix is called the kernel. The kernel is responsible for the allocation of resources and the management of the memory. The software connection between the user and the kernel is called the shell. There are several different shells in Unix systems, the most popular being the Cshell. Part of Unix's appeal and power is the generic nature of this operating system, which makes Unix independent of the language of the machine itself. It can run on virtually any computer equipped with a **C compiler**. A drawback to the more widespread popularity of Unix concerns the arcane nature of its command language and its general lack of user friendliness. These aspects reflect the origin of Unix—a system intended for a small cadre of specialists for whom the system's eccentricities posed no disadvantage. Now, Unix is adapting to a wider audience, with the development of graphical user interfaces such as MOTIF.

Another generic aspect of operating systems is their ability to perform a myriad of functions at the same time, staging these tasks so that the **CPU** is working on only one task at any particular time. Unix was designed to provide another level of multi-tasking capability. It was designed as a multi-user operating system, which allows more than one person to use the computer resources at the same time, and share resources with the other users on the system.

The multi-user nature of Unix is reflected by the login procedure, which typically requires a user to supply a name and a **password**. This allows users to differentiate their files from those of others. A Unix file is a collection of information, usually in text format, that is saved under a filename. Files are organized in a file system consisting of directories, which in turn are arranged under other directories, and so on. The organization has a **tree** structure. Related files can be grouped together in a common directory. An analogy for the organization of the files is a conventional file cabinet. The cabinet itself represents the main directory, the drawers represent subdirectories, the file folders in the drawers represent further subdirectories, and the actual report represents the file.

From its inception until about 5 years ago, Unix's popularity was centered principally around workstations—computers devoted to high-end computational tasks such as engineering **computer-aided design**, **desktop publishing**, manufacturing control, laboratory simulations, telephone communications, and software development. Now, the emergence of the Unix-based operating program called **Linux** is increasing the popularity of Unix for personal computers.

*See also* C; Telnet

# URL (Uniform Resource Locator)

The Uniform Resource Locator (URL) is the standard method of specifying the location (or "address") of an **object** (or "resource") on the **Internet**. The URL for a particular site on the **World Wide Web** (WWW or Web) can be compared to a postal address for a particular physical location. Typical objects located on Web pages include information and documents, and these objects usually also transport users to other pages on the Web. (In the past URL was the acronym for Universal Resource Locator, but has been generally replaced by the term Uniform Resource Locator.) URLs are used to specify the protocol (a standard procedure for regulating **data** transmission between computers) to be used. For example, URLs are used in the Web's protocol, called **HTTP (HyperText Transfer Protocol)**, where the resource can be an **HTML** (HyperText Markup Language) page, an image file, a program such as a **CGI (Common Gateway Interface)** application or **Java** applet (a small program sent along with a Web page), or any other file supported by HTTP. The resource can further specify the target of a hyperlink, often another HTML document stored on another computer system.

People who "surf" the Web use URLs to **access** resources by typing a **string** of characters that identifies the type of document, the computer the document is on, the directories and subdirectories the document is in, and the name of the document. To move within the Web, type the URL in the "address bar" on the Web **browser**, and press "enter" to begin surfing the Internet. For example, the URL of the home Web page for the United States's Library of Congress (LOC) is http://www.loc.gov/help/about.html.

Generally, the URL address is made up of these parts: *protocol://host.domainname/directory/filename.filetype*. The part of the URL before the colon represents the *(access) protocol* (the scheme, or set of rules for transporting and retrieving information); *http* means the document is on the WWW. But not all URLs use the HTTP protocol. Other **protocols** are possible, including (1) *ftp* (File Transfer Protocol) that allows the user to list files on, retrieve files from, and add files to another computer on the Internet, (2) *gopher* that consists of a menu-driven document delivery system for retrieving information from the Internet, (3) *news* that involves documents on a Usenet newsgroup (a forum for users to post and respond to **message**), (4) *Telnet* that is an access method in which users log on to a remote computer, (5) *mailto* (electronic mail, or **e-mail**), and (6) *WAIS* (Wide Area Information Server).

In general, two slashes after the colon introduces a *host.domainname*. Thus, the next part of the URL, in this case *www.loc.gov*, represents the specific computer (server) on which the document (file) is found: that is, *www* is the *host* and *loc.gov* is the *domainname*. (As a note, most people commonly use "URL" and "domain name" interchangeably.) The *.gov* extension identifies the computer as belonging to the United States government. Some other common extensions are: *.com* (commercial), *.net* (networking), *.mil* (military), *.org* (organization), and *.edu* (education, usually a college or university). A URL does not always have to be written with the complete address. If a user is already surfing within *http://*, for

instance, then that portion can be left off. For example, if a user wishes to go from the Library of Congress Web site to the White House Web site, and both reside in *http://*, then simply type in www.whitehouse.gov. This format is considered a "relative" or "partial" URL.

Following the *host.domainname* is the *directory*, or path on which the document is found. In the example above, the directory is *help*, which takes one from the Library of Congress's home page to the "Help and FAQs: General Information about the Library of Congress" page. The last item listed is the document *filename.filetype*, which in the example is *about.html*. This takes one to the "The Library of Congress: About this site" page. The *filename* is *about*, and the *filetype* is *html*. Filetype often includes text documents in html format, and images in gif and jpg format.

***See also*** E-mail; Gopher; HTML (HyperText Markup Language); HTTP (HyperText Transfer Protocol); Hypertext; Internet; Protocols; Telnet; WAIS; World Wide Web (WWW)

# Usability testing

Usability testing consists of a series of test methods used to measure a product's performance with respect to its audience. This testing allows the examiner to determine if the product satisfies the audience's needs, it also measures the product's ease of use.

This method of testing can be used to measure the performance of software **applications**, web applications, web pages, **hardware** or IT related instructions. The examiner or tester is usually called the designer, developer or software tester.

Although usability testing is used in different fields in the IT industry, it always requires the same preparation questions.

- What do you want the product to accomplish?
- What is the purpose of this testing?
- Who is the audience?
- Does this product fulfill the customer's needs? How usable is the product?
- What is the purpose of this testing? (What type of Answers am I looking for?)

These questions must be answered to conduct a good usability test. Then, it becomes the tester's responsibility to determine which test method or methods will best answer these questions and then **design** the test. In the usability test process the tester must identify the audience, determine the test design, determine the criteria for testing the audience and determine the tasks that the test audience will perform. The tester must acquire all materials needed to set up the test, obtain a sample audience, and either assign a person to run the test or observers to conduct **data** gathering.

These test methods, also refered to as experiments include prototype testing, thinking-out-loud protocol, questionnaires, observation testing, clustering and labeling exercises, and focus groups.

# USAGE

The term usage can take several meanings in the context of computer science and **programming**. First, usage refers to the **transition** from the development of an application with a software program to the deployment of the application in the computer's operating system. Put another way, usage is the execution of a software application.

An example is found in the **Java** programming language. There, the Java **Runtime** Environment (JRE) defines the core of the Java operating system. A critical subset of JRE **applications** can be bundled into a developed application to ensure that the application runs as it should when installed on another computer. The same principal applies to other operating languages. For example, in the **CGI** language, so-called scripts can be obtained, and the **code** used for the execution of tasks.

Usage also involves the use of the codes as they are supplied. If a code has been written for a set purpose—a certain font size or the specification of bolded text are two examples—then that usage is maintained.

Usage also refers to the extent to which the resources of one segment of an operating system are used by another segment of the system. The most common example of this type of usage is the usage of **memory** by a program or by a **function** operating within a program. This type of usage can be **static**, in the sense that a program requires a set portion of memory to run. Or, memory usage can be a shifting trait, as **data** is retrieved, stored, deleted or manipulated.

*See also* Programming; Software architecture

# USE CASE

Within the **UML** (Universal Modeling Language) a number of modeling techniques can be used to document knowledge needed to build a system. One type of model is a use case. A use case is a scenario that describes the interaction between an actor and the system being modeled. Actors are people or other systems that interact with the system to achieve a desired goal. This interaction is represented as a sequence of steps to carry out an **action**. Each interaction between actor and system is a separate use case.

Use cases are meant to capture what the system needs to do; other UML techniques illustrate how the system will meet these requirements. The purpose of use cases in the requirements stage is to build a system model that is understandable by both the developers and the customers.

Although use cases are initially developed to capture requirements for the system, they can be employed during several stages of development. Estimating the work effort, validating the system **design**, testing the system, and developing system documentation can all take advantage of the knowledge that use cases contain.

Use case diagrams visually illustrate the relationships between actors and the system. In UML a use case is drawn as an oval, and the actors are drawn as stick figures. Actors are connected to the use case with lines. Arrowheads on the lines are often used to indicate the initiator of the interaction. Use cases include a textual description of the scenario that describes the main flow of events, an exception flow that describes what could go wrong and how the system should handle the exception.

*See also* Abstract use case; Concrete use case; UML (Unified Modeling Language)

# USENET

USENET is an electronic discussion network that is disseminated worldwide. USENET is comprised of a set of newsgroups with names that are classified by subject. Messages can be sent to whatever newsgroup a user with a computer and the appropriate software wishes. These transmissions can then be broadcast via other networks to a wider audience.

The concept of a computer-networked newsgroup was proposed in 1977 by Tom Truscott and Jim Elis, then graduate students at Duke University in North Carolina. Afterwards, Steve Bellovin, also a graduate student at the University of North Carolina, wrote the first version of the news software. Further refinements increased the sophistication and the popularity of the newsgroup network. Rick Adams, then of the Center for Seismic Studies, took over coordination of the maintenance and enhancement of the news software in 1984. Under Adams' guidance, USENET took on its present form, with its greater diversity of newsgroups and hieratical structure, in late 1986.

The newsgroups are organized according to their specific areas of interest. Since the organization is a **tree** structure, the various groups are called hierarchies. There are seven major categories into which the newsgroups fit: comp (computer and computer science-related groups), misc (a general category for groups not fitting elsewhere), sci (science-related groups), soc (groups addressing social issues and socializing), talk (debate and discussion groups), news (news and software groups), and rec (recreation and hobby groups). Alternative hierarchies exist as well, among which are alt (a free form group), gnu (concerned with the GNU Project), and biz (business-related groups).

Some USENET newsgroups are moderated; postings are first vetted by a moderator for approval prior to their appearance in the newsgroup. Moderation is intended to keep newsgroup discussion focused on the relevant topics. Many other newsgroups are not moderated, and postings appear with no prior inspection.

The nature of the newsgroups that comprise the USENET is subject to debate. Definitions include those newsgroups listed in the "List of Active Newsgroups" or "Alternative Newsgroup Hierarchies" postings in news.lists.misc.

The free access to USENET has been maliciously exploited by some. As well, some un-moderated newsgroups have become chaotic and unfocussed. To counteract this behavior, USENET II has been created. Access to USENET II is more restricted than access to USENET, in an effort to promote more of an atmosphere of information exchange.

*See also* Bulletin board; E-mail; Internet

# USER-DEFINED FUNCTION

A user-defined **function** is a **code** created by a user that prompts the performance of an **action** and the computation of a **value**. The function can be programmed to activate via a designated keystroke. There are as many possible uses for user-defined function keys as there are keystrokes. An example of an user defined function is the **programming** of keys to trigger the activation or disabling of sound.

User-defined functions are subroutines, of which there are several **types**. An external function can be written using many operating languages, including **Java**. An SQL function is written entirely in SQL. A sourced function compliments and modifies an existing user-defined function.

In a spreadsheet program, a user-defined function can be applied to a cell, a region, defined by a column number and a row number, to which **data** is added. The function will occur when the data is entered. A user-defined function cannot alter the spreadsheet environment, such as by the selection, **deletion**, insertion, renaming, or formatting of existing data. The user-defined functions are the only function procedures that the Excel spreadsheet can use in a cell's formula.

Typically, a user-defined function manipulates or calculates a result based on the data, or on the arguments, that were specified as part of the defining of the function. The structure of a user-defined function, for a spreadsheet, consists of beginning and ending identifiers (Function and End Function, respectively) with so-called arguments forming the bulk of the function definition. Arguments are the qualifiers to the function, with criteria used in analyzing the data, and the order or hierarchy of analyses, as examples.

*See also* Commands; Computations

# V

## VALUE

With regards to computing, the term value is a quantity assigned to an element such as a **variable**, field, symbol, or label. The quantity involving a particular value can refer to (and be assigned to) alphabetic as well as numeric **data**.

Values within computers can be represented as alphabetic data, numeric data, or a combination of alphabetic and numeric data (commonly called alphanumeric data). Alphabetic data includes letters, control characters, punctuation marks, space characters, and other common symbols as well as the codes used to represent them.

Numeric data refers to numbers; more specifically numbers expressed in integer notation, fixed-point notation, and floating-point notation. Integer notation is a numeric format consisting of positive and negative whole numbers, such as 45, -87, and 125,953. Calculations involving integers are much faster than calculations involving floating-point numbers. As a result, integers are widely used in **programming** for purposes of counting and numbering. Fixed-point notation is a numeric format in which the decimal point has a specified position. Examples of fixed-point numbers with two digits to the left of the decimal point and one digit to the right are 48.5, -94.3, and 00.0. Floating-point notation, also called exponential notation, is a numeric format that is used to easily and efficiently represent very large and very small real numbers. This type of notation is stored in two parts, a mantisssa and an exponent. The mantissa consists of the significant digits in the number, and the exponent specifies the magnitude of the number (the position of the decimal point). For example, the number 532,000,000 can be expressed as 532E6 (commonly called "scientific floating-point notation"); that is, 532 with six zeroes to its right side. Used in a computer, the base for floating-point numbers is usually 2. Many microprocessors support **floating-point arithmetic**. For example, **Intel** Corporation's line of Pentium® microprocessors contains built-in math-coprocessors, also called FPUs, or Floating Point Units.

Alphanumeric data includes a combination of alphabetic and numeric data that was discussed earlier. The grouping of alphanumeric characters that have some relationship to one another is called a **character set**.

The general definition of *value* is fundamentally important to the precise set of mathematical rules for representing the interactions and relationships among words, numbers, symbols, and other data entered and stored in the **memory** of a computer. This set of rules is called digital logic, and is the basis for all operations within modern digital computers.

***See also*** Character sets; Digital logic; Floating-point arithmetic; Floating-point representation

## VALUE PARAMETER

A **value parameter** is a **variable** that is passed to a **function** when it is called. Value parameters are also called actual parameters. Given the function **call**:

pow(i, j);

i and j are both value parameters. The values of i and j at the time this call is made to the pow() function are the values passed into the formal parameters of the function. The formal parameters are the variables used in the definition of the function. Given the function definition:

int pow(int base, int exp) {...}

base and exp are the formal parameters of the function. The type of any value parameter needs to be the same type as the formal parameter, or a subtype of the formal parameter's type. The order in which value parameters are passed to a function call will correspond to the order in which the formal parameters will be assigned values when the function is evaluated. The function's definition determines its formal parameters. However, every time a function is called, it can have different value parameters.

# VARIABLE

A variable in a computer program is a symbol that identifies an area of the computer's **memory** where the program stores **data** it can modify. That is, a variable is a symbol that represents a **value**.

For example, in the **expression** "x + y" *x* and *y* are both variables. In computer **programming**, an expression is any valid combination of language symbols that represents a value. Each computer programming language has its own set of rules for what is and is not allowed in writing an expression. These rules are called the "syntax rules" of the language. For example, in **C**, **C++**, and **Java** "y = x + 6" is an expression, and so is the literal character **string** "this is an expression." Variables can represent numeric values, characters, character strings, or memory addresses.

Variables play an vital role in computer programming because they allow programmers to write programs in symbolic form instead of having to enter data into the program direct. The programmer uses variables to represent the data even if the values of the data are not known at the time the program is written. For example, in the expression above, y = x + 6, x may be a different value each time the program is run, and that means that y will be a different value each time the program is run, too. It is only when the program is actually run that the variables are replaced with genuine data. This means that any given program can process different sets of data.

Every variable in a program has two attributes associated with it: a name, called the variable name, and a data type. The "type" of a variable is a classification of what kind of data the variable can store. Computers use internal symbols and indicators to tell it that whether a variable is, say, an integer, like 1, 2, or 3; a floating point number, like 1.2 and 2.34, or a string of characters like "this is a string." Most **computer languages** allow programmers to create their own data **types** and then to declare variables that represent those types. Sometimes this can cause real problems when a two computers store the same data in different ways. A classic example of this is the "endian" issue, where computers read bits in the data bytes from right to left or left to right, depending on the computer, its **Central Processing Unit**, and the operating system.

Most programming languages demand that the programmer declares the type of every data **object** in the program at the time the program is turned into executable **code** by the **compiler**. Programming languages like C++, and Java are very strict about this and are particular in making sure that programmers do not do something they should not do with a variable of a given type. Other languages like **Perl** are much more relaxed and forgiving and will quietly allow the programmer to do the wrong thing and get unexpected results.

The opposite of a variable is a constant. A constant is a value that never changes once it is set. Some variables can have constant-like behaviour, too: in C and C++, something declared as "const" cannot be changed once it is set; similarly, in Java, something declared "final" is also unchangeable for the life of the program.

# VARIABLE DECLARATION

**Variable** declaration refers to the need to declare a variable before the variable can be used in a program. The declaration of variables is made via a variable declaration statement.

Variable declaration is a means of notifying the compiler—a program that translates source **code** into **object** code—about the existence and nature of a variable. Items of concern would include the type of variable, the variable name and information about the **memory** that has been allocated for the variable. A variable declaration tells the **compiler** to allocate enough memory to hold a **value** of this **data** type, and to associate the identified memory with the location.

The subsequent allocation of storage for the variable by the compiler represents another process often termed as variable definition. Although declaration and definition often occur almost simultaneously and cannot be distinguished, they are different functions. A variable declaration begins with "var." Then it declares a variable **identifier** whose type can be specified by a type identifier or a type definition. Various types of definitions are possible, including an **array**, a **record**, a set and a subrange. One example of a variable declaration would read as:

> var
> variable identifier: type identifier;
> ...
> variable identifier: type identifier

or a similar statement, except that the command phrase "type definition" is substituted for "type identifier."

Following its declaration, a variable is available for use in a program.

*See also* Programming; Variable

# VERIFICATION

A great deal of effort, money, and time are spent in the creation of software and **hardware**, and much also depends upon their correct performance. It is not at all uncommon for there to be situations where the loss of life and property would be the result of non-performance or incorrect performance of either hardware or software. Testing of the program or hardware prototype is not itself sufficient to guarantee correct behavior—how can we be certain it behaves correctly under all possible operating conditions? This can often be difficult to determine from testing alone, as operating conditions may vary widely, and sometimes may not be fully known in advance. It is also possible that certain very rare combinations of factors may occur to disrupt performance, but that these combinations may not be forecast in advance.

Thus, it becomes highly advisable to have a rigorous method by which one can be assured that an artifact will indeed work just the way it is required to. The application of such a method to one's design or ideas would enable there to be a formal assurance, for example, that a certain program is as correct in its behavior as is the statement of the Pythagorean theorem in geometry. Anyone who wished to verify this claim would be able to do so by following the formal proof, just as one could verify the **correctness** of the Pythagorean theorem.

The discipline by which one determines, in a mathematical fashion, the correctness of a **design** or concept, is called verification. "Verification' is a broad concept, covering both hardware and software verification, and it uses many distinct and important tools and techniques. In practice, most researchers in the field actually specialize in either software or hardware verification, and often use certain specific tools and techniques such as temporal logic, model checking, and so on.

Verification is obviously a concept much in demand for the sake of being able to produce sensible artifacts that do just what is desired of them and nothing else. It is also important in a legal sense, because issues of legal liability could be involved in case of artifacts that do not perform correctly and cause damage or injury. Verification is also important in an economic or financial sense, because investors may be unwilling to risk supporting a project about which there are no formal guarantees. Being able to formally verify that a certain concept is sound is also likely to help avoid blunders along the way that may lead to wastage of money and effort.

In order to verify that a certain program or a piece of hardware is going to perform as it should, it is necessary for one to first be able to describe it formally. Such specification of an artifact or a system should capture its essential characteristics in a sensible way, while leaving out inessential features that are not pertinent as to its design correctness. For example, for certain applications, the **memory** size and **CPU** speed of a computer may be relevant while its power consumption and external appearance may not be; accordingly, the former qualities should be included and the latter should not be, in the specification. Sometimes the determination of exactly what characteristics are essential for correct performance can be tricky to find out, for which reason formal verification can be a significant but incomplete step toward complete assurance. A well-known quote from the famous computer scientist **Donald Knuth** says, "Beware of bugs in the above **code**; I have only proved it correct, not tried it."

It is unfortunately also often the case that verification proofs are often tedious, involved, and difficult to understand; even if the program to be verified is not too long, it is likely as not that the proof of its correctness will be. For this reason, a major push in contemporary research is for tools to automate the obtaining of verification proofs, with human involvement being kept to a minimum. Major accomplishments have already occurred in this area, and it is now common practice to use an automated system that will mechanize many of the boring and routine aspects of verification.

Verification is thus an important part of software and hardware design. However, the state of the art in verification is yet a long way from being totally satisfactory. Much work needs to be done to enable the complete automation of verification proofs, and indeed, at this time the formal verification of complex systems is often so difficult that complete verification is considered to be too expensive and unjustifiable. Only partial verification, or verification of chosen parts or components, is attempted. Newer advances in the field should certainly help with these problems.

***See also*** Applications; Computer science and mathematics; Hardware; Invariants; Software; Temporal logic

# VIENNA DEFINITION LANGUAGE (VDL)

The Vienna Definition Language (VDL) is a language for defining **programming** languages. Specifically, VDL uses operational semantics to create a formal definition of a language. In operational semantics, programs are modeled using an abstract interpreter. If the program and the abstract program have equivalent properties and the abstract program is executed, the effects shown by the abstracted program will be reflected in the concrete program.

VDL was developed in the 1960s and 1970s in IBM's Vienna Laboratory. It was the first model of operational semantics. VDL was used in the 1970s to develop the **PL1 programming language**.

VDL evolved into a notation called the Vienna Development Method (VDM). VDM is a collection of techniques for the specification and development of systems. Its formal specifications use mathematical notation to provide a precise statement of the intended function of a system. VDM is still in use today, most commonly in Europe.

***See also*** PL1 programming language

# VIRTUAL MEMORY

It is common for modern processors to be running multiple processes at one time. Each process has an address space associated with it. To create a whole complete address space for each process would be much too expensive, considering that processes may be created and killed often, and also considering that many processes use only a tiny bit of their possible address space. Last but not least, even with modern improvements in **hardware** technology, machine resources are still finite. Thus, it is necessary to share a smaller amount of physical **memory** among many processes, with each process being given the appearance of having its own exclusive address space.

The most common way of doing this is a technique called virtual memory, which has been known since the 1960s but has become common on computer systems since the late 1980s. The virtual memory scheme divides physical memory into blocks and allocates blocks to different processes. Of course, in order to do this sensibly it is highly desirable to have a protection scheme that restricts a process to be able to **access** only those blocks that are assigned to it. Such a protection scheme is thus a necessary, and somewhat involved, aspect of any virtual memory implementation.

One other advantage of using virtual memory that may not be immediately apparent is that it often reduces the time taken to launch a program, since not all the program **code** and

**data** need to be in physical memory before the program execution can be started.

Although sharing the physical address space is a desirable end, it was not the sole reason that virtual memory became common on contemporary systems. Until the late 1980s, if a program became too large to fit in one piece in physical memory, it was the programmer's job to see that it fit. Programmers typically did this by breaking programs into pieces, each of which was mutually exclusive in its logic. When a program was launched, a main piece that would initiate the execution would first be loaded into physical memory, and then the other parts, called overlays, would be loaded as needed.

It was the programmer's task to ensure that the program never tried to access more physical memory than was available on the machine, and also to ensure that the proper overlay was loaded into physical memory whenever required. These responsibilities made for complex challenges for programmers, who had to be able to divide their programs into logically separate fragments, and specify a proper scheme to load the right fragment at the right time. Much of this work had to be done by guess and by God, as no formal tools existed that could allow for a clean solution to such problems. Thus, virtual memory came about as a means to relieve programmers creating large pieces of software of the wearisome burden of designing overlays.

Virtual memory automatically manages two levels of the memory hierarchy, representing the main memory and the secondary storage, in a manner that is invisible to the program that is running. The program itself never has to bother with the physical location of any fragment of the virtual address space. A mechanism called relocation allows for the same program to run in any location in physical memory, as well. Prior to the use of virtual memory, it was common for machines to include a relocation **register** just for that purpose. An expensive and messy solution to the hardware solution of a virtual memory would be software that changed all addresses in a program each time it was run. Such a solution would increase the running times of programs significantly, among other things.

Virtual memory enables a program to ignore the physical location of any desired block of its address space; a process can simply seek to access any block of its address space without concern for where that block might be located. If the block happens to be located in the main memory, access is carried out smoothly and quickly; else, the virtual memory has to bring in the block in from secondary storage and allow it to be accessed by the program.

The technique of virtual memory is similar to a degree with the use of processor caches. However, the differences lie in the block size of virtual memory being typically much larger (64 kilobytes and up) as compared with the typical processor cache (128 bytes and up). The hit time, the miss penalty (the time taken to retrieve an item that is not in the cache or primary storage), and the transfer time are all larger in case of virtual memory. However, the miss rate is typically much smaller. (This is no accident—since a secondary storage device, typically a magnetic storage device with much lower access speeds, has to be read in case of a miss, designers of virtual memory make every effort to reduce the miss rate to a level even much lower than that allowed in processor caches.)

Virtual memory systems are of two basic kinds—those using fixed-size blocks called pages, and those that use variable-sized blocks called segments.

***See also*** Central Processing Unit; Computer Architecture; Paging

# VIRTUAL-PRIVATE NETWORKS (VPNS)

Virtual-private networks or VPNs are public networks that function like private networks. VPNs operate by drawing on software-defined intelligence embedded at strategic points in a carrier network (such as those provided by AT&T, MCI Worldcom, or Sprint) forming part of the backbone of the **Internet**. In other words, VPNs use publicly shared facilities but allow for the creation of privacy over them. VPNs are usually Internet Protocol (IP)-based networks (i.e., using portions of the public Internet) that use encryption and tunnelling to achieve privacy of **data**. VPNs can also achieve privacy through a variety of intelligent mechanisms such as flexible routing of calls to different locations when nodes experience peak-hour traffic congestion, screening telephone numbers by location or by time of day, and automatically identifying telephone numbers. VPNs are becoming increasingly attractive to corporations, since they allow for private corporate data to be transmitted privately, while offering the cost effectiveness, network maintenance, network management, and diverse voice and data services that a large carrier network can provide.

Three kinds of VPNs currently exist: Remote Access VPNs, through which travelling corporate users can securely connect with their own corporate network; **Intranet** VPNs, where different branch offices can securely network with each other and connect to their corporate network; and Extranet VPNs, which extend an enterprise's corporate network to include partners, suppliers, and customers. VPNs are virtual because the network is dynamic, with connections set up and dissolved logically, as needed, over the physical infrastructure of the carrier network or Internet. There are no permanent, hard-wired, end-to-end connections in a VPN, as in a **Local-Area Network** (**LAN**) or **Wide-Area Network** (WAN). Instead, connections between corporate sites using a VPN are created and dissolved as needed, allowing bandwidth and other network resources to be utilized by other network users, when not in use by the corporation.

# VIRTUAL REALITY

A virtual reality (VR) system is one that creates an illusory environment for its user. The illusion may be valid in all directions, or limited to certain angles of view; it may substitute completely for the user's actual surroundings, or be superimposed over those surroundings; the senses affected may include vision, hearing, and touch. What distinguishes VR from three-dimensional video and from stereo sound, which create partial sensory illusions, is that the illusion created by a VR system reacts to the user's own movements. A VR user may have the sensation of moving through a space, of manipulating objects in that space, and so forth.

One way of classifying VR systems is by the completeness of the illusions they create. For example:

(1) Augmented reality. Some systems seek to enhance or augment what users can see with their own eyes. A brain surgeon looking through a special pair of goggles might be given the helpful illusion of seeing *through* a surgically exposed level of tissue to hidden neural structures. A pilot might look out the window of her or his aircraft and see, in addition to the visible sky and ground, what radar reveals about approaching aircraft or what a computerized map knows about the terrain below (boundaries, landmarks, targets). The problem of "dynamic registration" (that is, of the ever-changing alignment or "registration" of the virtual visual component with the real environment) looms large in the **design** of such systems.

(2) Caves. Large screens may be built to surround a user on anywhere from one to six sides (four walls plus floor and ceiling), presenting stereoscopic images of a virtual world. In such systems the user has some freedom of movement and can see their own body; however, they cannot approach the virtual world too closely without breaking the illusion. Applications of cave or "surround-screen" systems include telepresence or tele-immersion systems, which allow widely separated users to feel that they are occupying a common space. Such systems may also have augmented-reality features allowing the insertion of virtual objects (models, puppets, etc.) into the shared virtual space so that both users can manipulate them. Also classifiable as cave systems are training simulators for aircraft, spacecraft, trucks, and ships, all of which surround the user with a realistic set of physical controls and allow them to look out their "windows" at a virtual world.

(3) Immersive virtual environments. In a fully immersive virtual environment, the user wears a head-mounted display device that shuts out the real world and projects stereoscopic images onto miniature screens in front of the eyes. Intensive development effort is now being poured into "haptic" devices to extend a limited illusion to the sense of touch; these push against the user's hands to create the illusion of touching objects in the virtual world.

The possible applications of VR in education, medicine, science, engineering, and entertainment are too numerous to mention, but the number of actual applications remains modest due to technical obstacles. Cave systems, for instance, are by their nature large and expensive and suffer from mutual illumination of their screens, which reduces image contrast. Augmented-reality and immersive systems require users to wear irksome headsets that provide little or no peripheral vision, making it difficult to see where one is going in the virtual world. Further, the computational requirements of modeling an entire 3-D world in real time are intense, and expensive computers are needed for modeling all but the crudest worlds. Even after these technical problems have been solved, funda-

mental limits on VR will remain, such as those that arise from the biology of human beings. Kinesthesia, our sense of bodily movement, depends on nerves located in the inner ear and throughout the body and so cannot be fooled by lenses and speakers. The result is that a VR illusion of vigorous physical activity can never be totally convincing except in trivial special cases, such as walking or bicycling in a straight line.

Despite these problems, VR is already being applied to many tasks and is bound to be applied to many more. Several applications have been described above. Virtual environments have also been designed to help with the assessment and rehabilitation of mental disorders; VR can help test patients' powers of attention, memory, and spatial orientation, and virtual environments are being developed to teach patients such skills of daily living as driving cars or wheelchairs, crossing the street, cooking, and shopping. Architects and engineers designing very complex structures often use VR to visualize their works in progress, and VR is increasingly used to enable scientists to see and manipulate abstract relationships of **data**, equations, and the like. VR presents many obvious possibilities for the entertainment industry, but VR entertainment systems are still uncommon due to their high cost.

The National Aeronautics and Space Administration was an important early developer of VR techniques and recently has designed VR tools to aid in planetary exploration by wheeled rovers. (One such rover was successfully deployed on Mars in June 1995; others are scheduled to go to Mars in 2003 and 2004.) Rovers are equipped with some on-board **artificial intelligence** but still require human aid to navigate rocky alien landscapes. Since the round-trip radio time between Earth and Mars is many minutes, operators on Earth cannot simply drive such rovers by remote control; by the time the **driver** could see a problem, the rover might already be stuck or damaged. Therefore, before the rover is allowed to roll its movements are planned carefully in a three-dimensional virtual environment based on photographs taken by the lander spacecraft.

# Viruses

A virus in nature is a tiny organism that literally hovers at the edge of the living and the non-living. If it infects a host, it comes alive, using the host's resources to rapidly make many copies of itself, while possibly causing harm to the host. (There are some viruses that do no harm, or which might even benefit the host, living in a symbiotic relationship.) If it is not in a host and is left by itself, it is completely inert, consuming no resources and performing no actions indicative of life. In much the same way, a computer virus is a software program that is capable of infecting a host machine, and then making copies of itself while doing harm to the host.

Computer viruses have to be executable program **code**, and cannot be inert files that do not cause the computer to act. There are several common kinds of viruses: some can infect the "boot sector" of floppy disks or **hard drives**; others are called "**macro**" viruses because they infect other software that uses macros. Some viruses are spread as attachments to **e-mail**, while others are spread by sharing infected floppy disks and other media.

When a user tries to execute a program that has been infected, the virus is made active and becomes resident in the computer's primary storage or **random-access memory** (**RAM**). While the virus is active in the computer's RAM, any other program that is run will also become infected. If the computer is then shut off, re-starting it and invoking an infected program would cause the virus to become active again. If an infected program is used to write to a floppy disk or other medium, then the file written to is also infected, and will infect other computers if read on them. For this reason, it is commonly advised to do a "virus scan" on all unknown disks and other media before loading them on one's computer. A virus that is spread by e-mail is released when an attachment containing the virus's executable code is opened. The virus then causes a certain e-mail **message** to be sent to all the addresses stored in a user's online address book, and also does harm to the user's own machine. Persons who receive the infected e-mail from the user are safe if they do not open the attachment they receive. However, it is not uncommon for people to see a message from someone they know well and think the attachment must not be harmful, thus propagating the destructive chain further.

A computer virus has to have been created by deliberate effort; it doesn't arise by accident or just happen to be. Since computer viruses can severely damage software and **data** resulting in loss of information and much work for repair and restoration, they are threats to computer system security, and are thus taken seriously. In the United States, it is a felony under Federal law to create a virus that does serious damage to computer systems, and serious fines or imprisonment may result.

Unfortunately, a great many myths and hoaxes exist on the subject of computer viruses. It is not uncommon to find chain e-mail claiming to warn of some impending disaster due to a very severe virus outbreak. Some people even think that the harm caused in terms of lost productivity and such by virus hoaxes is even greater than that caused by real viruses. In this regard, we should note some common fallacies about viruses. Viruses are specific to certain operating systems, i.e., it is not possible for a virus to infect both a **Windows** machine and a **UNIX** machine, for example. Viruses also do not directly harm software, so if there is a "virus warning" about an online pathogen that would make one's computer explode, one knows it is false. One cannot also catch a virus simply by reading e-mail or performing other common, everyday tasks.

To reduce the chances of being exposed to and affected by viruses, everyone should adopt certain habits of safety. These include not opening any strange or unexpected attachments that show up in one's e-mail. If one is not sure why someone known to oneself is sending a certain message with an attachment, it is better to check with the sender whether the attachment was really purposeful. Reading the message itself is not risky, but opening the attachment might be. Another good measure is to avoid sharing files and programs without running a "virus scan" on them. In fact, there are specialized

"anti-virus" software programs that detect and remove many common viruses. Since viruses are created on an ongoing basis, it is necessary for one to be using the latest version of the anti-virus software in order to obtain the best possible protection. In order to obtain safety it is also a good idea to back up one's computer files on a regular basis. In case the files are lost due to a virus infection, or even due to any other cause, one would then be able to go to retrieve them from storage.

*See also* Applications; Computer crime

# VLIW (VERY LONG INSTRUCTION WORD) PROCESSOR

The Very Long Instruction Word (VLIW) processor consists of **CPU** (**central processing unit**) architecture that reads a relatively large group of instructions and executes them at the same time. VLIW architecture allows for an alternative way to organize microprocessors. In contrast to using **hardware** (e.g., the CPU's control unit) to perform complex decisions for the scheduling of machine-level instructions, VLIW architecture performs such scheduling at compilation time with the use of software. This transfer of operations from hardware to software (**microprocessor** to **compiler**) leads to easier designed and more efficient microprocessors. At the same time it takes advantage of the versatility of software to handle difficult tasks.

VLIW processing uses a set of instructions from **assembly language** that is implemented using horizontal microcode. (Horizontal microcode is a technique for implementing a set of instructions for a processor as a horizontal sequence of microcode instructions ("microinstructions"), each of which typically consists of a large number of **bit** fields and the address of the next microinstruction to execute.) A horizontally encoded instruction word that encodes four or more operations is normally considered "very long."

The VLIW processor combines many simple instructions into a single long instruction word that uses different registers (CPU **memory** devices). A language compiler or pre-processor separates program instructions into basic operations that are performed by the processor in parallel (that is, at the same time). These operations are placed into a "very long instruction word" that the processor can then disassemble, and then transfer each **operation** to an appropriate **functional unit**. For example, the group might contain four instructions, and the compiler ensures that those four instructions are not dependent on each other so they can be executed simultaneously. Otherwise, it places "no-ops" (blank instructions) in the group where necessary.

VLIW is sometimes seen as an improvement over the **reduced instruction set computer** (**RISC**) architecture, which also works with a limited set of relatively basic instructions and can usually execute more than one instruction at a time (a characteristic referred to as superscalar). A superscalar architecture is a processor that can execute two or more scalar operations in parallel. The main advantage of VLIW processors is that complexity is moved from the hardware to the software, which means that the hardware can be smaller, less expensive, and require less power to operate. The **design** of a compiler or pre-processor must determine how to build the very long instruction words. Producing **code** for VLIW machines is difficult, but can be made easier with trace scheduling, a compiler technique. Trace scheduling is a method of controlling and coordinating the operation of multiple hardware elements of a VLIW processor.

*See also* Compiler; Functional unit; Microprocessors; RISC (Reduced instruction set computer)

# VERY-LARGE-SCALE INTEGRATION (VLSI)

Very-large-scale integration, or VLSI for short, is a term related to integrated circuits. Integrated circuits are chips, such as the **Intel** Pentium chip, which reside inside a computer and function in the performance of the computer. A silicon chip consists of transistors, electrical gates that amplify an electrical signal and allow the current to flow. The transistors power the performance of other components of the chip, such as logic elements (also called **memory** cells). VLSI refers to an **integrated circuit** composed of hundreds of thousands of these memory cells

The first practical chip was made in 1959 by two companies, Fairchild and **Texas Instruments**. As with many technologies, advancements after this initial achievement produced products of improved performance and construction. In 1971, Intel was successful in combining logic elements, which formally were housed in several different chips, into a single chip. Subsequently, chips became smaller, faster, and less expensive over time. Engineers learned how to pack more and more logic elements into a single circuit. This effort gave rise to VLSI, where millions of transistors are packed onto a circuit.

VLSI technology has made today's portable and high-performance computers possible. Spin-off technologies directly attributable to VLSI include the Global Positioning System, which required a processor capable of performing billions of calculations per second. Commercial collaborations between companies engaged in VLSI research and network providers have produced home networks that are extremely fast and capable of many simultaneous functions.

Further developments are on the horizon. Within the next decade, a central feature controlling the size of integrated circuitry—metal-oxide **semiconductor** field-effect **transistor channel** length—will shrink into the range of 50 nanometers, a measurement less than 200 atoms in length. Such minuscule chips, on which will reside the entire operating information for a computer, will enable computer size to shrink. The manual dexterity and operating comfort of the user may well be the limiting factor determining how small computers become. And, for computers that operate within human input, molecular dimensions are conceivable.

*See also* Electric circuit; Intel; Nanotechnology

# VOICE RECOGNITION

Voice recognition or speech recognition is the capability of a computer to recognize spoken words. Speaking can be used in lieu of typing or **mouse** clicking to input information to the computer. There are two major types of speech recognition programs: speech-to-text and command-and-control. Speech-to-text systems transfer spoken words into written words for use in **applications** such as **word processing** programs. Command-and-control systems interpret spoken words as **commands**, for example, to open a new program or save a file.

Speech recognition research began in the 1950s. **IBM** demonstrated its first voice recognition device at the 1962 World's Fair in Seattle. Shoebox was a bulky arithmetic **calculator** that could recognize numerical digits spoken into a microphone. Computers that could converse with humans were popularized by science fiction during the 1960s, appearing in the movie *2001: A Space Odyssey* and the *Star Trek* television series. The actual computer technologies of the times lagged far behind.

In 1978 **Texas Instruments** introduced the *Speak & Spell* toy. This was one of the first consumer devices including a computer chip that could synthesize human speech. The first speech recognition systems for dictation purposes appeared in the 1980s. They were very expensive systems designed for specialized applications. Advances in computer processing speeds and digital signal processing brought the advent of general speech recognition software for the **personal computer** during the late 1990s.

Speech recognition by a personal computer requires a microphone for audio input, a sound card to process the input, and software including a speech engine. Speech sounds begin as vibrations in the throat that cause disruptions in the nearby air pressure. A graph of these changes over time is called a waveform. A microphone converts the pressure changes into electrical voltage changes (an analog signal). A computer sound card is an analog-to-digital converter that converts the voltage changes back into pressure changes and stores them as binary **code** on the **hard drive**.

The computer uses mathematical techniques such as Fourier analysis to break the digitized waveform into its frequency components. Speech sounds range in frequency from 30 to 20,000 Hertz (vibrations per second). Vowel sounds have lower frequencies, and consonant sounds have higher frequencies. A graph of frequency over time is called a spectrogram. The computer stores spectrograms as a two-dimensional **array** of energy values. Spectral analysis techniques include linear predictive coding, mel frequency cepstral coefficients, and cochlea modeling.

The computer reads the spectrogram patterns and compares them to known patterns for particular sounds or phonemes. A phoneme is a distinct speech sound. This includes individual letters, like "b" or "p" and sounds like "ch" or "ng." Vowels in particular can have different sounds depending on their usage, e.g., the words "book" and "boot" have two different "oo" phonemes. The computer uses pattern-matching **algorithms** and probability analysis to find the most probable match to phonemes, groups of phonemes, and words built into the software. Common recognition processes include the Gallager Tanner Wiberg (GTW) algorithm, the Hidden Markov Model (HMM), **neural networks**, and **expert systems**. HMM systems are the most widely used. Many of these systems also rely on linguistics information, such as **syntax** and grammar rules, to improve their word matching abilities.

Some speech recognition programs require discrete speech, i.e., a pause after each and every word. Others are natural language systems that allow a speaker to speak continuously. They use contextual information to choose which words make sense and to distinguish homophones such as "to," "too," and "two." The programs store frequently used words in an active vocabulary list or dictionary in the computer's **random-access memory**. A larger back-up dictionary, which can contain hundreds of thousands of words, is stored on the hard drive.

Some programs are speaker dependent. They are designed to become familiar with one particular speaker's voice and language patterns. The user initially trains the program by reading exercises and identifying mistaken identifications. Eventually the program develops a reliable voice file for that individual. Although the training can be time consuming, a large vocabulary is possible with this type of program. A speaker independent system requires no initial training. It comes equipped with a limited vocabulary and can conceivably recognize any person's speech.

The best speech recognition programs on the market achieve word recognition rates of approximately 90 percent. Roughly this means one mistaken word per sentence. Voice tone, pitch, inflection, and rate of speaking are all determining factors. Speakers with voice disorders, colds, or heavy accents can easily be misunderstood. Best performance is obtained when the program vocabulary is limited, background noise is minimized, and the speaker has a clear consistent voice with good articulation and enunciation.

Speech recognition technology is improving quickly and has become an area of focus for many software designers. The latest innovations are **Internet** voice portals. These systems use Voice Extensible Markup Language (VXML) to direct web browsers to **URL** addresses that are spoken rather than typed. Many experts predict that the keyboard and mouse will be obsolete within a decade. Growing consumer demand for voice responsive computers and technological advances in neural networks and **artificial intelligence** are expected to result in computers that not only recognize spoken words, but comprehend their meaning and can communicate with their human counterparts.

# VON NEUMANN, JOHN (1903-1957)

*American computer scientist and mathematician*

John von Neumann, considered one of the most creative mathematicians of the twentieth century, made important contributions to quantum physics, game theory, economics, meteorology, the development of the atomic bomb, and computer **design**. He was known for his problem-solving ability, his encyclopedic **memory**, and his ability to reduce complex problems to a mathematically tractable form. Von Neumann served as a consultant to the United States government on scientific and military matters, and was a member of the Atomic Energy Commission. According to mathematician Peter D. Lax, von Neumann combined extreme quickness, very broad interests, and a fearsome technical prowess; the popular saying was, "Most mathematicians prove what they can; von Neumann proves what he wants." The Nobel Laureate physicist Hans Albrecht Bethe said, "I have sometimes wondered whether a brain like von Neumann's does not indicate a species superior to that of man."

Max and Margaret von Neumann's son Janos was born in Budapest, Hungary, on December 28, 1903. As a child he was called Jancsi, which later became Johnny in the United States. His father was a prosperous banker. Von Neumann was tutored at home until age ten, when he was enrolled in the Lutheran Gymnasium for boys. His early interests included literature, music, science and psychology. His teachers recognized his talent in mathematics and arranged for him to be tutored by a young mathematician at the University of Budapest, Michael Fekete. Von Neumann and Fekete wrote a mathematical paper which was published in 1921.

Von Neumann entered the University of Budapest in 1921 to study mathematics; he also studied chemical engineering at the Eidgenössische Technische Hochschule in Zurich, receiving a diploma in 1925. In those same years, he spent much of his time in Berlin, where he was influenced by eminent scientists and mathematicians. In 1926 he received a Ph.D. in mathematics from the University of Budapest, with a doctoral thesis in set theory. He was named *Privatdozent* at the University of Berlin (a position comparable to that of assistant professor in an American university), reportedly the youngest person to hold the position in the history of the university. In 1926 he also received a Rockefeller grant for postdoctoral work under mathematician David Hilbert at the University of Göttingen. In 1929 he transferred to the University of Hamburg. By this time, he had become known to mathematicians through his publications in set theory, algebra, and quantum theory, and was regarded as a young genius.

In his early career, von Neumann focused on two research areas: first, set theory and the logical foundations of mathematics ; and second, Hilbert space theory, **operator** theory, and the mathematical foundations of quantum mechanics. During the 1920s, von Neumann published seven papers on mathematical logic. He formulated a rigorous definition of ordinal numbers and presented a new system of axioms for set theory. With Hilbert, he worked on a formalist approach to the foundations of mathematics, attempting to prove the consistency of arithmetic. In about 300 B.C., Euclid 's *Elements of Geometry* had proved mathematical theorems using a limited number of axioms. Between 1910 and 1913, Bertrand Russell and Alfred North Whitehead had published *Principia Mathematica,* which showed that much of the newer math could similarly be derived from a few axioms. With Hilbert, von Neumann worked to carry this approach further, although in 1931 **Kurt Gödel** proved that no formal system could be both complete and consistent.

Hilbert was interested in the axiomatic foundations of modern physics, and he gave a seminar on the subject at Göttingen. The two approaches to quantum mechanics—the wave theory of Erwin Schrödinger and the particle theory of Werner Karl Heisenberg—had not been successfully reconciled. Working with Hilbert, von Neumann developed a finite set of axioms that satisfied both the Heisenberg and Schrödinger approaches. Von Neumann's axiomatization represented an abstract unification of the wave and particle theories.

During this period, some physicists believed that the probabilistic character of measurements in quantum theory was due to parameters that were not yet clearly understood and that further investigation could result in a deterministic quantum theory. However, von Neumann successfully argued that the indeterminism was inherent and arose from the interaction between the observer and the observed.

In 1929 von Neumann was invited to teach at Princeton University in New Jersey. He accepted the offer and taught mathematics classes from 1930 until 1933, when he joined the elite research group at the newly established Princeton Institute for Advanced Study. The atmosphere at Princeton was informal yet intense. According to mathematician Stanislaw Ulam, writing in the *Bulletin of the American Mathematical Society,* the group "quite possibly constituted one of the greatest concentrations of brains in mathematics and physics at any time and place." During the 1930s von Neumann developed algebraic theories derived from his research into quantum mechanics. These theories were later known as von Neumann algebras. He also conducted research into Hilbert space, ergodic theory, Haar measure, and non-commutative algebras. In 1932 he published a book on quantum physics, *The Mathematical Foundations of Quantum Mechanics,* which remains a standard text on the subject. After becoming a naturalized citizen of the United States, von Neumann became a consultant to the Ballistics Research Laboratory of the Army Ordnance Department in 1937. After the attack on Pearl Harbor in 1941, he became more involved in defense research, serving as a consultant to the National Defense Research Council on the theory of detonation of explosives, and with the Navy Bureau of Ordnance on mine warfare and countermeasures to it. In 1943 he became a consultant on the development of the atomic bomb at the Los Alamos Scientific Laboratory in New Mexico.

At Los Alamos, von Neumann persuaded J. Robert Oppenheimer to pursue the possibility of using an implosion technique to detonate the atomic bomb. This technique was later used to detonate the bomb dropped on Nagasaki. **Simulation** of the technique at the Los Alamos lab required extensive numerical calculations which were performed by a staff of twenty people using desk calculators. Hoping to speed up the work, von Neumann investigated using computers for the calculations and studied the design and **programming** of **IBM** punch-card machines. In 1943 the Army sponsored work at the Moore School of Engineering at the University of Pennsylvania, under the direction of **John William Mauchly** and **J. Presper Eckert**, on a giant **calculator** for computing firing

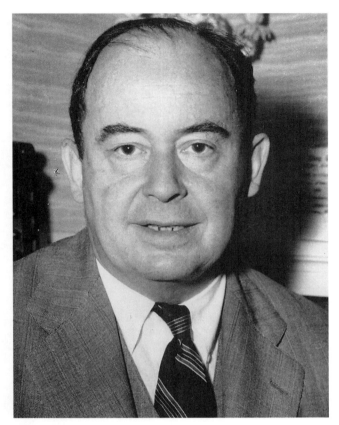

**John von Neumann**

tables for guns. The machine, called **ENIAC (Electronic Numerical Integrator and Computer)**, was brought to von Neumann's attention in 1944. He joined Mauchly and Eckert in planning an improved machine, **EDVAC (Electronic Discrete Variable Automatic Computer)**. Von Neumann's 1945 report on the EDVAC presented the first written description of the stored-program concept, which makes it possible to load a computer program into computer memory from disk so that the computer can run the program without requiring manual reprogramming. All modern computers are based on this design.

Von Neumann's design for a computer for scientific research, built at the Princeton Institute for Advanced Study between 1946 and 1951, served as the model for virtually all subsequent computer **applications**. Those built at Los Alamos, the RAND Corporation, the University of Illinois and the IBM Corporation all incorporated, besides the stored program, the separate components of arithmetic **function**, central control (now commonly referred to as the **central processing unit** or **CPU**), **random-access memory** (or **RAM**) as represented by the **hard drive**, and the **input and output** devices operating in serial or parallel mode. These elements, present in virtually all personal and **mainframe** computers, were all pioneered under von Neumann's auspices.

In addition, von Neumann investigated the field of neurology, looking for ways for computers to imitate the operations of the human brain. In 1946 he became interested in the challenges of weather forecasting by computer; his Meteorology Project at Princeton succeeded in predicting the development of new storms. Because of his role in early computer design and programming techniques, von Neumann is considered one of the founders of the computer age.

While in Germany, von Neumann had analyzed strategies in the game of poker and wrote a paper presenting a mathematical model for games of strategy. He continued his work in this area while he was at Princeton, particularly considering applications of game theory to economics. When the Austrian economist Oskar Morgenstern came to Princeton, he and von Neumann started collaborating on applications of game theory to economic problems, such as the exchange of goods between parties, monopolies and oligopolies, and free trade. Their ambitious 641-page book, *Theory of Games and Economic Behavior,* was published in 1944. Von Neumann's work opened new channels of communication between mathematics and the social sciences.

Von Neumann and Morgenstern argued that the mathematics as developed for the physical sciences was inadequate for economics, since economics seeks to describe systems based not on immutable natural laws but on human action involving choice. Von Neumann proposed a different mathematical model to analyze strategies, taking into account the interdependent choices of "players." Game theory is based on an analogy between games and any complex decision-making process, and assumes that all participants act rationally to maximize the outcome of the "game" for themselves. It also assumes that participants are able to rank-order possible outcomes without error. Von Neumann's analysis enables players to calculate the consequences or probable outcomes of any given choice. It then becomes possible to opt for those strategies that have the highest probability of leading to a positive outcome. Game theory can be applied not only to economics and other social sciences but to politics, business organization and military strategy, to mention only a few areas of its usefulness.

After the war, von Neumann served as a scientific consultant for government policy committees and agencies such as the CIA and National Security Agency. He advised the RAND Corporation on its research on game theory and its military applications, and provided technical advice to companies such as IBM and Standard Oil. Following the detonation of an atomic bomb by the Soviets in 1949, von Neumann contributed to the development of the hydrogen bomb. He believed that a strong military capacity was more effective than a disarmament agreement. As chairman of the nuclear weapons panel of the Air Force scientific advisory board (known as the von Neumann committee), his recommendations led to the development of intercontinental missiles and submarine-launched missiles. Herbert York, the director of the Livermore Laboratory, said, "He was very powerful and productive in pure science and mathematics and at the same time had a remarkably strong streak of practicality [which] gave him a credibility with military officers, engineers, industrialists and scientists that nobody else could match."

In 1954 President Eisenhower appointed von Neumann to the Atomic Energy Commission. Von Neumann was hopeful that nuclear fusion technologies would provide cheap and plentiful energy. According to the chairman of the Commission, Admiral Lewis Strauss, "He had the invaluable faculty of being able to take the most difficult problem, separate it into its components, whereupon everything looked brilliantly simple, and all of us wondered why we had not been able to see through to the answer as clearly as it was possible for him to do." He received the Enrico Fermi Science Award in 1956, and in that same year the Medal of Freedom from President Eisenhower.

Von Neumann has been described as a genius, a practical joker, and a raconteur. Laura Fermi, wife of the associate director of the Los Alamos Laboratory, wrote that he was "one of the very few men about whom I have not heard a single critical remark. It is astonishing that so much equanimity and so much intelligence could be concentrated in a man of not extraordinary appearance."

Von Neumann married Mariette Kovesi, daughter of a Budapest physician, in 1929. Their daughter, Marina, was born in 1935. Mariette obtained a divorce in 1937. The following year, von Neumann married Klara Dan, from an affluent Budapest family. In 1955, von Neumann was diagnosed with bone cancer. Confined to a wheelchair, he continued to attend Atomic Energy Commission meetings and to work on his many projects. He died in 1957 at the age of fifty-three.

# VON NEUMANN ARCHITECTURE

Von Neumann architecture describes a general framework, or structure, that a computer's **hardware**, **programming**, and **data** should follow. Although other structures for computing have been devised and implemented, the vast majority of computers in use today operate according to the von Neumann architecture.

The "von Neumann" in von Neumann architecture refers to Hungarian-American mathematician **John von Neumann** (1903–1957). Von Neumann was initially interested in access to the fastest computers available (of which there were few) during World War II in order to perform complex computations for a variety of war-related problems. In 1944, Von Neumann became a consultant to the **ENIAC (Electronic Numerical Integrator and Computer)** project, which upon its completion in 1945 became the world's first general purpose, electronic computer. Even before ENIAC's completion, von Neumann and several members of the team constructing ENIAC proposed building a more advanced computer, which would eventually become known as **EDVAC (Electronic Discrete Variable Automatic Computer)**. In 1945 von Neumann wrote a landmark paper entitled "The First Draft of a Report on the EDVAC," which encapsulated his ideas concerning the fundamental structure that a computer should follow. That report, which Von Neumann originally intended to be seen by a limited group of associates, nevertheless became widely disseminated and had an immediate impact on computer development in the United States and abroad.

Von Neumann followed up on his first report by producing two more papers coauthored with colleagues from the

ENIAC team. What emerged from these three papers was an overall structure, or architecture, which is by-and-large followed to this day by the vast majority of electronic, digital computers. Von Neumann envisioned the structure of a computer system as being composed of the following components: (1) the central arithmetic unit, which today is called the arithmetic logic unit (**ALU**). This unit performs the computer's computational and logical functions; (2) *memory*; more specifically, the computer's main, or fast, **memory**, such as RAM (**random access memory**); (3) a *control unit* that directs other components of the computer to perform certain actions, such as directing the fetching of data or instructions from memory to be processed by the ALU; and (4) *man-machine interfaces*; i.e., **input and output** devices, such as a keyboard for input and display monitor for output. Of course, computer technology has developed extensively since von Neumann's time. For instance, due to integrated circuitry and miniaturization the ALU and control unit have been integrated onto the same **microprocessor** "chip," becoming an integrated part of the computer's **central processing unit** (**CPU**).

The most noteworthy concept contained in von Neumann's first report was most likely that of the "**stored-program principle**." This principle holds that data, as well as the instructions used to manipulate that data, should be stored together in the same memory area of the computer. This idea deviated from the structure of previous computers. For example, ENIAC's numeric data was stored in its vacuum tube memory, while the instructions that directed the processing of that data was provided by certain hardware settings. That is to say, before each new computation with ENIAC, an **operator** set various dials, connected and disconnected various electric plugs, and so forth. Those particular hardware settings represented ENIAC's programming. It seemed obvious to von Neumann (as it did to several other people working on the ENIAC project) that to have a flexible, truly general-purpose computer meant that the stored program principle should be implemented.

One ramification of storing data and programming in the same general area of the computer's main memory is the need to distinguish between the two. The contents of the typical computer's main memory is "seen" by the computer as a series of zeroes and ones (i.e., binary digits, or "**bits**"). The computer needs direction in order to determine whether a particular block of information is data or instructions. Von Neumann's control unit is the mechanism used to make the data-versus-instruction determination. When the control unit initiates a **call** for an instruction to be fetched for processing, a unit called the *program counter* "points" to the instruction's

location in memory (i.e., its **address** in memory). The instruction is then fetched for execution by the processor. The address in memory of any data that is required is provided by the instruction itself. During this fetching and execution of an instruction, the program counter is incremented so that the next instruction can be found and executed. This process is sequential, meaning that instructions are executed in an ordered, sequential fashion, one instruction at a time. This *serial* execution of instructions is a hallmark of the von Neumann **computer architecture**. It is in contrast to *parallel processing* architectures in which multiple instructions are executed in tandem. A true **parallel processing** computer is considered a "non-von Neumann architecture" machine.

To summarize the main characteristics of the von Neumann architecture, it is noted that, first of all, such a computer is composed of distinct components, which are the ALU, control unit, input/output devices, and a single memory unit for storing both data and instructions (i.e., the stored-program principle). Secondly, instructions are carried out sequentially, one instruction at a time. As von Neumann himself recognized, the sequential execution of programming imposes a sort of "speed limit" on program execution since only one instruction at a time can be handled by the computer's processor. Computer pioneer **John Backus** called this the "von Neumann bottleneck." This bottleneck can manifest itself when the computer's CPU processes at a rate faster than information can be delivered from main memory. There have been a plethora of techniques devised to make the most of the sequential nature that von Neumann architecture places on computers by reducing any information bottlenecks. The development of faster processors has meant that programs are executed more quickly. Processing speed has also been increased by modifying the memory side of the equation, as in the case of cache memory (which basically provides a way of transferring information from main memory into a smaller, faster memory device). Other techniques include wider data buses to carry information more quickly between memory and the CPU; reduction of wait states (i.e., reduction of the time the CPU is required to suspend processing while waiting for information from auxiliary storage); and many other speed-enhancing strategies. It must be pointed out, however, that despite these advances and enhancements one is still left with the fundamental von Neumann architecture, which is followed in the overwhelming majority of computers in use today.

***See also*** EDVAC (Electronic Discrete Variable Automatic Computer); ENIAC (Electronic Numerical Integrator and Computer); Parallel processing; Stored-program principle

# WAIS

The Wide Area Information Server (WAIS) is a system on the **Internet** that searches and retrieves text and multimedia documents on **databases**. Thinking Machines Corporation, **Apple** Computers, and Dow Jones originally developed WAIS in the mid-1980s. In order to fully use WAIS the user must have access to a **TCP/IP** (Transmission Control Protocol/Internet Protocol) network on the Internet. Even without access to the Internet, users can still use WAIS on a limited basis. There are many free WAIS programs for several operating systems (such as **UNIX**, MS-**DOS** (**Microsoft** Disk Operating System), and Mac OS (Macintosh Operating System), and for specific environments (such as X-Windows, NeXT, and MS-**Windows**). WAIS uses the Z39.50 standard (a specification for a **query language** based on SQL (structured query language)) to process natural language queries.

There are over 400 WAIS libraries throughout the world. A server computer that contains files indexed to match keywords supports each library. Each server concentrates on a particular subject, such as physics, computers, or agriculture. A directory of server databases is available at several sites that can locate what databases are available on a particular subject. The different databases used within the WAIS system are organized in different ways but the user does not need to learn the differences of the different databases. The "natural language" used by WAIS accommodates those differences.

In general, the user inputs an inquiry as a natural language question. The server does not understand the question, but it is capable of taking certain important words and phrases in order to perform its search. For the inquiry "What is the history of the American Revolutionary war?" the search would concentrate on the important words "history," "American," "Revolutionary," and "war." The other words ("What," "is," "the," and "of") are called "stop words," words that are so common that they are eliminated from the search because they appear so frequently in every document. A completed search returns a list of documents (called "sources") that are ranked on the frequency of occurrence of the keyword(s). A score from 1 to 1,000 helps determine the ranking based on how well it matches the user's question (e.g., how many words it contains, its importance in the document). The more frequent the occurrence, the higher up on the list it appears. A "relevance feedback" feature allows the results of initial searches to help in future related searches. WAIS is also capable of being used as a search engine on a Web site. Other important features of the WAIS search engine include fielded search, right truncation (wildcard **searching**), and relevance ranking. Even though a search produces many valid responses, there are usually also many false matches as well. With today's ever-expanding and ever-improving search engines on the Internet, WAIS is considered a primitive search engine with only limited capabilities.

*See also* Query language; TCP/IP protocol

# WAIT STATE

A wait state is a processing cycle of a **microprocessor** during which it briefly waits for an **operation** to occur and complete before resuming activity. A program or process in a wait state is inactive for the duration of the wait state. For example, the **central processing unit** (**CPU**) working with a **word processing** program might communicate with main **memory** (sometimes called **random access memory** or **RAM**) for a particular instruction, and then go into a wait state until it receives a **message** back from memory. A wait state may refer to a "variable" length of time that a program has to wait before it can be processed, or to a "fixed" duration of time, such as one or more machine cycles. Wait state is also called a "time-out" period during which the CPU (often interchangeably called a microprocessor) or **bus** (the collection of wires through which **data** is transmitted from one part of a computer to another) remains idle. When memory is too slow to respond to the CPU's request for it, wait states are introduced until the memory can catch up. Normally the CPU works at a faster clock speed (usually expressed in megahertz (MHz) or millions of cycles per second) than RAM. So it may need to sit idle during some clock cycles (the oscillation speed of the computer's internal clock that determines execution times of instructions) in order for RAM to catch up. When this happens the CPU is automatically set to a wait state for one or more clock cycles so that it can synchronize with RAM speed. A delay of one or more clock cycles added to the execution time of a microprocessor's instruction allows it to communicate with slower external devices (such as printers and scanners). In addition, wait states are sometimes required because different components function at different clock cycles.

Likewise, buses sometimes require wait states if expansion boards (a printed circuit board that is inserted into a computer for added capabilities, such as a sound card) run slower than the bus. While one wait state is not perceptible, the cumulative effect of many wait states is to slow system performance.

An example of how a wait state affects computers is seen with Dynamic RAM (DRAM), which is a form of **semiconductor** RAM. DRAMs store information in integrated circuits that contain capacitors. Because capacitors lose their charge over time, DRAM boards must include the ability to repeatedly "refresh" (recharge) the RAM chips. While a DRAM is being refreshed, it cannot be read by the microprocessor. If the microprocessor must read the RAM while it is being refreshed, one or more wait states occur. Because their circuitry is relatively simple (a DRAM chip can hold approximately four times as much data as a comparable **static** RAM chip) DRAMs are more commonly used than static RAMs, even though they are slower. But there is a trade-off with using more DRAM memory, because wait state times are increased (versus if static RAM was used instead).

On the opposite side of a wait state is a *zero wait state*. A zero wait state system refers to high-speed memory that does not wait for machine cycles to respond before transferring data. In a zero wait state the microprocessor runs at the maximum speed without any "time-outs" to compensate for slower memory. Zero wait states are desirable because the more a microprocessor spends in wait states, the slower its processing performance. Wait states can be avoided, and moved into zero wait states, by using a variety of techniques, including burst mode, page-mode (RAM) memory, interleaved memory, and CPU cache.

*See also* Cycle time; Microprocessor

# WANG, AN (1920-1990)

*American computer scientist*

An Wang, a computer scientist and commercial computing executive, is best remembered for founding Wang Laboratories, a prominent manufacturer of office wordpro-

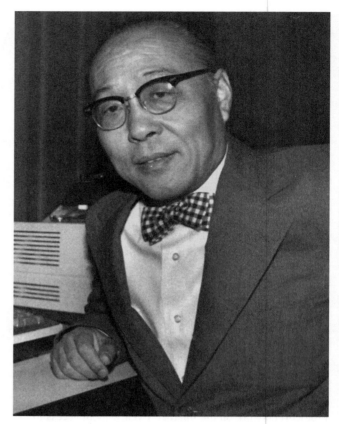

An Wang

cessing and dataprocessing computers in the 1970s and 1980s. His early work as a computer scientist focused on the development of magnetic core memories for computers in the late 1940s and early 1950s.

Wang, whose name means "Peaceful King" in Chinese, was born in Shanghai, China, on February 7, 1920. Because of its strategic location at the mouth of the Yangtze River, Shanghai was often a war zone during Wang's youth. Other areas of China were also at war: Japan captured the Chinese province of Manchuria in 1931. Wang's father, Yin Lu Wang, taught English in a private school and practiced traditional Chinese herbal medicine. Wang's mother was Zen Wan Chien. In elementary school, Wang excelled in math and science, but his grades in other subjects were so bad that he almost did not graduate. In high school some of his textbooks were written in English, which was to help him later when he moved to the United States.

Wang entered the prestigious Chiao-Tung University after high school and was elected class president. He studied electrical engineering, but spent more time competing at table tennis than studying. During this time, the Japanese began to conquer more and more of China. Wang managed to stay safe because the fighting was usually far away from him. He received his Bachelor of Science degree from Chiao-Tung University in 1940, remaining at the university as a teaching assistant from 1940 to 1941. As his part in the

Chinese war effort against Japan, he designed and built radio transmitters at the Central Radio Works in China from 1941 to 1945.

In April of 1945, Wang left China for America with some fellow engineers on a two-year apprenticeship. They were to learn about Western technology so they could rebuild China after the war. Wang, however, did more to build Western technology than to rebuild China. After arriving in the United States, Wang decided to apply to Harvard, where some of his teachers at Chiao-Tung University had studied. Many American men were still at war (Japan would not surrender until August, 1945), and Harvard needed students, so they admitted Wang. He performed well in Harvard's electrical engineering courses because he already had years of experience designing radios for the Chinese government. He received his Master of Science in electrical engineering in 1946.

Wang intended to return to China after he got his degree, but he had no money for the transportation. Through a school friend, he obtained a job with the Chinese Government Supply Agency in Ottawa, Ontario, Canada, where he worked from 1946 to 1947. The job was clerical, and he found it very boring. He decided to return to Harvard for a Ph.D., and he was accepted into the Applied Physics Department. He completed his program quickly and wrote his doctoral dissertation on nonlinear mechanics. Late in 1948, he finished his doctorate in applied physics.

Wang got his start in applied computer electronics when he went to work as a research fellow for **Howard Aiken** at the Harvard Computation Laboratory in May of 1948. Aiken, a computer pioneer, had developed the Mark I, the first automatic binary computer, in 1944. Wang did his most important work at Harvard in computer memories. Computer memories are essential to the development of computers as we know them today. Without computer memories, stored programs cannot exist, nor can **programming** languages or computer **applications**. When Wang went to work in the Harvard Computation Lab, there were already several kinds of memories: magnetic drums, punched cards, vacuum tubes, electromechanical relays, mercury delay lines, and cathode ray tubes. Each kind of **memory** had its disadvantages. Magnetic drums and punched cards were too slow, vacuum tubes burned out too often, and electromechanical relays were too noisy. Mercury delay lines made it hard for users to retrieve specific bits of **data** in a larger data set, and cathode ray tubes required a constant source of power or the data were lost.

Howard Aiken wanted Wang to invent a memory that would let a computer read and record data magnetically without the mechanical movement involved in a relay or rotating drum. Wang was perplexed for a while, because he found that when magnetic data were read, the process of reading the data destroyed them. But Wang soon discovered that he could use the data to rewrite the information in magnetic cores immediately after he destroyed it in the process of reading. Wang's ideas were used extensively in computers until magnetic core memories were replaced in the late 1960s by silicon chips. In 1955 Wang patented his ideas about reading and rewriting the information in magnetic memory cores.

In 1948, Wang met Lorraine Chiu, who was also from Shanghai, though her parents had been born in Hawaii. She was in the United States studying English at Wellesley College. They married in 1949. In September, 1950, their first child, Frederick, was born. A second son, Courtney, and a daughter, Juliette, were to follow. In April of 1955, both Wang and his wife became naturalized American citizens.

Harvard preferred to sponsor basic research and decreased its work in computers when they started to be developed commercially. Aware of this, Wang began thinking about starting his own company. On June 22, 1951, he founded Wang Laboratories in Cambridge, Massachusetts, to manufacture magnetic core memories. He had $600, and, as he said in his autobiography, "I had no orders, no contracts, and no office furniture." He subsisted for a while on contracts for manufacturing memories, on teaching, and on consulting. In November, 1953, Wang began a consulting contract with **IBM** for a thousand dollars a month that was to bring him some financial stability. In March of 1956 Wang sold his patent on magnetic core memories to IBM for $500,000.

In the early 1960s, Wang Laboratories developed a popular **typesetting** system that would justify and hyphenate text on a page. By 1964 the company had sales of more than $1,000,000 for the first time. Then Wang began to develop desktop calculators. One of these, the Model 300, was very successful because it was user friendly, small, and relatively cheap at $1,695. By 1967, Wang's sales were up to $6.9 million per year. To raise money and eliminate some of its debt, Wang Labs publicly offered its stock for sale in August of 1967. The stock was so popular that the value of the company soared. Before the sale of stock, on August 22, Wang Labs was worth about one million dollars. One day later, after its stock went on sale, it had a market capitalization of $70,000,000.

Wang began to realize that the future of the company was not in desktop calculators but in computers. He feared that desktop calculators would become lower-valued commodities because of increasing competition. In 1971 the first pocket **calculator** was manufactured by Bowmar Instruments, and in the following decades, the appliances became even smaller and less expensive. Wang Laboratories began producing its first word processors, the Wang 1200s, in 1972. The Wang 1200 was very primitive by today's standards. It stored data on a tape cassette and had no means of displaying text. Wang decided on some major improvements, and Wang Labs caused a sensation when it demonstrated its first CRT (cathode ray tube)-based word processor in June of 1976. In two years it was the largest distributor of such systems in the world. By 1982, Wang Laboratories had over a billion dollars in sales a year. By 1989, sales were $3 billion a year.

Wang received over a dozen honorary doctorates for his accomplishments, and, among other honors, was a fellow of the American Academy of Arts and Sciences. He underwent surgery to remove a cancerous tumor of the esophagus in 1989. He was readmitted to Massachusetts General Hospital in March of 1990 and died of cancer at the age of 70 on March 24, 1990.

# WATERFALL MODEL

The creation of large software **applications** is rarely, if ever, a simple and straightforward business. There are all the problems associated with vanilla **programming**, as also those associated with running a successful business, as well as the need to function in an environment where the competition is always fierce. There is not a great deal of scope for trial and error, and it is necessary to use a well-defined and rigorously enforced process model for software development that would form the basis for the creation of high quality software.

The standard life-cycle model of software is called a "waterfall model," because it is supposed to go down through a series of steps, reminding one of the route a natural waterfall takes over a series of rocks at different levels.

In the traditional waterfall model, the first step in the software life-cycle is requirements analysis—this is the stage where the customers are queried for their needs, and a formal description of the software requirements is created. The next step is **design**, where the software that is to meet the requirements is planned. The third stage is implementation, where teams of developers create the software. The fourth step is testing, at which time developers, as well as representatives of the user community, are allowed to use the software and are asked to report any bugs they find. Upon completion of this step, the software is declared operational, and only maintenance tasks are required thereafter.

The traditional waterfall model is much too simplistic, however, because each of the distinct steps it asks for is really itself a broad phase consisting of many sub-steps. To give a better perspective of what these smaller steps are, a more detailed waterfall model is usually described.

In the detailed waterfall model, the requirements analysis step is extremely important. It is necessary to understand the customer's needs and to translate them into appropriate desired system behaviors. Any miscommunication with the customer could be fatal to the project as a whole, as it could result in a product that does not meet the customer's expectations, thus giving the company a bad reputation—a real disaster in the competitive software vendor's marketplace. Yet, communicating with the customer is not always easy either, because the customer may have only vaguely-formulated objectives; or may have objectives that aren't vocalized very well and remain in the background for too long; or may have unrealizable or conflicting objectives. In some cases, it is necessary for the software development team to tell the customer exactly what he wants based on his vague utterances, and also whether he can get it—needless to say, this involves a fair amount of skill at diplomacy and personal communication, in addition to knowledge of software engineering. Once the customer's requirements are understood, it is then necessary to document those requirements in a formal manner and reach an agreement with the customer about them (this is most often done in the form of a legally binding contract).

Once the requirements analysis is over, design must happen. This itself has to have at least two distinct stages, system or architectural design at the large scale, and detailed design of modules, objects, and the like at the small scale.

After the design steps, module designs are coded by programmers, and are individually tested against their specifications. Such testing is usually called unit testing of modules. After the modules have been unit tested individually, they are put together as a functioning system in a step called system integration, and the system as a whole is tested to see if it meets behavior and performance requirements.

The customer cannot be left with just the system, of course—he will also want very detailed documentation that shows him how to use the system, what things to do or not do, and the like. The customer may also need special training in the system. For this reason, the finished product must be delivered to the customer with documentation, and possibly with training support as well. This documenting of the system and creation of training resources is considered to be part of the delivery step, but actually goes on from almost the very beginning of the software life-cycle, right in parallel with the development effort itself.

The waterfall model is conceptually simple to understand and is useful to explain the basics of software development, but even with the added detail, it is highly limited in its application as a practical method for managing such development. It is much too simplistic in its view of the software life-cycle, and focuses largely on creation of software as though it were a physical product or fixed artifact, rather than the result of incremental problem solving by a large group of diverse people. In practical software development, there are also numerous feedback loops that arise between stages—for example, a problem with the design may be discovered during implementation, leading to a reversion to the design step. The waterfall model also does not deal with **hardware** upgrades (a constant feature in contemporary information technology practice), incremental development, or development of later versions of software based on earlier ones.

The term "process maturity" refers to the effectiveness and comprehensiveness of an organization's software engineering practices. The widely accepted standard in this regard is the Capability Maturity Model (CMM) developed by the Software Engineering Institute at Carnegie-Mellon University in Pittsburgh, Pennsylvania. The CMM defines five levels of process maturity and has an associated assessment process to determine an organization's level of maturity in software engineering practice, with level five being the highest. An organization wishing to achieve the higher levels would probably do very well to avoid using the waterfall model of development and instead use an advanced model such as Boehm's Spiral Life-Cycle Model.

*See also* Object-oriented programming; Program design

# WATSON, THOMAS JOHN (1874-1956)

*American corporate executive*

American business executive Thomas J. Watson assumed management of the **International Business Machines** Corporation (**IBM**) in 1924 and built it into one of the world's largest and most respected corporations. As a manufacturer of business machines and computers, IBM under Watson's innovative and inspired supervision led a revolution in the business world that heralded the information age. By the end of 1955, Watson's last full year as IBM's chief executive officer, he had guided his company from debt to having total assets of $630 million and from fewer than 4,000 employees to 41,000. IBM was poised to dominate the emerging computer market, and by the 1960s and 1970s it controlled 80 percent of the U.S. market. Due to Watson's effective leadership, IBM had become a model for corporate planning, research, and customer and employee loyalty.

Thomas John Watson was born February 17, 1874, in Campbell, New York. He was descended from a Scottish-Irish family who had moved to upstate New York in the 1840s. Watson's father, Thomas, was a lumber dealer. Young Tom Watson was educated at Addison (New York) Academy. His father urged him to study law when he graduated and offered to pay his college expenses, but Watson was anxious to pay his own way and to begin his business career. Watson took a year-long course at the Elmira (New York) School of Commerce and, at the age of 17, found a job as a bookkeeper in Clarence Risley's market in Painted Post, New York. Soon bored, he took a job as a peddler selling organs and sewing machines.

From such a modest start, Watson would eventually emerge as one of America's greatest and most influential business executives. He married Jeanette Mary Kittridge of Dayton, Ohio in 1913, and they had two sons and two daughters. Two of their sons, Thomas J. Watson, Jr. and Arthur K. Watson, followed their father to work at IBM. Thomas J. Watson, Jr. became president of the company in 1952 and was chairman from 1961 to 1971.

A Presbyterian and a Democrat, Watson was a strong supporter of Franklin Roosevelt and Harry Truman. Dignified and conservative in his dress and manner, Watson neither smoked nor drank, nor did he take vacations, working 16-hour days and spending most of his evenings at the functions of his many employees' clubs. Watson's personality and manner defined the IBM corporate identity that extended to its severely conservative dress code and the ever-present stimulating signs that graced IBM offices such as "Aim High and Think in Big Figures," "Serve and Sell," and IBM's trademark, a Watson creation: "Think." Although Watson has been called "Salesman Number 1," his manner was the opposite of the typical salesman. While talking to Watson, who was bashful and soft spoken, most people forgot their sales resistance and succumbed to his quiet charm and integrity.

Watson's principal interest outside of business was as a patron of the arts. He began acquiring paintings when he was only 24, and was an outspoken advocate of the mutual benefit in joining the world of art with business. At the 1939 New York World's Fair he exhibited paintings by artists from 75 countries and a collection by American artists that IBM had acquired. For many years he served as a trustee at Columbia University and as the president of the International Chamber of Commerce. An adviser to several U.S. presidents, Watson, who never graduated from college, was the recipient of 32 honorary degrees. For offering IBM's considerable research

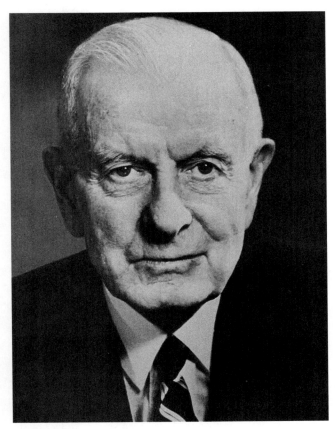

**Thomas J. Watson**

and production capacity for the war effort during World War II, Watson was given the U.S. Medal of Merit. He also received numerous decorations from several foreign countries, including the Merit Cross of the German Eagle, which Watson returned to Hitler in 1940, stating that the policies of the Nazis were contrary to the causes for which he worked.

In 1895 Watson joined the fast-growing National Cash Register (NCR) Company as a salesman. At first the company manager was uninterested in hiring him, but Watson persisted, making numerous trips to the company's Buffalo office. After several months he was finally offered a position. The United States was in the midst of a depression, and Watson sometimes went many weeks without a single sale. He sustained himself by quoting the tried-and-true slogans and homilies that he later would use at IBM. Despite his early lack of success, he received encouragement from his superiors, and, within two years, Watson had become the top salesman in the Buffalo office. He moved steadily up the company ladder to become general sales manager and was given a position in NCR's Dayton home office in 1903. Watson's aggressive assault on NCR's competition, the creation of a company to undercut competitor's prices on second-hand cash registers, was illegal, although it is unclear whether Watson was aware of this. Watson, along with NCR's president and 28 others, was indicted and convicted for the scheme. An appeals court later ordered a new trial, but it was never held. In 1913, in a dispute over an antitrust legal issue, Watson was fired from NCR, though he was presented with a $50,000 parting gift.

Watson was selected to head the Computing-Tabulating-Recording Company of Elmira, New York, a small holding company that controlled four small firms that produced punch-card tabulators, time clocks, and other business machines. As company president, Watson acted to secure loans to finance expansion. The move helped the company's gross sales increase from $2 million in 1914 to more than $33 million by 1949. Personnel increased from 235 to 12,000 during the same period. Watson was committed to research and development, and much of the borrowed funds went into engineering laboratories that produced new machines such as the key punch, card sorters, tabulators, and eventually the computer. In 1924 the firm merged with International Business Machines Corporation and took its name. The business he had taken over had by then more than doubled in terms of plant size, number of employees, and volumes of sales. As the head of IBM, Watson helped those figures double yet again about every five years during his reign.

In the 1930s, a new engineering laboratory was built in Endicott, New York, and IBM entered the electrical typewriter business with the purchase of Electromatic Typewriters, Inc. of Rochester, New York. As the holder of more than 1,400 patents as of 1941, IBM held a virtual monopoly in the field of business machines. IBM would maintain its dominance through the inspired leadership of Watson. Having been a salesman, Watson devoted considerable effort in training his sales force, insisting that IBM salesmen should know how to install, operate, and repair all the equipment that they sold. Working out the three basic steps in the selling technique: the approach, the demonstration, and the closing, Watson insisted that his salesmen stress that IBM sold not machines but service. Extremely concerned about IBM's corporate image, Watson was rigid in his hiring and personnel practices. Before World War II, employees at IBM were exclusively male and white Anglo-Saxon Protestants. Jews, Catholics, blacks, and women were unacceptable. All employees were expected to have a copy of *Men, Minutes and Money*, a collection of Watson's speeches and essays. Employees were expected to be freshly shaved, wearing daily shined shoes, and to follow their chairman's dress style—dark suits, quiet ties, and white shirts—whether in the main New York office or in the Endicott factory. The IBM image virtually defined the corporate concept of the "organization man." Yet the benefits of conforming to IBM's image were many. Forbes declared in a 1948 article that Watson had created "the nearest to ideal working conditions." Watson paid higher rates than his competition did. There were few firings, and benefits included health and life insurance, a rarity at the time. The company also maintained at Endicott a country club for all employees. IBM workers were made to feel that they were members of a special group who were encouraged in their innovations and originality and were expected to carry a THINK notebook to record their inspirations.

The benefits of Watson's emphasis on understanding the market and encouraging innovation are best demonstrated in IBM's entry into the electronics field. After World War II, IBM held off producing electronic computers, continuing to produce only its electromechanical machines in the early 1950s. Sperry Rand's development of **UNIVAC** in 1948, the first electronic computer, however, prompted IBM to accelerate its own electronic development. Though IBM had brought out its first electronic **calculator** in 1946, it was not until 1952 that IBM produced its first large-scale electronic **data** processing system. By 1956, the year of Thomas J. Watson's death, IBM had leaped far ahead of its competitors due to its superior software packages and worldwide marketing **operation**. IBM won the battle for dominance in the early years of the electronic revolution because of its considerable commitment to research and because its sales force knew what businesses needed for **information processing** and accounting. IBM therefore designed its machines to fit the needs of its customers, a successful strategy that Watson had spent his lifetime promoting.

By 1955, Watson's last full year as IBM's chief executive, the company's total assets were $630 million with a domestic work force of 41,000, with branch offices in 189 cities, and plants in six cities. The IBM World Trade Corporation had 19,000 employees, 11 plants, and 208 branch offices in 82 countries. Watson had seen his struggling company grow into a world giant that would continue to dominate the business machine market and the rapidly developing computer industry under the direction of his son.

During his tenure as head of IBM, Watson created one of the world's largest and most influential corporations. Dominating its markets, IBM supplied the business machines upon which American business depended by creating new products to meet customers' needs. Through the development of data processing equipment and a successful computer line, IBM changed the very nature of modern business itself. Through his years at IBM's helm, Watson managed to make IBM the gold standard for product reliability and innovation. He also forged the dominating principles of the corporate culture with its emphasis on company loyalty and team spirit, accomplishing the difficult task of simultaneously encouraging employee uniformity and innovation and individuality.

It may well be that Watson, described in a *Saturday Evening Post* article as a striking example of "one-man rule in business," was one of the last of the breed of dominating personalities whose identity became inseparable from that of his company.

The machines and devices that IBM pioneered changed modern culture in essential ways. From the calculator to the computer, IBM has been in the forefront of the information and electronic explosion in the second half of the twentieth century, a future that Thomas J. Watson anticipated and helped to create.

# WIDE-AREA NETWORK

**Data** networks that reach across large distances (across states or even continents), known as wide-area networks or WANs, have different requirements and network packet-switching technologies than those that span much shorter distances (within a single building or room) characterized by local-area networks or LANs. The differentiating factor separating the two types of networks is more of technology than distance, because there is no set maximum distance for WANs. WANs, therefore, are usually maintained by public telecommunication companies in countries around the world where WANs are in place. WAN technologies function at the lower three layers of the OSI reference model: the physical layer, the data-link layer, and the network layer.

WANs operate at slower speeds than LANs. Typical data passthrough rates range from 1.5 Mbps to 155 Mbps, and seem like a snail's pace compared to **LAN** speeds of up to 2 Gbps for a typical LAN network. LANs and WANs provide a balance in data networks because the advantage of one is a disadvantage in the other, and vice-versa. For example, while LANs send data at much faster rates, they cannot span large distances; WANs can span great distances, but send data at much slower rates (and with delays of up to several tenths of a second due to the need for WANs to bounce signals off of earth-orbiting satellites).

WANs are designed to provide reliable, fast, and secure communication between nodes on the network. Companies with locations all over the globe can have one integrated network by using various communication strategies and technologies. Because the public telecommunications organization of each country is heavily involved with WAN development, one cannot discount the political, technological, and strategic decisions that can and do influence WAN development.

### Basic WAN Varieties

The most fundamental type of WAN is called the leased line, which is a telephone line that has been leased for private use. In some contexts it is referred to as a dedicated line. A leased line is usually contrasted with a switched line or dial-up line.

Companies rent leased lines from the telephone company to interconnect different geographic locations in their company. The alternative is to buy and maintain their own private lines or, increasingly perhaps, to use the "public switched telephone network," or PSTN, with secure **message protocols**. (This is called tunneling, and it uses the **Internet** as part of a private secure network.)

### Packet-Switched WANs

First appearing in the 1960s, the Packet-Switched WAN is the foundation for all contemporary communication networks. Packet-Switched Data Networks, or PSDNs, transfer data between network nodes in small packets (a packet contains a few hundred bytes of data and carries information that informs the network **hardware** where to send it), where software at the receiving **node** re-assembles the packets into a file. However, overloaded packet-switched networks force computers on the network to wait before they can send additional packets. Despite this problem, PSDNs are very popular because of their low cost (many computers sharing bandwidth, thus requiring fewer connections) and performance.

### Frame Relay and Integrated Services Digital Network (ISDN)

Frame Relay is thought to be the next major leap in the X.25 packet-switching protocol. Frame Relay offers faster communication, equivalent to a T-3 line (44.736 Mbps compared to a T-1 line at 1.544 Mbps), and an overall better communication protocol. Frame Relay is a point-to-point service that replaces leased lines.

Integrated Services Digital Network, or ISDN, is a fully digital network service that can send most types of data (voice, image, information) to every node in an ISDN (meaning every house). This service is more popular in Europe than in the U.S.

### WAN Devices

A WAN switch is a multi-port **internetworking** device used in carrier networks. These devices typically switch traffic such as Frame Relay, X.25, and SMDS and operate at the data link layer of the OSI reference model.

A **modem** is a device that interprets digital and analog signals, allowing data to be transmitted over voice-grade telephone lines. At the source, digital signals are converted to a format designed for transmission over analog communication facilities. At the destination, these analog signals are returned to their digital form.

A **channel** service unit/digital service unit, or CSU/DSU, is a digital-interface device that adapts the physical interface on a data **terminal** to the interface of a data circuit-terminating switch in a switched-carrier network. The CSU/DSU also provides signal timing for communication between these devices.

An ISDN terminal adapter connects ISDN Basic Rate Interface (BRI, which is a level of ISDN service intended for the home and small enterprise) connections to other interfaces. A terminal adapter is essentially an ISDN modem.

### The Future of WAN

Since the world's largest WAN is the Internet, it only seems natural to assume that the future of WAN lies with a wireless Internet. Indeed, the current hype about wireless Internet does exceed the reality, but the next generation of wireless devices, called 3G (for 3rd generation), will combine voice and Internet capabilities into wireless handsets, promising faster **access** and increased capacity for many wireless products.

# WIENER, NORBERT (1894-1964)
*American mathematician*

Norbert Wiener was one of the most original mathematicians of his time. The field concerning the study of automatic control systems, called **cybernetics**, owes a great deal not only to his researches, but to his continuing efforts at publicity. He wrote for a variety of popular journals as well as for technical

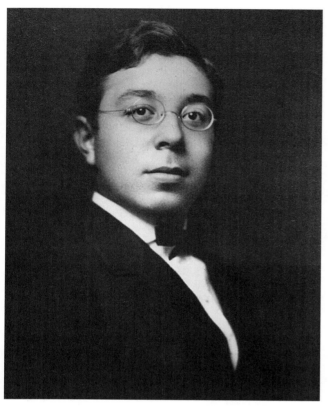

**Norbert Wiener**

1906 he entered Tufts University, as the family had moved to the Boston area, and he graduated four years later.

Up until that point Wiener's education had clearly outrun that of most of his contemporaries, but he was now faced with the challenge of deciding what to do with his education. He enrolled at Harvard to study zoology, but the subject did not suit him. He tried studying philosophy at Cornell, but that was equally unavailing. Finally, Wiener came back to Harvard to work on philosophy and mathematics. The subject of his dissertation was a comparison of the system of logic developed by Bertrand Russell and Alfred North Whitehead in their *Principia Mathematica* with the earlier algebraic system created by Ernst Schröder. The relatively recent advances in mathematical research in the United States had partly occurred in the area of algebraic logic, so the topic was a reasonable one for a student hoping to bridge the still-existent gap between the European and American mathematical communities.

Although Wiener earned a Harvard travelling fellowship to enable him to study in Europe after taking his degree, his father still supervised his career by writing to Bertrand Russell on Norbert's behalf. Wiener was in England from June 1913 to April 1914 and attended two courses given by Russell, including a reading course on *Principia Mathematica*. Perhaps more influential in the long run for Wiener's mathematical development was a course he took from the British analyst G. H. Hardy, whose lectures he greatly admired. In the same way, Wiener studied with some of the most eminent names in Göttingen, Germany, then the center of the international mathematical community.

Wiener returned to the United States in 1915, still unsure, despite his foreign travels, of the mathematical direction he wanted to pursue. He wrote articles for the *Encyclopedia Americana* and took a variety of teaching jobs until the entry of the United States into World War I. Wiener was a fervent patriot, and his enthusiasm led him to join the group of scientists and engineers at the Aberdeen Proving Ground in Maryland, where he encountered Oswald Veblen, already one of the leading mathematicians in the country. Although Wiener did not pursue Veblen's lines of research, Veblen's success in producing results useful to the military impressed Wiener more than mere academic success.

After the war two events decisively shaped Wiener's mathematical future. He obtained a position as instructor at the Massachusetts Institute of Technology (MIT) in mathematics, where he was to remain until his retirement. At that time mathematics was not particularly strong at MIT, but his position there assured him of continued contact with engineers and physicists. As a result, he displayed an ongoing concern for the applications of mathematics to problems that could be stated in physical terms. The question of which tools he would bring to bear on those problems was answered by the death of his sister's fiancé. That promising young mathematician left his collection of books to Wiener, who began to read avidly the standard texts in a way that he had not in his earlier studies.

The first problem Wiener addressed had to do with Brownian motion, the apparently random motion of particles in substances at rest. The phenomenon had earlier excited Albert Einstein's interest, and he had dealt with it in one of his

publications and was not reluctant to express political views even when they might be unpopular. Perhaps the most distinctive feature of Wiener's life as a student and a mathematician is how well documented it is, thanks to two volumes of autobiography published during his lifetime. They reveal some of the complexity of a man whose aspirations went well beyond the domain of mathematics.

Wiener was born in Columbia, Missouri, on November 26, 1894. His father, Leo Wiener, had been born in Bialystok, Poland (then Russia), and was an accomplished linguist. He arrived in New Orleans in 1880 with very little money but a great deal of determination, some of it visible in his relations with his son. He met his wife, Bertha Kahn, at a meeting of a Browning Club. As a result, when his son was born, he was given the name Norbert, from one of Browning's verse dramas. In light of the absence of Judaism from the Wiener home (Norbert was fifteen before he learned that he was Jewish), it is surprising that one of Leo Wiener's best-known works was a history of Yiddish literature.

As the title of the first volume of his autobiography *Ex-Prodigy* suggests, Wiener was a child prodigy. Whatever his natural talents, this was partly due to the efforts of his father. Leo Wiener was proud of his educational theories and pointed to the academic success of his son as evidence. Norbert was less enthusiastic and in his memoirs describes his recollections of his father's harsh disciplinary methods. He entered high school at the age of nine and graduated two years later. In

1905 papers. Wiener took the existence of Brownian motion as a sign of randomness at the heart of nature. By idealizing the physical phenomenon, Wiener was able to produce a mathematical theory of Brownian motion that had wide influence among students of probability. It is possible to see in his work on Brownian motion, steps in the direction of the study of **fractals** (shapes whose detail repeats itself on any scale), although Wiener did not go far along that path.

The next subject Wiener addressed was the Dirichlet problem, which had been reintroduced into the mathematical mainstream by German David Hilbert. Much of the earliest work on the Dirichlet problem had been discredited as not being sufficiently rigorous for the standards of the late nineteenth century. Wiener's work on the Dirichlet problem produced interesting results, some of which he delayed publishing for the sake of a couple of students finishing their theses at Harvard. Wiener felt subsequently that his forbearance was not recognized adequately. In particular, although Wiener progressed through the academic ranks at MIT from assistant professor in 1924 to associate professor in 1929 to full professor in 1932, he believed that more support from Harvard would have enabled him to advance more quickly.

Wiener had a high opinion of his own abilities, something of a change from colleagues whose public expressions of modesty were at odds with a deep-seated conviction of their own merits. Whatever his talents as a mathematician, Wiener's expository standards were at odds with those of most mathematicians of his time. While he was always exuberant, this was often at the cost of accuracy of detail. One of his main theorems depended on a series of lemmas, or auxiliary propositions, one of which was proven by assuming the truth of the main theorem. Students trying to learn from Wiener's papers and finding their efforts unrewarding discovered that this reaction was almost universal. As Hans Freudenthal remarked in the *Dictionary of Scientific Biography,* "After proving at length a fact that would be too easy if set as an exercise for an intelligent sophomore, he would assume without proof a profound theorem that was seemingly unrelated to the preceding text, then continue with a proof containing puzzling but irrelevant terms, next interrupt it with a totally unrelated historical exposition, meanwhile quote something from the 'last chapter' of the book that had actually been in the first, and so on."

In 1926 Wiener was married to Margaret Engemann, an assistant professor of modern languages at Juniata College. They had two daughters, Barbara (born 1928) and Peggy (born 1929). Wiener enjoyed his family's company and found there a relaxation from a mathematical community that did not always share his opinion of the merits of his work.

During the decade after his marriage, Wiener worked in a number of fields and wrote some of the papers with which he is most associated. In the field of harmonic analysis, he did a great deal with the decomposition of functions into series. Just as a polynomial is made up of terms like $x$, $x^2$, $x^3$, and so forth, so functions in general could be broken up in various ways, depending on the questions to be answered. Somewhat surprisingly, Wiener also undertook putting the operational calculus, earlier developed by Oliver Heaviside, on a rigorous basis. There is even a hint in Wiener's work of the notion of a distribution, a kind of generalized **function**. It is not surprising that Wiener might start to move away from the kind of functions that had been most studied in mathematics toward those that could be useful in physics and engineering.

In 1926 Wiener returned to Europe, this time on a Guggenheim fellowship. He spent little time at Göttingen, due to disagreements with Richard Courant, perhaps the most active student of David Hilbert in mathematical organization. Courant's disparaging comments about Wiener cannot have helped the latter's standing in the mathematical community, but Wiener's brief visit introduced him to Tauberian theory, a fashionable area of analysis. Wiener came up with an imaginative new approach to Tauberian theorems and, perhaps more fortunately, with a coauthor for his longest paper on the subject. The quality of the exposition in the paper, combined with the originality of the results, make it Wiener's best exercise in communicating technical mathematics, although he did not pursue the subject as energetically as he did some of his other works.

In 1931 and 1932 Wiener gave lectures on analysis in Cambridge as a deputy for G. H. Hardy. While there, he made the acquaintance of a young British mathematician, R. E. A. C. Paley, with whom a collaboration soon flourished. He brought Paley to MIT the next academic year and their work progressed rapidly. Paley's death at the age of twenty-six in a skiing accident early in 1933 was a blow to Wiener, who received the Bôcher prize of the American Mathematical Society the same year and was named a fellow of the National Academy of Sciences the next. Among the other areas in which Wiener worked at MIT or Harvard were quantum mechanics, differential geometry, and statistical physics. His investigations in the last of these were wide ranging, but amounted more to the creation of a research program than a body of results.

The arrival of World War II occupied Wiener's attention in a number of ways. He was active on the Emergency Committee in Aid of Displaced German Scholars, which began operations well before the outbreak of fighting. He made proposals concerning the development of computers, although these were largely ignored. One of the problems to which he devoted time was antiaircraft fire, and his results were of great importance for engineering applications regarding filtering. Unfortunately, they were not of much use in the field because of the amount of time required for the calculations.

Weiner devoted the last decades of his life to the study of statistics, engineering, and biology. He had already worked on the general idea of information theory, which arose out of statistical mechanics. The idea of entropy had been around since the nineteenth century and enters into the second law of thermodynamics. It could be defined as an integral, but it was less clear what sort of quantity it was. Work of Ludwig Boltzmann suggested that entropy could be understood as a measure of the disorder of a system. Wiener pursued this notion and used it to get a physical definition of information related to entropy. Although information theory has not always followed the path laid down by Wiener, his work gave the subject a mathematical legitimacy.

An interdisciplinary seminar at the Harvard Medical School provided a push for Wiener in the direction of the interplay between biology and physics. He learned about the complexity of feedback in animals and studied current ideas about neurophysiology from a mathematical point of view. (Wiener left out the names of those who had most influenced him in this area in his autobiography as a result of an argument.) One area of particular interest was prosthetic limbs, perhaps as a result of breaking his arm in a fall. Wiener soon had the picture of a computer as a prosthesis for the brain. In 1947 he agreed to write a book on communication and control and was looking for a term for the theory of messages. The Greek word for messenger, *angelos,* had too many connections with angels to be useful, so he took the word for helmsman, *kubernes,* instead and came up with *cybernetics.* It turned out that the word had been used in the previous century, but Wiener gave it a new range of meaning and currency.

Cybernetics was treated by Wiener as a branch of mathematics with its own terms, like signal, noise, and information. One of his collaborators in this area was John Neumann, whose work on computers had been followed up much more enthusiastically than Wiener's. The difference in reception could be explained by the difference in mathematical styles: von Neumann was meticulous, while Wiener tended to be less so. The new field of cybernetics prospered with two such distinct talents working in it. Von Neumann's major contribution to the field was only realized after his death. Wiener devoted most of his later years to the area. Among his more popular books were *The Human Use of Human Beings* in 1950 and *God and Golem, Inc.* in 1964.

In general, Wiener was happy writing for a wide variety of journals and audiences. He contributed to the *Atlantic, Nation,* the *New Republic,* and *Collier's,* among others. His two volumes of autobiography, *Ex-Prodigy* and *I Am a Mathematician,* came out in 1953 and 1956, respectively. Reviews pointed out the extent to which Wiener's **memory** operated selectively, but also admitted that he did bring the mathematical community to life in a way seldom seen. Although Wiener remarked that mathematics was a young man's game, he also indicated that he felt himself lucky in having selected subjects for investigation that he could pursue later in life. He received an honorary degree from Tufts in 1946 and in 1949 was Gibbs lecturer to the American Mathematical Society.

In 1964 Wiener received the National Medal of Science. On March 18, while travelling through Stockholm, he collapsed and died. A memorial service was held at MIT on the June 2, led by Swami Sarvagatananda of the Vedanta Society of Boston, along with Christian and Jewish clergy. This mixture of faiths was expressive of Wiener's lifelong unwillingness to be fit into a stereotype. He was a mathematician who talked about the theology of the Fall. He did not discover that he was Jewish until he was in graduate school but found great support in the poems of Heinrich Heine. Nevertheless, his intellectual originality led him down paths subsequent generations have come to follow.

## WILKES, MAURICE (1913- )
### *English computer engineer*

Maurice Wilkes developed an interest in radio as a child and specialized in radar research during World War II. After the war, Wilkes became involved in pioneering research on the development of computers and is best known for his development of **EDSAC**, the **Electronic Delay Storage Automatic Calculator**, the first computing machine to make use of the concept of a stored program. Over the last five decades, Wilkes has been actively involved in the formation of a number of computer organizations and associations.

Maurice Vincent Wilkes was born on June 26, 1913, in Dudley, England. His father, Vincent J. Wilkes, was employed at the time on the South Staffordshire estate of the Earl of Dudley. His mother's name is not mentioned in the usual biographical records nor in Wilkes's own autobiography *Memoirs of a Computer Pioneer.* She is described in the latter reference, however, as "one of a pioneering band of women who went into offices in their hobble skirts and worked the new-fangled type-writing machines."

Wilkes's early education in Dudley was interrupted by severe bouts of asthma, which he apparently inherited from his mother's side of the family. While he was still young, Wilkes's father moved the family to nearby Stourbridge in order to find a more congenial environment for his mother's health. Wilkes entered the King Edward VI Grammar School in Stourbridge at the age of eight and quickly developed an interest in science and mathematics. He was later to report in his *Memoirs,* "I think it was already clear to me [in the Sixth Form] that my life would be in physics or in physics-based engineering. I had seen enough to realize that there was a magic power in mathematics and I burned to be initiated fully into that mystery."

The other field that attracted Wilkes's interest at an early age was radio. The early 1920s were an era when "the wireless" was just becoming popular, with small amateur stations and crystal sets beginning to proliferate. Wilkes subscribed to *Wireless World* while he was still a teenager and a short time later was asked to build some equipment for station G6OJ, operated by the chemistry master at King Edward VI. In 1931 Wilkes applied for and received his own amateur radio operator's license.

Also in 1931 Wilkes graduated from King Edward VI and was accepted as a student at St. John's College, Cambridge. He concentrated in mathematics there and in June 1934 graduated with honors. He then applied for and received a research grant from the department of scientific and industrial research. He chose to use that grant to continue his studies at the Cavendish Laboratories at Cambridge, where he began work with the radio group in July 1934.

The first topic on which Wilkes was asked to work at the Cavendish involved a study of long radio waves. As he completed this project, the future direction of his career became more clear to him. He found that he was not particularly interested in pure or theoretical mathematics itself, but math "as application to any sort of physics was concerned. I did not have," he later wrote, "and indeed have never had, that interest in mathematical puzzles and fine points that characterize the natural theoretician. I looked forward to being able to apply the math I had learnt to physical problems."

An important turning point in Wilkes's life came in March 1936 when he attended a lecture given by D. R. Hartree of Manchester University. Hartree's lecture involved the demonstration of a differential analyzer, a mechanical device for solving differential equations. Wilkes says that he found the machine "irresistible," and, more than that, exactly the tool he needed to solve some of the mathematical problems involved in his study of long waves. His future in the computing sciences appears to have been set.

Before long, Wilkes was involved in the **operation** of Cambridge's own differential analyzer and, in later 1937 he was asked to join the university's newly established "Mathematical Laboratory," which was, in fact, a "computing laboratory." (The facility's name was actually corrected thirty-three years later.) Wilkes's official appointment at the time was as university demonstrator. In early 1938 he was awarded his M.A. degree and in October of the same year, his Ph.D.

The year of Wilkes's graduation was one of profound unrest in Great Britain and across Europe. Some observers expected the outbreak of war momentarily and were encouraging preparation for that event. Others held to the hope that peace could still be salvaged. Within a year of receiving his degree, Wilkes had been drafted into the program for the development of radarlike devices for the detection of, at first, submarines, and, later, surface ships and aircraft. His first assignment was at the radar station at Dunkirk, where he reported on August 28, 1939. Within a short time he was back in Cambridge, working on antisubmarine devices before returning to Dunkirk and, later, to other stations along the coast.

By 1941 Wilkes had been assigned to the Operations Research Group (ORG) headquartered in Petersham. Most of his work with the ORG involved the development of ten-centimeter radar instruments and, in particular, of the GL Mark I, II, and III detection systems. In 1943 Wilkes moved on to a new assignment in Malvern, where he worked on the development of the Oboe system. In his autobiography, Wilkes describes Oboe as a "blind-bombing system that depended on measurement of range from two land-based stations to the bombing aircraft."

At the war's conclusion, Wilkes volunteered for an assignment in Germany interviewing captured German scientists. His account of the two months he spent in Germany is an equal mix of new information gained from his interviewees, sparkling travelogue about the German countryside, and ongoing complaints about endless bureaucratic confusion. Wilkes returned to Cambridge from his Germany assignment on August 1, 1945, to an offer of a university lectureship and the post of acting director of the mathematical laboratory. In May 1946 Wilkes was given a copy of **John von Neumann**'s "Draft Report on EDVAC." The report contained, Wilkes later wrote, "the principles on which the development of the modern digital computer was to be based." "I recognized this at once as the real thing," he went on, "and from that time on never had any doubt as to the way computer development would go." In October 1946 Wilkes was given the title of director of the laboratory.

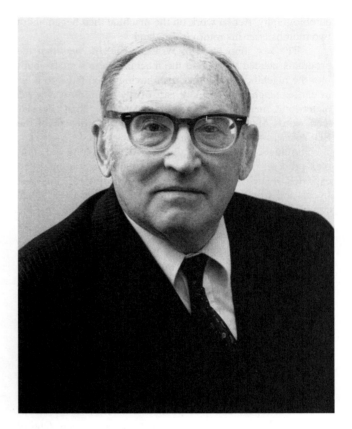

**Maurice Wilkes**

Wilkes's interest in computers had not precluded his continued research on atmospheric physics begun before the war. Indeed, this topic was one to which he kept returning for many years, even after he had earned his reputation in computer science. One of his accomplishments in the immediate postwar period was to confirm, using the differential analyzer, a prediction by C. L. Pekeris regarding factors affecting resonance in the atmosphere.

In early 1946 Wilkes was invited to attend a course on Electronic Computing to be held at the Moore School of Electrical Engineering in Philadelphia on August 8–31. Travel was still difficult in the postwar year of 1946, and Wilkes actually arrived two weeks late for the class. However, he had an opportunity to see the world's first electronic computer, the **ENIAC**, which, although it had already become something of a dinosaur in the computer world, still provided the standard for the future of computer development.

During this visit to the United States—the first of many over the next forty years—Wilkes spoke with most of the pioneers of computer science in the United States, including **Howard Aiken** at Harvard, S. H. Caldwell at the Massachusetts Institute of Technology (MIT), and **John William Mauchly** and H. H. Goldstine at the Moore School. It was during this visit that Wilkes "first began to sketch out the **design** of the machine that finally became the EDSAC," he states in his autobiography. Actual work on the machine then began about two months after his return to England.

The key innovation in Wilkes's EDSAC was that the programs needed to operate the machine were actually built into the machine itself rather than having to be fed into it, as in earlier machines. The key part of the machine was a 1.5 meter-long, mercury-filled tank, called a "tube," that held sixteen words of thirty-five bits each. The final design of the EDSAC was to consist of thirty-two such tubes.

Actual construction of the EDSAC was a long and complex process, filled with the problems and frustrations to be expected of such an undertaking. At a key point, officials of J. Lyons and Company offered an infusion of cash that made completion of the computer possible and at the same time led to the development of the first commercial versions of EDSAC, LEO 1, LEO 2, and LEO 3.

The first successful run of EDSAC took place on May 6, 1949. The machine read a program tape for computing a table of squares and correctly printed out the results. In a short period of time, researchers were making use of the powerful new computing tool. In early 1949, for example, the eminent statistician Ronald A. Fisher inquired about the use of EDSAC in the solution of a second-order nonlinear differential equation. A year later, Wilkes provided him with the results, results about which Wilkes later wrote, "I do not think that he had for one moment expected that we would produce." In 1950 Wilkes wrote a report describing the development and uses of EDSAC, a report that was published in 1951 by Addison-Wesley as *Preparation of Programs for an Electronic Digital Computer, with Special Reference to the EDSAC and the Use of a Library of Subroutines*. The book was reissued in 1982 as volume 1 of the Charles Babbage Institute reprint series on the history of computing. In July 1950 Wilkes left for his second visit to the United States, one that was to last for two months and was to include stops at every major computing center in the country. He visited the Institute for Advanced Studies in Princeton, New Jersey; the Eckert-Mauchly Corporation in Philadelphia; the National Bureau of Standards in Washington, D.C.; the U.S. Army proving ground in Aberdeen, Maryland; Harvard and MIT in Cambridge, Massachusetts; **IBM** World Headquarters in New York City; the navy proving ground in Dahlgren, Virginia; the University of Illinois; and the University of California at Berkeley.

Less than six months after his return from the United States, Wilkes had become deeply involved in the planning for the next stage in computing machinery, EDSAC 2. He recognized that the time had come to move from the experimental level represented by EDSAC 1 to a fully operational working machine that could begin to take on many of the research projects already envisioned by university researchers in many departments. By June 1951 funding had been obtained from the Nuffield Foundation, and construction was under way by the summer of 1953. An intermediary model, EDSAC 1.5, passed initial tests, and early in 1958 EDSAC 2 was formally put into operation. A few months later, on July 11, 1958, EDSAC 1 was formally closed down and dismantled, its parts sold for scrap.

In very little time, EDSAC 2 proved its worth to the scientific community. Its first notable success was in connection with the work of John Kendrew, who was working on the molecular structure of myoglobin. Kendrew had used EDSAC 1 to help analyze four hundred X-ray diffraction patterns in the early part of his research and had then turned to EDSAC 2 to examine ten thousand more photographs when that machine became available. In his 1962 Nobel lecture, Kendrew acknowledged the role of the EDSAC machines in facilitating the research for which he had received that coveted prize.

At nearly the same time, astronomer Martin Ryle found another use for EDSAC 2. Ryle was working on the problem of creating a radio telescope with a very large aperture capable of obtaining resolutions far better than any existing instruments. Ryle's approach was to construct the telescope of movable sections whose individual photographs could then be analyzed and combined by means of complex computer programs. The EDSAC 2 provided the technology that made that approach workable and that brought to Ryle the 1974 Nobel Prize in physics.

By the time EDSAC 2 was powered down on November 1, 1964, Wilkes had become a senior statesman in the field of computer **hardware**. Although he continued to be active in research, he also began to assume more responsibility in professional organizations. For example, in 1957 he was elected the first president of the British Computer Society, a post he held for three years. In 1965 he was appointed chairman of the Computer Advisory Committee of the Agricultural Research Council, a post he held for ten years. After 1950 Wilkes made many trips to the United States; when he reached mandatory retirement age at Cambridge in 1980, he moved to Maynard, Massachusetts, and took a job as staff consultant at the **Digital Equipment Corporation**. A year later he was also appointed adjunct professor at MIT. In 1986 Wilkes returned to Cambridge, where he became a consultant for the Olivetti Research Board.

Wilkes was married to Nina Twyman in 1947. They have three children, Margaret, Helen, and Anthony. Among his many awards have been the Harry Goode Memorial Award (1968) and the Eckert-Mauchly Award (1980) of the American Federation of Information Processing Societies, the McDowell Award of the Institute of Electrical and Electronics Engineers (1981), the Pender Award of the University of Pennsylvania (1982), the C and C Prize (Tokyo, 1988), and the Italgas Prize (Turin, 1991). He has also received honorary doctorates from eight universities.

# WIMP (WINDOWS, ICONS, MENUS, AND POINTING DEVICES)

WIMP stands for Windows, Icons, Menus, and Pointing. Most personal computers in use today provide a WIMP interface for their users. WIMP interfaces allow the user to exchange information with the computer by means of a pointing device (often a **mouse**) and a video monitor.

The pointing device referred to in the WIMP acronym enables the user to select images, words, and the like on the display screen. The pointing device can be any one of a number of devices, such as a touch-pad or trackball, but is most often a mouse. By manipulating the pointing device the user sends information to the computer, which in turn directs movement of a pointer (or cursor) on the monitor. The pointer is a symbol such as a small angled arrow or a figure shaped like the letter I. By moving the pointer over a word or image and then pressing a button, the user sends a command to the computer to mark that **object** for movement, activation, or the like. The user can then command the computer (using either an other cursor action or a keyboard action) to save a file to **disk drive**, launch a program, or whatever action might be appropriate for the selected object. The windows in WIMP refers to the discrete rectangular areas that appear on the computer's monitor, inside each of which are images and texts generated by the computer's software. As a program runs, its output is, usually, updated in its associated window. By using the pointing device, **windows** can be opened, closed, or re-sized. The icons of WIMP are small pictures that represent things like programs, folders, and individual files. Pointing and clicking on an **icon** directs the computer to perform a particular action, such as opening a window to display the contents of a file or the output of an application. WIMPs **menus** are lists of **commands** displayed optionally on the screen. A menu command can be activated by placing the cursor over it and then clicking a button.

The advent (and continued dominance) of the WIMP interface is due to a variety of historical events. One of these was the introduction of the microcomputer in the 1970s, which soon led to the development of personal computers (general-purpose microcomputers intended for use by a single user). The microcomputer was made possible by the development of the **microprocessor** (a computer-on-a-chip minus **memory**). The first commercial microprocessor was the **Intel** 4004, first produced in 1971 for use in electronic calculators. Computers that used microprocessors for their **central processing unit** were called microcomputers. By the mid-1970s, many companies were offering microcomputers or personal computers for sale. For example, in 1975 the company MITS introduced the **Altair** 8800 kit, which hobbyists purchased to assemble into their own microcomputer. However, these early consumer microcomputers did not offer a WIMP interface between the user and computer; indeed, the Altair 8800 had no monitor, keyboard, or **printer**! In 1977, **Apple** computer introduced what many consider to be the first successful **personal computer**, the Apple II. The Apple II had a keyboard and monitor, but no WIMP capabilities. In 1984 Apple introduced its highly successful Macintosh line of computers, which were the first commercial personal computers with a full WIMP interface.

The interactive capabilities of the Macintosh were borrowed from the creators of the first **graphical user interface** (**GUI**, pronounced GOO ee). The first GUI was demonstrated on a microcomputer called the Alto in 1973. The Alto was created at **Xerox Corporation's Palo Alto Research Center** in Palo Alto, California. The Alto had many features in common with today's WIMP systems, combining a mouse with a point-and-click GUI. This prototype computer system was demonstrated to Xerox management for possible commercial development, but management failed to grasp the enormous potential of such a system and declined to develop it further. However, **Steve Jobs**, co-founder of Apple Computers, did recognize the potential benefits offered by Alto's graphical interface, and incorporated its features into the company's Lisa and Macintosh computer lines.

The Apple Macintosh was a stunning commercial success. Its many fans were enamored with its WIMP features, which made computing seem much more natural than previous user interfaces such as command-line interfaces employing typed-in text commands or menu-based interfaces that offered lists or arrays of commands that the user activated by pressing keys on the keyboard. Others, however, were content with less intuitive input systems. For instance, users of **Microsoft** Corporation's disk operating system (**DOS**), which provided users a command-line interface, used the acronym WIMP in a derisive manner when referring to the Macintosh operating system. In spite of this cadre of loyal users, Microsoft Corporation decided that it, too, needed an operating system with GUI capabilities. Microsoft introduced its first GUI-capable operating system, Windows 1.0, in late November, 1985. Though rather crude compared to the rival Macintosh operating system, Microsoft's Windows, through repeated release of upgraded versions, would eventually become the world leader in operating system sales.

*See also* Apple; Graphical user interface (GUI); Icon; Mouse; Microprocessor

# WINDOWS

Windows are the rectangular areas used for displaying information in computer **graphical user interfaces** (**GUI**). Designed in the late 1960s as part of the first personal, graphical computer interface, windows remain a key element of most GUIs.

**Douglas Engelbart** and his team of researchers at the Stanford Research Institute (SRI) designed the first personal, graphical computer interface for their innovative computer system called the oN-Line System (NLS). The NLS interface was called a **WIMP** interface, which stands for windows, icons, menus, and pointers. (Engelbart is also famous for inventing the most commonly used pointing device—the mouse.) Engelbart and his researchers gave a legendary demonstration of NLS and the WIMP interface at a conference in 1968. Those who attended the NLS demonstration and saw the WIMP interface got a glimpse of what computing would look like in the future, especially personal computing.

Several SRI researchers went to work at the Xerox Palo Alto Research Center (PARC) in 1970. At **Xerox PARC** these researchers, along with other PARC researchers, further developed windows and the WIMP interface. PARC researchers specifically aimed to build a **personal computer** that a typical office worker could easily learn and use for everyday tasks. To promote ease of learning and use, **Alan Kay** designed an interface that he called a "desktop."

The desktop interface advanced the WIMP interface by using more icons and by treating the windows as sheets of paper that could be stacked on top of one another. The original windows had been "tiled," displayed all at once, next to one another. In this use of windows it is difficult to know which window is active, and the windows must be limited in number and small in size in order to fit on the screen. With stacked windows, it is clear which window is active—the one on top—and the computer screen area is used more efficiently.

In 1974 Xerox PARC developed the Alto. Although the Alto was originally conceived of as a computer for personal use and everyday work, its eventual **design** did not meet the original intent. The Xerox Star, introduced in the late 1970s, was based on the Alto and was a true personal computer for everyday use. The Star was the first computer to make use of Alan Kay's desktop interface. Due to its high cost and slow performance, the Star did not sell well. **Steve Jobs** of **Apple** computer saw a demonstration of the Alto in 1976 and used it as a basis for the Lisa computer. The Lisa was expensive and slow, like the Star, and did not sell well either. However, the Apple Macintosh, introduced in 1984, was hugely successful. Its attractive and elegant implementation of the WIMP desktop interface made it the first computer that was truly easy for non-computer literate people to learn and use.

Apple was not the only company to successfully capitalize on the interface developments pioneered at SRI and PARC. **Microsoft** developed software **applications** for the Macintosh and obtained a license for certain aspects of its interface. By 1990 Microsoft released Windows 3.0, its first successful version of its operating system with a GUI for the operating environment. Apple sued Microsoft for copyright infringement of its GUI but did not prevail in court. By the time Windows was released, Microsoft had already obtained a dominant position in the operating system market with MS-DOS, which had a command line interface. The success of the Windows operating environment strengthened and continued that dominance.

Companies that create operating systems with windows-based interfaces have established guidelines for the appearance and behavior of windows in their operating systems. Because Microsoft Windows is the most common operating system, Microsoft standards are the ones most other software developers follow. While types of windows vary from one operating system to another, in general, there are two types of windows: primary and secondary. Primary windows can appear independent of other windows. Examples of primary windows include application windows and directory ("folder") windows. Primary windows usually contain these elements:

- Title bar: Contains application and document titles on the left and maximize, minimize, and close buttons on the right
- Menu bar: Contains menu options
- Tool bar: Contains icons ("buttons") representing functions ("tools") users may access in the application
- Display area: Displays document, web site, directory contents, etc.

- Primary windows may also contain additional elements such as horizontal and vertical scroll bars and status bars.

Secondary windows can appear only within a main window. Examples of secondary windows include dialog boxes, document windows, and **message** boxes. The elements of secondary windows vary widely, depending on the purpose of the window.

# WIRELESS NETWORKS

Wireless communication networks have been around for centuries: the use of smoke signals from mountain tops to alert tribal members of impending danger; waving lanterns at night to signal neighbors of the arrival of unexpected or uninvited visitors. Broadcast radio and television are more contemporary examples of wireless communication, as are cellular and cordless telephones, garage door openers, and automobile car locks. Some of these examples use radio frequencies (RF), some use "invisible" light in the infrared (IR) spectrum.

### Wireless Network Infrastructures

The wireless **data** industry is still working out the bugs in developing and building data transmission networks and agreeing on standards and **protocols**. While there are several competing visions, many experts believe that the growing market for wireless data will support many networks and protocols, such as the following:

- Global Systems for Mobile (GSM) Communication is a digital cellular or Personal Communications Services (PCS) standard used throughout the world and is the de facto standard in Europe. GSM is used in Asia (except Japan) and is being used as the PCS standard in the United States at 1900 MHz (GSM and PCS1900 are the same standard; PCS is a two-way, 1900 MHz digital offering now being rolled out across the United States). GSM is based on Time Division Multiple Access (TDMA) technology (a digital air interface technology used in cellular and personal communications services), and includes a data-only **channel** used for Short **Message** Service (SMS). GSM is also referred to as "2G" technology, or "second-generation." 2G cell phones have a clearer signal (audio converted to digital **code**) that can also be encrypted. Data-only services, such as Palm, are considered second generation.

- Cellular Digital Packet Data (CDPD) is a packet data protocol designed to work over the Advanced Mobile Phone System, or AMPS (the original cellular network) or as a protocol for TDMA. The AMPS standard is referred to as first generation, or 1G, and any AMPS-based networks are analog. Such networks can be used only for voice transmission and suffer from interference, which greatly varies the quality of the transmission. There is little to no security with 1G networks as anyone with a radio tuner can eavesdrop on calls.

- Code Division Multiple Access (CDMA) is a spread spectrum air interface technology used in some digital cellular, personal communications services, and other wireless networks. The idea of spread spectrums was developed during World War II in an effort to thwart the enemy's attempt to listen to or jam radio signals. CDMA was thought to be too complicated for use in wireless networks until the late 1990s when it was resurrected by Qualcomm.

Two types of spread spectrum are in use today: Frequency Hopping Spread Spectrum (FHSS), which uses rapidly alternating FM signals known in advance by the sender and receiver, and Direct Sequence Spread Spectrum (DSSS), which covers a wide range of frequencies transmitting simultaneously. DSSS requires high bandwidth, usually in the megahertz (MHz) range. As an interesting side note, 1940s actress Heddy Lamarr is co-holder of the patent (issued in 1942) for FHSS, which was originally invented as a concept for using radio waves to control torpedo navigation during World War II.

### *Bluetooth™: A Global Wireless Communications Specification*

The term *Bluetooth™* refers to an open specification for a technology that enables short-range wireless voice and data communications anywhere in the world. The Bluetooth specification, referred to as [BTSIG99] after the Bluetooth Special Interest Group that created the Version 1 spec in 1999, explicitly defines a method for wireless transports to replace serial cables that would be used with modems, digital cameras, personal digital assistants (PDAs), keyboards, printers, external zip drives, scanners, mice, and many other **peripherals**.

Bluetooth wireless communication uses radio frequency technology to communicate through the air in basically the same way as broadcast radio or television. Because there is a limit to the usable bandwidth for radio frequency, it is highly regulated and licensed by government agencies. Frequencies in the 900 MHz and 2.4 GHz frequency range are unlicensed in the United States and throughout the world (though there are some rules in place for its use). Bluetooth wireless communication will operate in the 2.4 GHz frequency range. For additional information on the Bluetooth Open Specification, go to www.bluetooth.com. [Note: Bluetooth is a trademark of Telefonaktiebolaget L M Ericsson, Sweden.]

# WIRTH, NIKLAUS (1934-    )

*Swiss computer programmer*

Computer language pioneer Niklaus Wirth is well-known to anyone who has studied even the basics of computer **programming** and technology. His contributions to the field of computer language development—in particular, the creation of the programming language PASCAL—have played an important role in shaping the arts of computer **design** and programming.

Wirth was born on February 15, 1934 in Winterthur, Switzerland, to Walter, a geography professor, and Hedwig (Keller) Wirth. He attended the Federal Institute of

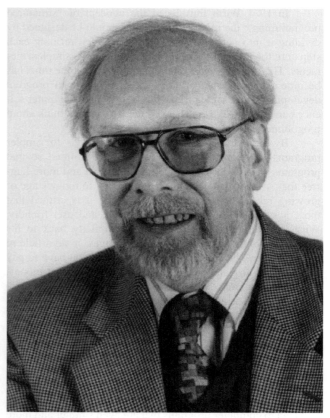

**Niklaus Wirth**

Technology (known by the initials ETH) in Zurich, Switzerland, receiving his bachelor's degree in 1958. Moving to Canada, he continued his education with a Master of Science degree in 1960 from Laval University in Quebec. Moving once again, this time to California, he received his doctorate from the University of California at Berkeley in 1963. At the time Wirth received his Ph.D. from Berkeley, nearby Stanford University was assembling its Computer Science Department, and Wirth was offered a position as an assistant professor in the department. There, Wirth and his colleagues developed a host of **computer languages**, including PL360 and Algol-W. Soon, Wirth had established himself as an expert in computer language development.

In 1967 Wirth moved back to his native Switzerland as an assistant professor of computer science at the University of Zurich. One year later, he accepted a position as a professor of computer science at ETH, his alma mater. Between 1968 and 1970 he developed the computer language **PASCAL**. Initially, Wirth had not intended for PASCAL to have commercial applications; because the language is so well suited for the microprocessors of today's computer systems, however, it has seen widespread use and development. Phillipe Kahn, an ETH graduate, formed his California-based computer software company around Wirth's language, selling more than a million copies of a modified PASCAL.

In 1971 Wirth introduced the concept of "structured programming," the idea that a program should be designed by dividing it into general but distinct steps, then refining each step until the final product is stripped down to its simplest elements. This concept, while creating quite a stir at the time, has become a standard methodology for most computer program development, and is taught in today's university computer science curriculums. Wirth "changed the way people think about programming," Kahn said in *Business Week.*

By design, **structured programming** leads to simpler programs. Similarly, Wirth's languages are defined so that programs written with them are easier to read and more bug-free than systems coded in other languages. In today's age of growing reliance upon computer systems, it is critical that those systems be both extremely reliable and user-friendly. Wirth himself traces his respect for simplicity back to his childhood hobby of building model airplanes; in an article in *Business Week,* he was quoted as saying, "If you have to pay [for a model airplane repair] out of your own pocket money, you learn not to make the fixes overly complicated." The journal of the Association of Computing Machinery said in a recent article that Wirth "has established a foundation for future research in the areas of computer language, systems, and architecture."

Beginning in 1979, Wirth developed the language **Modula**–2 and later a high-performance computer workstation called "Lilith," designed to utilize Modula–2. More recently, he has finished a new language called Oberon, which he hopes will lead to computer programs that are even simpler and more powerful than those created using PASCAL.

Wirth was the chairman of ETH's computer science division from 1982 until 1984 and again from 1988 through 1990; he was also appointed to lead the Institute of Computer Systems at ETH. He holds honorary doctorates from the University of York (England) and the Institute of Technology in Lausanne, Switzerland. He received the Emanuel Priore award from the Institute of Electrical and Electronics Engineers (IEEE) in 1983 and the coveted A. M. Turing award from the Association of Computing Machinery (ACM) in 1984. In 1987 Wirth received the Outstanding Contributions to Computer Science Education award from the ACM. In 1988 he was named a Computer Pioneer by the IEEE Computer Society and he was nominated as a Distinguished Alumnus of the University of California at Berkeley in 1992. Wirth and his wife, Nani Tucker, have three children, Carolyn, Christian, and Tina.

# WORD PROCESSING

Word processing software is, and has been for decades, among the most common of **applications** utilized for both commercial and home computing. It is interesting to note, then, that the history and development of word processing has had very little in common with the development of practical computing.

A simple definition of word processing might be the application of technology to manipulate printed text. That said, the lineage of word processing must be traced to the invention of both the printing press and of movable type—both arguably dating from around the end of the Middle Ages. These earliest systems were as costly as they were cumbersome, which caused the printed page to be held in widespread imagination as high art indeed. The result was that hand lettering, with all its inherent risks for errors and illegibility, remained the norm for the vast majority of text, for several hundred years.

It was not until the late eighteenth century that an inventor addressed the problem. Henry Mill constructed a portable **typesetting** system that can probably be considered the world's first typewriter. However, it was difficult to manufacture, difficult to use and was subject to frequent malfunction. It was not commercially successful.

Mill's endeavor was followed by that of William Burt, who patented a slightly more marketable "typographer" in 1829. But it was Christopher Sholes's invention, in 1867, that brought affordable typing to the world. Sholes also developed the familiar "QWERTY" keyboard, so configured to reduce the probability of jammed **hardware** by placing most common consecutive letters far apart. Sholes's typewriter was marketed worldwide by the Remington Company, best known for the rifles and six-shooters of the same name, and remained the standard for printed text production until well into the twentieth century.

The next logical step in the development of word processing was the application of electricity. Although Thomas Edison patented an electric typewriter as early as 1872, it was not until the 1930s that electrically assisted typing became common. The first commercially successful system was the **IBM** Electromatic. This model was the standard for business usage until its successor, the IBM Selectric, was introduced in 1961. The Selectric marked a notable advance as its "type-ball," which replaced the earlier configuration of numerous single-letter plates, could be easily and economically replaced. This made for quick, simple alterations between fonts, type-faces and point sizes.

Meanwhile, **data** management systems such as punch cards—originally developed for military use during World War II—found their way into business applications. The first true word processor, the Repetitive Typewriter marketed by the M. Shultz Company in the 1950s, utilized punch-code roll paper, not unlike those used by player pianos, to quickly replicate common letters and forms. Entire paragraphs could be manipulated within a document, by "cutting and pasting" the roll paper—which is how this common word processing term originated.

IBM entered the word processing market by introducing, in 1964, a version of the Selectric that included a magnetic tape drive for **data storage**. This model was also the first device to be commercially identified as a "word processor"; a term that originated as the direct translation of the German word for "typing."

Ensuing technical advances, for the next decade or so, mostly involved improved data storage capabilities. Magnetic storage remained the norm, although the various cards and tapes in use rarely had capacities beyond a page or two of printed text. The development of the floppy disk, in the early 1970s, marked a major advance in their ability to hold 100 or more pages of text. It was also in the early '70s that the first CRT screen word processor was marketed, the Lexitron. This was the first system that allowed for examination of an entire document without printing out a hard copy.

Floppy disks brought a second major development in word processing: loadable software. For the first time, word processing programs could be added to existing computer systems, making text manipulation capabilities available to most any user.

Throughout the '80s and '90s, upwards of 60 commercial word processing programs became available, each more user friendly and with more time-reducing features than the last. Spell checking, grammar checking and mail list managers became industry norms, and add-ons such as platform translators (to allow for document sharing among Mac and PC users) made word processing invisibly commonplace among home and business users, and requisite throughout the publishing world. Dozens of available fonts and colors, as well as stylization and formatting capabilities, has helped word processing evolve into **desktop publishing**, which has made the traditional roles of typesetters and printers all but obsolete.

The future of word processing remains tied to emerging technology. The **internet** has made document sharing global, and nearly instantaneous. **Voice recognition** software might one day replace the keyboard. The integration of word processing with functions such as bookkeeping and inventory management has even given rise to an entirely new software category: **information processing**.

However word processing evolves, it is unlikely to ever impact the cognitive methods that lies behind the act of composition. An author, in other words, will always be required to create the ideas that appear first on a screen, and then on paper. Word processing is not, and will never be, anything more than a writer's tool. But as it is a tool that has vastly reduced time spent on functions such as editing, proofreading and formatting, it is a tool that has irrevocably changed how we produce the printed word, both now and for decades to come.

## WORLD WIDE WEB

The World Wide Web is an information system that makes the **Internet** easier to use. While the Internet is a physical entity (a vast network of computers), the World Wide Web is more of a concept. It is a special way to encode, retrieve, and navigate many resources that are stored on Internet-linked computers. Such resources include **e-mail**, file transfer protocol, real-time communications, electronic bulletin boards, newsgroups, and **Telnet**. Each of these **applications** has a different set of communication rules that allows it take place. The World Wide Web makes all of these applications accessible through one interface.

The Internet has been evolving since the 1960s. Early users could send text messages to each other and store files so that others could access them, but the process was complicated and required knowledge of **computer languages**. In order for the Internet to become useful to the average person, an easier search and retrieval system was needed. In 1991 researchers at the University of Minnesota developed an internet navigation system (or **browser**) called **Gopher**. Although Gopher was menu-driven and featured point-and-click ease, it was still text based.

Around the same time a young man named **Tim Berners-Lee** developed a combination editor/browser called World Wide Web that included a **graphical user interface** (**GUI**). Berners-Lee worked for CERN, a European organization conducting advanced physics research. CERN had a large internal computer network on which researchers stored **data** and information in a variety of formats. The World Wide Web browser provided a single interface for downloading and displaying all these different resources. It featured a navigational tool called **hypertext** that allowed immediate jumping from one resource to another, even if they were stored on different computers.

Berners-Lee openly shared his computer **code** with others on the Internet, and its usefulness was immediately recognized. He developed a new communications protocol called **HyperText Transfer Protocol** (**HTTP**) for traversing hypertext links. He used elements of a markup language called **SGML** (**Standard Generalized Markup Language**) to format information and include hypertext links in documents. This eventually evolved into the more user-friendly HyperText Markup Language (**HTML**) widely used today to write and encode Web documents.

Throughout the 1990s, other browsers were released, including ViolaWWW, Erwise, Midas, and **Mosaic**. Mosaic was a graphical browser developed at the National Center for Supercomputing Applications at the University of Illinois. Released in 1993, it became very popular and was the precursor for the NetScape Navigator browser. By this time, the ideas behind the World Wide Web code had become more preeminent than the program itself. Berners-Lee changed the program's name to Nexus to distinguish it from what he called the "abstract space" on the Internet now known as the World Wide Web.

Today's World Wide Web is based on **client-server interaction**. A Web server is a computer that knows where to find resources (given their address) and how to extract them when someone asks. The asking is done through a client, which is a computer program such as Netscape, Internet Explorer, or Lynx, that presents the resources retrieved from the server. Berners-Lee developed an addressing **syntax** now called **Uniform Resource Locator** (**URL**) to specify the location and name of each resource. Every Web address has a syntax like http://www.webpage.com, where http identifies the protocol of the resource and the remaining portion tells the client which server to contact for its retrieval.

The World Wide Web is possible because of common use of the HTTP, URL, and HTML standards. In 1994 the World Wide Web Consortium (W3C) was formed to ensure that compatible specifications are used by the various parties involved in web technology. Developers, vendors, and web-based business leaders from around the world obtain a consensus on which specifications, **protocols**, and data formats should be used for the common good. However, there is no central authority that controls who can start a server or what type of resources are available on the World Wide Web.

Although it is not the only Internet resource tool, the World Wide Web is the most popular. In 1994 there were approximately 3,000 Web sites. By the end of 2000 there were more than 10 million web sites, representing a cross-section of global society. The Web made the internet accessible to average people who didn't know computer **programming**. It is used not only by businesses, educational institutions, and organizations, but by individuals. Many people have their own personal web pages on which they post information and photos.

The World Wide Web provides a single easy-to-use interface for accessing Internet resources in a variety of media, including programs, data, pictures, sound and video. Future trends for the World Wide Web include improved markup languages, such as **XML**, **voice recognition**, scalable vector **graphics**, and Web pages designed to be read by computer programs (rather than humans) using a technology called Resource Description Framework. All of these technologies are designed to improve resource sharing over the Internet and enhance the interactivity of the World Wide Web.

# WOZNIAK, STEPHEN (1950-    )

*American electronics engineer*

Stephen Wozniak, along with **Steven Jobs**, cofounded **Apple** Computer, Inc., and developed one of the most popular personal computers ever marketed. His contributions to Apple were almost exclusively technical—Jobs pushed the marketing potential of the Apple, while Wozniak provided the engineering know-how.

Wozniak's father, Jerry, was a Lockheed engineer, and his mother, Margaret, was president of a local Republican women's club. Young Wozniak grew up in Sunnyvale, a suburban development located in the Santa Clara Valley, now known as Silicon Valley. He was surrounded by the technological wizardry that grew out of Sputnik and the race for space. His parents provided a stable, close-knit environment.

Wozniak was an early devotee of electronics and in the fifth grade created a voltmeter from a kit. His interest in science and engineering led to a number of homemade devices: a ham radio, a makeshift electronic tic-tac-toe game, a **calculator**. By the time he entered Homestead High School, Wozniak had learned so much about the theory and practice of electronics that he became a prize student in the school's electronics courses.

When Wozniak met Steven Jobs in 1968, Wozniak was an accomplished student of electronics, although largely self-taught. Having flunked out of the University of Colorado, he was back home constructing a computer with a friend who also knew Jobs. Both Wozniak and Jobs took summer jobs at **Hewlett-Packard**, and Wozniak later returned to Hewlett-Packard after dropping out of Berkeley.

Together with Jobs, Wozniak spent the early years of the 1970s heavily immersed in the burgeoning computer culture of Silicon Valley, particularly among the hobbyists and video

game enthusiasts who were to become the first market for the **personal computer**. Both young men belonged to the Homebrew Computer Club, a Bay Area users' group that sprang up during the personal computer revolution of the mid-seventies.

This revolution would not have been possible without the development of the **microprocessor** in 1970 and the later discovery by hobbyists that this inexpensive silicon chip not only shrank the size of the computer but also shrank its price tag. The January 1975 issue of *Popular Electronics* announced the first computer kit, the **Altair** 8800, using an **Intel** 8080 microprocessor. Orders from hungry computer enthusiasts poured in—despite the fact that there seemed to be little to do with the computer once it was assembled.

In 1976, Wozniak, who was unable to afford the Altair, took the personal computer revolution a step further by constructing a computer out of a cheaper microprocessor and adding several chips for **memory**. The result was a naked circuit board, without case, keyboard, or screen, which was able to outperform the Altair. The Apple I formed the basis for the future Apple Computer, Inc. Steven Jobs marketed the crude computer through contacts from the Homebrew club.

The next step was the construction of a computer with a keyboard and color video display. Wozniak's engineering emphasized power and meticulous **design**. He was able to extract both speed and power out of relatively few chips. By fall 1976, Wozniak and Jobs were able to display their newest computer at a national computer fair. Their new machine attracted attention, although it clearly needed refinement. With Jobs's marketing efforts, Apple Computer, Inc., began to grow. In 1977, Wozniak, who had left Hewlett-Packard to work full time at Apple, completed the technical design of the Apple II.

The Apple II was the first personal computer that could be bought ready-made "off the shelf." Its success was due in part to its sleek design and its ability to accept "add-ons," such as music synthesizers, modems, and enhanced **graphics**. By 1978, Wozniak had incorporated a floppy **disk drive** into the Apple II, replacing the cassette tapes that had previously stored information. Using a floppy drive, the user could retrieve information in seconds. With this addition, and the availability in 1979 of VisiCalc, a spreadsheet program, the Apple II became a multimillion dollar success. In 1980, when Apple Computer, Inc., went public, sales stood at $117 million; in 1983, they reached $985 million.

Although Wozniak's association with Apple Computer left him a multimillionaire (in 1980, his stock in Apple was worth $88 million), his interest never wavered from the electronics and technical side of the business. He shared with Jobs a vision of democratic computing and believed that computers should be accessible to ordinary people. Early in his design career, he recognized the need for user-friendly software; by the late 1970s, the Apple II provided a growing market for software programs, especially in the educational field.

In 1981, Wozniak was piloting a single-engine plane near his home when it crashed on take-off. He was hospitalized and suffered amnesia. His convalescence lasted two years, during which time he became involved in New Age ventures, providing financial backing for two large music festivals near Los Angeles.

He returned to Apple in 1983, working as an engineer in the Apple II division. Despite the company's successes, its position within the personal computer market was being threatened by **IBM**. In the next tempestuous years at Apple, Wozniak remained aloof from corporate infighting. In January 1985, he (along with Jobs) was presented with the National Technology Award by President Reagan for his work at Apple. During that month, he resigned from the company to found a new **operation** called "CL–9 Inc." ("Cloud 9"), which produced remote control devices. The operation shut its doors in 1989.

Wozniak's life after Apple included several business ventures. He became involved in the Electronic Frontier Foundation, founded by Mitch Kapor (developer of Lotus), a user group dedicated to preserving First Amendment rights in the computer and communications fields. With his third wife and their six children, he built an elaborate home with mock caverns and prehistoric carvings in Los Gatos, California. After his retirement from Apple, he returned to the University of California at Berkeley and attained his bachelor's degree in **computer science and electrical engineering**.

# X

# X WINDOWS

X **Windows** is a system providing for the display and management of graphical information, in much in the same way as Microsoft's Windows Graphic Device Interface (GDI) and IBM's Presentation Manager.

The "X Org," a non-profit consortium comprising several members, developed the X Protocol in the mid-1980s to offer a **graphical user interface** that is transparent to the network, chiefly for the **UNIX** operating system. It is often said in the UNIX world that "the network is the computer," and the X protocol personifies this.

The chief difference between X and other graphical environments is the way the X Protocol has been designed as a true client-server system, meaning that it comprises two separate parts or processes that communicate in some way. **Microsoft** Windows and IBM's Presentation Manager merely display graphical information on the machine on which they are running, but the X Protocol breaks this **binding** by allowing **applications** to run in a more distributed fashion. It does this by creating a true client-server relationship at the program level.

The part of the application that decides what should be displayed is called the "X client." The X client is logically and, typically, physically separated from the part of the application that actually does the drawing, or the display.

The display is the "X server." X clients usually run on a machine that has spare computing power and displays the results on a slower machine using an X server. This is a real client-server relationship between an application and its display, and gives all the advantages of this kind of relationship.

To realize this separation, the application (running or incorporating the X client) is logically and often physically detached from the display (running the X server), and the two entities exchange **data** using a socket-based asynchronous protocol that works transparently over the network. A socket is merely a number or "handle" that describes a "log-ical channel" into the computer. It is rather like a telephone number in that information meant for that **channel** will be associated with that number. The protocol being "asynchronous" means that the X clients and servers exchange items of information or "packets" when the need arises rather than on a strict timed basis.

One of the quirks in some "flavors" of UNIX is that sometimes it is actually faster to use a deliberate physical separation of the X clients and X servers than to use both on the same machine, and it is not unknown for colleagues sitting next to one another to each run their X clients on the other's computer, and their X servers on their own computers. The reason this configuration is sometimes faster is that some computers treat network data with a higher priority than normal data, meaning that the network stuff is considered more important.

X also provides a "common windowing system" by specifying both device-dependent and device-independent layers. What this means is that the X Protocol theoretically hides the quirks and anomalies of the operating system (and the **hardware** underneath it all) from the applications using them. This is counted as a good thing because different hardware sets will present a common software inter-face yet have very different construction; this is the intention, at any rate.

Theoretically this would make the X Protocol the ideal windowing solution. In practice, however, the actual **function library**, called the "XLib API" (written in **C**), is very complicated indeed, and X **programming** is generally considered by most programmers as something best left to someone else.

Various layers have been written on top of XLib over the years to attempt to simplify X programming, but these attempts, most conspicuously Motif and its free counterpart, LessTif, are only partly successful because the **API** is still very complicated.

Much more recently developments like GTK++, wxWindows, and TrollTech's Qt have gone a long way to providing very much improved APIs on top of XLib, making the X windowing system a much less painful proposition.

# XEROX PARC

Xerox PARC is one of the research and technology laboratories of Xerox Corporation, specializing in networks and documents, smart matter, and knowledge ecologies. During the mid-1960s Xerox Corporation began to investigate ways to extend beyond its paper copier business. A few years later a plan was established for a scientific laboratory to develop advanced physics, materials science, and computer science technologies. The region around Palo Alto, California, was earmarked after nearby Stanford University showed a commitment to work with electronics and computer companies. This region is now collectively known as Silicon Valley.

Headed by **Robert Taylor**, former deputy director of the agency that established **ARPAnet** (the precursor to the **Internet**), Xerox organized in 1970 a team of renowned researchers at the Palo Alto Research Center (PARC) to specialize in computer and electronics research with the mandate of "creating the architecture of information." Some of the more important innovations that PARC scientists have developed are the first **personal computer**, the laser **printer**, Ethernet **local-area network**, network architecture, client/server architecture, **object-oriented programming**, and Internet standards and **protocols**.

Among the early inventions of PARC, one of the most important was the Xerox Alto. Developed in 1973, it is commonly considered the first personal computer (PC), though it was never released to the consumer market. The Alto contained a number of firsts, including the a WYSIWYG ("what-you-see-is-what-you-get") editor, **mouse**, **graphical user interface** (**GUI**; with **windows**, **icons**, pull-down menus, and pointers), and PC bit-mapped display. Xerox management believed it was too expensive to market to private and small-business owners; Steve Jobs, however, after visiting PARC, "borrowed" ideas like the mouse and the GUI for his new company **Apple**. Today's computers contain the same kinds of components that were developed by the Alto project. By the time its successor, the Xerox Star, was commercially released, other companies had introduced more affordable computers. Xerox soon exited the PC market and up-and-coming PC manufacturers assimilated their innovative features.

Another early invention of PARC was the laser printer. Gary Starkweather, who realized the importance of the laser for improving the traditional copier light source, created the technology at Xerox. Starkweather also believed that a laser-driven copier could function as a printer, transferring an image from a computer screen and posting its precise image on paper. Unfortunately Xerox management did not realize the importance in changing from their tried-and-true copiers. Luckily, one top-level Xerox researcher saw the importance in Starkweather's idea and transferred him to PARC in 1971. By 1972 Starkweather developed a working prototype, but Xerox did not introduce it until 1977. The laser printer soon became a best-selling product, and PARC's leadership in laser research (including laser diodes, multi-beam lasers, and blue lasers) became the key to early and recent Xerox's successes.

Another PARC breakthrough was the Ethernet, the global standard for connecting computers on local-area networks (**LAN**). Proposed by **Robert Metcalfe** and jointly developed with **Intel** and Digital in the mid-1970s, this networking standard increased the speed and reliability of **data** exchanges over LANs. The Ethernet created a series of sophisticated networking protocols that not only enabled distributed computing but led to a remodeling of internal computer-to-computer communications.

The development of Ethernet, Alto, and distributed computing prototypes of networking protocols led to XNS, Xerox's leading-edge network architecture. This in turn led to the Corporate Internet, a company-wide area-enterprise network that was well ahead of its time in allowing employees to easily exchange formatted documents. In fact, users of Xerox's 1981 STAR system were able to **access** file servers and printers around the world through simple point-and-click actions. This client/server architecture approach was an important PARC project that transferred **information processing** from centralized mainframes downloading to dumb terminals, to a more distributed access to intelligent computers.

PARC researcher **Alan Kay** created a computer **programming** language in 1972 called SmallTalk (complete with bitmap display, windowing system, and mouse) that was critical in creating the graphical user interface for the Alto. SmallTalk was the first true object-oriented programming language that allowed objects within programs to be individually described, addressed, and linked together with other objects without the necessity of rewriting an entire program. This PARC research revolutionized **the software industry**.

PARC scientists were also instrumental in designing and implementing the Internet standards and protocols that governed and defined how the Internet would operate. A partnership between PARC and several universities around the world created the "M-Bone" multicast backbone that was first implemented at PARC and has been delivering real-time video over the Internet since 1992. Currently, a PARC research team has been selected by the **World Wide Web** Consortium (W3C) to lead the development of HTTP-NG (**Hypertext Transfer Protocol Next Generation**), the new protocol that will improve performance and add features such as security to the transfer of information back and forth between Internet browsers and servers.

Other major PARC innovations are glyphs, information visualization, collaborative tools, flat panel displays, page description languages (PDL), device independent imaging, DocuPrint, integrated AI environments, BITblt, Mesa/Cedar, **expert systems**, **VLSI design** methodologies, linguistic compression technology, constraint-based scheduling, and SmartService.

PARC performs research, in unison with other Xerox research groups, along three major themes: (1) Networks and Documents, which deals with digitally stored document techniques and services, and helps define the standards and protocols for the Internet; (2) Smart Matter, which uses physical and computational sciences to reduce mechanical complexity in design and manufacturing through the use of computational sensing and controls; and (3) Knowledge Ecologies, which examines how to effectively extract meaningful knowledge, sometimes unwritten knowledge, and informally shared knowledge from organizations and documents.

The PARC ended up functioning more like a federal computer laboratory or an educational research center because many of its successes ended up accessible to all companies. These lost opportunities were often directly the result of missed chances by Xerox management in identifying their own innovative research and development activities. Many of PARC's researchers ended up forming their own Silicon Valley start-up companies using the technologies that Xerox failed to act upon. Unfortunately for Xerox, the PARC was a place where brilliant ideas often ended up outside of its control.

# XML (EXTENSIBLE MARKUP LANGUAGE)

XML is an acronym for Extensible Markup Language. A markup language is a means of identifying structured information in a document. Structured information contains content, such as words and pictures, and some indication of the role of the content (section heading, footnote, figure caption, as examples). Examples of structured information include entries in spreadsheets, address books, financial transactions, and technical drawings. A markup language like XML identifies the structured elements in a document. XML defines a way putting such structured information meaningfully into a text file.

The XML language enables the **design** of **data** format in a way that produces files that are easy to generate and read (by a computer—the text is not meant to be read by the user), unambiguous, and independent of any particular operating platform. Thus, XML can operate using a variety of computer operating systems.

Prior to the development of XML, the increasing complexity of documents taxed the ability of the medium to facilitate large-scale commercial publishing. The principle languages used to design documents for **Internet** exchange were **HTML** (HyperText Markup Language) and its **parent SGML** (**Standard Generalized Markup Language**). Each language has similar and unique features, and is not meant to replace one another. For example, while XML was designed to deliver structured format over the Web, some of the features the language lacks to make this goal practical are necessary for the creation and long-term storage of complex structured documents. For such storage purposes, SGML is preferred. Development efforts are underway to permit a seamless connection of SGML and XML.

XML was developed to allow documents having a great deal of structure to be usable on the Internet. The language

was developed by the **World Wide Web** Consortium, which itself was founded in 1994 by Web creator **Tim Berners-Lee** to provide common **protocols** for Web management and use. The language was developed for **applications** that could not be adequately handled by HTML or SGML. Such applications include a user's need to work between multiple and different **databases**, off-loading of processing tasks from the server to the user's computer, diverse representations of the same data, and the tailoring of information to the needs of multiple and simultaneous users. In HTML, these applications can be addressed, but by a proprietary **code** known as "script elements," delivered with proprietary **browser** features or **Java applets** (programs designed to be executed from within another program). The philosophy driving XML development is that the data is not bound to the tools of any particular vendor.

A real example of the difference in the **operation** of HTML and XML concerns the handling of health care information. A semi-automatic "drag and click" type of exchange of patient information between heterogeneous databases is not possible with HTML. Rather, printout of a **record** must be followed by the manual key entry of the information to the new database. Semi-automatic information transfer and exchange is possible using XML, because of the way that the structured elements in the document have been identified. The practical operation of this scenario requires an industry-standard interchange format. Such formats have been used for years by a umber of industries, including the aerospace, automotive, telecommunications, and computer software industries.

Future envisioned commercial efforts, such as the interactive, user-specified tailoring of television options, would require XML. Presently, operating languages that have been designed for Internet applications, such as Java, reply heavily upon XML.

*See also* HTML (HyperText Markup Language); Java; SGML (Standard Generalized Markup Language); World Wide Web

# X TERMINAL

An X **terminal** is a computer that lacks a disk. Accordingly, X terminals do not have (house) resident **applications**. X terminals are designed to connect a user to **network applications** that are running in an X server; a server operating in a network that uses the X Window system. In turn the X Window system is a network of interconnected **mainframe** computers, minicomputers, and workstations.

X terminals are usually connected to a server whose operating system is a **Unix**- or **Linux**-based system. They are thought of as being a predecessor of today's network computers. Because the computational power resides in the server rather than in the X terminal, these terminals can, in many cases, be old computers that as stand alone systems do not have the capacity to run the programs being used. The server powers the programs and the display is exported to the X terminal monitor.

Older computers are able to function as X terminals because only the minimum amount of **commands** for the display of the operative program are actually sent to the terminal. The terminal needs only the ability and capacity to request information from the displayed program in a point and click fashion. An X terminal is thus a way to utilize a computer that would be independently nonfunctional for complex computational procedures.

Use of X terminal allows a multiple user network to be constructed relatively inexpensively. For home, telecommuting, or small office applications, this often an attractive option to more expensive network capable computers.

*See also* Network applications

# Y

## YEAR-2000 BUG

The Year 2000 bug, also known as the Y2K or Millenium **bug**, was the anticipated inability of many computer programs and embedded devices to handle year-dates later than Dec. 31, 1999. Many such programs and devices were constructed to interpret dates as running between 1900 and 1999, inclusive, and so lacked any way to represent years after 1999. Computer experts forewarned that when January 1, 2000 arrived, computers that were not "Y2K-compliant" would read the year 2000 as the year 1900. This was deemed likely to adversely affect huge amounts of software, particularly accounting and database systems, thus generating expensive errors or even shutting down systems. Since banks, power grids, nuclear power plants, water-treatment systems, and other industries were almost entirely computerized by 1999, it was feared that the Y2K bug might even trigger widespread societal breakdown.

No one knew exactly how serious or widespread the Y2K bug would be. Predictions ranged from "no big deal" to worldwide crisis. The general consensus was that the worst problems would occur outside the United States, and would most adversely affect communications, financial systems, air transportation, and oil supplies. Within the United States, the least-prepared sectors were small businesses, state and local governments, and the health-care industry.

In the 1950s, **mainframe** computers (i.e., those shared by multiple users via **terminal** connections) were bulky, slow, and expensive to operate. Computer **memory** was especially expensive: an amount of memory that in 1999 would cost less than $10 then cost hundreds of thousands of dollars. For this reason, programmers shaved down memory requirements by recording only the last two digits of the year: that is, 1959 was saved as 59. This became a common required practice in software development.

In the 1970s Robert Bemer, a programmer for **IBM**, was one of the first to warn about the Y2K problem. Few listened.

When the Y2K bug was at last perceived widely as a problem, many experts agreed that it had been greatly exacerbated by the unwillingness of organizations to identify a technical problem that had no short-term impact on financial reports prior to 1999. Once the use of the two-digit standard became widespread, the change to a four-digit **code** became surprisingly difficult and expensive. Organizations had to evaluate their computer systems, identify those threatened by the Y2K bug, and either repair them (at high cost) or replace them (at higher cost).

Computers were not the only machines that contained two-digit year dates. Embedded devices, such as sensors inside machines, were one of the most difficult aspects of the Y2K bug because these were difficult to locate and fix, yet controlled key products and services such as utilities, telecommunications, banking, and sewage.

Personal computers were also at risk for Y2K problems. The Basic Input/Output System (**BIOS**), critical boot-up software in all personal computers, contained information the machine needed each time it was turned on. When the year changed to 2000, many personal computers that were not Y2K-compliant read the BIOS clock as 1900 or defaulted to the operating system (OS) start date, such as 1980 for the **Windows** OS.

Other calendar dates besides January 1, 2000 were also seen as potential Y2K problems. April 1, 1999 (99th day of the 99th year) and September 9, 1999 (9/9/99) were listed as potential problems because many programmers used 9999 or 9/9/99 to represent a file's termination date or an unknown date. February 29, 2000 was seen as a potential problem because year 2000 was a leap year; it was thought that some computers might fail to interpret the year as having 366 days rather than 365. These problems, however, did not materialize.

Because not all companies expected to be fully Y2K-compliant by January 1, 2000, and since disruptions might occur, executives drew up contingency plans. The United States Social Security Administration estimated that it would need to review about 50 million lines of code to correct its system's problems, while the United States Treasury Department installed emergency generators. The American Red Cross advised citizens to stockpile food, water, and money. A common estimate predicted that one trillion dollars in total worldwide damages could result from the Y2K problem. In the US, a law was even enacted to encourage companies to share Y2K-compliance information about their products with customers and other companies.

A small economic boom occurred in the late 1990s as companies spent many billions of dollars to "repair" or "upgrade" computers that had no real defect or shortcoming other than possible vulnerability to the Y2K bug. Businesses and individuals stockpiled goods, fearing computer glitches would halt everyday services. Some analysts predicted an economic slowdown in early 2000 caused by Y2K-related problems. In reality, only minimal disruptions and minor problems were experienced on and after January 1, 2000.

# Z

## ZADEH, LOTFI ASKER (1921-    )

*Russian American electrical engineer*

Lotfi Asker Zadeh, who described himself in an interview with Jeanne Spriter James as an "American, mathematically oriented, electrical engineer of Iranian descent, born in Russia," is responsible for the development of **fuzzy logic** and fuzzy set theory. Zadeh is also known for his research in system theory, **information processing, artificial intelligence, expert systems**, natural language understanding, and the theory of evidence. His first two papers that set forth the fuzzy theories, "Fuzzy Sets" and "Outline of a New Approach to the Analysis of Complex Systems and Decision Processes," have been listed as "Citation Classics" by the *Citation Index,* a publication that counts and lists those papers which have been cited most often in the writings of others. Zadeh received the prestigious Honda Prize—an award that was introduced in 1977 to honor technology that advances a "humane civilization"—from the Honda Foundation in Japan in 1989. That same year Japan's Ministry of Trade and Industry, along with almost fifty corporate sponsors, opened a laboratory for International Fuzzy Engineering Research (LIFE) with a budget of approximately $40 million for a six-year period. Six months after its initiation, Zadeh became an advisor to LIFE. Although fuzzy theory has received less attention in the United States, industrial applications have begun to appear in U.S. organizations as well.

Zadeh was born February 4, 1921, in Baku, a city on the Caspian Sea in the Soviet Republic of Azerbaijan. Originally named Lotfi Aliaskerzadeh, he simplified his name to Lotfi Asker Zadeh when he arrived in the United States. His father, Rahim Aliaskerzadeh (Asker), was a correspondent for Iranian newspapers and also an importer-exporter; his mother, Fannie (Fania) Koriman Aliaskerzadeh (Asker), was a pediatrician. Zadeh and his parents settled in Teheran (TehrÄn), the capital city of Iran, in 1931, when he was ten years old. Zadeh explained in an interview that the culture shock he felt as a result of this move was caused by the change from a school which promoted "atheism and the persecution of anyone religiously oriented, to a religious school run by American missionaries where he attended chapel every morning." Zadeh was taught in Persian—a language he had to learn after his arrival in Iran—at American College, the Presbyterian missionary school. He attended this school for eight years and then took the entrance exams for the University of Teheran, scoring third in the country. As an electrical engineering major he was first in his class his freshman and sophomore years. However, the disruption of World War II was felt at the university and in the electrical engineering department, which graduated only three students, Zadeh among them, in 1942.

During the year after his graduation, Zadeh worked with his father supplying construction materials to the U.S. Army in Iran. His contacts with Americans made him decide to move to the United States in 1943. Arriving in 1944, he enrolled at the Massachusetts Institute of Technology (MIT), which awarded him an M.A. in electrical engineering in 1946. During his years at MIT, the university was abuzz with excitement over developments in **cybernetics**, information and communication theory, and advances in computer applications. Zadeh caught the excitement as well and enrolled in the doctoral program at Columbia University. At the same time he was appointed an instructor there. He received his Ph.D. in 1949. Rising from instructor to professor of electrical engineering, he was on staff at Columbia from 1946 to 1959, when he moved on to the University of California at Berkeley.

In 1963 Zadeh was appointed chairman of the electrical engineering department at Berkeley. It was in the following years that he developed the first outlines of fuzzy theory. Fuzzy logic is the logic that underlies inexact or approximate reasoning, and it is most usefully seen as a branch of set theory. While traditional set theory works with sets of clearly defined objects, fuzzy theory deals with objects that belong to sets with what has been called varying degrees of membership. The set of tall trees, for instance, comprises trees that are tall, trees that are very tall, and trees that are not quite so tall. While the human mind can swiftly make qualitative—and therefore to some extent subjective—judgments of what is tall, machines, particularly computers, could traditionally be programmed only to deal with quantitative measures. Fuzzy logic as Zadeh developed it, however, prescribes the rules by which linguistic models containing qualitative judgments are translated into computer **algorithms**. In effect, machines can then be programmed to process "approximate" **data** and deal with the gray areas of life.

Although fuzzy theory was enthusiastically received and applied in Japan, China, and several European countries, it was greeted with a great deal of skepticism in the United States. Many scientists claimed that probability theory was already successfully being used to tackle the same problems that fuzzy theory solved. However, probability theory deals with uncertainty arising in a quantitative, mechanistic universe, while fuzzy theory clarifies uncertainty that follows from the subjective aspects of human cognition. Recently, fuzzy theory has gained a foothold in the United States as well. The most important application of the theory to be developed in the United States is AT&T's expert system on a chip. Hiroyuki Watanabe, the computer scientist who built the "first known expert system on a chip" with Masaki Togai, said in an interview with Jeanne Spriter James that manipulation of information is easier with fuzzy logic, which he described as a sophisticated method that allows for a minimum of engineering time to develop applications. Daniel McNeill and Paul Freiberger, in their book *Fuzzy Logic,* sum up Zadeh's contribution to the world of science as follows: "Fuzzy logic is practical in the highest sense: direct, inexpensive, bountiful. It forsakes not **precision**, but pointless precision. It abandons an either/or hairline that never existed and brightens technology at the cost of a tiny blur. It is neither a dream like AI [artificial intelligence] nor a dead end, a little trick for washers and cameras. It is here today, and no matter what the brand name on the label, it will be here tomorrow."

In 1968 Zadeh took a sabbatical from Berkeley. He spent half a year at **IBM** and another six months at MIT. When he returned from his leave, he began teaching only computer science courses at Berkeley. Since then he has spent periods as a visiting scientist at the IBM Research Laboratory in San Jose, California, in 1973 and 1978, as a visiting scholar at the Artificial Intelligence Center of SRI International at Menlo Park, California, in 1981, and as a visiting member of the Center for the Study of Language and Information at Stanford University in 1988.

Zadeh's research has earned him many honors and awards, including the Congress Award from the International Congress on Applied Systems, Research and Cybernetics (1980), the Outstanding Paper Award from the International Symposium on Multiple-valued Logic (1984), and the Berkeley Citation, from the University of California at Berkeley (1991). Zadeh is a member of many organizations, including the American Association for Artificial Intelligence, the World Council on Cybernetics, the American Mathematics Society, the National Academy of Engineers, and the Russian Academy of Natural Sciences. He has received honorary doctorates in the United States and Europe, from universities including the State University of New York in Binghamton,

Paul Sabatier University in France, Dortmund University in Germany and the University of Granada in Spain. Zadeh still supervises doctoral dissertations at Berkeley and keeps a busy calendar of speaking engagements. He founded the Berkeley Initiative in Soil Computing (called the BISC group) in 1991 and serves as its director, and is a member of the editorial boards of forty journals.

Zadeh married Fay Sand, his childhood sweetheart from Iran, on March 21, 1946, and they have two children, Stella and Norman. He is an accomplished amateur photographer, specializing particularly in portraiture, and has made portraits of many famous scientists and artists.

## ZONE PUNCH

The term zone punch relates to the use of punch cards, which was a means of recording **data** in a storable form prior to the advent of keying or scanning data into a computer's database. The pattern of punch card coding derived from a system proposed by **Herman Hollerith** in 1890. With punch cards, the pattern of punched-out holes denoted numbers or letters. The holes could act as areas where an electrical circuit could be completed. The electrical pattern could be further used to record and transfer the information contained on a punch card into the computers of the time.

A aspect of the punch card technology was termed a zone punch. A zone punch was a hole punched in one of the upper three rows of a twelve-row punch card. A zone punch could also be done in the eighth or ninth rows in **EBCDIC** (Extended Binary **Code** Decimal Interchange Code) coded cards.

In the Hollerith punch card system each card consisted of 80 columns of 12 rows each. The bottom ten holes of each column were used to record numbers of 0 through 9. The top two holes in each column were used for out-of-band, or zone, punches. Each column could hold one of the numeric symbols required as a hole punched in the column. The symbol denoted depended upon the distance from the top that to where the hole was punched.

The top three rows of a punch card were termed the punch rows. A punch in the top-most row of a column represented a plus sign, while a punch in the second row from the top represented a minus sign. A punch in the third row from the tope represented a zero and so on; the bottom row was used to represent a nine. As an example, a comma was typically encoded as 0-8-3, or punches in rows 0, 8 and 3 of one card column.

Zone punches—punches made in one of the columns of the top three rows of the punch card—in combination with a punch made elsewhere on the card denoted letters of the alphabet in the so-called punched card code and in the Hollerith code. For example, a punch in the top (or plus) zone row and a punch in one of the 1 to 9 rows would represent the upper case letters from A to I. A punch in the second zone row from the top (the minus) and in one of the other 1 to 9 rows represented an upper case letter from J to R. Finally, a punch in the zero zone row an a punch in one of the 2 to 9 rows represented an upper case letter from S to Z.,

Punch cards are no longer used. However, their use is still significant, as the company founded by Hollerith evolved into the International Business Machine Corporation.

*See also* BCD (Binary Coded Decimal); EBCDIC (Extended Binary Code Decimal Interchange Code)

# ZUSE, KONRAD (1910-1973)
*German computer scientist*

Konrad Zuse was one of the most honored figures in the history of computing, with his influence on computing in Britain and America abated only because of World War II. In 1938, in Germany, Zuse built a binary **calculator**, the Z1. A young engineering student without knowledge of similar inventions being built simultaneously in other parts of the world, Zuse created several computers that equaled in some respects and surpassed in many ways the capabilities of American-built computers of the same generation. With the war intervening, it was not until several years later that Zuse's inventions were known outside Germany.

Born in 1910 in Berlin-Wilmersdorf, Zuse grew up in East Prussia, where his family moved shortly after his birth. He attended school in Braunsberg, experiencing an early education that revolved around a curriculum based on the classics and Latin. By his mid-teens he had developed a fascination for engineering and in 1927, at the age of seventeen, he enrolled at the Technical University (Technische Hochschule) in Berlin. He graduated eight years later with a degree in civil engineering.

While at engineering school, Zuse became disillusioned by the "long and awful" calculations he had to perform, according to David Ritchie in *The Computer Pioneers*. Some equations were so tedious it would take the better part of a year to solve on a desktop calculator. Upon graduation he went to work at the Henschel Flugzeugwerke (aircraft factory) in Berlin, where he was a stress analyst, studying the amount of stress an airplane in flight could stand before it began to break apart. Because of the extreme difficulty Zuse came across working with differential equations, he knew he would have to build a machine that could automatically do his calculations.

The biggest problem Zuse found when making the initial sketches for his machine was not in the calculations themselves, but in the steps in between—the recording and transferring of intermediate results. And, as the equations became larger, the transfer became more difficult. Getting those intermediate results from one part of a problem to another was Zuse's main task. He considered several options before arriving at the idea of creating a calculator with a mechanical keyboard. In fact, twenty years after the war, Zuse admitted in a speech which is quoted in *The Computer Pioneers,* "I did not know anything about computers, nor had I heard about the early work of Charles Babbage." Babbage

was a contemporary of Zuse who also made early discoveries in the field of computing.

Zuse's ideal computer contained an arithmetic unit and storage unit, a selection mechanism to link the two, and a control unit that would be directed by punched tape and would deliver instructions to the selection mechanism and arithmetic unit. Once he had finalized his computer **design**, he devoted full time to its realization, using his parents' living room as his workshop.

Although he was a competent draftsman and skilled mechanic, he was relatively ignorant when it came to electrical engineering. He also knew very little about how to go about constructing a mechanical calculator. With his lack of knowledge Zuse was able to approach his project without the burden of conventional ideas. Later, after the war, he said, "Thus—unprejudiced—I could go new ways," according to Ritchie in *The Computer Pioneers*.

Since Zuse was more familiar with **binary arithmetic**—math based on a two digit system rather than ten—he decided to make his machine a binary device. Zuse's reasoning was that if he didn't have to represent ten numbers when two would work, why should he? A major influence on him was the writings of Gottfried Wilhelm Leibniz, who several centuries earlier imagined the entire universe reduced to binary values. In fact, one of Zuse's reports about his work was entitled, "Hommage to Leibniz."

The computer that Zuse designed and built, with the help of friends, had a mechanical **memory** unit that used movable pins in slots to indicate, by their position, zeroes and ones. Because of his use of the binary approach, the memory space was surprisingly compact, occupying about a cubic meter. Zuse's first computer was produced in 1938 when he connected his mechanical memory with a crude mechanical calculating unit.

With the help of friends and a supply of secondhand telephone relays, Zuse built his second computer, the Z2 computer, using electromechanical relays. Although the Z2's relays were problematic, making it less reliable than the Z1, it sparked the interest of the German Experimental Aircraft Institute, or Deutsche Versuchanstalt für Luftfahrt (DVL). The problem of trying to overcome flutter, a shivering of aircraft wings, demanded extensive calculations and the DVL was not equipped to handle the tasks. The Z2 was seen as a possible solution to the DVL's perplexing problem.

Zuse received money from the DVL for the design and manufacture of a relay computer. He began work on the Z3 while still using his parents' living room. The Z3, with two thousand relays and the capability to multiply, divide, or extract a square root in only three seconds, was completed in 1941. The Z3 was extremely compact (occupying only the volume of a closet) and had a sophisticated push-button control panel enabling the user to carry out operations with the touch of a finger. A single keystroke would convert decimal numbers into binary and, with another keystroke, switch them back again.

Zuse even created an innovative **programming** notation that included the now familiar symbols $\geq$ (greater than or equal to) and $\leq$ (less than or equal to). He used punched motion picture film for input. In addition to designing and building a sophisticated yet compact computer, Zuse, with the Z3, also created the first computer to achieve automatic control of a sequence of calculations. A person was no longer needed to continually punch in numbers. Zuse's computer could automatically carry out a **string** of calculations.

In fact, Zuse became a software pioneer before the concepts of software and **hardware** were fully developed. As noted in *The Computer Pioneers,* Zuse remarked in a postwar speech to an American audience, "In the early forties nobody knew the difference between hardware and software. We concentrated ourselves on purely technological matters, both logical design and programming."

Although the Z3 was totally destroyed in 1944 when an Allied bomb fell on the apartment building where the Zuses lived, he did produce another computer, the S1, that was a non-programmable version of the Z3 that was used to design German glider bombs, unmanned aircraft that carried high explosives and were carried aloft by bombers. Directed to their targets by radio control, the bombs were usually dropped on British ships. In fact, the British feared glider bombs more than almost any other aerial weapon because, since it was pilotless, it could not be disabled. During the last two years of the war, glider bombs were used against Allied shipping in the Mediterranean. Zuse's S1 assisted in plotting a glider bomb's actual flight path as well as its deviations. With those factors in place the control surfaces on the glider bomb's wings and tail could be adjusted to ensure a steady flight and a direct hit.

With the Allied armies moving toward Germany from the west and the Russians advancing from the east, Zuse finished the Z4 an even more advanced mechanical computer. To escape damage from Allied bombs he kept moving the Z4 around Berlin. By 1945 Zuse moved the Z4 to the university town Göttingen, a fair distance west of Berlin. The computer was left with the Experimental Aerodynamics Institute, or Aerodynamische Versuchanstalt (AVA). As the Allies contin-

ued to advance, Zuse, once again, moved the Z4, this time to Hinterstein, a small Alpine village, where he hid it in a barn.

Although Zuse felt he needed to keep his computer from harm's way, his brilliant work was also hidden from the rest of the world until years after Germany surrendered. In fact, it wasn't until French troops discovered Zuse and the Z4 in Hinterstein that word of the computer reached the British and Americans.

Observers who saw the Z4 in **operation** were amazed at what Zuse had accomplished. Without any knowledge of other, previous computer designs to assist him, as well as no information about contemporaneous computer projects in the United States and Britain, Zuse had designed and built his computers practically from scratch. In 1951, Zuse demonstrated the Z4 in Zurich, where one observer, quoted in *The Computer Pioneers,* wrote, "I could not believe it."

There were several contributing factors in addition to the isolation of his work at Hinterstein as to why Zuse's wartime achievements took so long to be recognized. The Z4 looked more like a **typesetting** machine than the huge American machines. Also, Zuse resented the Allies so he did not cooperate with their inquiries about his machines.

It was only well after the war that Zuse learned about other computer scientists such as **Howard H. Aiken** and his team at Harvard, who worked extensively on technological development during the war years. Although they had constructed computers larger than Zuse thought possible, it was Konrad Zuse who had brought computer design farther than they had.

After the war Zuse continued to design calculating machines and in 1949 established a small computer company, Zuse KG, that developed into a leading manufacturer of small scientific computers. He remained with the firm until 1966. After retirement, he remained as a consultant to the firm but devoted most of his remaining years to painting, his lifelong hobby. He died in 1973.

Abbate, Janet. *Inventing the Internet*. Cambridge: MIT Press, 1999.

"Data abstraction in C++." About.com (July 2, 2001). <http://cplus.about.comcompute.cplus/library/weekly/aa032299.HTM>.

"Inventors of the Modern Computer Mouse and Windows, Douglas C. Engelbart." About.com. <http://inventors.about.com/science/inventors/library/weekly/aa081898.htm>.

Abrams, Marc. *World Wide Web: Beyond the Basics*. Upper Saddle River, NJ: Prentice Hall, 1998.

"Choose Ada." Ada Information Clearinghouse (June 5, 2001). <http://www.adaic.org>.

"Introducing Ada." Adahome.com (June 5, 2001). <http://www.adahome.com/articles/1998-01/ar_intro.HTML>.

Adler, Irving. *Mathematics*. New York: Doubleday, 1990.

"Point to Point Protocol (PPP)." Advanced Computer Communications (August 9, 2001). <http://www.rgb.co.uk/support/guides/ppp.HTM>.

"An Information System for Sharing Experiences between Cities." Agencedesvilles.org (August 14, 2001). <http://agencedesvilles.org/anglinfsys.HTML>.

Agrawal, R., et al. "Mining Association Rules between Sets of Items in Large Databases." *Proceedings of the ACM-SIGMOD International Conference on the Management of Data,* May 1993: 207-216.

"RS232 Data Interface—A Tutorial." AirBorn Electronics (July 3, 2001). <http://www.arcelect.com/rs232.HTM>.

"Computer Security: A Practical Definition." Albion.com (August 1, 2001). <http://www.albion.com/security/intro-4.HTML>.

Albitz, Paul. *DNS and BIND*. Sebastopol, CA: O'Reilly, 1998.

Alcock, David. "Links to EBCDIC." <http://www.planet-mvs.com/links/ebcdic.html>.

Alexander, David C. *Machine & Assembly Language Programming*. Blue Ridge Summit, PA: Tab Books, 1982.

Alexandridis, Nikitas A. *Microprocessor System Design Concepts*. Rockville, MD: Computer Science Press, 1984.

*All about Personal Computer Peripherals*. Delran, NJ: Datapro Research Corporation, 1984.

Allen, J. F. "Maintaining Knowledge about Temporal Intervals." *Communications of the Association of Computing Machinery* 26 (1983): 832-843.

Allen, John. *Anatomy of LISP*. New York: McGraw-Hill, 1978.

Altman, Laurence, editor. *Large Scale Integration*. New York: McGraw-Hill, 1976.

"Digital Signature Guidelines—Free Download." American Bar Association (July 16, 2001). <http://www.abanet.org/scitech/ec/isc/dsgfree.HTML>.

"ANSI Online." American National Standards Institute. <http://www.ansi.org>.

"RISC and CISC." Amiga Interactive Guide. <http://www.inf.fh-dortmund.de/person/prof/si/risc/intro_to_risc/irt0_index.html>.

Amos, S. W. *Principles of Transistor Circuits: Introduction to the Design of Amplifiers, Receivers, and Digital Circuits*. Oxford: Newnes, 2001.

Anderson, Ronald E., et al. "Using the New ACM Code of Ethics in Decision Making." *Communications of the ACM* 36, no. 2, February 1993: 98-106.

Andrews, Paul. *How the Web Was Won: Microsoft from Windows to the Web.* New York: Broadway Books, 1999.

"The Unicode Character Encoding Standard." The Arabic Scientific Alliance (August 9, 2001). <http://www.asca.com/unicode.HTML>.

"BBS." EMC300: Arizona State University. <http://seamonkey.ed.asu.edu/emc300/help/B>.

Asimov, Isaac. *An Easy Introduction to the Slide Rule.* Boston: Houghton Mifflin, 1965.

"Introduction to the ASCII table." ASPfree.com (June 7, 2001). <http://www.aspfree.com/authors/robert/view.asp?aid=17>.

"ACM Code of Ethics and Professional Conduct." Association for Computing Machinery. <http://www.acm.org/constitution/code.html>.

"Annual Symposium on Computational Geometry." Association for Computing Machinery (August 15, 2001). <http://www.acm.org/pubs/citations/proceedings/compgeom/98524/p332-skiena/>.

"Software Engineering Code of Ethics and Professional Practice." Association for Computing Machinery and Institute of Electrical and Electronic Engineers. <http://www.acm.org/serving/se/code.htm>.

"A Query Language for XML." AT&T (June 7, 2001). <http://www.research.att.com/~mff/files/final.HTML>.

"The Turing Test." Badpen.com (August 10, 2001). <http://www.badpen.com/turing/>.

Bains, Sunny. "Analog Computer Trumps Turing Model." *EETimes,* November 3, 1998. <http://www.eetimes.com/story/OEG19981103S0017>.

Band, Jonathon, and Masanobu Katoh. *Interfaces on Trial: Intellectual Property and Interoperability in the Global Software Industry.* Boulder: Westview Press, 1995.

Bangert-Drowns, R. L., et al. "Effectiveness of Computer-based Education in Secondary Schools." *Journal of Computer-Based Education* 12 (March 1985): 59-68.

Bank, D. "The Java Saga." *Wired* (December 1995): 30-38.

Bardini, Thierry. *Bootstrapping: Douglas Engelbart, Coevolution, and the Origins of Personal Computing.* Stanford: Stanford University Press, 2000.

"Replacing Your Front End Processor." Barr Systems. <http://www.barrsys.com/news/whitepaper/fepwhite.asp>.

Bates, Clare. "Emergence of the Computer." Bryn Mawr College. <http://mainline.brynmawr.edu/~ccongdon/cs110fall97/Termpapers/jose-ivanina.html>.

"Fuzzy Logic." Battelle Memorial Institute (June 15, 2001). <htpp://www.emsl.pnl.gov:2080/proj/neuron/fuzzy/what.HTML>.

"An Introduction to Programming: Programming Loops." BBC On-line (July 5, 2001). <http://www.bbc.co.uk/h2g2/guide/A520895>.

"Handshaking." Beaglesoft (June 22, 2001). <http://www.beaglesoft.com/Manual/page33.HTM>.

Beakley, George C. *The Slide Rule, Electronic Hand Calculator, and Metrification in Problem Solving.* New York: Macmillan, 1975.

Becker, Ralph. "ISDN Definitions." <http://www.ralphb.net/ISDN/defs.html>.

Beckman, Mel. "An Introduction to ISDN." <http://www.jet.net/isdn/isdnintro.html>.

"What Are MOOs/MUDs/MUSHes?" Bedford St. Martins (July 24, 2001). <http://www.bedfordstmartins.com/english_research/internet/com2c2.HTM>.

Bemer, Bob. "EBCDIC and the P-Bit (The Biggest Computer Goof Ever)." <http://www.bobbemer.com/P-BIT.HTM>.

"My APL Tutorial." Ben Gurion University (June 14, 2001). <http://www.cs.bgu.il/~gmaprogramming-languages/apl/tutorial/intro.HTML>.

Bernardi, Vincent. "ACM Turing Awards Quotations." École normale supérieure de Lyon. <http://www.ens-lyon.fr/~vbernard/TAQuots.html>.

Berners-Lee, Tim. "The World Wide Web: Past, Present and Future" (August 1996). The World Wide Web Consortium (August 8, 2001). <http://www.w3.org/People/Berners-Lee/1996/ppf.html>

"Dynamic Programming: All Over Bioinformatics." BiBiServ (June 9, 2001). <http://bibiserv.techfak.uni-bielefeld.de/dynprog/tutorial/node2_ct.HTML>.

Birnes, William J., editor. *Microcomputer Applications Handbook.* New York: McGraw-Hill, 1989.

Blotnick, Srully. *Computers Made Ridiculously Easy.* New York: McGraw-Hill, 1984.

Blum, Bruce I. *Software Engineering: A Holistic View.* New York: Oxford University Press, 1992.

Boehm, Barry W. "Software Engineering." *Milestones in Software Evolution,* edited by Paul W. Oman and Ted G. Lewis. Los Alamitos, CA: IEEE Computer Society Press, 1990.

Bohme, Frederick G. *100 Years of Data Processing: The Punchcard Century.* U. S. Department of Commerce, Bureau of the Census, Data User Services Division, 1991.

Boire, Richard Glen. "Banning Books in the Digital Age." *Extra!,* March-April 2001, 27-28.

Boniface, Douglas M. *Micro-electronics: Structure and Operation of Microprocessor-based Systems.* Chichester, England: Albion Publishers, 1996.

Boyd, Ida Mae. "The Fundamentals of Computer Hacking." SANS Institute (July 11, 2001). <http://www.sans.org/infosecFAQ/hackers/fundamentals.htm>.

Boylestad, Robert L. *Introductory Circuit Analysis.* Columbus, OH: Merrill Publishing Company, 1987.

"Point of Sale (P.O.S.) Systems." Bret A. Bennett Automated Data Solutions. <http://www.bretabennett.com/babrwc/ps-va.htm>.

"An Introduction to DOS." Brighton University, BURKS (Brighton University Resource Kit for Students) (July 10, 2001). <http://burks.brighton.ac.uk/burks/pcinfo.osdocs/dosinfo.HTM>.

"Donald Knuth." Brighton University, BURKS (Brighton University Resource Kit for Students) (July 10, 2001). <http://burks.brighton.ac.uk/burks/foldoc/21/33.htm>.

Bromley, A. G. "Difference and Analytical Engines." In *Computing Before Computers,* edited by W. Asprey. Ames, IA: Iowa State University Press, 1990.

Bronson, Richard. *Matrix Methods: An Introduction.* New York: Academic Press, 1969.

Brooks, Jr., F. P. "What's Real about Virtual Reality?" *IEEE Computer Graphics and Applications* 19, no.6 (1999):16-27.

"Class Structure—Categorizing Methods." Bucknell University (July 22, 2001). <http://www.eg.bucknell.edu/~cs203/subpages/Slides/SI.20/node4.HTML>.

Burnham, David. *The Rise of the Computer State.* New York: Random House, 1984.

"Take Precautions to Prevent Computer Hacking." The Business Journal (July 11, 2001). <http://portland.bcentral.com/portland/stories/1998/07/27/focus8.HTML>.

Byman, Jeremy. *Andrew Grove and the Intel Corporation.* Greensboro, New Carolina: Morgan Reynolds, 1999.

Cajori, Florian. *A History of Mathematical Notations.* Chicago: The Open Court Publishing Company, 1928.

"Advanced: Superscalar and VLIW." Calvin College, Grand Rapids, MI. <http://www.calvin.edu/academic/rit/webBook/computer/hardware/cpu/adv_superscalar.htm>.

Campbell-Kelly, Martin, and William Aspray. *Computer: A History of the Information Machine.* New York: Basic Books, 1996.

Campbell, Todd. "The First E-Mail Message." *Pretext Magazine* (March 1998). <http://www.pretext.com/mar98/features/story2.htm>.

"Concurrent Programming in C under the UNIX Operating System." Canisius University (August 10, 2001). <http://barada.canisius.edu/~meyer/OLDCOURSES/FALL00/CSC330/OTHER/IPC/concurrency.HTML>.

"Donald E. Knuth." Carleton University, School of Computer Science. <http://www.scs.carleton.ca/~csgs/turing/knuth.html>.

Carlson, David. "Heaps and Heapsort." Computing and Information Sciences Department, Saint Vincent College. <http://cis.stvincent.edu/carlsond/swdesign/heaps/heaps.html>.

———. "Heapsort." Computing and Information Sciences Department, Saint Vincent College. <http://mcs.une.edu.au/~comp282/Lectures/Lecture_17/lecture_17/>.

Carmell, Tim. "Spectrogram Reading." Center for Spoken Language Understanding at Oregon Graduate Institute of Science and Technology (June 5, 2001). <http://cslu.cse.ogi.edu/tutordemos/SpectrogramReading/waveform.html>

"Backtracking Algorithm." Carnegie Mellon University (August 9, 2001). <http://www.cs.cmu.edu/afs/cs/project/jair/pub/voulme4/vanbeek96a-html/node6.HTML>.

"PERL—Practical Extraction and Report Language." Carnegie Mellon University (June 23, 2001). <http://www.cs.cmu.edu/cgi-bin/perl-man>.

"The Personal Software Process (PSP)." Carnegie Mellon University, Software Engineering Institute. <http://www.sei.cmu.edu/tsp/psp.html >.

"Phase the Firewall System into Operation." Carnegie Mellon University (June 11, 2001). <http://www.cert.org/security-improvement/practices/p063.HTML>.

Carr, William N. *MOS/LSI Design and Application.* New York: McGraw-Hill, 1972.

"A Closer Look at DVD." CD-Info (June 17, 2001). <http://cd-info.com?CDIC/Technolgy/DVD/dvd.HTML>.

"Compound Statement." Cee (July 22, 2001). <http://www.cee.hw.ac.uk/~rjp/Coursewww/CPPwww/compound.HTML>.

"Functions—Constant Reference Parameters." Central Queensland University (July 10, 2001). <http://www.infocom.cqu.edu.au/Staff/Mike_Turnbull/Home_Page/Lecturetts/Sect6.HTM>.

"A Short Introduction to Quantum Computing." Centre for Quantum Computing (July 29, 2001). <http://www.qubit.org/intros/comp/comp.HTML>.

Ceruzzi, Paul E. *A History of Modern Computing.* Cambridge, MA: The MIT Press, 1998.

Chambers, Catherine. *Computer.* Des Plaines, IL: Heinemann Interactive Library, 1998.

"Burroughs Corporation Records, Edsger W. Dijkstra Papers, 1971-1979." Charles Babbage Institute: Center for the Information Processes, University of Minnesota, Twin

Cities. <http://www.cbi.umn.edu/collections/inv/burros/dijkstra.htm>.

Chen, J., et al. "Large On-Off Ratios and Negative Differential Resistance in a Molecular Electronic Device." *Science* 286 (November 1999): 1550-52.

Chester, A., Hanes, R., and J. Cheshire. "Service Creation Tools for Speech Interactive Services." *BT Technology Journal* 14 (April 1996): 43-51.

"So You're Buying a New Computer? An Introduction to Computer Hardware." Chicago Kent College of Law (July 20, 2001). <http://ck.kentlaw.edu/support/intro.hardware.HTML>.

"Jim W's APL Information." Chilton (June 14, 2001). <http://www.chilton.com/~jimw/Welcome.HTML>.

Choi, Joongmin. "Theories, Principles, and Guidelines." Department of Computer Science and Engineering, Hanyang University. <http://cse.hanyang.ac.kr/~jmchoi/class/1997-1/hci/classnote/node2.html>.

Chomsky, Noam. *Aspects of the Theory of Syntax*. Cambridge, MA: M.I.T. Press, 1965.

Ciminiera, Luigi. *Advanced Microprocessor Architectures*. Reading, MA: Addison-Wesley Pub. Co., 1987.

Cipra, B. "The FFT: Making Technology Fly." *SIAM News*, no. 3 (1993): 1-4.

"Internetworking Basics." Cisco Systems Inc. (September 13, 2000). <http://www.cisco.com/univercd/cc/td/doc/cisintwk/ito_doc/introint.htm#xtocid130451>.

"Increment (++) and Decrement (--) Operators." City University of New York (August 10, 2001). <http://163.238.35.140/klibaner/incrdecr.htm>.

Clapes, Anthony Lawrence. *Softwars: The Legal Battle for Control of the Global Software Industry*. Westport, CT: Quorum Books, 1993.

"Creating a Compound Condition." Clemson University (August 12, 2001). <http://people.clemson.edu/~awoszcz/PA-3/tsld005.HTM>.

"Petri Nets." Clemson University (July 16, 2001). <http://taylor.ces.clemson.edu/1e340/files/340-16.HTM>.

"Napster Filters Clean House." Cnet.com (June 20, 2001). <http://news.cnet.com/news/0-1005-202-5753132.HTML>.

"Is COBOL Dying . . . or Thriving?" The COBOL Newswire (June 7, 2001). <http://www.infogoal.com/cbd/cbdz009.HTM>.

"Bill Klein's COBOL FAQ." COBOL Report.com (June 7, 2001). <http://www.cobolreport.com/faqs/cobolfaq.HTM>.

Colomb, S., and L. Baumert. "Backtrack Programming." *Journal of the Association of Computing Machinery* 12 (1965): 516-24

Comer, Douglas. *The Internet Book: Everything You Need to Know about Computer Networking and How the Internet Works*. Upper Saddle River, NJ; Prentice-Hall, 1997.

*Computer Basics*. Alexandria, VA: Time-Life Books, 1989.

Computer Knowledge. <http://www.cknow.com>.

"Beginning Computer Hardware Guide." The Computer Technology Documentation Project (June 6, 2001). <http://ctdp.tripod.com/hardware/pc/begin.HTML>.

ComputerProblems.com. <http://www.computerproblems.com>.

Computeruser.com. <http://www.computeruser.com>.

"VLIW Microprocessors." *ComputerWorld*, <http://careers.computerworld.com/home/print.nsf/(frames)/000214qs?OpenDocument&~f>.

"Compound Assignment." Contactor Data (July 7, 2001). <http://www.contactor.se/~dast/fpl-old/language/compoundassign.HTML>.

Cooley, J. W., and J. W. Tukey. "An Algorithm for the Machine Calculation of Complex Fourier Series." *Mathematics of Computation* 19 (1965): 297-301.

Copi, Irving M. *Symbolic Logic*. Fifth Edition. New York: Macmillan Publishing Co., 1979.

"Menus." Corel Corporation (August 12, 2001). <http://www.corel.com/partners_developers/ds/CO328DK/docs/pfit7/_F1MENUS.HTM>.

Cortada, James W. *Historical Dictionary of Data Processing: Biographies*. Westport, CT: Greenwood Press, 1987.

"Technical Data and Computer Software." Council on Governmental Relations (June 8, 2001). <http://www.cogr.edu/data.HTM>.

Cover, Robin. "SGML: General Introductions and Overviews." Oasis: XML Cover Pages. <http://www.sgmlsource.com/history/index.htm >.

Cowart, Robert. *Mastering Windows 95: The Windows 95 Bible*. San Francisco: Sybex, 1995.

Cragon, Harvey G. *Computer Architecture and Implementation*. New York: Cambridge University Press, 2000.

Crook, Welton Joseph. *Abacus Arithmetic: How to Perform Some Calculations on the Chinese Abacus*. Palo Alto: Pacific Books, 1958.

Crowder, Norman A. *The Arithmetic of Computers: An Introduction to Binary and Octal Mathematics*. Garden City, NY: Doubleday, 1960.

"Internet and the New Business Connectivity." Foundation Report 106, CSC Index Research and Advisory Services. <http://www.cscresearchservices.com/foundation/library/106/RP22.asp>.

"FORTRAN 90 in Scientific Computing." CSC Mathematical Topics (June 17, 2001). <http://www.csc.fi/math_topics/Publ/f90.HTML>.

"Microsoft Excel Binary File Format." Cubic (July 1, 2001). <http://www.cubic.org/source/archive/fileform/misc/excel.txt>.

"From the Abacus to Wintermute: Fragments from a History of Computing." Culture.com (July 4, 2001). <http://www.culture.com.au/brain_proj/babbage.HTM>.

"Message-Oriented Middleware." Cutter Consortium (August 14, 2001). <http://cutter.com/itgroup/reports/message.HTML>.

"POS Systems." Data Efficient Systems. <http://www.attheforefront.com/dataefficientsystems/Definition.htm>.

"A Characterization of Data Mining Technologies and Processes." Datamining.com (July 11, 2001). <http://www.datamining.com/dm-tech.HTM>.

Davis, Martin D., et al. *Computability, Complexity, and Languages*. Boston: Harcourt, Brace, & Company, 1994.

"Using Object Modeling CASE Tools." *Dbms Magazine* (June 30, 2001). <http://www.dbmsmag.com/9707d16.HTML>.

Deboo, Gordon J. *Integrated Circuits and Semiconductor Devices: Theory and Application*. New York: Gregg Division: McGraw-Hill, 1977.

"DARPATech 2000 Symposium Presentations." Defense Advanced Research Projects Agency. <www.darpa.mil/DARPATech2000/presentation.html>.

Deitel, Harvey M., and Barbara Deitel. *Computers and Data Processing*. Orlando: Academic Press, 1985.

"Napier's Rods, Abacus, and Slide Rule." Delft University of Technology, Mathematical Geodesy and Positioning. <http://www.geo.tudelft.nl/mgp/people/gerold/indnap.htm#napier>.

Dennis, Jason M. "Secondary Storage Devices and Technologies." CDA 5155 Computer Architecture Project, Department of Computer and Information Science and Engineering, University of Florida. <http://www.cise.ufl.edu/~jmd/storage.html>.

"Women in Information Technology." DeSai Institute. <http://www.desai.com/articles/new_women_in_IT_101998.htm>.

Dessauer, John H. *My Years with Xerox: The Billions Nobody Wanted*. Garden City, NY: Doubleday, 1971.

"DIGITAL Computer Timeline." Digital Equipment Corporation's Information Research Services. <http://www.montagar.com/dfwcug/VMS_HTML/timeline/1957.htm>.

"CP/M Operating System Manual." Digital Research. <http://museum.sysun.com/museum/cpm/>.

Dijkstra, Edsger W. "From my Life." Department of Computer Sciences, The University of Texas at Austin. <http://www.cs.utexas.edu/users/almstrum/cs373/general/EWD1166.html>.

Dilson, Jesse. *The Abacus: A Pocket Computer*. New York: St. Martin's Press, 1968.

"Introduction to CD-ROM." Disctronics (June 18, 2001). <http://www.disctronics.co.uk/cdref/cd-rom/cd-romintro.HTM>.

"Bar Code History" and "Using Bar Code Technology." Doublecam: Bar Code Solutions. <http://www.barcodingsolutionsinc.com/bar_code_history.html> and <http://www.barcodingsolutionsinc.com/bar_code_technology.html>.

Doyle, Leo F. *Computer Peripherals*. Upper Saddle River, NJ: Prentice Hall, 1999.

"Implementing Assertions for Java." *Dr. Dodd's Journal* (August 9, 2001). <http://www.ddj.com/articles/1998/9801/9801d.htm?topic=testing>.

"It's Not Easy Being Green (or 'Red'): The IBM Stretch Project." *Dr. Dobb's Journal: The History of Computing*. <http://www.ddj.com/articles/2000/0085/0085b/0085b.htm>.

Drake, Jim, editor. *What Is a Computer?* Des Plaines, IL: Heinemann Library, 1999.

"Unix Introduction." Drexel University (June 23, 2001). <http://www.drexel.edu/irt/helpcentral/unixintro.HTML>.

"Memory Technology." Drix (June 9, 2001). <http://www.drix.be/ram.HTM>.

"The Scientist and Engineer's Guide to Digital Signal Processing." Dsp Guide (July 7, 2001). <http://www.dspguide.com/datacomp.HTM>.

"Imagesetters on the Desktop?" DtpJournal.com (June 5, 2001). <http://www.dtpjournal.com/archives/9604d05.HTML>.

"Distributed Concurrency Control." Dublin City University (July 21, 2001). <http://www.compapp.dcu.ie/databases/f463.HTML>.

"ASCII and EBCDIC Compared." Dynamoo.com. <http://www.dynamoo.com/technical/ascii-ebcdic.htm>.

"FAT: File Allocation Table." Easy Desk Software (July 11, 2001). <http://www.easydesksoftware.com/fat.HTM>.

"IBM 7030—'Stretch.'" Ed Thelen's Nike Missile Web Site. <http://ed-thelen.org/comp-hist/vs-ibm-stretch.html>.

"Chemical Researchers Design Molecular Computer." EE Times (July 05, 2001). <http://www.eetimes.com/story/OEG19991109S0036>.

"Holographic Storage Nears Debut." EE Times (July 04, 2001). <http://www.eetimes.com/story/OEG20010423S0113>.

Egan, Janet I. *Writing a UNIX Device Driver.* New York: Wiley, 1988.

Entacher, Karl. "A Collection of Selected Pseudorandom Number Generators with Linear Structures." <http://random.mat.sbg.ac.at/~charly/server/server.html>.

"Creating Your Own Function." Envar.com (June 24, 2001). <http://www.envar.com/udf.HTM>.

"Character Input and Output." Eskimo.com (July 10, 2001). <http://www.eskimo.com/~scs/cclass/int/sx2c.HTML>.

Esteller, Rosana, et al. "A Comparison of Waveform Fractal Dimension Algorithms." *IEEE Transactions on Circuits and Systems—I. Fundamental Theory and Applications,* 48, no. 2 (February 2001): 177-83.

Evans, Christopher. *The Making of the Micro: A History of the Computer.* New York: Van Nostrand Reinhold, 1981.

Fahie, J. J. *A History of Wireless Telegraphy.* New York: Arno Press and *The New York Times,* 1971.

"National Computer Crime Squad." Federal Bureau of Investigation (July 07, 2001). <http://www.emergency.com/fbi-nccs.HTM>.

"Fighting computer espionage." Federal Computer Week (July 07, 2001). <http://www.few.com/print.asp>.

Ferguson, Charles H. *High St@kes, No Prisoners: A Winner's Tale of Greed and Glory in the Internet Wars.* New York: Times Business: Random House, 1999.

Ferry, Steven. *The Story of Microsoft.* New York: Warner Books, 2000.

"An Introduction to ASCII." FidoNews (June 07, 2001). <http://www.holysmoke.org/wb/wb0013.HTM>.

Fielding, R., et al. "Request for Comments: 2068, Hypertext Transfer Protocol—HTTP/1.1." Network Working Group. <http://www.cis.ohio-state.edu/cgi-bin/rfc/rfc2068.html>.

"What in the World Is an X Terminal?" Firstsol (August 10, 2001). <http://www.firstsol.com/xterm.HTML>.

Fitts, P. M. "The Information Capacity of the Human Motor System in Controlling the Amplitude of Movement." *Journal of Experimental Psychology* 47 (1954): 381-91.

Flamm, Kenneth. *Creating the Computer: Government, Industry, and High Technology.* Washington, D.C.: The Brookings Institution, 1988.

———. *Targeting the Computer: Government Support and International Competition.* Washington, D.C.: The Brookings Institution, 1987.

Flores, Ivan, *The Logic of Computer Arithmetic.* Englewood Cliffs, NJ: Prentice-Hall, 1963.

Floyd, Thomas L. *Electronics Fundamentals: Circuits, Devices, and Applications.* New York and Toronto: Maxwell Macmillan International Publishing Group: Collier Macmillan Canada, 1991.

"DLT handbook." Focused Distribution Concept (June 18, 2001). <http://www.fdeint.com/products/dlt/dlthandbook/chapter02.asp>.

FOLDOC: Free On-Line Dictionary of Computing <http://foldoc.doc.ic.ac.uk/foldoc/foldoc.cgi?FOLDOC>.

Foster, David. *Intelligent Universe: A Cybernetic Philosophy.* New York: Putnam, 1975.

Freedman, Alan. *The Computer Desktop Encyclopedia.* New York: American Management Association, 1996.

"PPP Protocol Overview." Freesoft (August 09, 2001). <http://www.freesoft.org/CIE/Topics/65.HTM>.

Freiberger, Paul. *Fire in the Valley: The Making of the Personal Computer.* Berkeley: Osborne/McGraw-Hill, 1984.

Friedman, John. "Hitler's Willing Executives." *The Nation* (May 21, 2001): 40-3.

Fuhs, Howard. "Password Security." Fuhs Security Consultants (August 17, 2001). <http://www.fuhs.de/fachartikel/Password_Security.htm>.

Gao, H. J., et al. "Reversible, Nanometer-Scale Conductance Transitions in an Organic Complex." *Physical Review Letters* 84 (February 2000): 1780-3.

"Scientists Flip Molecular Switch." Goecities (July 16, 2001). <http://www.geocities.com/Area51/Shadowlands/6583/project256.HTML>.

"VLSI—Very Large Scale Integration." Geocities (June 8, 2001). <http://www.geocities.com/CapeCanaveral/4466/vlsi.HTML>.

Gilbert, Howard. "Introduction to TCP/IP." PCLT. <http://www.yale.edu/pclt/COMM/TCPIP.HTM

"GNU Advanced Monitoring and Control Structure." GNU's Not Unix!—The GNU Project and the Free Software Foundation (FSF) (July 10, 2001). <http://www.gnu.org/software/awacs/>.

Goldfarb, Charles F. "A Brief History of the Development of SGML." SGML Source Home Page. <http://www.sgml-source.com/history/sgmlhist.htm>.

Goldwasser, Sam. "Robot Mechanics." *Poptronics* 2, no. 3 (March 2001): 57-9.

Gouyet, Jean-François. *Physics and Fractal Structures.* Paris: Springer, 1996.

Gray, George T., and Ronald Q. Smith. "Sperry Rand's Third-Generation Computers, 1964-1980." *IEEE Annals of the History of Computing* 23, no. 1 (January-March 2001). <http://www.computer.org/annals/an2001/a1003abs.htm/>.

Green, Cliff. "An Introduction to Internet Protocols for Newbies." <http://www.halcyon.com/cliffg/uwteach/shared_info/internet_protocols.html>.

Greenia, Mark W. *History of Computing: An Encyclopedia of the People and Machines that Made Computer History.* Lexikon Services (CD), 1998.

Gregg, John. *Ones and Zeros: Understanding Boolean Algebra, Digital Circuits, and the Logic of Sets.* New York: IEEE Press, 1998.

Groover, Mikell P. *CAD/CAM: Computer-aided Design and Manufacturing.* Englewood Cliffs, NJ: Prentice-Hall, 1984.

Gustafson, John L. "An FPS Forerunner: The Atanasoff-Berry Computer." Ames Laboratory, Department of Energy, Iowa State University. <http://www.scl.ameslab.gov/Publications/A%2DBComputer.html>.

Hahn, Harley. *The Internet Complete Reference.* Berkeley: Osborne McGraw-Hill, 1994.

Halbert, Debora J. *Intellectual Property in the Information Age: The Politics of Expanding Ownership Rights.* Westport, CT: Quorum Books, 1999.

Halliday, David, and Robert Resnick. *Physics.* New York: John Wiley & Sons, 1978.

Hamming, Richard. *Introduction to Applied Numerical Analysis.* New York: Hemisphere Publishing, 1989.

Hanegraaff, Hank. *The Millennium Bug Debugged: The Facts Behind All the Y2K Sensationalism.* Minneapolis: Bethany House, 1999.

Hansen Media Knowledge Base: Digital Media and the Internet. <http://www.hansenmedia.com>.

Hanson, Peggy L. *Keypunching.* Englewood Cliffs, NJ: Prentice-Hall, 1984.

Hazen, Robert M. *The Breakthrough: The Race for the Superconductor.* New York: Summit Books, 1988.

Helander, Martin, editor. *Handbook of Human-Computer Interaction.* New York: Elsevier Science Publishing Company, 1988.

"Conditional Control Structures." Heriot-Watt University (August 12, 2001). <http://www.cee.hw.ac.uk/~pjbk/pathways/cpp1/node73.HTML>.

"Increment and Decrement Operators." Heriot-Watt University (August 10, 2001). <http://www.cee.hw.ac.uk/~pjbk/pathways/cpp1/node65.HTML>.

Herrick, Clyde N. *Basic Electronics Math.* Boston: Newnes, 1997.

Hetzel, Bill. *The Complete Guide to Software Testing,* Second Edition. Wellesley, MA: QED Information Sciences, Inc., 1988.

"About HP." Hewlett-Packard Company. <http://www.hp.com/hpinfo/abouthp/main.htm>.

"History and Facts." Hewlett-Packard Company. <http://www.hp.com/hpinfo/abouthp/histnfacts.htm>.

Hiltzik, Michael A. *Dealers of Lightning: Xerox PARC and the Dawn of the Computer Age.* New York: Harper Business, 1999.

Hinden, Robert. "IP Version 6 (IPv6)." Nokia Inc. (April 12, 2001). <http://playground.sun.com/pub/ipng/html/ipng-main.html>.

Hirsh, Michael. "Dark Questions for IBM." *Newsweek* (February 19, 2001): 38.

Hodges, Andrew. *Turing.* New York: Routledge, 1999.

"Introduction to Intranet." Hong Kong University of Science and Technology (June 08, 2001). <http://www.cyber.ust.hk/handbook3/01_hb3.HTML>.

Hopkins, Ken. "Compatibility of Architectures." Newman College Technology Department, Newman College. <http://www.newman.wa.edu.au/technology/12infsys/html/2_10.htm>.

"How BIOS Works." How Stuff Works (June 16, 2001). <http://www.howstuffworks.lycos.com/bios.HTM>.

"How Computer Memory Works." How Stuff Works (June 9, 2001). <http://www.howstuffworks.com/computer-memory.HTM>.

"Contracts for Abstract and Polymorphic Functions." How to Design Programs.org (July 22, 2001). <http://www.htdp.org/2001-01-18/Book/node111.HTM>.

Hsu, John Y. *Computer Architecture: Software Apects, Coding, and Hardware.* Boca Raton, FL: CRC Press, 2001.

Hunter, William L. *Getting the Most Out of Your Electronic Calculator.* Blue Ridge Summit, PA: Tab Books, 1974.

"Member Functions." Ibiblio (August 12, 2001). <http://www.ibiblio.org/obp/thinkCScpp/chap11.HTM>.

"XML, Java, and the Future of the Web." Ibiblio (July 16, 2001). <http://www.ibiblio.org/pub/sun-info/standards/xml/why/xmlapps.HTM>.

"From Analytical Engine to Electronic Digital Computer: The Contributions of Ludgate, Torres, and Bush." *IEEE Annals of the History of Computing* 4, no. 4 (October 1982) <http://www.computer.org/annals/an1982/a4327abs.htm>.

"Petri Net Models." Imperial College (July 16, 2001). <http://www.doc.ic.ac.uk/~nd/surprise_97/journal/vol2/njc1/>.

"FAQs about Solid State Disk (SSD)." Imperial Technology (June 16, 2001). <http://www.imperialtech.com/faqsol-id.HTM>.

"Data Mining—Association Rules." Indian Institute of Science (July 11, 2001). <http://dsl.serc.iisc.ernet.in/~vikram/mining.HTML>.

"Binary File." Indiana State University (July 1, 2001). <http://ase.isu.edu/ase01_07/ase01_07/bookcase/ref_sh/foldoc/58/11.HTM>.

"Top-Down Design Approach." Indiana State University (July 4, 2001). <http://www.cs.indiana.edu/hyplan/asengupt/thesis/oral/subsubsecton3.2.2.1.HTML>.

"Computer Crime: An Emerging Challenge for Law Enforcement." Info-sec.com (August 8, 2001). <http://www.info-sec.com/access/infoseczh.html-ssi>.

"A Short History of CP/M." Information Center: Everything about the Amstrad PCW. <http://www.joyce.de/english/cpmstory.htm>.

"Password Protection." Information Services. <http://www.comedition.com/Computers/InformationServices/passwordprotect.htm>.

"Attribute." Information Technology Service (June 8, 2001). <http://www.its.bldrdoc.gov/fs-1037/dir-003/_0417.HTM>.

"Magnetic Disk Recording." Integrated Publishing (July 24, 2001). <http://www.tpub.com/neets/book23/103.HTM>.

"Octal Number System." Integrated Publishing. <http://www.tpub.com/neets/book13/53e.htm>.

"SGML: Answers to Basic Questions." International SGML/XML Users Group (July 29, 2001). <http://www.isgmlug.org/whatsgml.HTM>.

"Context Sensitive Situations." Iowa State University (July 20, 2001). <http://www.cs.iastate.edu/~leavens/FoCBS/bespalko-node3.HTML>.

Ismail, Amin R. *Microprocessor Hardware and Software Concepts.* New York: Collier Macmillan, 1987.

Jackson, Tim. *Inside Intel: Andy Grove and the Rise of the World's Most Powerful Chip Company.* New York: Dutton, 1997.

Jacobson, Gary, and John Hillkirk. *Xerox: American Samurai.* New York: Macmillan Publishing Company, 1986.

James, Kevin. *PC Interfacing and Data Acquisition: Techniques for Measurement, Instrumentation, and Control.* Boston: Newnes, 2000.

"Kludge." The Jargon Dictionary. <http://info.astrian.net/jargon/terms/k/kludge.html>.

"About the Java Technology." Java.Sun.com (July 11, 2001). <http://java.sun.com/docs/books/tutorial/getStarted/intro/definition.HTML>.

"JRE Usage Example." Java.Sun.com (August 18, 2001). <http://java.sun.com/products/jdk/1.1/jre/example/>.

"Learning the Java Language: What Is a Class?" Java.Sun.com (July 21, 2001). <http://java.sun.com/docs/books/tutorial/java/concepts/class.HTML>.

"Learning the Java Language: What Is an Object?" Java.Sun.com (July 29, 2001). <http://java.sun.com/docs/books/tutorial/java/concepts/object.HTML>.

"Abstract Classes vs. Interfaces." Java World (July 22, 2001). <http://www.javaworld.com/javaqu/2001-04/03-qa-0420-abstract.HTML>.

"Inheritance vs. Composition: Which One Should You Choose?" Java World (August 17, 2001). <http://www.javaworld.com/javaworld/jw-11-1998/jw-11-techniques.html>.

"Object-Oriented Language Basics, Part 3: Composition—Build Objects from Other Objects." Java World (August 17, 2001). <http://www.javaworld.com/javaworld/jw-06-2001/jw-0608-java101.html>.

"Using Menus and Menu Bars in Applets." Java World (August 12, 2001). <http://www.javaworld.com/jw-11-1966/jw-11-menubars.HTML>.

"DOS Commands." Jegsworks (July 10, 2001). <http://www.jegsworks.com/Lessons/reference/doscommands.HTM>.

Jha, A. R. *Superconductor Technology: Applications to Microwave, ElectroOptics, Electrical Machines & Propulsion Systems.* New York: John Wiley & Sons, 1998.

"Glossary for Information Retrieval." Johns Hopkins University (July 5, 2001). <http://www.cs.jhu.edu/~weiss/glossary.HTML>.

"Information Retrieval and the Internet." Johns Hopkins University (July 5, 2001). <http://milton.mse.jhu.edu:8001/research/education/retrieval.HTML>.

Johnson, Deborah, and Helen Nissenbaum, editors. *Computers, Ethics, and Social Values.* Englewood Cliffs, NJ: Prentice Hall, 1995.

Johnson, Keith, with Philip Baczewski and Melody Childs. *Using Gopher.* Indianapolis: Que, 1995.

Johnson, Steven. "Paradigm Shtick—Steven Johnson Takes a Hard Look at the Promise of 'Push.'" *FEED Magazine.* <http://www.feedmag.com/97.02johnson/97.02johnson.html>.

Jones, Arnita A. and Philip L. Cantelon. *Corporate Archives and History: Making the Past Work.* Malabar, FL: Krieger Publishers, 1993.

Jones, R., and R. Lins. *Garbage Collection: Algorithms for Automatic Dynamic Memory Management.* New York: John Wiley & Sons, 1996.

Jortberg, Charles A. *The First Computers.* Minneapolis: Abdo & Daughters, 1997.

Kaye, H. S. *Computer and Internet Use Among People with Disabilities*. Disability Statistics Report (13). Washington DC: U.S. Department of Education, National Institute on Disability and Rehabilitation Research, 2000.

Kessler, Gary C. "An Overview of TCP/IP Protocols and the Internet." <http://www.garykessler.net/library/tcpip.html>.

Khare, Rohit, and Ian Jacobs. "W3C Recommendations Reduce 'World Wide Wait': Tired of Having to Make Coffee While You Wait for a Home Page to Download?" <http://www.w3.org/Protocols/NL-PerfNote.html>.

Kit, Edward. *Software Testing in the Real World: Improving the Process*. New York: Addison-Wesley Publishing Company, 1995.

Klein, Naomi. "Computer Hacking: New Tool of Political Activism." *The Toronto Star* (July 23, 1998). (July 11, 2001). <http://www.cultdeadcow.com/news/newspapers/toronto_star72398.txt>.

Knuth, Donald E. "The Art of Computer Programming (TAOCP)." Stanford University. <http://www-cs-faculty.stanford.edu/~knuth/taocp.html>.

Kochan, D., editor. *CAM: Developments in Computer-Integrated Manufacturing*. New York: Springer-Verlag, 1985.

Koved, L., and B. Shneiderman. "Embedded Menus: Selecting Items in Context." *Communications of the American Association of Computing Machinery* 29 (April 1986): 312-18.

"How to Use a Search Engine Efficiently." Kreskus (July 22, 2001). <http://keskus.hut.fi/opetus/s38118/s00/tyot/28/use.shtml>.

Lancaster, Don. *The Hexadecimal Chronicles*. Indianapolis: H. W. Sams, 1981.

"Parsing: In Depth." Lancaster University (June 19, 2001). <http://www.ling.lancs.ac.uk/monkey/ihe/linguistics/corpus2/2full.HTM>.

Landow, George P. *Hypertext: The Convergence of Contemporary Critical Theory and Technology*. Baltimore: Johns Hopkins University Press, 1992.

Lanier, Jaron. "Virtually There." *Scientific American* (April 2001): 66-75.

"Dense Holographic Storage Promises Fast Access." Laser Focus World (July 4, 2001). <http://silver.neep.wisc.edu/~lakes/hoStorage.HTML>.

"The OPM Query Language and Translator—Version 4.1." Lawrence Berkeley National Laboratory (June 07, 2001). <http://gizmo.llbl.gov/DM_TOOLS/OPM/OPM_4.1/OPM_QLT/QLT.HTML>.

"Declaration." Learnthat (August 12, 2001). <http://www.learnthat.com/define/d/declaration.shtml>.

Leiner, B., V. Cerf, D. Clark, R. Kahn, L. Kleinrock, D. Lynch, J. Postel, L. Roberts, and S. Wolff. *A Brief History of the Internet*. The Internet Society (May 22, 2001). <http://www.isoc.org/internet/history/brief.html>.

Levitz, Kathleen. *Logic and Boolean Algebra*. Woodbury, NY: Barron's Educational Series, 1979.

Levy, Steven. *Insanely Great: The Life and Times of Macintosh, the Computer that Changed Everything*. New York: Viking, Penguin Group, 1994.

Lewin, Morton H. *Logic Design and Computer Organization*. Reading, MA: Addison-Wesley, 1983.

Lienhard, John H. The Engines of Our Ingenuity. University of Houston. <http://www.uh.edu/engines/epi360.htm>.

"Larry Wall, the Guru of Perl." Linux Journal (June 23, 2001). <http://www2.linuxjournal.com/lj-issues/issues61/3394.HTML>.

"An Introduction to RAID." Linux Step X Steps (June 10, 2001). <http://sxs.sandbox.dynip.com/raidintro.HTML>.

"What Is a Device Driver?" Linuxdoc (July 23, 2001). <http://www.linuxdoc.org/LDP/khg/HyperNews/get/devices/whatis.HTML>.

"Case Sensitivity." Linuxguruz (July 22, 2001). <http://www.linuxguruz.org/foldoc/foldoc.php?case-sensitive>.

"Address Resolution Protocol." Linuxports (June 10, 2001). <http://linuxports.com/howto/intro_to_networking/c7198.HTM>.

Linzmayer, Owen W. *Apple Confidential: The Real Story of Apple Computer, Inc.*, San Francisco: No Starch Press, 1999.

Lockman, Darcy. *Computers*. New York: Benchmark Books, 2000.

Logsdon, Tom. *Computers: Today and Tomorrow, The Microcomputer Explosion*. Rockville, MD: Computer Science Press, 1985.

Long, Larry, and Nancy Long. *Computers*. Second Edition. Englewood Cliffs, NJ: Prentice-Hall, 1990.

Loshin, David. *Efficient Memory Programming*. New York: McGraw-Hill, 1999.

Lowe, Doug. *Networking for Dummies*. Foster City, CA: IDG Books Worldwide, 2001.

Lynch, Danial C., editor. *Internet System Handbook*. Reading, MA: Addison-Wesley, 1993.

Lynn, M. Stuart, and the Technology Assessment Advisory Committee to the Commission on Preservation and Access. "The Relationship Between Digital and Other Media Conversion Processes: A Structured Glossary of Technical Terms." Conservation OnLine (CoOL), Preservation Department of Stanford University

Libraries. <http://palimpsest.stanford.edu/byauth/lynn/glossary/term3-3.html>.

Malone, Michael S. *Infinite Loop: How Apple, the World's Most Insanely Great Computer Company Went Insane.* New York: Currency Book: Doubleday, 1999.

Manger, Jason J. *The World-Wide-Web, Mosaic, and More.* New York: McGraw-Hill, 1995.

Mann, Charles C. "Electronic Paper Turns the Page." *Technology Review* (March 2001). <http://www.techreview.com/magazine/mar()1/mann.asp>.

Masci, David. *Artificial Intelligence.* Washington, DC: Congressional Quarterly, 1997.

"Classifier." Massachusetts Institute of Technology (August 12, 2001). <http://www.pdos.lcs.mit.edu/click/doc/Classifier.n.HTML>.

"Classifier System." Massachusetts Institute of Technology (August 12, 2001). <http://www.media.mit.edu/~rich/memory/SIU00/node15.HTML>.

"What the Heck Does that Mean? An Overview of Functional Programming." Massachusetts Institute of Technology (July 24, 2001). <http://www.csg.lcs.mit.edu/Users/earwig/fp-overview.HTML>.

Maxfield, Clive. *Bebop to the Boolean Boogie: An Unconventional Guide to Electronics.* Eagle Rock, VA: LLH Technology Publishing, 1995.

"Charles Babbage's Difference Engine." Maxmon (July 4, 2001). <http://www.maxmon.com/1822ad.HTM>.

McCarthy, John. "History of LISP." <http//:www-formal.stanford. edu/jmb/history/lisp/>.

"Data Structures and Algorithms. Topic #9: Binary Search Trees." McGill University (July 15, 2001). <http://www.cs.mcgill.ca/~cs251/OldCourses/1997/topic9/>.

Mead, Carver, and Mohammed Ismail, editors. *Analog VLSI Implementation of Neural Systems.* Boston: Kluwer Academic Publishers, 1989.

*Memory and Storage.* Alexandria, VA: Time-Life Books, 1990.

"Information Hiding." Mephzara.com (August 12, 2001). <http://www.mephzara.com/techzone/programming-hints/information_hiding_e.php>.

"Terminal and Non-Terminal Symbols." Merlyn.net (August 13, 2001). <http://www.merlyn.net:457/tools/Yacc_specs_symbols.HTML>.

Michael, George A. "An Oral and Pictorial History of Large-Scale Scientific Computing as it Occurred at the Lawrence Livermore National Laboratory." National Energy Research Scientific Computing Center. <http://www.nersc.gov/~deboni/Computer.history/GAM.Intro.5.html>.

"BASE—Baseline Table." Microsoft (July 3, 2001). <http://www.microsoft.com/OpenType/OTSpec/base.HTM>.

"MOF Boolean Data Type." Microsoft. <http://msdn.microsoft.com/library/psdk/wmisdk/mof_24px.htm.>.

"9.5 Hand Tracing." Minnesota Community and Technical College (August 17, 2001). <http://www.mctc.mnscu.edu/~tollerev.faculty.mctc/c1500/c1500chap9.htm>.

Mitoraj, Lisa. "Artificial Engineering: Find Out How You Can Use Artificial Intelligence in Your Engineering Applications." Office.com (Winstar). <http://www.office.com/global/0,2724,209-161,FF.html>.

"VLSI: Very Large Scale Integration: Where Small Is Getting Smaller Fast!" Mitre (June 08, 2001). <http://www.mitre.org/jobs/features/vlsi.shtml>.

Molich, R., and J. Nielsen. "Improving a Human-Computer Dialogue." *Communications of the Association of Computing Machinery* 33 (March 1990): 338-48.

"Compound Assignment Statements." Montana State University (July 07, 2001). <http://www.cs.montana.edu/cimo/120/C_examples/assignment.HTML>.

Moon, Parry Hiram. *The Abacus: Its History, Its Design, Its Possibilities in the Modern World.* New York: Gordon and Breach Science Publishers, 1971.

Morgan, Eric Lease. *WAIS and Gopher Servers: A Guide for Internet End-Users.* Westport, CT: Mecklermedia, 1994.

Moschovitis, Christos J. P. *History of the Internet: A Chronology, 1843 to the Present.* Santa Barbara: California, ABC-CLIO, 1999.

Muller, Nathan J. *Desktop Encyclopaedia of Telecommunications.* 2nd edition. New York: McGraw-Hill Telecommunications, The McGraw-Hill Companies, 2000.

Murdocca, Miles, and Vincent P. Heuring. *Principles of Computer Architecture.* Upper Saddle River, NJ : Prentice Hall, 2000.

"DEC C Language Reference Manual." Myths.com (August 13, 2001). <http://www.myths.com/pub/doc/openvms/decc/6180p003.HTM>.

Nance, Berry. *Introduction to Networking.* Indianapolis: Que, 1994.

Narayan, Rom. *Data Dictionary, Implementation, Use and Maintenance.* New Jersey: Prentice Hall, 1988.

"Theoretical Research: Intangible Cornerstone of Computer Science." National Academy Press (August 12, 2001). <http://www.nap.edu/readingroom/books/far/ch8_bl.HTML>.

"Fundamentals of Data Storage." National Center for Geographic Information and Analysis (June 16, 2001).

<http://www.ncgia.ucsb.edu/education/curricula/giscc/units/u037.HTML>.

"About Us." National Center for Supercomputing Applications (NCSA), University of Illinois, Champaign-Urbana, Illinois. <http://www.ncsa.uiuc.edu/About/NCSA/>.

"Array." National Institute of Standards and Technology (June 30, 2001). <http://hissa.nist.gov/dads/HTML/array.HTML>.

"Data Structure." National Institute of Standards and Technology (July 22, 2001). <http://hissa.nist.gov/dads/HTML/datastructur.HTML>.

"Node." National Institute of Standards and Technology (July 24, 2001). <http://hissa.nist.gov/dads/HTML/node.HTML>.

"The Digital Dilemma: Intellectual Property in the Information Age." National Research Council, Committee on Intellectual Property Rights in the Emerging Information Infrastructure. 2000. <http://www.nap.edu/books/0309064996/html>.

"Mask." National Telecommunications and Information Administration, Institute for Communication Sciences. <http://www.its.bldrdoc.gov/fs-1037/dir-022/_3224.htm>.

"Overflow." National Telecommunications and Information Administration, Institute for Communication Sciences. <http://www.its.bldrdoc.gov/fs-1037/dir-026/_3799.htm>.

"History of Hypertext Systems" and "History of Web Hypertext." National University of Singapore, University Scholars Programme. <http://www.thecore.nus.edu.sg/writing/ccwp10/rina/new_system.html> and <http://www.thecore.nus.edu.sg/writing/ccwp10/rina/new_web-hyper.html>.

Naughton, Patrick, and Herbert Schildt. *Java: The Complete Reference.* Berkely: McGraw-Hill, 1997.

"The Internet and Music Technology." Nbnet (June 20, 2001). <http://www.nb.net/~mycall/Info.HTML>.

"The Fast Fourier Transform Demystified." NegativeZero.org (June 7, 2001). <http://www.foo.tho.org/charles/fft.HTML>.

"The Case for Government Promotion of Open Source Software." Netaction (July 2, 2001). <http://www.netaction.org/opensrc/oss-whole.HTML>.

"TCP/IP Network Concepts." Network Gods (June 07, 2001). <http://proxyfaq.networkgods.com/prxdocs/htm/prenet.HTM>.

"Network Applications." *Network Magazine*, January 1, 1999. <http://www.networkmagazine.com/article/NMG20000724S0017/1

"A Look Back at the Very First Laser Printer." New Media News, Jones Computer Network. <http://www.newmedianews.com/tech_hist/dover.html>.

"Memory Allocation." New Mexico State University (June 9, 2001). <http://www.cs.nmsu.edu/~ekerriga/presentation/>.

Norberg, Arthur L. and Judy E. O'Neill. *Transforming Computer Technology: Information Processing for the Pentagon, 1962–1986.* Baltimore: The Johns Hopkins University Press, 1996.

"Password Issues." North Carolina State University. <http://uni22ws.unity.ncsu.edu/PG/pg_data_public/csc379/web-search/39/>.

Northrup, Nancy. *American Computer Pioneers.* Springfield, NJ: Enslow Publishers, 1998.

"Computer-Assisted Instruction." Northwest Regional Educational Laboratory (Jun 10, 2001). <http://www.nwrel.org/scpd/sirs/5/cu10.HTML>.

"Abstract Class." Object-Arts.com (July 22, 2001). <http://www.object-arts.com/Lib/EducationCentre4/htm/abstractclass.HTM>.

"The Open Source Initiative." Open Source.org (July 2, 2001). <http://www.opensource.org/>.

"Blaise Pascal (1623-1662)." Oregon State University (June 22, 2001). <http://www.orst.edu/instruct/phl302/philosophers/pascal.HTML>.

"A Bluetooth Primer." The O'Reilly Network (June 7, 2001). <http://www.oreillynet.com/lpt/a/wireless/2000/11/03/bluetooth.HTML>.

"Components of Object-Oriented Programming." The O'Reilly Network (July 21, 2001). <http://www.oreillynet.com/lpt/a//mac/2001/04/20/cocoa.HTML>.

"The Programming Research Group." Oxford University, Computing Laboratory. <http://web.comlab.ox.ac.uk/oucl/about/prg/overview.html>.

Packard, David. *The HP Way: How Bill Hewlett and I Built Our Company.* New York: Harper Business, 1995.

Palfreman, Jon. *The Dream Machine: Exploring the Computer Age.* London, England: BBC Books, 1991.

"Win2K/Stream: A New Virus that Runs on Windows 2000." Panda Security (August 18, 2001). <http://www.pandasecurity.com/pressrelease09-04-00B.htm>.

Parker, D. Stott, et al. "Monte Carlo Arithmetic: How to Gamble with Floating Point and Win." *Computing in Science and Engineering* (July-August 2000): 58-68.

Patterson, D. A., et al. "A Case for Redundant Array of Inexpensive Disks (RAID)." *University of California at Berkley Report No. UCB/SCD/87/391* (December 1987).

   

Patterson, David A. *Computer Architecture: A Quantitative Approach.* San Francisco: Morgan Kaufmann Publishers, 1996.

"How a CD-ROM Works and How to Make it Faster." PC Improvements (June 17, 2001). <http://www.pcin.net/help/articles/printout/cdromspeed.shtml>.

"Solid-State Storage: Memory on the Go." *PC Magazine* (June 16, 2001). <http://www.zdnet.com/filters/printerfriendly/0,6061,2344720-50,00.HTM>.

"High Performance Debugging Standards Effort." PCTools (July 6, 2001). <http://www.pctools.org/hpdf/article.HTML>.

Peeters, Alex. "Protocols and Protocol Stacks." <http://citap.freeservers.com/publications/tcp-ip/tcpip008.htm>.

"Aggregate Data Types." Penn State University (July 2, 2001). <http://www.personal.psu.edu/staff/j/b/jbc103/ist240web/lecure14.HTML>.

"Perl History." Perl Mongers Press Room (June 23, 2001). <http://www.perl.org/press/history.HTML>.

Peterson, Gerald R. *Basic Analog Computation.* New York: Macmillan, 1967.

Peterson, Larry L. *Computer Networks: A Systems Approach.* San Francisco: Morgan Kaufmann Publishers, 2000.

Petzold, Charles. *Code: The Hidden Language of Computer Hardware and Software.* Redmond, WA: Microsoft Press, 1999.

"On-line Education Can Get You There, from Here." Pittsburg Business Times (July 29, 2001). <http://pittsburg.bcentral.com/pittsburg/stories/1997/03/24/focus1.HTML>.

Poor, Alfred, Bruce Brown, Diane Jecker, and John Morris. "Speech Recognition." *PC Magazine* (May 17, 2001). <http://www.zdnet.com/pcmag/features/speech/intro.html>

"The Art of Pattern Matching." Prefab.com (July 7, 2001). <http://www.prefab.com/textmachine/docs/chapter5theartof.HTML>.

"The History of Computer Programming Languages." Princeton University (August 17, 2001). <http://www.princeton.edu/~ferguson/adw/programming_langauges.shtml>.

"Serving the Suits: Xerox PARC." Public Broadcasting Service (PBS) Online. <http://www.pbs.org/opb/nerds2.0.1/serving_suits/parc.html>.

"Big Numbers." Public Logica Server (July 22, 2001). <http://public.logica.com/~stepneys/cyc/b/big.HTM>.

"The History of Shareware & PSL." Public Software Library (June 12, 2001). <http://www.pslweb.com/history.HTM>.

"Molecular Memory for Computers." Punjabilok.com (July 16, 2001). <http://www.punjabilok.com/scince/molecular_mem.HTM>.

Ralston, Anthony, editor. *Encyclopedia of Computer Science and Engineering.* New York: Van Nostrand Reinhold Company, 1983.

Raymond, Eric S. "Kludge." <http://www.tuxedo.org/~esr/jargon/html/entry/kludge.html>.

"Email: Using Signature Files." Reinet (July 16, 2001). <http://www.reinet.com/library/computers/file33.HTM>.

"Member Functions and Interfaces." Relisoft.com (August 12, 2001). <http://www.relisoft.com/book/lang/scopes/5memberi.HTML>.

Riley, H. Norton. "The von Neumann Architecture of Computer Systems." Computer Science Department, California State Polytechnic University. <http://www.csupomona.edu/~hnriley/www/VonN.html/>.

Ritchie, David. *The Binary Brain: Artificial Intelligence in the Age of Electronics.* Boston: Little, Brown, 1984.

————. *The Computer Pioneers.* New York: Simon and Schuster, 1986.

"How the Internet Browser Works." The River Internet Access Company (June 22, 2001). <http://info.theriver.com/workbook/Workbook/browser_works.HTM>.

Rojas, Raul, and Ulf Hashagen. *The First Computers: History and Architectures.* Cambridge: MIT Press, 2000.

Rothman, Milton A. *Cybernetics: Machines that Make Decisions.* London England: Franklin Watts, 1972.

"Information about Programming in C or Pascal." Royal College of Technology (June 22, 2001). <http://cit.rcc.on.ca/pascal/howtopro.HTM>.

Ruble, David A. *Practical Analysis and Design for Client/Server and GUI Systems.* Upper Saddle River, NJ: Prentice Hall PTR, 1997.

"Overview of Nanotechnology." Rutgers University (July 5, 2001). <http://nanotech.rutgers.edu/nanotech/intro.HTML>.

"Criteria for CASE Tools." Rutherford Appleton Laboratory (July 5, 2001). <http://hepunx.rl.ac.uk/atlas/oo/tools/critieria.HTML>.

"Mind Machine Museum: A Virtual Museum and Gallery of Vintage Computers." San Francisco State University. <http://online.sfsu.edu/~hl/mmm.html/>.

Sander, Leonard M. "Fractal Growth." *Scientific American* (January 1987): 94-100.

Sanders, G. Lawrence. *Data Modeling.* Danvers, MA: Boyd & Fraser Publishing Company, 1995.

"Configuring the Serial Line Internet Protocol (SLIP)." The Santa Cruz Operation (August 9, 2001). <http://uw7doc.sco.com/NET_tcpip/slipN.intro.HTML>.

Saxon, James A. *The Slide Rule.* Englewood Cliffs, NJ: Prentice-Hall, 1966.

Schmidt, David A. *Denotational Semantics—A Methodology for Language Development.* Boston: Allyn and Bacon, 1986.

Schueller, Ulrich, and Hans-Georg Veddeler. *Upgrading and Maintaining Your PC.* Grand Rapids, MI: Abacus, 1996.

Schuler, Charles A. *Electric Circuit Analysis.* Glencoe, NY: 1993.

"Avoiding a Data Crunch." *Scientific American* (June 16, 2001). <http://www.sciam.com/2000/0500issue/0500toig.HTML>.

"On the Horizon: Holographic Storage." *Scientific American* (July 4, 2001). <http://www.sciam.com/0500issue/0500toigbox5.HTML>.

"Quantum Computing with Molecules." *Scientific American* (July 29, 2001). <http://www.sciam.com/1998/0698issue/0698gershenfeld.HTML>.

Scott, Phil. "I, Robonaut." *Scientific American* 284, no. 4 (April 2001): 27.

Scrivener, Stephen A. R., and Sean Cooper. "Introducing CSCW—What it Is and Why We Need It." *Computer-Supported Cooperative Work,* edited by Stephen A. R. Scrivener. Brookfield, VT: Avebury Technical, 1994.

Searle, Steven J. "A Brief History of Character Codes." TRON Web. <http://tronweb.super-nova.co.jp/characcodehist.html>.

Sears, A. "Layout Appropriateness: A Metric for Evaluating User Interface Widget Layout." *IEEE—Transactions on Software Engineering,* 19 (1993): 707-19.

"Fuzzy Logic—An Introduction." Seattle Robotics (June 15, 2001). <http://www.seattlerobotics.org/encoder/mar98/fuz/fl_part1.HTML>.

Seth, Anuj. "The Data Encryption Page." <http://www.geocities.com/SiliconValley/Network/2811/intro.htm

Sevenich, Richard A. "Compiler Construction Tools." *Linux Gazette* 39 (March 25, 1999). <http://www.linuxgazette.com/issue39/sevenich.html>.

Shasha, Dennis E., and Cathy A. Lazere. *Out of Their Minds: The Lives and Discoveries of 15 Great Computer Scientists.* New York: Copernicus, 1995.

Siepel, A., et al. "ISYS: A Decentralized, Component-Based Approach to the Integration of Heterogeneous Bioinformatics Resources." *Bioinformatics* 16 (2000): 1-12.

"Selectors." The Slackers Guide to Style Sheets (August 13, 2001). <http://slackerhtml.tripod.com/stylesheets/selectors.HTML>.

"The Mouse: A Virtual Unknown." Silicon Valley.com. <http://www0.mercurycenter.com/svtech/news/special/engelbart/ >.

Sleurink, H. *The Multimedia Dictionary.* San Diego: Academic Press, 1995.

Smith, Douglas K., and Robert C. Alexander. *Fumbling the Future: How Xerox Invented, then Ignored, the First Personal Computer.* William Morrow & Co., 1988.

"The Object at Hand." *Smithsonian Magazine* (July 4, 2001). <http://www.smithsonianmag.si.edu/smithsonian/issue96/feb96/object.HTML>.

Snoeyink, Jack. "IEEE 754 Floating Point Standard." Department of Computer Science, The University of North Carolina at Chapel Hill. <http://www.cs.unc.edu/~snoeyink/c/c205/ho3.htm>.

Softky, Marion. "Building the Internet: Bob Taylor won the National Medal of Technology 'For visionary leadership in the development of modern computing technology.'" *The Almanac* (October 11, 2000). <http://www.almanac-news.com/morgue/2000/2000_10_11.taylor.html>.

Sommers, Hobart H. *The Slide Rule and How to Use It.* New York: Follett Publishing Company, 1964.

Sommerville, Ian. *Software Engineering,* Fourth Edition. New York: Addison-Wesley Publishing Company, 1992.

"Top-Down Design." South Dakota State College (July 4, 2001). <http://step.sdsc.edu/s95/design/top_down/>.

"Routine and Subroutine." Southeast University (August 10, 2001). <http://iroi.seu.edu.cn/books/whatis/routine.HTM>.

"Executable and Nonexecutable Statement Classification." Southwest Cyberport (June 22, 2001). <http://kumo.swcp.com/walt/fortran/F77_std/rjcnf0001-sh-7.HTML>.

"Port-Mapped vs. Memory-Mapped I/O." Speedhost (August 1, 2001). <http://www.hive.speedhost.com/code3.HTM>.

"Bit Slice." Spots Interconnect, Inc. <http://spots.ab.ca/~sarah/gloss/gloss_b.htm#bitslice>.

Srihari, Sargur N. *Computer Text Recognition and Error Correction.* Silver Spring, MD: IEEE Computer Society Press, 1985.

Stallman, Richard. "The GNU Project" (July 2, 2001). <http://www.gnu.org/gnu/the-gnu-project.HTML>.

"Chapter Three: The Bridge between Two Centuries." Stanford University. <http://www.stanford.edu/group/mmdd/SiliconValley/Augarten/Chapter3.html>.

"Xerox PARC." Stanford University, Stanford Business School. <http://gobi.stanford.edu/computer_history/xerox2.htm>.

"Donald E. Knuth: Professor Emeritus." Stanford University: Department of Computer Sciences. <http://soe.stanford.edu/compsci/faculty/Knuth_Donald.html>.

Stanley, A. E. *HyperTalk & HyperText.* Boston: Newtech, 1992.

Steele, Heidi. *How to Use the Internet.* Emeryville, CA: Ziff-Davis Press, 1996.

Stoddard, S., Jans, L., Ripple, J. and Kraus, L. *Chartbook on Work and Disability in the United States, 1998.* An InfoUse Report. Washington, D.C.: U.S. National Institute on Disability and Rehabilitation Research.

Stojanovski, Toni, and Ljupco Kocarev. "Chaos-Based Random Number Generators—Part I: Analysis." *IEEE Transactions on Circuits and Systems—I: Fundamental Theory and Applications* 48, no. 3 (March 2001): 281-8.

Stoy, Joseph E. *Denotational Semantics: The Scott-Strachey Approach to Programming Language Theory.* Cambridge, MA: MIT Press, 1977.

Streater, Jack W. *How to Use Integrated-Circuit Logic Elements.* Indianapolis: H.W. Sams, 1979.

Stremler, Ferrel G. *Introduction to Communication Systems.* Reading, MA: Addison-Wesley, 1982.

Stross, Randall E. *The Microsoft Way: The Real Story of How the Company Outsmarts its Competition.* Reading, MA: Addison-Wesley Publishing Company, 1996.

Sze, S. M. *Physics of Semiconductor Devices.* New York: Wiley, 1981.

Taylor, Ashley George. "WIMP Interfaces." <www.cc.gatech.edu/classes/cs6751_97_winter/topics/dialog-wimp>.

"Types of Animation Systems." Taylor University (June 20, 2001). <http://www.css.taylor.edu/instrmat/graphics/hypergraph/animation/anim1.HTM>.

"Lucent unit takes storage into third dimension." TechWeb. July 4, 2001. <http://content.techweb.com/wire/story/TWB20010130S0017>.

Tennant, Roy, John Ober, and Anne G. Lipow. *Crossing the Internet Threshold: An Instructional Handbook.* Berkeley, CA: Library Solutions Press, 1994.

Terrell, David L. *Microporcessor Technology.* Reston, VA: Reston Publishing Company, 1983.

Tesler, Pearl. "Universal Robots: The History and Workings of Robotics." The Tech Museum of Innovation (March 3, 2001). <http://www.thetech.org/robotics/universal/index.html>.

"Algorithm Choices Give Pattern Matching an Edge." Test & Measurement World (July 7, 2001). <http://www.tmworld.com/articles/2000/09_algorithm.HTM>.

"Cond." Texas A&M University (August 12, 2001). <http://grimpeur.tamu.edu/~colin/lp/node23.HTML>.

"Software for Graphics and Data Analysis." Texas A&M University (July 24, 2001). <http://stommel.tamu.edu/~baum/ocean_graphics.HTML>.

"File Manipulation (Output File Stream)." Thames Valley District School Board (August 13, 2001). <http://www.tvdsb.on.ca/saunders/courses/DSC4a/Cplusplus/ostreams.HTM>.

"The Motherboard and its Components." ThinkQuest. <http://library.thinkquest.org/3308/mother.htm>.

Thompson, Robert Bruce. *PC Hardware in a Nutshell: A Desktop Quick Reference.* Cambridge, MA: O'Reilly, 2000.

Thompson, William J. *Computing in Applied Science.* New York: John Wiley & Sons, 1984.

"Retrieving a Subset of Rows: Compound Conditions." Thunderstone (August 12, 2001). <http://www.thunderstone.com/site/texisman/node40.HTML>.

Thurston, Hugh Ansfrid. *The Number System.* New York: Interscience Publishers, 1956.

"Canada Probing Alleged Computer Spying." *The Times of India On-line* (July 7, 2001). <http://www.timesofindia.com/270800/27info11.HTM>.

"Object-Oriented Programming." TooDarkPark (July 21, 2001). <http://www.toodarkpark.org/computers/objc/oop.HTML>.

"Turing's Claim." Turing.org (August 10, 2001). <http://www.turing.org.uk/turing/scrapbook/test.HTML>.

"Types of Spread Spectrum Communications." (June 12, 2001). <http://murray.newcastle.edu.au/users/staff/eemf/ELEC351/SProjects/Morris/types.htm>.

"A&M Records v. Napster: MP3 File Sharing Disputes Continue in the Aftermath of Recent Court Rulings." The UCLA Online Institute for Cyberspace Law and Policy. <http://www.gseis.ucla.edu/iclp/napster.htm>.

"The Digital Millennium Copyright Act." The UCLA Online Institute for Cyberspace Law and Policy. <http://www.gseis.ucla.edu/iclp/dmca1.htm>.

Uddin, M. Saleh. *Digital Architecture.* New York: McGraw-Hill, 1999.

*Understanding Solid-State Electronics: A Self-Teaching Course in Basic Semiconductor Theory.* Texas Instruments Incorporated Learning Center. Dallas: The Center, 1978.

"System Memory Allocation." Unet (Jun 9, 2001). <http://www.unet.univie.ac.at/aix/aixprggd/genprogc/sys_mem_alloc.HTM>.

"What Is Unicode?" Unicode.org (August 9, 2001). <http://www.unicode.org/unicode/standard/WhatIsUnicode.HTML>.

"Data Mining, Data Warehousing and Knowledge Discovery." United States Department of Defense, Information Analysis Center, Data & Analysis Center for Software. <http://www.dacs.dtic.mil/databases/url/key.hts?keycode=222/>.

"Computer Crime and Intellectual Property Section." United States Department of Justice (August 8, 2001). <http://www.usdoj.gov/criminal/cybercrime/cclaws.HTML>.

"Fibre Channel." United States Navy (July 5, 2001). <http://www.nswc.navy.mil/cosip/feb98/tech0298-1.shtml>.

"Variable Declaration." Universität GH Essen (August 13, 2001). <http://didaktik.physik.uni-essen.de/~gnu-pascal/gpc_109.HTML>.

"UML semantics." l'Universite de Haute-Alscace (August 12, 2001). <http://www.uml.crespim.uha.fr/documentation/version1.0/semantics/semantics_ch6.HTML>.

"Pattern Matching and Text Compression Algorithms." Université de Marne-la-Vallée (July 7, 2001). <http://www.dcs.kel.ac.uk/teaching/units/csmtsp/B5.HTML>.

"Notation for Hand Tracing." University of Alberta (August 17, 2001). <http://www.cs.alberta.ca/~zaiane/courses/cmput102/slides/Tpoic5/sld008.htm>.

"Unconditional State Transition." University of Alberta (August 13, 2001). <http://sheerness.cs.ualberta.ca/~pawel/SIDE/man_sicle/node22.HTM>.

"The VLIW Approach." The University of Arizona, Computer Architecture and Design. <http://www.ece.arizona.edu/~ece462/Lec05F00/tsld011.htm>.

"Accessors and Modifiers." University of Bordeaux (July 22, 2001). <http://www.ufr-mi.u-bordeaux.fr/~papanik/C++/lecture/html/node27.HTML>.

"Primer on Object-Oriented Programming." University of Bradford (July 29, 2001). <http://www.eimc.brad.ac.uk/java/tutorial/Project/1/ooprim.HTM>.

"Guide to Faster, Less Frustrating Debugging." University of California at Davis (July 6, 2001). <http://heather.cs.ucdavis.edu/~matloff/UnixAndC/Clanguage?Debug.HTML>.

"How a Web Browser Works." University of California at Davis (June 22, 2001). <http://arbor.ucdavis.edu/resources/internet/browsers/browser.HTML>.

"Evolution of Computer Code for Controlling Agents: v1." University of California at Los Angeles (July 21, 2001). <http://www.bol.ucla.edu/~bredelin/Essays/evolveRed.HTML>.

"Art of Assembly Language." University of California at Riverside (June 8, 2001). <http://webster.cs.ucr.edu/Page_asm/ArtofAssembly/CH01/Ch01-1.HTML>.

"New Technology, Old Vision." University of California at Riverside (June 30, 2001). <http://www.cmp.ucr.edu/essays/edward_earle/millenium/08_new_old.HTML>.

"Spinning a Web Search." University of California at Santa Barbara (July 5, 2001). <http://www.library.ucsb.edu/untangle/lager.HTML>.

"Heapsort." University of Canterbury, Computer Science Department. <http://www.cosc.canterbury.ac.nz/teaching/classes/cosc122/Book/node79.html>.

"Part XIII—File and String Streams." University College London (August 13, 2001). <http://www.cs.ucl.ac.uk/staff/G.Roberts/c.html/c__bo_15.HTM>.

"Clarence (Skip) Ellis, Professor." University of Colorado at Boulder, Department of Computer Science. <http://www.cs.colorado.edu/~skip/Home.html>.

"Computer-Supported Cooperative Learning in a Virtual University." University of Exeter (August 8, 2001). <http://www.media.uwe.ac.uk/masoud//author/jcal.HTM>.

"Object-Oriented Programming: What the Heck Is Analysis?" University of Florida (August 15, 2001). <http://www.cise.ufl.edu/~jnw/cop4331sp00/Lectures/17.HTML>.

"User Interface Management Systems: The CLIM Perspective." University of Hamburg (July 16, 2001). <http://kogs-www.informatik.uni-hamburg.de/~moeller/uims-clim/clim-intro.HTML>.

"Variable Definition vs. Declaration." University of Hawaii (August 13, 2001). <http://www-ee.eng.hawaii.edu/Courses/EE150/Book/chap14/subsection2.1.1.4.HTML>.

"Illinois and the Birth of a Technology: Anderson Reflects on the Origins of the Computer." University of Illinois, Department of Computer Science. <http://www.cs.uiuc.edu/whatsnew/newsletter/interim93/>.

"A Gentle Introduction to SGML." University of Illinois at Chicago (July 29, 2001). <http://www.uic.edu/orgs/tei/sgml/teip3sg/SG.HTM>.

"Theorist Applies Computer Power to Uncertainty in Statistics." University of Illinois at Urbana-Champaign (July 2, 2001). <http://www.mste.uiuc.edu/stat/bootarticle.HTML>.

"Punched Card Codes." University of Iowa (August 10, 2001). <http://www.cs.uiowa.edu/~jones/cards/codes.HTML>.

"PSP Resources Page." University of Karlsruhe (August 9, 2001). <http://wwwipd.ira.uka.de/PSP/>.

"On-Line Education: A Paper about the Need for and Applications of Internet-Based Education in Distance Education and Classroom-Based Learning." University of Liverpool (July 29, 2001). <http://www.socio.demon.co.uk/on-line-ed.HTML>.

"The History of Computer Animation in Film." University of Maryland (June 20, 2001). <http://www.wam.umd.edu/~danf/engl/>.

"Personal Software Process." University of Massachusetts. <http://www2.umassd.edu/swpi/PersonalSoftwareProcess/psp.html>.

"Desktop Publishing." University of Memphis (June 5, 2001). <http://www.msci.memphis.edu/~rybrnp/cl/wp/dtp.HTML>.

"Tree Data Structures." University of Michigan (July 24, 2001). <http://hpcc.engin.umich.edu/CFD/users/charlton/Thesis/html/node28.HTML>.

"An Introduction to File Input/Output." University of Mississippi (August 18, 2001). <http://tdlee.ncpa.olemiss.edu/~clt/cs178/Lectures/cs178.lect27.html>.

"Definition—Z39.50 Gateway." University of Missouri. <http://web.missouri.edu/~mulvsha/webpacdesign/sld006.htm>.

"A GTK+ Binding for Haskell." University of New South Wales (August 9, 2001). <http://www.cse.unsw.edu.au/~chak/haskell/gtk/>.

"Bit-Slice Processor." University of North Florida, Jacksonville. <http://www.unf.edu/~swarde/Execution_Units/Bit-Slice_Processor/bit-slice_processor.html>.

"A Brief History of Spreadsheets." University of Northern Iowa (June 22, 2001). <http://dss.cba.uni.edu/dss/sshistory.HTML>.

"Hardware Conflict Issues." University of Oregon (August 12, 2001). <http://www.uoregon.edu/~dalbrich/conflict.HTML>.

"Roles of IT in Improving Our Educational System. Part 7: Highly Interactive Computing in Teaching and Learning." University of Oregon (July 16, 2001). <http://www.uoregon.edu/~moursund/D.A.V.E./highly_interactive.HTM>.

"Proving Programs Correct." University of Rochester (August 12, 2001). <http://www.cs.rochester.edu/u/leblanc/csc173.94/correctness.HTML>.

"The DEC PDP Family: The First Minicomputers." University of Science and Technology at Manchester, United Kingdom. <http://hoc.co.umist.ac.uk/storylines/compdev/industrialisation/pdp.html>.

"Functional Programming." University of St. Andrews (July 24, 2001). <http://www-fp.dcs.st-and.ac.uk/introduction.HTML>.

"Hashing." University of St. Andrews (July 15, 2001). <http://www-theory.dcs.st-and.ac.uk/~mda/cs2001/hashing/genral.HTML>.

"John Backus." University of St. Andrews, School of Mathematical and Computational Sciences. <http://www-groups.dcs.st-and.ac.uk/~history/Mathematicians/Backus.html>.

"John Napier." University of St Andrews, School of Mathematical and Computational Sciences. <http://www-history.mcs.st-and.ac.uk/history/Mathematicians/Napier.html>.

"John von Neumann." University of St Andrews, School of Mathematical and Computational Sciences. <http://www-groups.dcs.st-andrews.ac.uk/~history/Mathematicians/Von_Neumann.html >.

"Photonic Networks? . . . What Are They?" University of Strathclyde (July 16, 2001). <http://www.opto.eee.strath.ac.uk/Networks/networks_2.HTML>.

"Introduction to RAID Technology." University of Texas (June 10, 2001). <http://www.utexas.edu/cc/vms/about/raid.HTML>.

"Donald Knuth." University of Texas at Austin. <http://laurel.actlab.utexas.edu/~cynbe/muq/muf3_20.html>.

"Edsgar Wybe Dijkstra." University of Texas at Austin, Department of Computer Sciences. <http://www.cs.utexas.edu/users/UTCS/report/1997/dijkstra.html> and <http://www.cs.utexas.edu/users/UTCS/report/1994/profiles/dijkstra.html>.

"Unix (Basic Introduction)." University of Toronto (June 23, 2001). <http://www.scar.utoronto.ca/~ccweb/manuals/unixintro.HTML>.

"Attribute-List Declarations." University of Waterloo (July 20, 2001). <http://web.ajk.its-sby.edu/archives/Introduction_XML/attribute_decl.HTML>.

"FAT—File Allocation Table." University of Western Australia (July 11, 2001). <http://www.cs.uwa.edu.au/undergraduate/units/231.316/fat.HTML>.

"History and Timeline." Unix-systems (June 23, 2001). <http://www.unix-systems.org/what_is_unix/history_timeline.HTML>.

"The History of the Development of Parallel Computing." Virginia Polytechnic Institute and State University, Department of Computer Science. <http://ei.cs.vt.edu/~history/Parallel.html>.

"Control Structure." The Voice Response Development Environment Organization (July 9, 2001). <http://www.vorde.org/voiceProcessing/mb-cti-thesis/node11.HTML>.

"Selectors." W3.org (August 13, 2001). <http://www.w3.org/TR/REC-CSS2/selector.HTML>.

"XBL-XML Binding Language." W3.org (August 9, 2001). <http://www.w3.org/TR/xbl/>.

Waggoner, Shelly Cashman. *Discovering Computers 98: A Link to the Future.* Cambridge, MA: Course Technology, 1998.

"NeuroShell Classifier." Ward Systems (August 12, 2001). 2001. <http://www.wardsystems.com/products.asp?p-classifier>.

Warshofsky, Fred. *The Patent Wars: The Battle to Own the World's Technology.* New York: John Wiley & Sons, Inc., 1994.

Waters, John K. *The Everything Computer Book.* Holbrook, MA: Adams Media, 2000.

Watson, Clyde. *Binary Numbers.* New York: Crowell, 1977.

Watson, Des. *High-level Languages and their Compilers.* Reading, MA: Addison-Wesley, 1989.

Web Dictionary of Cybernetics and Systems. Principia Cybernetica Web. <http://pespmc1.vub.ac.be/ASC/indexASC.html>.

"Intro to the If Statement." Web Dreamland (July 10, 2001). <http://www.webdreamland.com/articles/scripting/if_intro.HTML>.

"Site Usability Heuristics for the Web." Web Review (July 24, 2001). <http://www.webreview.com/1997/10_10/strategists/10_10_97_2.shtml>.

Weber, Nico. "Computers and Linguistics: Computers and Translation." <http://www.sp.fh-koeln.de/Personen/Weber/Tomsk%20Lectures/Syntax.html>.

Webopedia: Online Computer Dictionary for Internet Terms and Technical Support. Internet.com Corp. <http://webopedia.internet.com>.

Wegenkittle, Stefan. "Empirical Testing of Pseudorandom Number Generators." <http://crypto.mat.sbg.ac.at/~ste/dipl/>.

Weinberg, Neal. "Networks of the Future." Network World (May 3, 1999). <http://www.nwfusion.com/news/1999/0503future.html>.

White, Bebo. "The World Wide Web and High-Energy Physics." *Physics Today* 51, no. 11 (November 1998): 30-6.

White, Ron. *How Computers Work.* Hemel Hempstead: Indianapolis: Que, Prentice Hall, 1999.

"Leonardo Torres y Quevedo." Williamette University. <http://www.willamette.edu/~sosorio/lab0.html >.

Williams, Michael R. *A History of Computing Technology,* Second Edition. IEEE Computer Society, 1997.

Williams, Scott. "Computer Scientists of the African Diaspora." State University of New York at Buffalo. <http://www.math.buffalo.edu/mad/computer-science/computer_science.html>.

Wilson, Paul. "Introducing Computer-Supported Cooperative Work." *Computer-Supported Cooperative Work,* edited by Stephen A. R. Scrivener. Brookfield, VT: Avebury Technical, 1994.

Winston, Patrick Henry. *LISP.* Reading, MA: Addison-Wesley, 1989.

Winters, Paul A., editor. *The Information Revolution: Opposing Viewpoints.* San Diego: Greenhaven Press, 1998.

Wolinsky, Art. *The History of the Internet and the World Wide Web.* Berkeley Heights, NJ: Enslow Publishers, 1999.

"Combinations." Wollongong University (July 9, 2001). <http://engineering.uow.edu.au/Courses/Stats/File2419.HTML>.

"Permutation." Wollongong University (July 9, 2001). <http://engineering.uow.edu.au/Courses/Stats/File2418.HTML>.

"Survey of Grammar Models." Worcester Polytechnic Institute (July 20, 2001). <http://www.cs.wpi.edu/~jshutt/thesis/survey.HTML>.

"HyperText Markup Language Home Page." World Wide Web Consortium (August 1, 2001). <http://www.w3.org/MarkUp/>.

"XML in 10 Points." World Wide Web Consortium (July 16, 2001). <http://www.w3.org/XML/1999/XML-in-10-points>.

Wyatt, Allen. *Using Assembly Language.* Carmel, IN: Que, 1992.

"Palo Alto Research Center." Xerox Corporation. <http://www2.xerox.com/go/xrx/xrx_research/AX_6_1.jsp?id=48660>.

"Xerox PARC." Xerox Palo Alto Research Center. <http://www.parc.xerox.com/parc-go.html>.

"Functional Programming and XML." XML.com (July 24, 2001). <http://www.xml.com/lpt/a/2001/02/14/functional.HTML>.

"What Is XML?" XML.com (July 16, 2001). <http://www.xml.com/lpt/a/98/10/guide1.HTML>.

"High-Level Language." Xrefer.com. <http://www.xrefer.com/entry/641770>.

"Integrated Circuit (IC, microchip)." Xrefer (August 10, 2001). <http://www.xrefer.com/entry/622964>.

Yang, Edward S. *Fundamentals of Semiconductor Devices.* New York: McGraw-Hill, 1978.

Yanowitz, Jason. "Under the Hood of the Internet: An Overview of the TCP/IP Protocol Suite." <http://info.acm.org/crossroads/xrds1-1/tcpjmy.html>.

Young, Neville W. *A Complete Slide Rule Manual.* New York: Drake Publishers, 1973.

Yu, Albert. *Creating the Digital Future: The Secrets of Consistent Innovation at Intel.* New York: Free Press, 1998.

Zadeh, L. "Fuzzy Sets." *Information and Control* 8 (1965): 338-53.

Zamir, Saba, editor. *Handbook of Object Technology.* Boca Raton: CRC Press, 1999.

"How to Determine If You Have a Hardware Conflict." Zoltrix (August 12, 2001). <http://www.zoltrix.com/support/CONFLICT.HTM>.

**c. 1500 B.C.**

Stone tablets found at Nippur (Iraq) in the 1930s by Otto Neugebauer (1899–1990) suggest that the Babylonians are using the abacus at this time—some of the pictographs are reminiscent of the form of an abacus; see also c. 75 AD.

**c. 800 B.C.**

The *I Ching* is used in China—it is based on binary principles. The *I Ching* (meaning Book of Changes) is one of the Five Classics of Confucianism (though it has traditionally been attributed to Wen Wang of the 12th century B.C.). It discusses the religious system used during the Chou dynasty, and a section of "commentaries" (written later) represents a philosophical examination of life and ethics. It contains numerous pictographs that many modern researchers argue represent a system of binary numbering and arithmetic.

**c. 400 B.C.**

The Spartans employed a cipher device called the *scytale* to ensure secure communications between their commanders. This is the first recorded use of cryptography in the field of communications.

**c. 300 B.C.**

A symbol is used by the Babylonians to indicate a gap between numbers, this is an early form of positional notation and the use of a symbol for zero.

**c. 240 B.C.**

The Sieve of Eratosthenes is used to determine prime numbers.

**c. 87 B.C.**

It is believed the Antikythera mechanism is manufactured around this time and lost in the sea shortly afterwards. It is an early analog astronomical computer.

**c. 75**

Writings by Pan Ku (c. 32–92) in China describe the workings of the abacus, made from bamboo; see also 1500 B.C..

**595**

In India, the first known use of our number system, with base ten and positional notation.

**820**

Muhammad ibn Musa Al'Khowarizmi, a Tashkent cleric and mathematician, develops the concept of a written process that delineates the steps needed to achieve a goal; his book on the subject gives this process its modern name—algorithm.

**960–1279**

During the Sung dynasty in China, a complex counting board is developed to handle massive calculations, including simultaneous linear and quadratic equations; interest in magic squares is also high in China at this time.

**1202**

Leonardo of Pisa (1170–1250)—better known as Fibonacci (son of Bonacci)—publishes *Liber Abbaci* (which is subsequently updated and re-released in 1228). This is the work that first gives us Fibonacci numbers (largely ignored for the next three centuries), it also includes methods of calculation and multiplication. This book also marks the beginning of the use of the modern number system.

**1274**

Raymond Lull (1235–1316) invents his logic machine—a series of disks containing numbers or symbols that can be combined to give statements by rotating the disks.

**c. 1300**

The abacus, in the form that we now know it (wire and beads), was first used in China at this time; it replaced the previously used calculating rods.

**1430**   Leon Baptista Alberti invents his cipher machine—a polyalphabet system utilizing a cipher disk to encode and decode messages.

**1492**   Francesco Pellos (Pellizzati) publishes a work that gives us the first printed example of the decimal point.

**1494**   Luca Pacioli publishes *Summa de Arithmetica*, which popularizes the work of Fibonacci (1170–1250) as well as dealing with general remarks on numbers, proto-algebra, and specifics of double entry book keeping.

**1500**   Drawings indicate that Leonardo Da Vinci (1452–1519) invented a 13-wheel counter.

**Mid 16th century**
The use of Hindu Arabic numerals overtakes the use of Roman numerals in the United Kingdom and Europe.

**1585**   *De Thiende* ("The Tenth") and *La Pratique d'arithmetique* by Simon Stevin (1548–1620) are both published. These works introduce a form of decimal notation in which the decimal point is indicated by a zero in a circle, with units to the right-hand side shown with corresponding locators; for example, 15.421 would be shown by 15(0)4(1)2(2)1(3). Stevin also suggests the decimal system for measurement.

**1614**   John Napier (1550–1617) publishes his first table of logarithms (an abbreviation of *logos arithmos*—the number of the expression) in *Mirifici logarithmorum canonis descriptio* (Descriptions of the Marvelous Rule of Logarithms). An early calculator called Napier's rods (or bones) is used to calculate the values.

**1620**   Edmund Gunter (1581–1626) invents a basic slide rule that is well received, particularly for navigation at sea. While publishing mathematical tables he invents the word cosine.

**1622**   William Oughtred (1575–1660) creates a circular slide rule based on the logarithms of Napier. In 1654 he makes the horizontal version with which we are more familiar.

**1623**   Wilhelm Schickard (1592–1635) designs a calculating machine using rotating cylinders and linking mechanisms; it is called Schickard's calculating clock. His work is lost until 1956 when it is rediscovered by Franz Hammer (who had discovered and lost it again in 1935); credit for designing a mechanical calculator often went to later figures such as Pascal (1642) or Leibniz (1671).

**1624**   Henry Briggs (1561–1630) in *Arithmetica logarithmica* (The Arithmetic of Logarithms) publishes the first table of common (or Briggsian) Logarithms.

**1631**   The work of Thomas Harriot (c. 1560–1621) is published posthumously; *Artis analyticae praxis* considers some calculations using base 2 or binary arithmetic. It is not until the development of computers that the binary number system becomes widely used.

**1642**   Blaise Pascal (1623–1662) invents one of the first calculating machines (based on rotating discs)—it is called the numerical wheel or the Pascaline and it is essentially a mechanized abacus.

**1646**   Sir Thomas Browne describes a person who computes as a computer—he is the first known person to use this word.

**1668**   Samuel Morland (1625–1695) produces a non-decimal adding machine for use in England.

**1671**   Gottfried Willhelm von Leibniz (1646–1716) invents a calculating machine (the mechanical multiplier or the stepped reckoner) that can carry out addition and multiplication. The most complex calculating machine to this date, it could also extract square roots. The machine was lost and rediscovered in 1879.

**1673**   René Grillet invents an adding machine—his obsession with secrecy means we know nothing about it today other than it existed.

**1679**   Gottfried Willhelm von Leibniz (1646–1716) gives a generalized treatment of positional number systems and introduces a binary system where 1 represents God and 0 a void.

**1714**   Henry Mill invents the earliest known typewriter.

**1736**   Jacques Vaucanson (1709–1782) builds his first automaton (a mechanized man)—a flute player.

**1774**   Philipp Matthaus Hahn builds calculating machines that are accurate to 12 decimal places.

**1777**   Charles Mahon (1753–1816), the third Earl of Stanhope, produces a mechanical logic machine—the Stanhope Logic Demonstrator, a multiplying calculator.

**1786**   J. H. Mueller articulates the idea of the first difference engine—a machine for calculating values of a polynomial. He is, however, unable to raise funds for its manufacture.

**1790**   Thomas Jefferson (1743–1826) invents a wheel cipher for encoding messages. His device is used as late as World War II.

**1801**   Joseph-Marie Jacquard (1752–1834) invents an automatic loom that uses punched cards to control the patterns—this is the Jaquard loom.

**1809**   A number of patents were given for devices to help the blind read—after much evolution these devices eventually become the OCR systems used by computers.

**1813** The Analytical Society is founded by Charles Babbage (1791–1871), John Herschel (1792–1871), and George Peacock (1791–1858) at Cambridge University, England. Their aim is to push forward the acceptance of LaGrange's algebra.

**1814** Johann H. Hermann (1785–1842) produces his planimeter—a device utilizing a disk-and-wheel system for integrating measurements to calculate the area under a curve on a graph.

**1820** Charles Xavier Thomas de Colmar (1785–1870) invents the first mass-produced calculator, the Arithmometer.

**1822** Charles Babbage (1791–1871) works on the first mechanical computers, initially the difference engine and subsequently the analytical engine (from 1834 to his death). Due to circumstances beyond his control Babbage never completes working models of any of his machines; however, in 1991 the Science Museum in London built the difference engine.

**1829** William Austen Burt invents a difficult-to-use version of the typewriter—the first patented typewriter in the United States.

**1829** Charles Wheatstone (1802–1875) uses punched paper tape to store data.

**1838** Samuel Finley Breese Morse (1791–1872) and Alfred Vail (1807–1859) unveil their telegraph system.

**1842** Ada Augusta King (1815–1852) (Countess of Lovelace) translates Menabrea's pamphlet on the Analytical Engine, adding her own notes and becomes the world's first programmer.

**1843** Georg Scheutz (1785–1873) of Stockholm produces a small difference engine in 1834 (after reading a description of Charles Babbage's work). The Swedish government funds development that leads to a device with a fitted printer in this year—the first of its kind.

**1847** George Boole (1815–1864) publishes *A Mathematical Analysis of Logic* in England. This is the forerunner of Boolean logic and the binary number system that is basis of modern computer design.

**1850** Victor Mayer Amedee Mannheim (1831–1906) invents the logarithmic slide rule that would dominate mechanical calculation until the middle of the 20th century.

**1853** Georg Scheutz (1785–1873) and Edvard Scheutz (1821–1881) produce a Tabulating Machine. Based on Georg Scheutz's designs, this version was capable of processing 15-digit numbers.

**1858** A telegraph cable is made to cross the Atlantic Ocean. It functions for only a few days, but it is the first successful attempt at real-time trans-Atlantic communication.

**1867** Charles Wheatstone (1802–1875) produces his clock-like cipher machine, which he called a crytpograph.

**1868** Christopher Latham Sholes (1819–1890) invents the first commercial typewriter.

**1872** William Thomson, Lord Kelvin (1824–1907) invents a large-scale analog computer to predict tide heights—the harmonic analyzer.

**1874** Émile Baudot (1845–1903) devises the Baudot code—a system of transmitting information in which five equal-length bits represent one character, it is initially used in telegraph communication.

**1876** Alexander Graham Bell (1847–1922) invents the telephone.

**1880** Ramon Verea (1838–1899) produces a calculator that is the first to multiply rather than merely repeat additions.

**1884** The American Institute for Electrical Engineering (AIEE) is formed. This is the first of the organizations that will eventually merge to produce the IEEE in 1963.

**1885** Allan Marquand (1853–1924) produces a mechanical logic machine.

**1886** Herman Hollerith (1860–1929) invents a machine that can record data by punching holes in small cards; the cards are read when passed through a device that makes electrical contacts through the holes. The company Hollerith forms to make this device eventually becomes International Business Machines, IBM.

**1886** Dorr Eugene Felt (1862–1930) produces the comptometer—the first machine into which numbers can be entered via keys rather than dials; he produces the first version with a printer in 1889.

**1888** William Seward Burroughs (1857–1898) is granted a patent for his calculating machine (invented in 1884); this lays the foundation for the subsequent formation of the Burroughs Adding Machine Corporation in 1905 (a renamed version of the American Arithmometer Company).

**1890** The punch cards of Herman Hollerith (1860–1929) are first used in tabulating the American census. Hollerith won a government-sponsored competition for the delivery of data-processing equipment to assist in the processing of the census data.

**1890** Leonardo Torres y Quevedo (1852–1936) builds the world's first chess computer—limited in use, it can only solve certain endgame problems.

**1893** Charles Proteus Steinmetz (1865–1923) develops law of hysteresis, which eventually become the basis of magnetic core memory.

**1893** A four-function calculator—called "The Millionaire"—is invented in this year by Otto Schweiger.

**1895** Guglielmo Marconi (1874–1937) transmits the first radio signal.

**1896** The Tabulating Machine Company is founded; it eventually changes its name to International Business Machines (IBM).

**1901** Off the Greek island of Antikythera, a barnacle-encrusted machine is found, which, when cleaned up, is determined to be an early analog astronomical calculator (manufactured c. 87 B.C.). It is now known as the Antikythera mechanism.

**1904** John Ambrose Fleming (1850–1934) invents the diode vacuum tube.

**1906** The International Electrotechnical Commission is founded to standardize work and definitions in the electrotechnical field.

**1906** The electronic tube (valve) or triode vacuum tube is invented by Lee De Forest (1873–1961); this is constructed by adding a third valve to control current flow to the diode vacuum tube of John Ambrose Fleming (1850–1934).

**1908** Campbell Swinton (1863–1930) of the UK describes an electronic scanning method that is basically the forerunner of the cathode ray tube for TVs and computer monitors.

**1908** Percy E. Ludgate (1883–1922) produces his analytical engine, which is very similar to the machines of Charles Babbage (1791–1871).

**1911** The Calculating Tabulating Recording Company is formed (a merger of the Hollerith Tabulating Machine Company of 1896 with the Computing Scale Company and the International Time Recording Company).

**1912** The Institute of Radio Engineers is founded—the second organization that will form IEEE in 1963.

**1912** Emmanuel Goldberg patents a machine to recognize printed text and then convert it into telegraph messages—this is an early example of OCR (Optical Character Recognition).

**1915** Manson Benedicks discovers that germanium crystals can be used to convert alternating current to direct current—an important aspect of microchips.

**1918** The American National Standards Institute (ANSI) is founded to facilitate the voluntary adoption of standards and systems.

**1918** The Enigma Machine—a cipher or encryption device that makes written communications extremely difficult to understand by third parties (who don't know the "key" to the "code")—is invented by Arthur Scherbius (1878–1929). It is used extensively by the Germans during the Second World War.

**1919** W. H. Eccles and F. W. Jordan produce the first flip-flop circuit design—a switching circuit critical to high speed electronic counting systems.

**1920** The word *robot* is coined by Czech playwright Karel Cápek (1890–1938) in his play *RUR (Rossum's Universal Robots)*; the word is derived from the Czech for "compulsory labor."

**1921** Edith Clarke (1883–1959) patents a graphical calculator.

**1924** The Calculating Tabulating Recording Company is renamed (after some mergers) International Business Machines (IBM); the first chairman is Thomas John Watson (1874–1956).

**1925** Bell Telephone Laboratories is formed.

**1925** Vannevar Bush (1890–1974) at the Massachusetts Institute of Technology builds a large-scale differential analyzer. For several years this is the largest computational device in the world.

**1926** The International Federation of the National Standardizing Associations (ISA) is founded; it is concerned primarily with producing and maintaining standards in mechanical engineering.

**1927** The first demonstration of television occurs in the United States; President Herbert Hoover's face is seen and the voice component is provided over a telephone wire.

**1927** J. A. O'Neill patents magnetic tape as a storage device.

**1930** The company Geophysical Services is founded. In 1951 it changes its name to Texas Instruments.

**1931** Kurt Friedrich Gödel (1906–1978) publishes his incompleteness theorems, which prove (in part) that a computer can never be programmed to answer all mathematical problems.

**1933** IBM produces the first electric typewriter.

**1934** Alonzo Church (1903–1995) develops a branch of mathematical logic know as lambda calculus; it deals with the applications of functions to their arguments.

**1934** Rósa Péter (1905–1997) publishes the first article on recursive theory.

**1935** Konrad Zuse (1910–1995) develops his Z 1 computer in his parents' living room in Berlin. The Z 2 comes in 1938, helped by Helmut Schreyer. These are binary arithmetic computers.

**1935** IBM introduces the IBM 601–a punch card machine that can perform multiplication operations in 1 second.

**1936** Alan Turing (1912–1954) theorizes a computer capable of complex serial calculations—the Turing Machine.

**1937** The notebooks and works of Charles Babbage (1791–1871) are rediscovered.

**1937** Alan Turing (1912–1954) lays down the foundations of automata theory with this work *On Computable Numbers*.

**1937** Claude Elwood Shannon (1916–2001) links Boolean logic to digital circuit design.

**1939** The Hewlett Packard Company is founded by David Packard (1912–1996) and William Redington Hewlett (1913–2001).

**1939** George Robert Stibitz (1904–1995) (with Samuel Williams) builds his Complex Number Calculator (retrospectively this device was called the Bell Labs Model 1); it is the first full-scale electromagnetic relay calculator. A demonstration version was previously constructed in 1937.

**1939** John Atanasoff (1903–1995) and Clifford Berry (1918–1963) produce their prototype of the Atanasoff-Berry Computer. Although a full-size production model is made in 1942, the Second World War halts further development.

**1940** George Robert Stibitz's (1904–1995) Complex Number Calculator was the first device to be used remotely over telephone lines.

**1940** John William Mauchly (1907–1980) announces he has constructed his harmonic analyzer—an analog processor built to analyze weather data.

**1941** During the development of the Atanasoff-Berry Computer, memory is added that is made from capacitors—these contain refresh circuits that are the first practical example of regenerative memory.

**1941** Helmut Hoezler invents the first all-electronic general-purpose analog computer.

**1941** Konrad Zuse completes the Z3—this is the first fully functional program-controlled electromechanical digital computer.

**1943–1959**
Computers manufactured during this period are usually regarded as first-generation computers (some regard the start date as 1951).

**1943** Warren Sturgis McCulloch (1898–1972) and Walter Pitts (1923– ) advance automata theory in *A Logical Calculus Immanent in Nervous Activity*; they model their work on animal nervous systems.

**1943** The chairman of IBM, Thomas John Watson (1874–1956), estimates that the world market for computers is perhaps as high as five units.

**1943** Alan Turing (1912–1954), Tommy Flowers (1905–1998), Harry Hinsley (1922–1998), and M. H. A. Newman at Bletchley Park, England, construct a device called Colossus to crack the German encryption codes created by their Enigma Machine; Colossus becomes fully operational in 1944 but remains top secret until 1970—the decryption algorithms have never been released.

**1943** Howard Aiken (1900–1973) constructs his Harvard IBM Automatic Sequence Controlled Calculator (the Mark I)—a 35 ton general-purpose electromechanical computer; subsequent work with IBM produces several more versions, up to the mark IV.

**1945** Kay McNulty Mauchly Antonelli (1921– ), after working as a human computer calculating ballistic tables, starts work as one of the first programmers of ENIAC (a computer completed in 1946).

**1945** Grace Murray Hopper (1906–1992) at Harvard, working with the Harvard IBM Mark II computer, examines a halted machine to find that a dead insect in the relays is jamming the operation. The notation in the logbook includes the bug (which is dutifully glued to the page), and subsequent repairs of the machine are referred to as "debugging." The logbook and bug are on display at the National Museum of American History at the Smithsonian Institution.

**1945** Konrad Zuse (1910–1995) flees to Zurich at the end of WWII and constructs his Z4 computer; he forms a computer company that eventually becomes part of the Siemens Corporation.

**1945** Vannevar Bush (1890–1974), then science adviser to the president, speculates about "a future device for individual use ... in which an individual stores all his books, records, and communications, and which is mechanized so that it may be consulted with exceeding speed and flexibility. It is an enlarged intimate supplement to his memory."

**1945** John von Neumann (1903–1957) writes the *First Draft of a Report on the EDVAC*, a ground-breaking work on the architectural design of computers; this design becomes know as von Neumann architecture. The report, though widely read by computer scientists, is never published.

**1945** John von Neumann (1903–1957), working on the EDVAC, is the first person to implement the merge-sort algorithm.

**1945** Alan Turing (1912–1954) describes a system of sub-routines that we now recognize as sub programs.

**1946** John W. Mauchly (1907–1980) and J. Presper Eckert (1919–1995) complete the Electronic Numerical Integrator and Calculator (ENIAC), designed to calculate artillery-firing tables. It covers 15,000 square feet and weighs 30 tons.

**1946** Adele Goldberg writes the manual for ENIAC based on her extensive experience as its main programmer.

**1946** The first computer meeting takes place at the University of Pennsylvania where delegates are told about ENIAC and the plans for EDVAC.

**1946** J. Presper Eckert Jr. (1919–1995) and John W. Mauchly (1907–1980) leave the University of Pennsylvania to establish the first computer company, the Electronic Control Corp. They plan to build the Universal Automatic Computer (UNIVAC); the company eventually becomes part of Remington Rand.

**1946** Electronic Research Associates (ERA) is created in Minneapolis to make computers. It eventually becomes part of Remington Rand.

**1946** Arthur Burks, John von Neumann (1903–1957), and Herman Goldstine write *A Preliminary Discussion of the Logical Design of an Electronic Computing Instrument.*.

**1947** The work of the ISA and the IEC is combined into one organization—the International Organization for Standardization (ISO) whose role is to facilitate the international coordination and unification of industrial standards.

**1947** Transistors are invented by William Bradford Shockley (1910–1989), John Bardeen (1908–1991), and Walter H. Brattain (1902–1987) of Bell Laboratories. They will eventually lead to smaller, more efficient, and faster computers.

**1947** Thomas M. Kilburn (1921–2001) designs and extends the memory storage capacity of the Williams Kilburn tube—an electronic memory storage device.

**1947** The Association for Computing Machinery (ACM) is formed.

**1948** Claude Elwood Shannon (1916–2001) publishes *A Mathematical Theory of Communication* and founds the subject of information theory.

**1948** Max Herman Alexander Newman (1897–1984) at Bletchley Park, Manchester (UK), builds his machine nicknamed "Baby." This is actually one of the first machines that is a computer rather than a calculator (it utilizes a stored program as its operating system), and it stores both program and data in a primitive type of random access memory (RAM).

**1948** Thomas John Watson (1874–1956) oversees the building of the Selective Sequence Control Computer at IBM. This is IBM's first move away from punched card machines and toward real computers.

**1948** Norbert Wiener (1894–1964) founds the field of cybernetics with his publication *Cybernetics, or Control and Communication in the Animal and the Machine*.

**1948** Magnetic drum memory is introduced as a data storage device for computers.

**1948** A device utilizing both electronic and relay switches is created, the SSEC (Selective Sequence Electronic Calculator).

**1949** John W. Mauchly (1907–1980) develops Short Order Code—the first high-level programming language.

**1949** Theories for self-replicating programs are first put forward—these are the basis for what become known as computer viruses.

**1949** Norman Joseph Woodland (1921– ) and Bernard Silver take out a patent on an article classification system based on identifying patterns using light—the bar code is born.

**1949** An Wang (1920–1990) files a patent for his pulse transfer-controlling device.

**1949** Jay W. Forrester (1918– ) invents magnetic core memory. Working independently, so does An Wang (1920–1990).

**1949** The Electronic Delay Storage Automatic Computer (EDSAC) becomes operational—it is the world's first large-scale, fully functional, stored-program electronic digital computer and it was designed by Maurice Vincent Wilkes (1913– ) and his colleagues at the Mathematical Laboratory, Cambridge, England.

**1949** Sam Alexander builds the Standards Eastern Automatic Computer (SEAC) and Harry Douglas Huskey (1916– ) builds the Standards Western Automatic Computer (SWAC) for the United States National Bureau of Standards.

**1950** K. H. Davis produces the first speech recognition machine, though it is capable of recognizing only the numbers zero through nine.

**1950** The floppy disk is invented at the Imperial University in Tokyo by Yoshiro Nakamatsu (1928– ); the sales license is sold to IBM.

**1950** Richard Wesley Hamming (1915–1998) publishes a paper on error-detecting and error-correcting codes; they become known as Hamming codes. This starts a new subject in the field of information theory.

**1950** EDVAC (Electronic Discrete Variable Automatic Computer) is completed at the University of Pennsylvania based on ideas outlined by John von Neumann (1903–1957).

**1950** Alan Turing (1912–1954), in a paper entitled "Computing Machinery and Intelligence," argues that computers will, in time, be programmed to acquire abilities that rival human intelligence. He devises a test—the Turing test—for such machines: An investigator poses a series of questions to a human being and a computer, neither of which he can see. If, based solely on the answers to his questions, the investigator can not distinguish between the human and the computer, the machine is considered to have passed the test.

**1951** Jay Forrester (1918– ) and Robert Rivers Everett (1921– ) of MIT finish work on a simulator for the Air Force. This real-time processing digital computer is known as Whirlwind.

**1951** The Professional Group on Electronic Computers (PGEC) of the Institute of Radio Engineers is formed (a forerunner of the Computer Society). This group organizes a number of computer conferences and provides specialist computer journals for publication.

**1951** A machine based in part on the plans of Alan Turing (1912–1954) is completed at the University of Manchester by Harry Huskey. Called Pilot ACE (Automatic Computing Engine), the machine is believed by many to be the world's first programmable digital computer.

**1951** The Ferranti Mark I and the Univac I are delivered to customers—these are regarded as the first commercially available computers.

**1951** An Wang (1920–1990) forms Wang Laboratories.

**1951** Howard Aiken's (1900–1973) Mark III is the first full-scale machine to operate with a drum memory system; this machine is also featured on the cover of *Time* magazine (the first computer to have this honor).

**1951** Polish mathematician and logician Jan Lukasiewicz (1878–1956) proposes a prefix and a postfix mathematical system; these become accepted as polish notation and reverse polish notation.

**1951** Jay Wright Forrester (1918– ) is granted a patent on matrix core memory.

**1951** Betty Holberton manufactures a soft merge generator; future developments of this technology yield the compiler.

**1951** David John Wheeler (1927– ), Maurice Vincent Wilkes (1913– ), and Stanley Gill (1926–1975) introduce sub programs (subroutines) and add the Wheeler jump to allow these programs to be implemented.

**1951** Maurice Vincent Wilkes (1913– ) devises microprogramming—a method for designing a computer system's control section.

**1952** Grace Murray Hopper at Remington Rand (working on UNIVAC) describes a compiler and language translation for the first time. This is the birth of the so-called automatic programming system. A-O is the first compiler.

**1952** UNIVAC is used by CBS to predict the results of the presidential election based on a return of 5% of the counted votes; CBS did not believe the landslide result that UNIVAC predicted for Eisenhower and withheld the results until a higher percentage of returns was available.

**1952** Autocode—the first high-level computer language—is developed by Alick Glennie.

**1952** Illiac I at the University of Illinois and Ordvac (for the United States Military) are the first computers built using von Neumann architecture.

**1953** It is estimated that there are 100 computers in the world.

**1953** IBM produces the Type 701 EDPM; called the defense calculator, this was IBM's first real computer and its successors sealed the success of IBM in the mainframe market.

**1953** IBM produces the IBM 650—the magnetic drum calculator; it is the first mass-produced computer.

**1953** Nathaniel Rochester produces an assembler—the first symbolic language translator written for a computer.

**1953** A commercial version of EDSAC, named LEO, is launched in the UK by the Lyons Company.

**1953** Ken Olsen (1927– ) uses ferrite core memory technology to build the Memory Test Computer.

**1954**    Earl Masterson unveils the Uniprinter (line printer); a printer developed specifically for computers, it is capable of printing at 600 lines per minute.

**1954**    Texas Instruments releases the silicon transistor, vastly reducing manufacturing costs of transistors.

**1955**    The first optical character reader (OCR) system is produced by the Intelligent Machines Research Corporation (IMR).

**1955**    SHARE is formed. This is a group dedicated to sharing computer programs and experiences in order to save people the time and effort of constantly reinventing particular ideas. Later the name is retroactively designated as an acronym for Society to Help Alleviate Redundant Effort. This was the first large-scale input of independent users into the way computers operate.

**1956**    Alan Newell (1927–1992) and Herbert Albert Simon (1916– ) provide a rule-based (heuristic) approach to proving theorems in logic; it is used in the design of their list processing language, IPL2.

**1956**    John McCarthy (1927– ) and Marvin Lee Minsky (1927– ) organize the first conference on Artificial Intelligence, at Dartmouth College, New Hampshire.

**1956**    The Livermore Atomic Research Computer (LARC) is developed by UNIVAC. This is the last large-scale machine made with decimal-only memory storage.

**1956**    Edsger Wybe Dijkstra (1930– ) invents an efficient algorithm for producing the shortest paths in graphs to demonstrate the abilities of the ARMAC computer.

**1956**    The first true operating system is developed by Gene Amdahl (for the IBM 704).

**1956**    Evelyn Boyd Granville (1924– ) starts to write programs for NASA for the Project Vanguard and Project Mercury Space programs. In 1949 she was the first African American woman to receive a Ph.D. in mathematics in the United States.

**1957**    Noam Chomsky (1928– ) publishes *Syntactic Structures*.

**1957**    William C. Norris (1911– ) forms Control Data Corporation (CDC), which begins manufacturing supercomputers.

**1957**    IBM produces the IBM 305 RAMAC (Random Access Method of Accounting and Control); the first computer with a disk memory system, it offers a semi random access to data.

**1957**    The USSR launches Sputnik I, the first artificial satellite in orbit.

**1957**    IBM markets the first dot matrix printer.

**1957**    John McCarthy founds MIT's Artificial Intelligence department.

**1957**    Digital Equipment Corporation (DEC) is founded by Ken Harry Olsen (1926– ) and Harlan Anderson.

**1957**    John W. Backus (1924–1988) releases FORTRAN (FORmula TRANslator), a programming language that allows users to express problems in terms of mathematical formulae.

**1958**    The first version of the programming language Algol (ALGOrithmic Language) is released.

**1958**    Bell Laboratories develops the modem data phone, which allows telephone lines to transmit binary data.

**1958**    The Advanced Research Projects Agency, ARPA, is formed for the American Department of Defense.

**1958**    Jack St. Clair Kilby (1923– ), Jean Hoerni (1924–1997), Kurt Lehovec, and Robert N. Noyce (1927–1990) (of Texas Instruments) produce the first monolithic integrated circuit—a transistor with capacitors and resistors on a single semiconductor chip, it is the first microchip. By 1960 transistors would replace the use of vacuum tubes in the manufacture of computers, and in 1961 integrated circuits would start to be used.

**1958**    Michael O. Rabin (1931– ) develops the idea of the one-way function (one that is easy to compute but one the inverse of which is very difficult to compute); this proves to be the basis of many systems of cryptography.

**1959–1964**
Computers produced during this time are regarded as second-generation computers.

**1959**    John W. Backus (1924–1988), at a UNESCO meeting, presents a formal notation of how to describe the syntax of a given computer language. The following year Peter Naur (1928– ) modifies this at the meeting where Algol60 is formulated. This is the Backus-Naur Form (BNF) notation.

**1959**    IBM manufactures the IBM 1401 and the IBM 1620 desk-size computers for business and science use, respectively.

**1959**    Xerox produces the first commercial copy machine.

**1959**    Jack St. Clair Kilby (1923– ) of Texas Instruments designs a flip-flop integrated circuit.

**1959**    General Electric produces a device to process checks using magnetic ink.

**1959**    Michael O. Rabin (1931– ) and Dana S. Scott (1932– ) publish a paper—*Finite Automata and Their Decision Problem*—that introduces the idea of nondeterministic machines. They are awarded the ACM Turing Award for this in 1976.

**1960**    Algol60 is released—the first structured procedural language.

**1960**    Paul Baran (1926– ) of the Rand Corporation publishes an 11 volume work on distributed communication via computers. It covered the idea of packet switching but the report was ignored.

**1960**    Frank Rosenblatt (1928– ) of Cornell University builds the Perceptron—a computer that can learn by trial and error through a neural network.

**1960**    The Conference on Data System Languages, led by Joe Wegstein and Grace Hopper (1906–1992), introduces the first exclusive business language—COBOL (Common Business Oriented Language).

**1960**    John McCarthy develops LISP (LISt Processing) programming, a pioneering programming language.

**1960**    The Tandy Corporation is founded by Charles David Tandy (1918–1978).

**1961**    IBM releases the Selectric range of typewriters, fitted with the innovative printer head the Selectric Ball, developed by Alvin A. Snaper.

**1961**    George C. Devol builds the first industrial robot for a company called Unimation; it is used in the manufacture of television tubes.

**1961**    Fernando Jose Corbató (1926– ) of MIT produces CTSS (Compatible Time Sharing System), allowing wide-spread remote accessing of computers.

**1961**    MIT sees the first attack by hackers—a group who borrowed their name from the terminology of model railway enthusiasts.

**1961**    Leonard Kleinrock (1934– ) publishes *Information Flow in Large Communication Nets*—this is the paper that launched the theory and practice of packet switching.

**1961**    IBM releases Stretch, the IBM 7030, which runs 30 times faster than the 704; this computer was first delivered to the Los Alamos National Laboratory.

**1961**    Univac releases LARC (The Livermore Advance Research Computer); this and the IBM 7030 are the first two successful supercomputers.

**1961**    Charles Anthony Richard Hoare (1934– ) publishes the quicksort algorithm.

**1962**    In his doctoral thesis Carl Adam Petri (1926– ) puts forward a theory of communication between asynchronous components of a computer system; subsequent work modifies this into the Petri net.

**1962**    Stanford and Purdue Universities both open departments of computer science—they are the first in the world.

**1962**    At the University of Manchester, UK, the Atlas computer is constructed; this is the first computer to use virtual memory and paging.

**1962**    Steve Russell (MIT) invents the first computer game (Space War) for the DEC PDP-1.

**1962**    Kenneth Eric Iverson (1928– ) releases A Programming Language (APL).

**1962**    Ivan Sutherland (1938– ) releases Sketchpad—the first system for interactive graphics.

**1963**    The programming language SNOBOL is released.

**1963**    The computer language Forth, developed by Charles H. Moore, is released.

**1963**    The Hewlett Packard 150 is the first computer to use a touch-screen.

**1963**    A code for information exchange between systems is standardized; this code is known as ASCII (the American Standard Code for Information Interchange).

**1963**    Formation of the IEEE by the merging of the AIEE (American Institute of Electrical Engineers) and the IRE (Institute of Radio Engineers).

**1964**    DEC launch the PDP-8 minicomputer, designed by Kenneth Harry Olsen (1926– ); this is the first minicomputer (at the time it cost $16,000).

**1964**    Douglas Englebart (1925– ) develops the mouse—it does not become popular until 1983 when it is used on Apple computers. IBM adopts it in 1987.

**1964**    Using the CTSS system developed in 1961, IBM produces the first on-line, real-time reservation system for American Airlines; it is called SABRE.

**1964**    BASIC, devised by John George Kemeny (1926–1993) and Tom Eugene Kurtz (1928– ), is used by the Dartmouth Time Sharing System (an operating system) as a language for students to develop their own programs.

**1964**    Gene Myron Amdahl (1922– ), working at IBM, leads the team that develops the IBM 360 (so numbered because it is an "all round" performer) series of mainframe computers.

**1964**    IBM develops a computer-aided design (CAD) system.

**1964**    The Programming language PL1 is developed by IBM; it is a combination of FORTRAN and COBOL. Its original name was to be NPL (New Programming Language).

**1964–1972**

Computers developed between this period are usually described as third-generation machines.

**1965**   Ivan Sutherland demonstrates the first head-mounted display; this is the first step on the way to virtual reality.

**1965**   Fuzzy set theory is proposed by Lotfi Asker Zadeh (1921– ); it is a mathematical representation of vagueness and uncertainty. Fuzzy logic is a sub set of fuzzy set theory.

**1965**   Maurice Wilkes (1913– ) and Gordon Scarott propose the idea of cache memory.

**1965**   Gordon E. Moore (1929– ), writing in *Electronics Magazine*, suggests that computer complexity doubles every year, this is revised in 1975 to state that a doubling in complexity occurs every 18 months.

**1965**   A new system of coding known as EBCDIC (Extended Binary Code Decimal Interchange Code) is introduced by IBM to use with their series of 360 mainframe computers.

**1965**   J. C. R. Licklider (1915–1990) of ARPA heads a group of researchers to produce a general-purpose shared-memory multiprocessing timesharing system. Work on ARPAnet commences in 1969.

**1965**   The ARPA experimental network is set up by linking a computer in California with another in the same laboratory and adding a third from DEC (the linkage is by a dedicated phone line.

**1965**   Gordon Bennett Bell (1934– ) designs the PDP 6 minicomputer for DEC (Digital Equipment Corporation); this is the first minicomputer released to the commercial data-processing market.

**1965**   The first true supercomputer—the Control Data Corporation CD6600—is developed by Seymour Cray (1925–1996).

**1965**   IBM produces diskettes for use with its 370 series of machines.

**1966**   Christopher Strachey (1916–1975) publishes his work *Towards a Formal Semantics,* founding the field of denotational semantics, which provides a mathematical basis for programming languages.

**1966**   IBM coins the phrase "word processing."

**1966**   Alan J. Perlis (1922–1990) is awarded the ACM Turing Award for his influence in the area of advanced programming techniques and compiler construction.

**1966**   The programming language Euler is developed by Niklaus Wirth (1934– ).

**1966**   The programming language Algol-W is released by Niklaus Wirth (1934– ); it is a modification of Algol 60.

**1967**   Ole-Johan Dahl (1931– ) and Kristen Nygaard (1926– ) of the Norwegian Computing Center (NCC) at Oslo launch Simula—the first object-oriented language.

**1967**   William W. Tunnicliffe (1922–1996) presents a talk on separating the contents of documents from their format—this eventually leads to the development of SGML in 1980 (via the production of GML in 1969).

**1967**   Jack Kilby, James Merryman, and James van Tassel (Texas Instruments) invent a four-function pocket calculator.

**1967**   Mac Hack VI—a chess program written by Richard Greenblatt—is made an honorary member of the US Chess Federation.

**1968**   Donald Ervin Knuth (1938– ) publishes the first volume of *The Art of Computer Programming.*

**1968**   The first computers using integrated circuits are released—the Burroughs 2500 and the Burroughs 3500.

**1968**   A NATO conference on software introduces the term software engineering.

**1968**   MIT develops the programming language LOGO—an educational tool designed by Seymour Papert (1928– ), Marvin Minsky, Daniel G. Bobrow, and Wallace Feurzeig.

**1968**   Alan Kay (1940– ) produces software for a prototype personal computer, called the Flex.

**1968**   A Federal Information Processing Standard promotes the use of a six figure format for dates, thus ensuring the year 2000 problem.

**1968**   Edsger Wybe Dijkstra (1930– ) describes semaphores and introduces the dining philosopher's problem, which later becomes a standard example in concurrency theory.

**1968**   Robert Noyce (1927– ), Gordon Moore (1929– ), and Andrew Grove (1936– ) found Intel (short for INTegrated ELectronics).

**1968**   An updated version of Algol is released—Algol68.

**1968**   Robert Heath Dennard (1932– ) invents random access memory (RAM).

**1968**   Vienna Definition Language (VDL) is designed by Heinz Zemanek (1920– ).

**1968**   Douglas C. Englebart (1925– ) demonstrates a microwave link between a computer in San Francisco and Stanford.

**1969**   Jack Schwartz publishes *Set Theory as a Language for Program Specification and Programming,* which introduces SETL as a programming language for sets.

**1969** Dennis MacAlister Ritchie (1941– ) and Kenneth Thompson (1943– ) of Bell Telephone Laboratories develop UNIX.

**1969** Marvin Lee Minsky (1927– ) is awarded the ACM Turing Award for form and content in computers and pioneering work on artificial intelligence.

**1969** ARPAnet is up and running with 4 nodes, utilizing packet switching and 50 kb/s phone lines; the network is funded by the US Department of Defense and is the forerunner of the Internet.

**1969** The RS 232 serial interface standard is accepted by the Electronic Industries Association to allow data exchange between computers and peripherals.

**1969** IBM starts to price software separately from hardware—a decision that essentially launches the software industry.

**1969** Gary Starkweather at Xerox PARC demonstrates how a laser beam working with a xerography process can be used to print.

**1969** General Markup Language (GML), designed by Charles Goldfarb at IBM, is released.

**1970** Lucifer is developed by Horst Feistel (1915–1990) of IBM. It is a conventional cryptosystem that will eventually transform into DES (Data Encryption Standard).

**1970** IBM markets the first floppy disk, it is 8 inches in diameter.

**1970** The first RAM chip is introduced by Intel—it is called the 1103 and has a capacity of 1024 bits.

**1970** SRI International develops Shakey—the first robot to use artificial intelligence to navigate around an area.

**1970** Winston Royce publishes *Managing the Development of Large Software Systems*, which outlines the waterfall development model.

**1970** Xerox Corporation opens a Research and Development center at Palo Alto, California—Xerox Palo Alto Research Center (or Xerox PARC for short).

**1970** Edgar F. Codd starts publishing his series of papers on database management systems. He is awarded ACM Turing Award in 1981 for this work.

**1970** James Hardy Wilkinson (1919–1986) is awarded the ACM Turing Award for his research in numerical analysis to facilitate the use of the high-speed digital computer; he also received special recognition for his work in computations in linear algebra and "backward" error analysis.

**1970** ALOHAnet is developed by Norman Abramson at Hawaii; this is a packet-switching radio network. It is connected to ARPAnet in 1972.

**1970** The Pascal language is defined by Niklaus Wirth (1934– ); it is a successor to the various forms of Algol.

**1970** Martin Davis and several others put forward a solution for the insolvability of Hilbert's tenth problem.

**1970** The programming language B is developed at Bell Laboratories by Ken Thompson and D. M. Ritchie.

**1971** Niklaus Wirth develops the programming language Pascal.

**1971** Don Hoefler, writing in *Electronic News,* creates a regular column entitled "Silicon Valley, USA"; this is the first appearance of the term that now identifies the area of northern California where many computer, software, and other high-technology businesses are located.

**1971** David Parnas first describes information hiding.

**1971** Working at Xerox Parc Alan C. Kay invents the Smalltalk programming language—the first object-orientated programming language.

**1971** Stephen Cook (1939– ) defines a new group of problems that are essentially not computable; this is a set of non-deterministic polynomial completeness.

**1971** Marcian (Ted) Hoff (1937– ), Stan Mazor (1943– ), and F. Fagin of Intel invent the first computer microprocessor, the Intel 4004; this single chip, easily examined in the palm of one's hand, was more powerful than the 1946 ENIAC, which was the size of a house, covering 1,800 square feet and weighing 30 tons.

**1971** Erna Schneider Hoover (1926– ), working at Bell Laboratories, is granted one of the first patents on software. This is for a computerized telephone switching system.

**1971** A new computer language, C, is developed and released by Dennis Ritchie (1941– ) of Bell Laboratories. It is named C simply because it is a successor to the B language, it was originally to be called B+.

**1971** John McCarthy (1927– ) is awarded the ACM Turing Award for his lecture "The Present State of Research on Artificial Intelligence" and his general work in the area of Artificial Intelligence.

**1971** Ray Tomlinson (1941– ), Bolt Beranek, and M. A. H. Newman invent an electronic mail program to send messages across a network; it starts being used extensively by ARPAnet in 1972.

**1971**  Stephen A. Cook publishes the paper *The Complexity of Theorem Proving Procedures*. This paper lays the foundations of NP-completeness and advances our understanding of the complexity of computation.

**1972**  The 5.25 inch floppy disk is first marketed.

**1972**  The Prolog logic programming language is developed by Robert A. Kowalski and Alain Colmerauer; it is often used for Artificial Intelligence programming.

**1972**  John T. Draper (aka "Cap'n Crunch") becomes the first of the so-called Phone Phreaks—a phone hacker. Using a toy whistle from a cereal box, Draper finds he can make free phone calls.

**1972**  The daisywheel printer is introduced by David Lee of Diablo Systems.

**1972**  Ray Tomlinson (1941– )—author of the first e-mail software—chooses the @ sign for e-mail addresses.

**1972**  Hewlett Packard releases the first scientific pocket calculator—the HP 35; it uses reverse polish notation.

**1972**  Lawrence (Larry) Gilman Roberts writes the first e-mail management program, which lists incoming emails and allows selection for reading, filing, forwarding, and responses.

**1972**  The Micro Instrumentation and Telemetry Systems (MITS) 816 becomes available; this is the first digital microcomputer for personal use.

**1972**  The ARPAnet is demonstrated for the first time in Washington, D.C.

**1972**  The computer company Atari is founded (it's original name is Syzygy) by Nolan Bushnell (1945– ); its first release is the popular arcade game Pong.

**1972**  Computers designed from this date on are regarded as fourth generation computers; the fifth generation of computers are yet to be seen.

**1972**  Wang, VYDEC, and Lexitron release word processing systems.

**1972**  Cray Research is formed.

**1973**  Vinton Grey Cerf (1943– ) coinvents the Internet and subsequently TCP/IP with Bob Kahn.

**1973**  The first local area network (LAN) system is put in place; this is Ethernet, developed by Robert Metcalf (1946– ) at Xerox PARC.

**1973**  Xerox PARC develops a computer called the Alto that uses a mouse, Ethernet, and a graphical user interface; this is an experimental personal computer.

**1973**  Charles W. Bachman is awarded the ACM Turing Award for his outstanding contributions to database technology.

**1973**  The specification for file transfer protocol (ftp) is laid down.

**1973**  IBM produces the first sealed hard disk drive; it is called the Winchester (after the rifle) and it uses two 30Mb platters.

**1973**  ARPAnet goes international with connections to London and Norway; France is working on its own system. It is believed that there are 2,000 users of ARPAnet, and 75% of the traffic is e-mail.

**1974**  Charles Simonyl (Xerox PARC) writes the first wysiwyg (what you see is what you get) program—Bravo.

**1974**  Bar codes are introduced on grocery store items; the first item (a pack of chewing gum) is scanned in an Ohio supermarket.

**1974**  The first computer-controlled robot is developed.

**1974**  Donald E. Knuth (1938– ) is awarded the ACM Turing Award for his major contributions to the analysis of algorithms, the design of programming languages, and for his contributions to the "art of computer programming" through his well-known books in the series by this title.

**1974**  BBN Technologies opens Telenet, a commercial version of ARPAnet; this is the first public packet data service.

**1974**  In the UK James Ellis, Clifford Cocks, and Malcolm Williamson invent a public-key cryptosystem, but for security reasons they are not allowed to publish it; it is based on the difficulty of factoring integers.

**1974**  CLIP 4, the first computer utilizing parallel architecture, is released.

**1975**  Michael Rabin (1931– ) produces an algorithm for finding large primes rapidly; this is the first use of randomization in a program.

**1975**  Allen Newell (1927–1992) and Herbert Alexander Simon (1916–2001) are awarded the ACM Turing Award for joint scientific efforts extending over twenty years; initially in collaboration with J. Cliff Shaw (1922–1991) at the RAND Corporation, and subsequently with numerous faculty and student colleagues at Carnegie-Mellon University, they receive the award for having made basic contributions to artificial intelligence, the psychology of human cognition, and list processing.

**1975**　H. Edward Roberts and MITS produce the Altair 8800, a mass-produced personal computer that could be bought as a kit (for $397) or fully assembled (for $497).

**1975**　IBM produced its first personal computer, the 5100; it proves too expensive for mass-market penetration, particularly when competing against products such as the Altair 8800 (which cost less than $500).

**1975**　Bill Gates (1955– ) and Paul Allen (1953– ) found Microsoft, initially to sell the software GW BASIC, at Albuquerque, New Mexico.

**1975**　The TCP/IP protocols for the Internet are laid down.

**1975**　The first mailing list is set up on ARPAnet; called MsgGroup, it is devoted to the discussion of science fiction.

**1975**　Whitfield Diffie and Martin Hellman develop their public-key cryptography system utilizing paired keys.

**1976**　The Data Encryption Standard (DES), a cryptosystem developed by IBM, is released; it is based on the 1970 Lucifer system.

**1976**　The Electric Pencil—the first word processor program—is written by Michael Shrayer for the Altair.

**1976**　Steve Wozniak (1950– ) and Steve Jobs (1955– ) sell circuit boards at a computer club convention; when assembled, the product is the Apple I computer.

**1976**　OnTyme becomes the first commercial provider of e-mail. There are too few users to make the service viable.

**1976**　IBM introduces ink jet printing.

**1976**　Steve Jobs (1955– ) and Steve Wozniak (1950–) form the company Apple.

**1976**　The CP/M operating system is designed by Gary Kildall (1942–1994) for use on systems utilizing the Intel 8080 processor; this was the first standard operating system.

**1976**　Cray 1, the first commercially developed supercomputer, becomes available; its speed becomes an informal benchmark for future supercomputers—for example, in the mid 1990s supercomputers were operating at 1,000 Cray's.

**1976**　Joan Margaret Winters joins the SHARE Human Factors project—a group dedicated to reminding software and hardware manufacturers that humans are the end users of their products.

**1977**　Steve Jobs (1955– ) and Steve Wozniak (1950–) produce the Apple II as a rival to the Altair 8800; it is an immediate success due to the easier data entry afforded by the addition of a keyboard.

**1977**　Ken Olson—chairman and founder of Digital Equipment Corporation (DEC) is quoted as saying "There is no reason anyone would want a computer in their home."

**1977**　Annie J. Easley (1933– ) at NASA develops a number of computer programs for various energy projects (measuring quantities such as the speed of solar wind and how long a battery will last).

**1977**　Niklaus Wirth develops and releases Modula—a successor to the programming language Pascal.

**1978**　Xerox releases the 9700 laser printer, the first commercially available laser printer; it is capable of printing 120 pages per minute.

**1978**　The ML Programming language is developed by M. Gordon, R. Milner, L. Morris, M. Newey, and C. Wadsworth.

**1978**　Robert W. Floyd is awarded the ACM Turing Award for having a clear influence on methodologies for the creation of efficient and reliable software. He also helped create several computing fields: the theory of parsing, the semantics of programming languages, automatic program verification, automatic program synthesis, and analysis of algorithms.

**1978**　Daniel Bricklin and Bob Frankston release Visicalc. This is the first spreadsheet aimed at the home computer user.

**1978**　Ronald L. Rivest, Adi Shamir (1952– ), and Leonard Adleman release their public-key cryptosystem; it is known by their initials, RSA.

**1978**　Stanley Mark Rifkin (using the alias Mike Hanson) commits one of the largest bank robberies ever, stealing $10,200,000 from Security Pacific National Bank in Los Angeles. He carries this out as an employee by moving the funds electronically.

**1978**　Intel releases the 8086 chip; this is the first commercially available 16-bit processor.

**1978**　The computer game Space Invaders is released, launching a craze and a major industry.

**1979**　The UNIX users network is set up allowing the creation of many discussion groups.

**1979**　The U.S. Department of Defense produces its draft document on a new, Pascal-based language called Ada (after Lady Ada Lovelace). The language is standardized in 1983, and in 1990 it is released to the public (prior to this it was for Defence projects only); development is by Jean Ichbiah.

**1979**　Robert M. Metcalfe (1946– ) founds the 3Com Corporation to promote Ethernet as the standard LAN.

**1979** Micropro International releases Wordstar, the first home PC word processor.

**1979** Kevin MacKenzie sends an e-mail message to a USENET discussion group suggesting a way of graphically representing emotion in typed messages; the "emoticon" is born: :) .

**1979** John Cocke and his team produce the IBM 801 Minicomputer; this is the first RISC machine (Reduced Instruction Set Computer).

**1979** The compact disk is invented. Initially used for audio, it comes to be used as a data-storage device.

**1980** David A. Patterson, as part of a DARPA-sponsored project, develops two machines called RISC I and RISC II, along with the IBM 801 and the Stanford MIPS machine of John L. Hennessy; these are among the first machines to be developed as reduced-instruction-set computers (RISC).

**1980** The first working draft version of SGML (Standard Generalized Markup Language) is published; the sixth version in 1983 is accepted as an industry standard. It is developed by Charles Goldfarb.

**1980** Tony Hoare is awarded the ACM Turing Award for his fundamental contributions to the definition and design of programming languages.

**1980** Wayne Ratcliff produces the first PC database program, dbase II.

**1980** Sony releases the first 3.5-inch floppy disk.

**1981** Bill Gates (1955– ) is asked in an interview about computer memory—he states that "640K ought to be enough for anybody." Typical home computers in 2001 have upwards of 128 megabytes of RAM.

**1981** IBM introduces its personal computer for the home and office.

**1981** The MS DOS operating system is released with IBM PCs.

**1981** The Xerox 8010 System (The Star) is released; it utilizes a graphical user interface with windows, icons, menus, and pointing devices and is subsequently much copied (it also has a wysiwyg word processor).

**1981** A landmark in computer gaming is released: Pacman.

**1981** Some of the first viruses found outside of computer laboratories are found in the Apple II operating system; the viruses are called Apple 1, 2, 3, etc. These viruses are spread through pirated computer games.

**1982** The Byzantine Agreement (a model for fault finding in distributed processes) is proposed and accepted.

**1982** John Warnock releases the programming language PostScript and forms Adobe Systems with Charles Geschke.

**1982** David C. Plummer publishes the details and definition for the ARP (Address Resolution Protocol).

**1982** Benoit B. Mandelbrot (1924– ) writes *The Fractal Geometry of Nature,* which introduces the Mandelbrot set—a group of numbers following a particular pattern that can give complex pictures; he also coins the word *fractal.*

**1982** ARPA establishes the Transmission Control Protocol (TCP) and Internet Protocol (IP) as the protocol suite for ARPAnet; this combined suite is generally known as TCP/IP.

**1982** Bill Joy, Vinod Khosla, Scott McNealy, and Andy Bechtolsheim (1956– ) found Sun Microsystems.

**1982** Physicist Richard Feynman reports on the stimulation of quantum mechanical objects by other quantum systems, thus opening the door on the development of quantum computing.

**1982** The improved Intel chip—the 80286—is released; it has double the clock speed of the 8086 (20 MHz) and can access a greater amount of memory.

**1982** The Musical Instrument Digital Interface (MIDI) standard is published; it allows computers to be connected to musical instruments.

**1983** *Time* magazine unveils the microcomputer as its "Man of the Year."

**1983** Radio Shack/Tandy market the first portable computer (lap top), the TRS 80, designed by Kazuhiko Nishi.

**1983** The changeover from NCP to the TCP/IP system takes place on the Internet (the protocol is originally established in 1982 by DCA and ARPA).

**1983** Fred Cohen is the first to formally define a virus as "a computer program that can affect other computer programs by modifying them is such a way as to include a (possibly evolved) copy of itself."

**1983** The Microsoft Windows graphical user interface system is first announced; it is 1985 before the software actually ships.

**1983** Adele Goldberg writes the definitive book on the programming language Smalltalk, *Smalltalk-80: The Interactive Programming Environment;* she argued against it being given away free—thus ensuring the future success of JAVA.

**1983** ARPAnet is split into ARPAnet and MILNET, the latter is exclusively for the use of the Defense Data Network.

**1983**      The computer language C++ is released by AT&T Bell Laboratories.

**1983**      Commodore releases the SX 64, the first portable computer with a color monitor.

**1984**      VLIW (Very Long Instruction Word) processor is launched in the Trace/300 series of computers produced by Mulitflow Computers Inc.

**1984**      Author William Gibson (1948– ) coins the term *cyberspace* in his book *Neuromancer*.

**1984**      The Apple Macintosh range of computers is launched on the market; it is co-designed by Jef Raskin and Steve Jobs.

**1984**      Niklaus Wirth is awarded the ACM Turing Award for developing a sequence of innovative computer languages, Euler, Algol-W, Modula, and Pascal. Pascal has become pedagogically significant and has provided a foundation for future computer languages, systems, and architectural research.

**1984**      Jaron Lanier (1960– ) forms the company VPL Inc. and devises the term *virtual reality*. The company leads to many innovations in this new field.

**1984**      The DNS (Domain Name System) is introduced to the Internet.

**1984**      Richard Matthew Stallman (1953– ) develops the GNU project to rival the UNIX system; rapidly some 20 million users adopt GNU/Linux-based systems.

**1984**      The Post Office Protocol (POP) is proposed as a standard for downloading e-mail from a server.

**1984**      Hewlett Packard introduces the LaserJet laser printer; this is the first desktop device available and it can print at eight pages per minute.

**1984**      The 3.5-inch diskette is introduced as a medium of storage.

**1984**      MIT launches the Athena Project, a network that can run local applications as well as call on remote resources—an operating environment that is both hardware and software independent. It is later renamed X-Windows.

**1985**      The CD-ROM is produced jointly by Phillips and Sony.

**1985**      This year marks the first commercial release of the programming language C++, developed by Bjarne Stroustrup of Bell Laboratories.

**1985**      Leslie B. Lamport (1939– ) creates the LaTex typesetting system.

**1985**      Richard M. Karp is awarded the ACM Turing Award for his continuing contributions to the theory of algorithms, which include the development of efficient algorithms for network flow and other combinatorial optimization problems; the identification of polynomial-time computability with the intuitive notion of algorithmic efficiency; and, most notably, contributions to the theory of NP-completeness. Karp introduced the now standard methodology for proving problems to be NP-complete.

**1985**      Intel releases the 80386 chip.

**1985**      Microsoft release the first version of Windows; it is not, strictly speaking, an operating system because it needs MS DOS to run—it is merely a graphical user interface.

**1985**      Paul Brainard releases PageMaker for the Macintosh; this is the first desktop publishing software to be commercially available for a personal computer.

**1986**      NSFnet is created with a backbone speed of 56Kbs; the five super computing centers it establishes allows an explosion of connections, particularly with universities.

**1986**      The Unix users network is renamed USENET.

**1986**      Congress passes the Computer Fraud and Abuse Act, making it illegal to break into computer systems.

**1986**      John Hopcroft and Robert Tarjan are awarded the ACM Turing Award for fundamental achievements in the design and analysis of algorithms and data structures.

**1987**      Ronald Rivest devises the RC2 conventional cipher system; similar to the DES key, it utilizes a variable key length. (RC1 was never released and subsequent updates followed the same naming system.)

**1987**      Michael F. Barnsley works out the fractal image compression algorithm that allows much greater compression in the storage of images.

**1987**      RAID (Redundant Array of Independent Disks) mass-storage devices are developed at the University of California at Berkeley.

**1987**      John Cocke is awarded the ACM Turing Award for significant contributions in the design and theory of compilers, the architecture of large systems, and the development of reduced-instruction set computers (RISC).

**1987**      Larry Wall introduces the programming language Perl.

**1988**      DARPA sets up the Computer Emergency Response Team (CERT) to react to national computer security issues involving the Internet.

**1988** An optical chip—which uses light rather than electricity—is developed; it has much improved processing speeds when compared to conventional chips.

**1988** Alice Rowe Burks, who worked as a so-called human computer during WWII, publishes her first book, *The First Electronic Computer: The Atanasoff Story.*

**1988** This year marks the first record of a virus being transmitted by the Internet; this is the Morris worm (initially called the Internet worm), named after Robert T. Morris Jr. (1966– ), a graduate student at Cornell University who launches his worm on ARPANet to see what effect it has on UNIX machines.

**1988** As a response to the Morris worm the first Internet firewalls appear; at this time they are merely routers used to separate networks into smaller LANs.

**1988** The first color laser printers are released.

**1988** The first graphing calculator is produced by Texas Instruments.

**1989** Tim Berners-Lee invents the World Wide Web while working at CERN.

**1989** Marcus Hess (the so-called Hannover Hacker) and several others are arrested in Germany for hacking into American sites and selling coding information to the Soviet intelligence agency KGB.

**1989** William Kahan is awarded the ACM Turing Award for his fundamental contributions to numerical analysis and floating-point computations.

**1989** Phillip Emeagwali (1957– ) writes a formula that is used to perform the fastest computer computation in the world—3.1 billion calculations per second, this surpasses the theoretical maximum speed of the largest supercomputers in use in this year.

**1989** The Intel 80486 chip is released—it contains the equivalent of nearly one-and-a-half million transistors.

**1990** The first commercial provider of Internet dial-up access is premiered, it is called The World.

**1990** James Gosling (of Sun Microsystems) develops the programming language Oak, which is later renamed Java.

**1990** John V. Atanasoff is awarded the National Medal of Technology by George Bush for his invention of the electronic digital computer and for contribution toward the development of a technically trained U. S. workforce.

**1990** Fernando J. Corbato is awarded the ACM Turing Award for his pioneering work on the concepts and development of the general-purpose large-scale time-sharing and resource-sharing computer systems CTSS and Multics.

**1990** The ARPANet is decommissioned.

**1990** HTML (Hyper Text Markup Language) is developed by Tim Burners-Lee.

**1990** The URL (Uniform Resource Location) and http (Hyper Text Transfer Protocol) are developed by Tim Burners-Lee.

**1991** Linus Torvalds (1969– ) releases his freeware rival to the Unix operating system, Linux.

**1991** DEC provides the first commercially available firewall; it utilizes filters and application gateways (proxies) to provide protection.

**1991** The Difference Engine, designed by Charles Babbage (1791–1871) about 150 years earlier, is finally built by the Science Museum in London, England.

**1991** WAIS (Wide Area Information Servers) are invented by Brewster Kahle of the Thinking Machines Corporation.

**1991** Robin Milner is awarded the ACM Turing Award for three distinct achievements: 1) LCF, the mechanization of Scott's Logic of Computable Functions (a theoretically based yet practical tool for machine-assisted proof construction); 2) the computer language ML; 3) the development of CCS, a general theory of concurrency.

**1991** Gopher (an ftp search engine) is released from the University of Minnesota; it is the work of Paul Lindner and Mark P. McCahill.

**1991** Pretty Good Privacy (PGP) is released by Philip Zimmerman; it is a public-key cryptosystem.

**1992** Butler W. Lampson is awarded the ACM Turing Award for contributions to the development of distributed personal computing environments and the technology for their implementation: workstations, networks, operating systems, programming systems, displays, security, and document publishing.

**1992** The phrase "surfing the Internet" is used for the first time by author Jean Armour Polly.

**1993** Shafi Goldwasser is the recipient of the first Gödel prize of theoretical computer science for her work on interactive proofs.

**1993** Apple releases the Newton—the first personal digital assistant (PDA).

**1993** Juris Hartmanis and Richard E. Stearns are awarded the ACM Turing Award in recognition of their seminal paper establishing the field of computational complexity theory.

**1993** The internet browser Mosaic is released by Marc Andreesen (1971– ), Eric Bina, and Jim H. Clark (1944– ); it is instantly and widely popular.

**1993** Mary Shaw receives the Warnier Prize for contributions to software engineering—specifically for software architecture.

**1993** Intel releases the first of its Pentium chips, which contains more than twice the number of transistors than its previous release, the 80486.

**1993** Leonard Adleman demonstrates the computing potential of DNA (biological computing) by solving a previously unsolvable mathematical problem using sequences of DNA.

**1994** Edward Albert Feigenbaum and Raj Reddy are awarded the ACM Turing Award for pioneering the design and construction of large-scale artificial intelligence systems, demonstrating the practical importance and potential commercial impact of artificial intelligence technology.

**1994** Marc Andreesen (1971– ) and Eric Bina write Netscape based on their Mosaic program; they also set up the Netscape Communications Corporation.

**1994** First Virtual—the first cyberbank—opens for business.

**1995** Disney's animated film *Toy Story* becomes the first full-length feature movie to be created entirely with computers.

**1995** Windows 95 is released; this is the first version of Windows that is more like a self-contained operating system because, unlike previous versions, it does not require an existing installation of DOS. (Although Windows 95 does require many of DOS's system files, these come with it and are installed and run in the "background.")

**1995** Kevin D. Mitnick is arrested by the FBI for gaining illegal access to other peoples computer systems. He is the first person convicted under this law, and he carried out his theft of 20,000 credit card numbers while on the run for stealing software from DEC in 1989.

**1995** John Gage and Marc Andreesen (1971– ) announce that the Java programming language exists and that it will be incorporated into Netscape browsers (launch of Java is by Sun Microsystems).

**1995** Manuel Blum is awarded the ACM Turing Award for recognition of his contributions to the foundations of computational complexity theory and its application to cryptography and program checking.

**1995** World Wide Web meta-search engines are released. The content of the web is actively and automatically catalogued.

**1995** Richard White has an RSA file-security encryption program tattooed on his arm; due to U.S. arms-export control laws against taking such information out of the country, he becomes the first person to be classified as "munitions."

**1996** Amir Pnueli is awarded the ACM Turing Award for seminal work introducing temporal logic into computing science and for outstanding contributions to program and systems verification.

**1996** Internet phones become popular, though the technology has been available for a number of years; U.S. telecommunications companies ask Congress to ban the technology.

**1996** Web access via a television set is introduced.

**1997** Maurice Peter Herlihy (1954– ) devises the Aleph Toolkit system, a collection of Java programs that allow work to be carried out irrespective of the operating system used.

**1997** IBM computer Deep Blue becomes the first machine to beat a reigning World Chess Champion (Gary Kasparov).

**1997** Intel releases the Pentium II chip; it has much larger on chip cache memory than previous chips.

**1997** Sandia National Laboratories and France Telecom successfully apply for a patent on protonic memory—a memory system that uses embedded protons, which, unlike standard RAM, do not lose their data when the system is switched off.

**1997** Douglas Englebart is awarded the ACM Turing Award for an inspiring vision of the future of interactive computing and the invention of key technologies to help realize this vision.

**1997** Object Constraint Language—OCL—is developed by Jos Warmer of IBM; it is a language for business modeling.

**1998** The Bluetooth standard in wireless networks is agreed upon by Ericcson, Nokia, Intel, IBM, and others.

**1998** Windows 98 is released. Legal action is brought against Microsoft because various items of software—notably Microsoft's web browser, Internet Explorer—are intricately tied to the operating system; this is felt by many to be a restrictive, monopolistic practice.

**1998** Kevin Warwick, Professor of Cybernetics at the University of Reading in the U.K., becomes the first human to host a microchip. The approximately

23mm-by-3mm glass capsule containing several microprocessors stays in Warwick's left arm for nine days. It was used to test implant's interaction with computer-controlled doors and lights in a futuristic "intelligent office building."

**1998**   The World Wide Web Consortium (W3C) accepts the version-one specifications of Extensible Markup Language (XML).

**1998**   James Gray is awarded the ACM Turing Award for seminal contributions to database and transaction processing research and technical leadership in system implementation.

**1998**   Canada launches CA*net3, the first national optical Internet.

**1998**   An American court bans the practice of buying domain names that are copyrighted and then selling them to the original copyright holders for massive profits; the practice is called squatting, an example of which might be this: registering the domain name "coke.com" before the CocaCola Company and then selling the name to the corporation for much more than it cost to register.

**1999**   The mp3 audio compression technology system is unveiled.

**1999**   Frederick P. Brooks Jr. is awarded the ACM Turing Award for landmark contributions to computer architecture, operating systems, and software engineering.

**1999**   Intel and Hewlett Packard jointly develop a 600 MHz chip; this is the first 64-bit chip.

**2000**   With the change from 1999 to 2000, many people, encouraged by massive media attention, fear calamity as computer systems around the world confront a date they were never programmed to recognize; the Year 2000 (Y2K) Bug is expected to wreak havoc on commerce, hospitals, air traffic control systems, etc. Relatively speaking, nothing happens.

**2000**   Andrew Chi-Chih Yao is awarded the ACM Turing Award for recognition of his fundamental contributions to the theory of computation, including the complexity-based theory of pseudorandom number generation, cryptography, and communication complexity.

**2000**   Microsoft releases Windows 2000 and Windows ME.

**2000**   The love bug virus infects 45 million computers in over 20 countries in only 24 hours.

**2000**   Napster introduces a hugely popular system for sharing files (particularly mp3 music) over the Internet; court injunctions are taken out by the music industry and copyright holders, and legal action closes Napster in 2001.

**2000**   The World Wide Web is believed to have exceeded one billion indexable pages.

**2001**   Apple release the Macintosh OS X operating system; it extends the capabilities of the machine allowing greater Unix compatibility and preemptive multitasking.

**2001**   The Code Red Worm is launched: at a predetermined time and date it gets all commercial servers it has infected to bombard a number of US government sites. As with many viruses and their warnings, little effect is noticed, other than the clogging up of systems with repeated e-mail warnings.

**2001**   Forwarding e-mail is made illegal in Australia with the advent of the Digital Agenda Act; the rationalization is that it is an infringement of the personal copyright act.

# GENERAL INDEX

## A

Abacus, **I:1f–2,** I:98–99, II:375–76
Abstract and concrete use cases, **I:2**
Abstract class, I:2
Abstract data types, **I:2–3**
Abstract operation, **I:3,** II:502–4
Abstract syntax, **I:3–4**
Abstraction, **I:4–5,** II:455
    example via Phileas Fogg character in *Around the World in 80 Days,* I:4
    finite-state machines, **I:235–36**
    procedural, **II:455**
    Shaw's work in, II:502–4
Access and access mode, **I:5–6**
Accessors and modifiers, **I:6**
Accumulator, **I:6–7**
Action, **I:7**
Ada (programming language), **I:7–8,** I:363
Adder circuit, **I:8–9**
Adding machines, I:85, I:99
Address register, **I:10,** II:479
Addressing, **I:9**
Adleman, Leonard Max, **I:10–11,** I:70–71
Adobe Systems, II:451–52
Aggregate data types, **I:11**
Aiken, Howard, **I:11–12,** I:275–77
ALGOL 60/68, **I:12–13, I:13–14,** II:443
Algorithms, **I:14–15**
    analysis of, I:22–23, I:336, II:502–4
    backtracking, I:53–54
    combinatorial, I:327–29
    complexity theory, I:131–33
    computability, I:135–36, II:557
    computational geometry, I:136–37
    cryptography, I:174–75, II:469–70, II:471
    data relationship, I:42–43
    divide and conquer, **I:203–4**
    generic for automatic programming, I:49, II:506
    genetic, I:255–57, II:473
    graph, **I:265–66**
    greedy, **I:269,** II:506
    *Introduction to Algorithms* by Thomas Corman et.al., I:22
    learning, **I:345–46**
    permutation *vs.* combination, I:129
    randomized, **II:472–73**
    searching and sorting, **II:494–95,** II:518–19, **II:519–20**
Al-Khowarizmi, Mohammed ib-n Musa
    algorithms, I:14
Allen, Paul Garner (Microsoft cofounder), **I:15–17,** I:*18,* I:253–55
Allocation/deallocation of memory, **I:17**
Alphanumeric character, **I:18**
Altair, **I:18,** II:487–88
Amdahl, Gene M., **I:18–20,** I:*19*
Amdahl Corp., I:19
America Online, I:27
American Arithmometer company, I:85
American National Standards Institute (ANSI), **I:20–21**
    C language standard, I:91–93
    COBOL language standard, I:124–25
American Standard Code for Information Interchange (ASCII), I:18, **I:21–22.** *See also* Standards
Amortized analysis, **I:22–23**
Analog computers, I:23–24
    oldest computer, I:27
Analog *vs.* digital computing, **I:23–24**
Analysis class, **I:24**
Analytical engine, **I:24–25,** I:321–22
    Babbage's involvement in, I:51–53, II:463
    Lovelace's work with, **I:363–65**
Anderson, Harlan, I:196–97
Andor Systems Corp., I:20
Andreesen, Marc, **I:25–27,** I:*26,* II:391
Animation, I:151–52
Antikythera mechanism, **I:27**
Antonelli, Kay McNulty Mauchley, **I:28**
API (applications program interface), **I:28–29**
APL, **I:29–30,** I:319
Apollo Moon program, II:545
Apple Computer Inc., **I:30–32,** I:*31*
    Apple II, I:344, II:445
    Jobs, cofounder of, **I:323–25,** I:*324*

# B

# C

## E

## Q

## R

## S